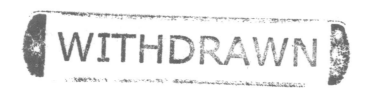

Therapeutic
Microbiology

PROBIOTICS AND
RELATED STRATEGIES

Therapeutic Microbiology

PROBIOTICS AND RELATED STRATEGIES

Edited by

James Versalovic
Department of Pathology,
Texas Childrens Hospital, Houston

Michael Wilson
Eastman Dental Institute,
University College London,
London, United Kingdom

ASM
PRESS

Washington, DC

Library of Congress Cataloging-in-Publication Data

Therapeutic microbiology : probiotics and related strategies / [edited by] James
Versalovic, Michael Wilson.
    p. ; cm.
Includes bibliographical references and index.
ISBN 978-1-55581-403-8
1. Probiotics. 2. Microorganisms—Therapeutic use. I. Versalovic, James. II. Wilson,
Michael, 1947 Apr. 12–
[DNLM: 1. Probiotics—therapeutic use. 2. Gastrointestinal Diseases—prevention &
control. 3. Gastrointestinal Diseases—therapy. 4. Intestines—immunology.
5. Intestines—microbiology.   QU 145.5 T398 2008]

RM666.P835T54 2008
615′.329—dc22   2008016646

Address editorial correspondence to: ASM Press, 1752 N St., N.W., Washington, DC
20036-2904, U.S.A.

Send orders to: ASM Press, P.O. Box 605, Herndon, VA 20172, U.S.A.
Phone: 800-546-2416; 703-661-1593
Fax: 703-661-1501
Email: Books@asmusa.org
Online: estore.asm.org

Contents

Contributors

STEVEN A. ABRAMS
USDA/ARS Children's Nutrition Research Center, and Dept. of Pediatrics, Texas Children's Hospital, Baylor College of Medicine, 1100 Bates St., Houston, TX 77030

COVADONGA BARBÉS
Área de Microbiología, Departamento de Biología Funcional, Facultad de Medicina, Universidad de Oviedo, 33006 Oviedo, Spain

STIG BENGMARK
Institute of Hepatology, University College London Medical School, 69-75 Chenies Mews, London WC1E 6HX, United Kingdom

JOHN BIENENSTOCK
The Brain-Body Institute and Dept. of Pathology and Molecular Medicine, McMaster University, and St. Joseph's Healthcare Hamilton, Hamilton, Ontario, Canada

ANTHONY R. BIRD
Commonwealth Scientific and Industrial Research Organization, Food Futures National Research Flagship, and CSIRO Human Nutrition, Adelaide, South Australia

DOUWINA BOSSCHER
BENEO-Orafti, Aandorenstraat 1, B3300 Tienen, Belgium

JEREMY P. BURTON
BLIS Technologies Ltd., Centre for Innovation, University of Otago, P.O. Box 56, Dunedin, New Zealand

PATRICE D. CANI
Université Catholique de Louvain, School of Pharmacy, MD/FARM/PMNT
7369 UCL, 73 Avenue Mounier, B-1200 Brussels, Belgium

XINHUA CHEN
Division of Gastroenterology, Dana 601A, Beth Israel Deaconess Medical
Center, Harvard Medical School, 330 Brookline Ave., Boston, MA 02215

CHRIS N. CHILCOTT
BLIS Technologies Ltd., Centre for Innovation, University of Otago, P.O. Box
56, Dunedin, New Zealand

DAVID P. A. COHEN
Laboratory of Virology, Wageningen University, Binnenhaven 11, 6709 PD
Wageningen, The Netherlands

GIOVANNI V. COPPA
Institute of Maternal-Infantile Sciences, Polytechnic University of Marche,
60123 Ancona, Italy

WILLEM M. DE VOS
Laboratory of Microbiology, Wageningen University, Dreijenplein 10, 6703 HB
Wageningen, The Netherlands

NATHALIE M. DELZENNE
Université Catholique de Louvain, School of Pharmacy, MD/FARM/PMNT
7369 UCL, 73 Avenue Mounier, B-1200 Brussels, Belgium

TRI DUONG
Genomic Sciences Graduate Program, Dept. of Food, Bioprocessing and
Nutrition Sciences, North Carolina State University, Raleigh, NC 27695

GEORGE FAHEY
Dept. of Animal Sciences, University of Illinois, 1207 W. Gregory Dr., Urbana,
IL 61801

ELENA FORONI
Dept. of Genetics, Biology of Microorganisms, Anthropology and Evolution,
University of Parma, Parma, Italy

PAUL FORSYTHE
The Brain-Body Institute and Dept. of Pathology and Molecular Medicine,
McMaster University, and St. Joseph's Healthcare Hamilton, Hamilton,
Ontario, Canada

ORAZIO GABRIELLI
Institute of Maternal-Infantile Sciences, Polytechnic University of Marche,
60123 Ancona, Italy

GLENN R. GIBSON
Dept. of Food Biosciences, The University of Reading, Whiteknights, Reading
RG6 6AP, United Kingdom

FRANCISCO GUARNER
Digestive System Research Unit, University Hospital Vall d'Hebron,
CIBEREHD, Passeig Vall d'Hebron, 119-129, 08035 Barcelona, Spain

DAVID HERNOT
Dept. of Animal Sciences, University of Illinois, 1207 W. Gregory Dr., Urbana,
IL 61801

KASIPATHY KAILASAPATHY
Probiotics and Encapsulated Functional Foods Research Unit, School of Natural
Sciences, Centre for Plant and Food Science, University of Western Sydney,
South Penrith DC, Locked Bag 1797, NSW 1797, Australia

CIARÁN P. KELLY
Division of Gastroenterology, Dana 601A, Beth Israel Deaconess Medical
Center, Harvard Medical School, 330 Brookline Ave., Boston, MA 02215

SAIJA KILJUNEN
Dept. of Virology, University of Turku, 00014 Turku, Finland

TODD R. KLAENHAMMER
Dept. of Food, Bioprocessing and Nutrition Sciences and Southeast Dairy Foods
Research Center, North Carolina State University, Raleigh, NC 27695

SERGEY R. KONSTANTINOV
Duke University Medical Center, 272 Jones Bldg., Durham, NC 27710

ANNE L. MCCARTNEY
Dept. of Food Biosciences, The University of Reading, Whiteknights, Reading
RG6 6AP, United Kingdom

J. H. MEURMAN
Institute of Dentistry and Dept. of Oral and Maxillofacial Diseases, Helsinki
University Central Hospital, PB 41, University of Helsinki, FI 00014 Helsinki,
Finland

AUDREY M. NEYRINCK
Université Catholique de Louvain, School of Pharmacy, MD/FARM/PMNT
7369 UCL, 73 Avenue Mounier, B-1200 Brussels, Belgium

EVA OGUÉ
Dept. of Food Biosciences, P.O. Box 226, The University of Reading,
Whiteknights, Reading RG6 6AP, United Kingdom

MARIA PAJUNEN
Institute of Biotechnology, University of Helsinki, 00014 Helsinki, Finland

HELENA M. R. T. PARRACHO
Dept. of Food Biosciences, The University of Reading, Whiteknights, Reading
RG6 6AP, United Kingdom

ROBERT A. RASTALL
Dept. of Food Biosciences, P.O. Box 226, The University of Reading,
Whiteknights, Reading RG6 6AP, United Kingdom

GREGOR REID
Canadian R&D Centre for Probiotics, Lawson Health Research Institute,
F2-116, 268 Grosvenor St., London, Ontario, N6A 4V2, Canada

ANGELA RIBBERA
Dept. of Genetics, Biology of Microorganisms, Anthropology and Evolution, University of Parma, Parma, Italy

ALEX RODRIGUEZ-PALACIOS
Dept. of Preventive Veterinary Medicine, Food Animal Health Research Program, Ohio Agricultural Research and Development Center, The Ohio State University, Wooster, OH 44691

G. A. W. ROOK
Centre for Infectious Diseases and International Health, Windeyer Institute of Medical Sciences, Royal Free and University College Medical School, 46 Cleveland St., London W1T 4JF, United Kingdom

IAN ROWLAND
Dept. of Food Biosciences, University of Reading, P.O. Box 226, Whiteknights, Reading RG6 6AP, United Kingdom

MARY ELLEN SANDERS
Dairy & Food Culture Technologies, International Scientific Association for Probiotics and Prebiotics, 7119 S. Glencoe Ct., Centennial, CO 80122

DELPHINE M. SAULNIER
Dept. of Food Biosciences, The University of Reading, Whiteknights, Reading RG6 6AP, United Kingdom

MICHAEL SCHULTZ
Dept. of Medical and Surgical Sciences, Medicine Section, University of Otago Medical School, P.O. Box 913, Dunedin, New Zealand

SHAYAN SHARIF
Dept. of Pathobiology, Ontario Veterinary College, University of Guelph, Guelph, Ontario, N1G 2W1, Canada

MIKAEL SKURNIK
Dept. of Bacteriology and Immunology, Haartman Institute, University of Helsinki, and Helsinki University Central Hospital Laboratory Diagnostics, 00014 Helsinki, Finland

JENNIFER K. SPINLER
Dept. of Pathology, Baylor College of Medicine, and Dept. of Pathology, Texas Children's Hospital, 6621 Fannin St., MC 1-2261, Houston, TX 77030

JOHN R. TAGG
Dept. of Microbiology and Immunology, University of Otago, P.O. Box 56, Dunedin, New Zealand

GERALD W. TANNOCK
Dept. of Microbiology and Immunology, University of Otago, Dunedin, New Zealand

DAVID L. TOPPING
Commonwealth Scientific and Industrial Research Organization, Food Futures National Research Flagship, Adelaide, South Australia

FRANCESCA TURRONI
Dept. of Genetics, Biology of Microorganisms, Anthropology and Evolution, University of Parma, Parma, Italy

JAN VAN LOO
BENEO-Orafti, Aandorenstraat 1, B3300 Tienen, Belgium

DOUWE VAN SINDEREN
Alimentary Pharmabiotic Centre and Dept. of Microbiology, Bioscience Institute, National University of Ireland, Western Road, Cork, Ireland

ELAINE E. VAUGHAN
Laboratory of Microbiology, Wageningen University, Dreijenplein 10, 6703 HB Wageningen, The Netherlands

MARCO VENTURA
Dept. of Genetics, Biology of Microorganisms, Anthropology and Evolution, University of Parma, Parma, Italy

JAMES VERSALOVIC
Dept. of Pathology, Baylor College of Medicine, and Dept. of Pathology, Texas Children's Hospital, 6621 Fannin St., MC 1-2261, Houston, TX 77030

J. SCOTT WEESE
Dept. of Pathobiology, Ontario Veterinary College, University of Guelph, Guelph, Ontario, N1G 2W1, Canada

JERRY WELLS
Host-Microbe-Interactomics Group, University of Wageningen, Marijkeweg 40, 6709 PG Wageningen, The Netherlands

PHILIP A. WESCOMBE
BLIS Technologies Ltd., Centre for Innovation, University of Otago, P.O. Box 56, Dunedin, New Zealand

MICHAEL WILSON
Division of Microbial Diseases, UCL Eastman Dental Institute, University College London, 256 Grays Inn Road, London WC1X 8LD, United Kingdom

N. WITT
Centre for Infectious Diseases and International Health, Windeyer Institute of Medical Sciences, Royal Free and University College Medical School, 46 Cleveland St., London W1T 4JF, United Kingdom

ERWIN G. ZOETENDAL
Laboratory of Microbiology, Wageningen University, Dreijenplein 10, 6703 HB Wageningen, The Netherlands

Preface

Currently there is enormous interest in the indigenous microbiota of humans and other animals, and significant advances are being made with regard to their composition and function. What has become clear is that these communities are not simply passive bystanders. On the contrary, they participate in a range of complex interactions with their host and vice versa. As the role of these microbial communities in maintaining animal health is increasingly being recognized, there has been a concomitant increase in our enthusiasm for manipulating their composition in order to promote the health of their host. The latter concept is central to "therapeutic microbiology." As editors of the first book on this subject, we feel obligated to at least attempt a definition of the term—but this is no easy matter. As a starting point, therapeutic microbiology may be defined as the use of microbes, or compounds other than antimicrobial agents, to confer some benefit on an animal by altering its indigenous microbiota, immunity, or physiology or else by eliminating a particular pathogen. As well as probiotics and prebiotics, such a definition encompasses replacement therapy—an approach with great potential that involves the use of a specific "effector organism" to eliminate, or control the growth of, a particular pathogen present in the host.

Although probiotics have a very long history, interest in manipulating the indigenous microbiota of animals has increased dramatically during the past few years, with the number of papers in this field in 2007 being fivefold greater than that published in 2000. There are several ways in which the indigenous microbiota of humans and other animals can be altered, and these include the use of probiotics, prebiotics, synbiotics, and bacteriophages. These approaches, together with replacement therapy, have been advocated not only as a means of promoting well-being in humans and other animals but also as a way of preventing or treating a range of disease conditions. It is only within recent years, however, that the results of a number of well-designed clinical studies have provided evidence, previously lacking, that such approaches can indeed be beneficial to humans and other animals in terms of disease prevention and remission.

This book contains chapters written by many of the leading researchers in the field of therapeutic microbiology. As can be appreciated from the Contents, it consists of sections dealing with the biological principles underlying the manipulation of the indigenous microbiota, the biology of the effector organisms that have been utilized for this purpose, and the use of probiotics, prebiotics, synbiotics, bacteriophages, and replacement therapy for the prevention and treatment of diseases as well as for conferring a range of other benefits on humans and other animals. It will serve as an important reference source for all those interested in this fast-moving field.

We would like to thank all of the authors for providing such excellent material for the book, Greg Payne at ASM Press for his invaluable input, and Tiffany Morgan for her skillful coordination of the project.

James Versalovic
Michael Wilson

Introduction

1

Therapeutic Microbiology: Probiotics and Related Strategies
Edited by J. Versalovic and M. Wilson
© 2008 ASM Press, Washington, DC

Mary Ellen Sanders

Introduction

1

Live microbes that when administered in adequate amounts confer a health benefit on the host are termed "probiotics" (FAO, 2001). The use of microbes to treat or prevent disease is a concept that has matured in recent years. Parallel avenues of research have converged to provide the mechanistic and clinical evidence to support emerging efficacious products in the marketplace. Important contributing research includes using modern molecular methods to refine our understanding of the types and activities of microbes colonizing healthy and diseased humans; identifying the way in which microbes dynamically interact with host cells and other commensal microbes; applying functional genomics and gene array techniques to better understand the genetic and metabolic capacity of therapeutic microbes; improving the technological approaches to identity, definition, composition, stability, and delivery of benefits; and perhaps most importantly, measuring in a controlled fashion the health effects of live microbes administered to animal or human hosts.

Concomitant, related advances have also been realized in the area of prebiotics. Prebiotics are nondigestible food ingredients that have a beneficial effect through their selective metabolism in the intestinal tract (Gibson et al., 2004). By nature of their ability to influence the intestinal microbiota and environment, their physiological effects are often complementary to probiotic influences.

Numerous are the types of health effects of probiotics and prebiotics supported by controlled (albeit some are preliminary) studies in the target host animal (humans, companion animals, or animals used in animal agriculture). When considering the breadth of such effects, it must be kept in mind that there are many different genera, species, and strains of microbes used as probiotics and many different biochemical compositions of prebiotics. The physiological effects of each of these different agents may be specific to the agent, the dose, and the physiological, nutritional, and immune status of the host. With regard to strain specificity of probiotic effects, the emerging evidence seems to be quite complicated. It is well accepted that different strains of even the same species express different functions in vivo (Maassen et al., 2000), but little is known about the effects of blending different strains which may lead to a final effect that is not predicted by results from using the strains

Mary Ellen Sanders, Dairy & Food Culture Technologies, International Scientific Association for Probiotics and Prebiotics, 7119 S. Glencoe Ct., Centennial, CO 80122.

singly (Bruno Pot, personal communication). For example, Collado et al. (2007) observed that probiotic strains used in combination had improved adherence in cell culture compared to when they were tested as single strains. The practical implications of such observations suggest the importance of testing blended strain products as they are in the final product formulation. However, these findings also may expand possibilities for applications that are not achievable by the use of single strains (Timmerman et al., 2007).

Another emerging observation is that the mode of delivery of the agents may be important for in vivo functionality. For example, probiotics delivered in fermented milk products compared to concentrated, dried preparations may have different in vivo effects. Delivery matrices may influence probiotic or prebiotic functionality in several ways: (i) by increasing the ability of the probiotic to survive or remain physiologically active in the product; (ii) by increasing the ability of the probiotic to survive and be effective at the site of action once in the host; and (iii) by delivering complementary functionality through components of the delivery system or from fermentation-derived active ingredients.

A few studies comparing the physiological effects generated by probiotics delivered in different product formats have been conducted. In an animal model of arthritis, Baharav et al. (2004) showed that consumption of live *Lactobacillus rhamnosus* GG in yogurt resulted in reduced severity of arthritis in rats compared to the same probiotic delivered in dried culture suspended in water. In humans, Chiang et al. (2000) found enhancement of natural killer cell activity induced by *Bifidobacterium lactis* HN019 when the probiotic was fed to healthy subjects in oligosaccharide-enriched milk compared to regular low-fat milk. However, *L. rhamnosus* GG was effective in promoting recovery from acute diarrhea in children when delivered at the same dose as either dried, concentrated powder or fermented milk (Isolauri et al., 1991). The delivery vehicle may also impact the physiological status of the probiotic as it is consumed. For example, resistance to host factors such as stomach acid and digestive enzymes depends on the physiological status of the strain.

Generalizations about the "health effects of probiotics or prebiotics" can be misleading if references to the strain or strains used, doses delivered, and product format are not integral to such discussions. With this caution in mind, it is of interest to note the list of health targets for the many different types of probiotics that have been tested in humans. This list includes improved immune function (with both increased response to nonself invaders and decreased autoimmune functions

and inflammation); improved colonic barrier integrity; decreased incidence, duration, or symptoms of intestinal, vaginal, and respiratory infections or ailments; improved intestinal regularity; reduced symptoms associated with and increased compliance with antibiotic treatment; improvement in some quality of life indicators such as absences from work or day care; and reduction of colic in infants. Controlled human studies for prebiotics are less numerous but add enhanced mineral absorption and reduction of cancer biomarkers to the list of potential targets. In animal models, the influences of probiotics and prebiotics include improved digestion, improved feed efficiency, improved ability to resist infections, and reduction in pathogen shedding. It is worthwhile in this context to note the publication of several well-controlled human trials showing no effect of probiotic and/or prebiotic intervention on a variety of clinical end points. Dissemination of such information is critical to providing a better understanding of the parameters for successful intervention for probiotics and prebiotics.

How these agents function in vivo is a largely unanswered question in many cases. But noteworthy progress has been made in recent years on recognizing the dynamic interactions among live microbes and their hosts. These observations have provided this field with important insights into how consumption of exogenous microbes may impact host health. Perhaps the most compelling means of probiotic function may be through interaction with host immune cells, which may occur during transit of the microbe through the sparsely colonized small intestine that is rich in immune sensing cells. Dendritic cells play a central role in regulating immune responses (Niess and Reinecker, 2006), and some probiotic microbes have been shown to stimulate dendritic cells selectively, facilitating their maturation and differentiation to effector cells (Foligne et al., 2007). Certain Toll-like receptors sense lipoteichoic acid from gram-positive bacteria, bacterial DNA, or viruses, leading to innate immune system cascade responses (Takeuchi and Akira, 2007). This mechanism has been shown to be responsible for the anti-inflammatory effects of probiotic bacteria (Rachmilewitz et al., 2004; Grangette et al., 2005).

Mechanisms other than response of immune system parameters have also been identified. Probiotics have been shown to stimulate mucin production in cell culture (Mack et al., 1999). Such intestinal epithelial cells were less likely to be invaded by infective *Escherichia coli*. Commensal microbes and probiotic bacteria have been shown to alter the glycosylation patterns of epithelial cells, thereby altering the ability of pathogens to adhere (Freitas et al., 2003). This strategy was exploited by Paton et al. (2000) to produce genetically altered live bacteria that effectively titrated pathogens from a mouse model of *E. coli* infection. Host-microbe communication also flows to the probiotic. Bron et al. (2004) documented genes that were induced in a strain of *Lactobacillus plantarum* in the intestinal tract of mice. The production of short-chain fatty acids by *Lactobacillus* and *Bifidobacterium* has long been thought to be an important contributor to a healthier intestinal environment, although these two genera are not the only intestinal microbes with this metabolic ability. Antimicrobial peptides produced by probiotics may also play a role in reducing the levels of pathogenic activity in vivo. Recently, Corr et al. (2007) were the first to confirm that a bacteriocin produced in vivo was responsible for antipathogenic effects. Their observations were made in an animal model of *Listeria* infection. Reinforcing epithelial barrier integrity has also been proposed as a mechanism by which probiotics can improve intestinal and systemic health (Luyer et al., 2005).

One commonly cited benefit of probiotics and prebiotics is that they "improve the balance of intestinal microbiota." The widespread use of this claim on commercial products notwithstanding, this claim should be rigorously considered. It is necessary to define what is meant by "improved balance." Some consider improved balance to be synonymous with increasing the levels of intestinal bacteria that are considered to be beneficial (e.g., lactobacilli or bifidobacteria). In fact, this may be considered an a priori principle of both probiotic and prebiotic interventions. However, strictly speaking, such intestinal microbial population changes have not been causally linked to health benefits. In most cases the link is correlational (www.usprobiotics.org/docs/AFFSA%20probiotic%20prebiotic%20flora%20immunity%202005.pdf). Scientists today have not defined an intestinal microbiota for optimum health, nor do they assert with certainty that increasing levels of intestinal lactobacilli or bifidobacteria will necessarily make a person healthier. Changes in the intestinal environment (such as alteration of levels of certain metabolic end products) may result from altering populations of colonizing microbes, but to what extent these population changes are directly responsible for health benefits must be more scrupulously studied. Levels of bifidobacteria and lactobacilli in the feces may be a biomarker of health, but as yet an unvalidated one. Fundamental to this hypothesis is that there is an inherent flaw to intestinal colonization of modern humans (presumably due to the diet and environment of modern times compared to most of human history) and striving to change the character of our intestinal microbiota colonization is a worthwhile goal. However, the gaps in knowledge regarding the actual composition of the human intestinal microbiota (Zoetendal et al., 2006) and the apparent nature of the microbiota that makes it refractory to alteration make it necessary to challenge the simplistic assertion that probiotics improve the balance of the intestinal microbial community. Furthermore, aside from increases in the microbes being fed, probiotics do not seem to have a large or predictable impact on populations of intestinal microbes, and the effect they exert is generally transient. Unless the microbes impacted are known pathogens, it is doubtful that demonstrating a probiotic- or prebiotic-induced impact on the gut microbiota is sufficient to convincingly substantiate a health effect.

Another approach to interpret the assertion of "improved balance" is that probiotics may help the intestinal microbiota recover from perturbations, such as those caused by antibiotic use. A few studies have assessed this concept (Madden et al., 2005; Engelbrektson et al., 2006) and have shown that probiotics can fortify the properties of the colonizing microbiota that enable it to resist change and recover from challenges. Dore and colleagues (De La Cochetiere et al., 2005) demonstrated that, in general, the dominant components of the human fecal microbiota recovered to pretreatment levels with no intervention after a short-course antibiotic challenge in most tested individuals. However, the authors noted that perturbed levels persisted in some subjects, suggesting that "strategies reinforcing the ability of the fecal microbiota to resist modifications would be of clinical relevance."

In addition to the composition of the intestinal tract microbiota, it is fruitful also to consider its biochemical nature. Largely influenced by the colonizing microbiota and the fermentation processes they undergo, the environment may be a more precise indicator of intestinal health. Commonly, the combined action of the gut microbiota is blamed for the production of a myriad of putatively dangerous metabolites such as amines, phenols, and thiols in the colon. De Preter et al. (2004) used stable isotope-labeled markers in a placebo-controlled human trial to demonstrate that a *Lactobacillus casei* strain or lactulose could impact end products of colonic bacterial metabolism. Inasmuch as these end products are implicated in the pathogenesis of some diseases, this is an indirect measure of the ability of probiotics and prebiotics to improve the intestinal environment. Molecular strategies promise to be fruitful in elucidating the character of the healthy human intestinal tract. Egert et al. (2006) suggest that "such research approaches could provide a basis for the definition of a healthy gut based on key properties of microbial functionality" and provide needed indicators to assess the value of dietary interventions on intestinal health.

This book serves a grand purpose of consolidating the range of information available on how microbes can be used to promote health and prevent or treat disease. It also highlights the most productive avenues of research that are under way to close the gaps in understanding the impact of probiotics and prebiotics on health and human physiology.

References

Baharav, E., F. Mor, M. Halpern, and A. Weinberger. 2004. *Lactobacillus* GG bacteria ameliorate arthritis in Lewis rats. *J. Nutr.* 134:1964–1969.

Bron, P. A., M. Marco, S. M. Hoffer, E. Van Mullekom, W. M. de Vos, and M. Kleerebezem. 2004. Genetic characterization of the bile salt response in *Lactobacillus plantarum* and analysis of responsive promoters in vitro and in situ in the gastrointestinal tract. *J. Bacteriol.* 186:7829–7835.

Chiang, B. L., Y. H. Sheih, L. H. Wang, C. K. Liao, and H. S. Gill. 2000. Enhancing immunity by dietary consumption of a probiotic lactic acid bacterium (*Bifidobacterium lactis* HN019): optimization and definition of cellular immune responses. *Eur. J. Clin. Nutr.* 54:849–855.

Collado, M. C., J. Meriluoto, and S. Salminen. 2007. Development of new probiotics by strain combinations: is it possible to improve the adhesion to intestinal mucus? *J. Dairy Sci.* 90:2710–2716.

Corr, S. C., Y. Li, C. U. Riedel, P. W. O'Toole, C. Hill, and C. G. Gahan. 2007. Bacteriocin production as a mechanism for the antiinfective activity of *Lactobacillus salivarius* UCC118. *Proc. Natl. Acad. Sci. USA* 104:7617–7621.

De La Cochetiere, M. F., T. Durand, P. Lepage, A. Bourreille, J. P. Galmiche, and J. Dore. 2005. Resilience of the dominant human fecal microbiota upon short-course antibiotic challenge. *J. Clin. Microbiol.* 43:5588–5592.

De Preter, V., K. Geboes, K. Verbrugghe, L. De Vuyst, T. Vanhoutte, G. Huys, J. Swings, B. Pot, and K. Verbeke. 2004. The in vivo use of the stable isotope-labelled biomarkers lactose-[^{15}N]ureide and [^{2}H$_{4}$]tyrosine to assess the effects of pro- and prebiotics on the intestinal flora of healthy human volunteers. *Br. J. Nutr.* 92:439–446.

Egert, M., A. A. de Graaf, H. Smidt, W. M. de Vos, and K. Venema. 2006. Beyond diversity: functional microbiomics of the human colon. *Trends Microbiol.* 14:86–91.

Engelbrektson, A. L., J. R. Korzenik, M. E. Sanders, B. G. Clement, G. Leyer, T. R. Klaenhammer, and C. L. Kitts. 2006. Analysis of treatment effects on the microbial ecology of the human intestine. *FEMS Microbiol. Ecol.* 57:239–250.

Foligne, B., G. Zoumpopoulou, J. Dewulf, A. Ben Younes, F. Chareyre, J. C. Sirard, B. Pot, and C. Grangette. 2007. A key role of dendritic cells in probiotic functionality. *PLoS ONE.* 2:e313

Food and Agriculture Organization of the United Nations (FAO). 2001. Health and Nutritional Properties of Probiotics in Food including Powder Milk with Live Lactic Acid Bacteria. http://www.who.int/foodsafety/publications/fs_management/en/probiotics.pdf. Accessed April 28, 2008.

Freitas, M., E. Tavan, C. Cayuela, L. Diop, C. Sapin, and G. Trugnan. 2003. Host-pathogens cross-talk. Indigenous bacteria and probiotics also play the game. *Biol. Cell* 95:503–506.

Gibson, G. R., H. M. Probert, J. A. E. van Loo, R. A. Rastall, and M. B. Roberfroid. 2004. Dietary modulation of the human colonic microbiota: updating the concept of prebiotics. *Nutr. Res. Rev.* 17:259–275.

Grangette, C., S. Nutten, E. Palumbo, S. Morath, C. Hermann, J. Dewulf, B. Pot, T. Hartung, P. Hols, and A. Mercenier. 2005. Enhanced antiinflammatory capacity of a *Lactobacillus plantarum* mutant synthesizing modified teichoic acids. *Proc. Natl. Acad. Sci. USA* 102:10321–10326.

Isolauri, E., M. Juntunen, T. Rautanen, P. Sillanaukee, and T. Koivula. 1991. A human *Lactobacillus* strain (*Lactobacillus casei* sp strain GG) promotes recovery from acute diarrhea in children. *Pediatrics* 88:90–97.

Luyer, M. D., W. A. Buurman, M. Hadfoune, G. Speelmans, J. Knol, J. A. Jacobs, C. H. Dejong, A. J. Vriesema, and J. W. Greve. 2005. Strain-specific effects of probiotics on gut barrier integrity following hemorrhagic shock. *Infect. Immun.* 73:3686–3692.

Maassen, C. B., C. van Holten-Neelen, F. Balk, M. J. den Bak-Glashouwer, R. J. Leer, J. D. Laman, W. J. Boersma, and E. Claassen. 2000. Strain-dependent induction of cytokine profiles in the gut by orally administered *Lactobacillus* strains. *Vaccine* 18:2613–2623.

Mack, D. R., S. Michail, S. Wei, L. McDougall, and M. A. Hollingsworth. 1999. Probiotics inhibit enteropathogenic *E. coli* adherence in vitro by inducing intestinal mucin gene expression. *Am. J. Physiol.* 276:G941–950.

Madden, J. A., S. F. Plummer, J. Tang, I. Garaiova, N. T. Plummer, M. Herbison, J. O. Hunter, T. Shimada, I. Cheng, and T. Shirakawa. 2005. Effect of probiotics on preventing disruption of the intestinal microflora following antibiotic therapy: a double-blind, placebo-controlled pilot study. *Int. Immunopharmacol.* 5:1091–1097.

Niess, J. H., and H. C. Reinecker. 2006. Dendritic cells: the commanders-in-chief of mucosal immune defenses. *Curr. Opin. Gastroenterol.* 22:354–360.

Paton, A. W., M. Renato, and J. C. Paton. 2000. A new biological agent for treatment of Shiga toxigenic *Escherichia coli* infections and dysentery in humans. *Nat. Med.* 6:265–270.

Rachmilewitz, D., K. Katakura, F. Karmeli, T. Hayashi, C. Reinus, B. Rudensky, S. Akira, K. Takeda, J. Lee, K. Takabayashi, and E. Raz. 2004. Toll-like receptor 9 signaling mediates the anti-inflammatory effects of probiotics in murine experimental colitis. *Gastroenterology* 126:520–528.

Takeuchi, O., and S. Akira. 2007. Signaling pathways activated by microorganisms. *Curr. Opin. Cell Biol.* 19:185–191.

Timmerman, H. M., L. E. Niers, B. U. Ridwan, C. J. Koning, L. Mulder, L. M. Akkermans, F. M. Rombouts, and G. T. Rijkers. 2007. Design of a multispecies probiotic mixture to prevent infectious complications in critically ill patients. *Clin. Nutr.* 26:450–459.

Zoetendal, E. G., E. E. Vaughan, and W. M. de Vos. 2006. A microbial world within us. *Mol. Microbiol.* 59:1639–1650.

Basic Biology

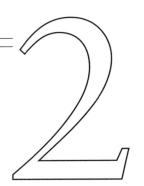

2

Therapeutic Microbiology: Probiotics and Related Strategies
Edited by J. Versalovic and M. Wilson
© 2008 ASM Press, Washington, DC

2.1. THE INDIGENOUS MICROBIOTA

Gerald W. Tannock

2

Role of the Indigenous Microbiota in Health and Disease

Philosophers and theologians regard humans as the crown of creation, but to the microbes we are no more—and no less—than the proverbial free lunch.

Abigail Salyers and Dixie Whitt,
microbiologists

There is no free lunch.

Milton Friedman, economist

It is a sobering thought that humans could be considered to be nothing more than a mobile buffet for microbes. Yet it is true that regions of the body that are superficial or accessible through exterior orifices (skin, respiratory tract, digestive tract, and vagina) are inhabited throughout our lives by microbial populations that form communities of characteristic sizes and biodiversities (summarized by Tannock, 1995, and Wilson, 2005). Lumped together, these communities constitute the indigenous microbiota of the human body. This chapter focuses on the indigenous microbiota of the human large bowel, arguably the best-known ecosystem of the body.

The study of microbial communities falls within the domain of microbial ecology—the study of the interrelationships that occur between populations within a community and between the community and the environment

in which it is located. Microbial ecology is about how ecosystems work and therefore details the functions of populations, individually and collectively, in nature. Sadly, the recent study of the microbial communities of the human body has almost exclusively involved compositional studies in which 16S rRNA gene clone libraries have been derived so as to prepare catalogues of microbes detected in various body sites (Bik et al., 2006; Eckburg et al., 2005; Hayashi et al., 2005; Wang et al., 2005). It has revealed little about how body ecosystems operate, since the vast majority of the body's inhabitants are uncultivated and unknown. It is clear from genetical studies, however, that there is tremendous variation in the composition of communities between individual humans when considered at the taxonomic level of species and strains (Lay et al., 2005; Kimura et al., 1997; McCartney et al., 1996). There is, though, a grand plan revealed in terms of higher-level phylogeny (Eckburg et al., 2005). Thus, the fecal bacterial community of humans sampled anywhere in the world is dominated by four phyla: *Firmicutes*, *Bacteroidetes*, *Proteobacteria*, and *Actinobacteria*. Curiously, there are two phyla of gram-positive and two of gram-negative bacteria. Especially common are members of three broad phylogenetic groups: the *Bacteroides-Prevotella* group, the *Eubacterium*

Gerald W. Tannock, Department of Microbiology and Immunology, University of Otago, Dunedin, New Zealand.

rectale-Clostridium coccoides group (Clostridium cluster XIVa), and the Clostridium leptum subgroup (Clostridium cluster IV) (Lay et al., 2005). The diversity of community compositions recognized among humans is evidence of functional redundancy in the microbial (especially bacterial) world. Many different types of bacteria can carry out the same metabolic function, and therefore, there is a choice as to which bacterial species can fill a specific ecological niche in an ecosystem. Which species fills a specific niche in a particular human may merely be the result of chance exposure, although it would be nice to think that species especially fitted to the physiological idiosyncrasies of the individual human are selected, each individual human supplying the "fertile soil" for particular microbes (Rawls et al., 2006). Since the physiological characteristics of the human host can be considered to reflect the constitution of the genome, it is reasonable to expect that, just as there is a "normal" range of blood chemistries in human populations, there is also a normal range of human indigenous microbiota.

One must consider, however, whether physiology solely reflects the genetic constitution of the human. Molecular biological studies of bowel bacteria-mouse relationships suggest that microbes impact importantly on murine physiology. Hence, Bacteroides thetaiotaomicron in the bowel, in relatively short-term gnotobiotic mouse experiments, influenced fucosylation of the enterocyte extracellular matrix, and up- or down-regulated murine genes whose products are associated with nutrition, epithelial integrity, and angiogenesis (Hooper et al., 1999, 2001; Stappenbeck et al., 2002). These are impacts on bowel mucosa, but a systemic effect on the deposition of fat has also been reported in relation to the bowel microbiota of mice. The latter work revealed that murine physiology is actually attuned to the down-regulation of fat storage after weaning but that the bowel microbiota negates the mouse regulatory mechanism by reducing the production of fasting-induced adipose factor (FIAF) in the intestinal mucosa that leads to a corresponding increase in the systemic activity of lipoprotein lipase (LPL). FIAF is an inhibitor of LPL, the latter influencing the uptake of triglycerides by adipocytes (Backhed et al., 2004). Whether this phenomenon is applicable to humans is unknown, but it certainly provides an excuse to the obese: "it's not the inappropriate food that I eat and the lack of exercise that make me fat; it's my bowel bacteria." Knowledge of the impressive impact of the indigenous microbiota on the physiology of experimental animals has, of course, been available for many decades. Comparisons of germfree animals and their conventional counterparts revealed differences in immunological structures, rates of epithelial cell turnover, blood

volume, and even sleep patterns among numerous other effects referred to as "microbe-associated characteristics" (summarized by Tannock, 1997). Molecular biological investigations enable the mechanistic details of these differences to be uncovered.

The bowel community is composed mostly of eubacterial species. Archaea and fungi may be present but form less than 1 and 0.05%, respectively, of the total community (Miller and Wolin, 1983; Simon and Gorbach, 1984). The bacterial community of the large bowel comprises about 2×10^{13} cells, based on about 10^{11} bacterial cells per g of contents and an average of 200 g of contents per large bowel. Nevertheless, these bacteriological figures pertain only to the distal large bowel since most bacteriological information is obtained from the examination of feces. It is somewhat distressing that hard data concerning the indigenous microbiota of humans are difficult to come by; estimates rule the day because the analytical methods that are used even in the 21st century are crude and, therefore, give approximate values. Indeed, it is unwise to consider data to be absolute in this work, and strictly controlled, comparative studies provide the best predictions of biological effects. We still do not have an accurate catalogue of the bacteria that can be encountered in human feces. This is because the results of high-throughput sequencing projects have polluted the DNA databanks with unreliable 16S rRNA gene sequences, making meaningful analysis of catalogues of bacterial inhabitants impossible to obtain (Ashelford et al., 2005, 2006). Do 400 bacterial species constitute the bowel community, as estimated in the 1970s, or do 1,000, as estimated recently (Moore and Holdeman, 1974; Eckburg et al., 2005)? As your children or undergraduate students may ask you, "What difference does it make?"

Does it really matter who lives in the bowel? "Who" as to what species. Even if we had the perfect taxonomic catalogue, about 75% of the bacteria in the large bowel are unknown and little can be inferred from their phylogeny as to what their functions are in nature (Suau et al., 1999). DNA-based methods of analysis that are used to define the composition of complex bacterial communities reveal "who has been there," but they tell us nothing about their status in the ecosystem. The DNA used in the analysis could have come from dead cells, lysed cells, living but metabolically quiescent cells, from dormant forms of cells (spores), from transient (allochthonous) bacteria, or from indigenous (autochthonous) species. We need to know more than this if we are to understand the microbial ecology of the bowel or of any other body site. The valid questions to ask are "whose habitat is this?," "what are the functional attributes of the inhabitants that permit life in this ecosystem?," and "how do these functions contribute to community structure?" Recognition of autochthonous species can only be achieved by temporal studies that provide information about population size, constancy of detection, and biomarkers of ecological function (Tannock, 2004). *Lactobacillus reuteri*, for example, is autochthonous to the digestive tract of mice because this species is detectable throughout the life of the animal, is present in predictable and constant numbers, and produces biofilms on forestomach epithelia (an ecological function). Molecular investigations are beginning to reveal the bacterial features that underpin *L. reuteri* autochthony in the murine digestive tract (Tannock et al., 2005; Walter et al., 2003, 2005, 2007).

The adherence of *Lactobacillus* cells to, and proliferation on, epithelial surfaces in anterior regions of the guts of rodents, pigs, horses, and poultry have tempted some researchers to consider that the same phenomenon occurs in the human bowel (Fuller and Brooker, 1974; summarized by Tannock, 1992; Yuki et al., 2000). This overlooks the differences in the anatomy and histology of the human digestive tract relative to that of other monogastric animals. The formation of *Lactobacillus* biofilms in the digestive tract is conditional on the presence of a nonsecretory squamous epithelium such as that of the rodent forestomach or avian crop. The gastrointestinal tract of humans lacks this prerequisite for biofilm formation because it is lined by an epithelium composed of columnar cells. Bacteria could, of course, become trapped and possibly multiply in the mucus layer that is continuously secreted onto the surface of the epithelium lining the human gastrointestinal tract. Biopsy specimens collected from human bowels at endoscopy have been used to detect the association of bacteria with mucosal surfaces (Bibiloni et al., 2006; Lepage et al., 2005; Prindiville et al., 2004; summarized by Tannock, 2005). However, these are not perfect samples for microbiological analysis because they consist of only a few milligrams of tissue that have been collected from subjects that have undergone bowel cleansing prior to endoscopy. Residual bowel cleansing solution, essentially a fecal solution, pools in the bowel and bathes the mucosal surfaces, in all likelihood contaminating it, as well as contaminating the endoscope and its mechanical parts that collect the sample. It is possible that the bacteria detected in association with biopsies are mostly contaminants from the fecal solution and that the reported differences in biopsy specimen profiles and fecal profiles resulting from nucleic acid analysis may be artifacts (Zoetendal et al., 2002). This view is supported by the outcome of microscope-based studies in which bacterial cells were not seen in close proximity to epithelial surfaces in bowel specimens collected from healthy humans (Swidsinski et al., 2002; Van der Waaij et al., 2005).

Molecular analysis of communities based on RNA rather than DNA can be helpful with respect to identifying bacteria that have a niche in the ecosystem because it is recognized that actively metabolizing bacterial cells contain more ribosomes than quiescent cells (Felske et al., 1997). Most of the RNA extracted from bacteria is rRNA, so analyses based on this nucleic acid, such as fluorescent in situ hybridization, are useful because they target rRNA and therefore detect cells that have some metabolic activity. RNA can also be extracted directly from samples collected from ecosystems and used in PCR/denaturing gradient gel electrophoresis (DGGE)/temporal temperature gel electrophoresis, which are electrophoretic methods that provide a snapshot of the community composition in the form of a genetic profile or fingerprint (Muyzer and Smalla, 1998). This analytical approach is extremely useful in screening community composition, especially in a comparative manner. For example, as reported by Tannock et al. (2004), RNA was extracted from the feces of humans who had consumed biscuits containing oligosaccharides originating in milk or inulin. RNA-DGGE profiles of the fecal microbiota were different from those prepared from control samples because of the detection or increased staining intensity (relative to an internal standard) of 16S rRNA gene sequences originating from *Bifidobacterium adolescentis* and/or *Collinsella aerofaciens*. This showed that the dietary oligosaccharides impacted on the metabolism of only certain bowel inhabitants. Altered profiles were not detected by DNA/DGGE, inferring that bacterial cell numbers did not increase. This was confirmed by enumeration of bifidobacterial populations, which remained unchanged during dietary manipulation. It could be argued, therefore, that metabolically quiescent bifidobacterial cells were present in the bowel prior to supplementation of the diet with oligosaccharides. When oligosaccharides were added to the diet, a substrate for metabolism became available, but because other nutrients were growth limiting in the highly regulated bowel community, an increase in bifidobacterial numbers did not occur. Hence, despite up-regulation of 16S rRNA production induced by the presence of novel substrates, increased metabolic activity was not translated into increased cell number. Increased metabolic activity without an increase in the number of bacterial cells is not contradictory because it has been shown in rumen studies that energy spillage (energy dissipation; futile cycles) occurs in bacterial communities where growth is limited by nutrients other than energy sources (Cook and

Russell, 1994; Russell and Cook, 1995). Expectations of altering the population size of selected bacteria in the human bowel by means of dietary supplementation (prebiotics) seem to overlook the complete nutritional package necessary for bacterial growth and the competitive nature of the bowel ecosystem. Nevertheless, it is amazingly easy to modify the composition of the cecal microbiota of rats, perhaps because the animals will eat anything at all, at concentrations that humans cannot tolerate (Snart et al., 2006).

Which brings us, reasonably logically, to the microbial dinner table. A chemostat is a culture apparatus that is used to maintain the growth of bacterial cultures continuously and at a constant rate under laboratory conditions. Culture medium is fed into a culture vessel containing the bacterial cells at a rate controlled by a flow regulator. The culture volume is held constant by means of an overflow tube that enables spent medium (effluent) to pass from the culture vessel. The human large bowel is the equivalent of a chemostat. It is fed with culture medium derived from the undigested components of the diet that pass from the small bowel, as well as substances produced endogenously by the human host. Hence, this culture medium is particularly rich in complex carbohydrates derived from plant cell walls and complex glycoproteins from mucus (Cummings and Macfarlane, 1991; Roberton and Corfield, 1999). The ileocecal valve regulates the flow of culture medium into the large bowel; feces are the effluent. Under these circumstances, a continuous fermentation of exogenous and endogenous substrates by consortia of bacteria proceeds, resulting in the formation of short-chain fatty acids (mainly acetic, propionic, and butyric), amines, phenols, indoles, and gases as the major products (Cummings and Macfarlane, 1991). Large-bowel biochemistry is similar from one person to the next, so regardless of phylogenetic composition, the bacterial communities carry out the same overall fermentation (summarized by Tannock, 2003). It is very similar to the fermentation that occurs in the rumen (Hungate, 1966; Russell, 2002). Whereas the structure and function of the rumen ecosystem are reasonably well understood (to the extent that energy balances can be calculated), knowledge of the flow of carbon from plant residues (dietary fiber) and endogenous substrates (such as mucins) through the community is in a pitiful state in the case of the human large-bowel fermentation. There is a desperate need to define the food-bacteria-mucosa webs that exist in the bowel because this knowledge will help us to understand the meaning of health and how maintenance of a healthy bowel is achieved.

Generously, but in fact unavoidably, we lay a banquet for the bowel bacteria. The groaning table of dishes of complex polysaccharides that our bowel provides is shared with the microbes that consequently have established themselves on the outside of the inside of our body. In sharing the table (*mensa*) with the microbes, we confer on them the title of "commensals." The predominant bowel commensals, as one would expect, are superbly adapted to munching on complex polysaccharides as revealed by glimpses of their collective metabolism under laboratory conditions, but also through analysis of a few representative fully sequenced genomes, as well as by a dip into community genetics (Flint et al., 2007; Gill et al., 2006; Schell et al., 2002; Xu et al., 2003). The bacteria are endowed with the ability to produce numerous hydrolytic enzymes and to regulate their use according to the kinds of substrates that they sense in their environment. Strict regulation of catabolic pathways must be an extremely important attribute in a habitat where the nutritional profile varies from day to day according to the omnivorous and varied dietary preferences of the human host, and this helps to explain the remarkable consistency in biochemistry and biodiversity of the human bowel (Lay et al., 2005; summarized by Tannock, 2003; Zoetendal et al., 1998).

"There is no free lunch": services rendered deserve payment in return. What do the commensals render unto us in return for three square meals a day? Probably the greatest benefit that they confer on the human host is "colonization resistance" ("competitive exclusion"), a phenomenon particularly well known in the case of the bowel community (Van der Waaij et al., 1971). Long ago demonstrated in gnotobiotic experiments, the presence of the indigenous microbiota enhances nonspecific resistance to infection. Germfree mice can be infected by the oral route by a dose of *Salmonella enterica* serovar Typhimurium as small as 10 cells; the infectious dose for conventional mice is about 10^9 cells. The self-regulated, homeostatic community already established in the conventional bowel provides a hurdle that only large numbers (a high dose) of pathogenic cells can surmount (summarized by Tannock, 1984). Moreover, competitive exclusion guarantees that probiotic organisms must be consumed each day in order to maintain their transient existence in the bowel (Tannock et al., 2000). How does competitive exclusion work? Explanations are vague but best summarized in the niche exclusion principle: two species cannot simultaneously occupy the same ecological niche (Hardin, 1960). Only the better adapted will be successful. This can easily be envisaged in the case of nutritional competition because the species/strain that best binds and transports a source of energy and carbon into its cells will outcompete a biochemically less capable organism. In nonhuman hosts, such as in the chicken crop, competition for epithelial locations could also be important (Hagen et al., 2005). Not to be forgotten, moreover, is the production of antimicrobial molecules that could give a competitive edge by altering the chemical environment, making it unsuitable for growth by other species. Short-chain fatty acids can be invoked in this respect, as can hydrogen sulfide and perhaps bacteriocins (summarized by Tannock, 1984; Corr et al., 2007). Multiple mechanisms must participate synergistically in the control of populations within such a complex community. It would be especially interesting to know how the minority populations are maintained at very low population levels, teetering on the brink of washout from the bowel. Probably, these are scavengers that feed on the crumbs left on the table by the obligately anaerobic, fiber-hydrolyzing bacteria. *Lactobacillus ruminis*, which is an autochthonous member of the human bowel community and which can ferment oligosaccharides but cannot degrade polysaccharides, may provide an example of this lifestyle (Snart et al., 2006). We know precious little of how competitive exclusion works in the case of the microbiota of experimental animals, let alone what happens in the human bowel. It is extremely difficult to define competitive mechanisms even using experimental animal models. Hentges and Freter (1962) found that the order in which bacterial strains were introduced into the experimental system ordained which of two organisms would eventually dominate the ecosystem numerically. Freter and colleagues (1973) and Ducluzeau and Raibaud (1979) showed that the diet fed to experimental animals influenced the outcome of competition experiments. By changing the diet, the number and types of available ecological niches are changed. The bowel community is composed of hundreds of species, which in turn implies that there are approximately that number of ecological niches in the ecosystem—the more niches, the more biodiversity. The diversity of bacterial types in the human bowel reflects, therefore, the intensely competitive nature of this ecosystem in which mutations and horizontal gene transfer have permitted adaptation of bacteria to fill diverse niches. The bowel has been, and perhaps still is, a hotbed of evolution.

Salyers (1982) calculated that it would require 30 to 45 g of carbohydrate to supply the energy and carbon sources of the human bowel community each day. The sources of these microbial nutrients have been alluded to earlier in the chapter, but we should return to this topic again because the fermentation of polysaccharides results in short-chain fatty acids, a proportion of which are absorbed from the bowel. In ruminants, which rely almost entirely on microbial activities for life, these microbial fermentation products provide the main energy and carbon sources for the animal (Russell, 2002). Monogastric animals with large ceca, such as rodents, pigs, horses, and chickens, must gain considerable nutritional value from the cecal fermentation because the organ comprises up to 5% of body weight (McBee, 1977). Such a large organ is not something that an animal seeking a quick exit from the proximity of predators would willingly carry without good reason. Perhaps primitive humans also derived benefit from the large bowel fermentation, but it is unlikely that it is of much significance today when, at least in the rich nations of the world, humans have overnutrition rather than malnutrition. Nutritionists continue to laud the role of butyric acid as an important source of energy and carbon for colonocytes lining the large bowel (Roediger, 1980).

The bowel of neonates resembles that of a germfree animal because it does not yet harbor a microbial community. This germfree state is short-lived because a characteristic succession of bacteria colonizes the bowel as the infant ages. The climax community is not reached until the child is about 4 years of age, when stability in community genetic fingerprints is achieved and the enterobacteria, enterococci, and bifidobacteria that were numerous in early life have subsided to minority membership of the community (Cooperstock and Zedd, 1983; Norin et al., 1985). Nucleic acid-based methods of analysis show that bifidobacteria form between 60 and 91% of the total bacterial community in the feces of breast-fed babies and 28 to 75% (average 50%) in formula-fed infants during early life (Harmsen et al., 2000). The infant during early life is therefore almost a monoassociated gnotobiote, and bifidobacterial antigens may be important instigators of immunological development. The lack of exposure of babies to particular bifidobacterial species and/or the elimination of bifidobacterial species from the bowel through the use of antibiotics might reduce the exposure of children in early life to important bacterial antigens at a critical time in the maturation of the immune system, for example in removing (immune deviation) the T helper 2 (Th2) skew characteristic of the newborn child (Prescott et al., 1998; Yabuhara et al., 1997). This immune deviation, or lack thereof, may have implications in dictating whether children are prone to allergies such as asthma and atopic eczema (Hopkin, 1997). The potential impact of the bowel bacteria of infants on the programming of the immune system invokes Dubos' concept of "biological Freudianism." Drawing on the results obtained from experiments with specific-pathogen-free mice, Dubos and colleagues (1966) concluded that "from all points of view, the child is father of the man, and for this reason we need to develop an experimental science that might be called biological Freudianism. Socially and individually the response of human beings to the conditions of the present is always conditioned by the biological remembrance of things past." The prescience of Dubos and colleagues in the development of experimental science based on the concept of biological Freudianism is remarkable and admirable. Freud postulated that an unconscious mental process or event was not just one that cannot, except through psychoanalysis, ever be brought to mind. The unconscious exerted a dynamic and determining influence upon the conscious mind: the past is alive in the present. Like an iceberg, the bulk of which is unseen below the surface of the sea, the bowel bacteria of early life, unseen and unfelt, just like the unconscious mind, may condition and shape the immune system for later life. Much research, both bacteriological and immunological, remains to be done on this topic.

The rest is doom and gloom. The indigenous microbiota is a potent source of opportunistic infections that arise when the mechanisms that normally confine the microbes to a particular site are disrupted. Anaerobic infections following bowel surgery, urinary tract infections, chronic respiratory tract infections, dental/gingival diseases, and annoying skin conditions come into this category (Finegold, 1977). Confinement of one's dinner guests to a corner of the house is not usual in an anthropomorphic sense, but it is the best solution in the case of commensals and their associated antigens. The maintenance of lotic environments (flows of secretions and digesta) and intact epithelial barriers are the main defenses. Leaky epithelia, probably a genetic predisposition activated by as yet unknown factors early in life, seem to be a critical feature of Crohn's disease in which a chronic immune inflammation of the bowel mucosa is apparently fueled by antigens derived from the bowel microbiota. Macdonald and Monteleone (2005) have proposed that, in Crohn's disease, bacterial cells and/or their antigens pass via M cells into Peyer's patches where CD4+ T cells are activated and migrate to the lamina propria. In healthy humans, because there is not an antigenic challenge in that site, the T cells die there by apoptosis. Increased epithelial permeability in Crohn's disease patients, compounded by a dysfunctional immune system, allows sufficient bacterial antigens to enter the lamina propria from the bowel lumen to trigger T-cell activation, breaking tolerance mediated by immunosuppressive cytokines and T regulatory cells. The immune cells pursue their normal policy of eradicating threatening bacteria and their components, but this is impossible to achieve because the antigenic sources are bacteria residing in the bowel. Hence, a chronic inflammation occurs because the antigenic fuel is supplied continuously from the bowel lumen through the defective

epithelial barrier. Thus, in Crohn's disease, the bowel microbiota acts as a surrogate pathogen. Much effort has been expended in searching for specific microbes to associate with the etiopathogenesis of Crohn's disease and ulcerative colits (Sartor, 2004), but it makes more sense to incriminate particular antigens with the capacity to drive the chronic inflammation. Powerful antigens produced by a wide range of microbial species could be responsible, one such being bacterial flagellin, which has a 13-amino-acid region that is highly conserved across the motile bacterial world, is required for protofilament formation and bacterial motility, and binds to Toll-like-receptor 5 and thereby activates a cascade of reactions within immune cells that may prove proinflammatory (Smith et al., 2003). A subset of Crohn's disease patients with complicated disease (fibrostenosis and small bowel involvement) have elevated levels of serum antibodies to bacterial flagellin relative to controls (Lodes et al., 2004; Targan et al., 2005). Elson's work with gene expression libraries offers an exciting approach to identifying further candidate proinflammatory antigens produced by the bowel microbiota (Konrad et al., 2006).

The list of maladies with which the human indigenous microbiota has been associated is of significant size. Sometimes disease is produced iatrogenically, such as in the case of antibiotic-associated colitis (proliferation and toxin production by *Clostridium difficile*) (Bartlett, 1983), sometimes in association with other diseases (for example, contaminated small-bowel syndrome and diverticulosis) (Gracey, 1983). In any case, life in association with microbes, as is life in general, is perilous, a delicate balance between health and disease. Humans do not need an indigenous microbiota for life, since germfree children have been delivered by sterile cesarean section and maintained in isolators until receipt of a bone marrow transplant to correct congenital immunological abnormalities. "David" lived gnotobiotically for 12 years and, although not germfree for the entire time, never harbored more than a simple collection of microbes in his body (Bealmear et al., 1985). A consequence of Pandora's curiosity, however, was to liberate untold evils into the world. Microbes must surely be counted among these evils when the huge toll of infectious diseases on humanity is considered. We have no choice, however, but to live in a microbe-colonized world. The indigenous microbiota, it seems, can be a force for good or for evil. We may not be getting good value in return for providing them nourishment. Fortunately, Pandora did not let *Hope* escape from her jar, so we have the prospect of conducting research that will enable us to better understand the indigenous microbiota. Medical science continues to be more concerned with defining the abnormal in order to find the means to heal. Medical knowledge focuses on the pathogenesis of diseases and the derivation of intervention strategies. We know a lot about diseases, but do we really understand health?

To understand health, we must learn about the mechanisms that operate in the healthy body by which stable ecosystems are sustained and maintained. We need to delineate the blueprints that underpin the microbial ecology of the healthy human body. Then, health might be guarded by reason, perhaps by interventions that would produce predictable outcomes on the basis of knowledge of molecular networks. Fortunately, the technological approaches to achieve these goals are at the fingertips of microbiologists: metagenomics to access and assess community genetics (Handelsman, 2004), and metabolomics to analyze functional attributes of the indigenous microbiota in concert with that of the host (Kell et al., 2005; Van der Werf et al., 2005). Drawing the blueprint of the microbial ecology of the body will require a systems biology investigation encompassing a diversity of scientists from different disciplines. A fusion of biological and computational expertise will clearly be required (Nicholson et al., 2004). The primary aim of the research will be to understand how all of the heterogeneous parts (dietary components, bacterial consortia, and human physiology and development) are integrated, with a supplementary aim of identifying biomarkers of health or disease. Assembling the results of fundamental analyses of the microbial ecology of the human body may enable us to govern our lives by reason and to support a realistic, holistic view of health (Dubos, 1959).

> This variable composition of man's body hath made it as an instrument easy to distemper; and, therefore, the poets did well to conjoin music and medicine in Apollo, because the office of medicine is but to tune this curious harp of man's body and to reduce it to harmony.
>
> Francis Bacon, 17th century scientist
> and statesman

References

Ashelford, K. E., N. A. Chuzhanova, J. C. Fry, A. J. Jones, and A. J. Weightman. 2005. At least 1 in 20 16S rRNA sequence records currently held in public repositories is estimated to contain substantial anomalies. *Appl. Environ. Microbiol.* **71:**7724–7736.

Ashelford, K. E., N. A. Chuzhanova, J. C. Fry, A. J. Jones, and A. J. Weightman. 2006. New screening software shows that most recent large 16S rRNA gene clone libraries contain chimeras. *Appl. Environ. Microbiol.* **72:**5734–5741.

Backhed, F., H. Ding, T. Wang, L. V. Hooper, G. Y. Koh, A. Nagy, C. F. Semenkovich, and J. I. Gordon. 2004. The gut microbiota as an environmental factor that regulates fat storage. *Proc. Natl. Acad. Sci. USA* **101:**15718–15723.

Bartlett, J. G. 1983. Pseudomembranous colitis, p. 447–479. *In* D. J. Hentges (ed.), *Human Intestinal Microflora in Health and Disease.* Academic Press, New York, NY.

Bealmear, P. M., M. A. South, and R. Wilson. 1985. David's story: the gift of 12 years, 5 months, and 1 day, p. 475–489. *In* B. S. Wostman and J. R. Pleasants (ed.), *Germfree Research: Microflora Control and Its Application to the Biomedical Sciences.* Alan R. Liss, New York, NY.

Bibiloni, R., M. Mangold, K. L. Madsen, R. N. Fedorak, and G. W. Tannock. 2006. The bacteriology of biopsies differs between newly diagnosed, untreated, Crohn's disease and ulcerative colitis patients. *J. Med. Microbiol.* **55:**1141–1149.

Bik, E. M., P. B. Eckburg, S. R. Gill, K. E. Nelson, E. A. Purdom, F. Francois, G. Perez-Perez, M. J. Blaser, and D. A. Relman. 2006. Molecular analysis of the bacterial microbiota in the human stomach. *Proc. Natl. Acad. Sci. USA* **103:**732–737.

Cook, G. M., and J. B. Russell. 1994. Energy spilling reactions of *Streptococcus bovis* and resistance of its membrane to proton conductance. *Appl. Environ. Microbiol.* **60:**1942–1948.

Cooperstock, M. S., and A. J. Zedd. 1983. Intestinal flora of infants, p. 79–99. *In* D. J. Hentges (ed.), *Human Intestinal Microflora in Health and Disease.* Academic Press, New York, NY.

Corr, S. C., L. Yin, C. U. Riedel, P. W. O'Toole, C. Hill, and C. G. M. Gahan. 2007. Bacteriocin production as a mechanism for the anti-infective activity of *Lactobacillus salivarius* UCC118. *Proc. Natl. Acad. Sci. USA* **104:**7617–7621.

Cummings, J. H., and G. T. Macfarlane. 1991. The control and consequences of bacterial fermentation in the human colon. *J. Appl. Bacteriol.* **70:**443–459.

Dubos, R. 1959. *Mirage of Health. Utopias, Progress, and Biological Change.* Rutgers University Press, New Brunswick, NJ.

Dubos, R., D. Savage, and R. Schaedler. 1966. Biological Freudianism: lasting effects of early environmental influences. *Pediatrics* **38:**789–800.

Ducluzeau, R., and P. Raibaud. 1979. *Ecologie Microbienne du Tube Digestif.* Masson, Paris, France.

Eckburg, P. B., E. M. Bik, C. N. Bernstein, E. Purdom, L. Dethlefsen, M. Sargent, S. R. Gill, K. E. Nelson, and D. A. Relman. 2005. Diversity of the human intestinal microbial flora. *Science* **308:**1635–1638.

Felske, A., H. Rheims, A. Wolerink, E. Stackebrandt, and A. D. L. Akkermans. 1997. Ribosome analysis reveals prominent activity of an uncultured member of the class Actinobacteria in grassland soils. *Microbiology* **143:**2983–2989.

Finegold, S. M. 1977. *Anaerobic Bacteria in Human Disease.* Academic Press, New York, NY.

Flint, H. J., S. H. Duncan, K. P. Scott, and P. Louis. 2007. Interactions and competition within the microbial community of the human colon: links between diet and health. *Environ. Microbiol.* **9:**1101–1111.

Freter, R., G. D. Abrams, and A. Aranki. 1973. Patterns of interaction in gnotobiotic mice among bacteria of a synthetic "normal" intestinal flora, p. 429–433. *In* J. B. Heneghan (ed.), *Germfree Research*. Academic Press, New York, NY.

Fuller, R., and B. E. Brooker. 1974. Lactobacilli which attach to the crop epithelium of the fowl. *Am. J. Clin. Nutr.* 27:1305–1312.

Gill, S. R., M. Pop, R. T. DeBoy, P. B. Eckburg, P. J. Turnbaugh, B. S. Samuel, J. I. Gordon, D. A. Relman, C. M. Fraser-Liggett, and K. E. Nelson. 2006. Metagenomic analysis of the human distal gut microbiome. *Science* 312:1355–1359.

Gracey, M. 1983. The contaminated small bowel syndrome, p. 495–515. *In* D. J. Hentges (ed.), *Human Intestinal Microflora in Health and Disease*. Academic Press, New York, NY.

Hagen, K. E., L. L. Guan, G. W. Tannock, D. R. Korver, and G. E. Allison. 2005. Detection, characterization, and in vitro and in vivo expression of genes encoding S-proteins in *Lactobacillus gallinarum* strains isolated from chicken crops. *Appl. Environ. Microbiol.* 71:6633–6643.

Handelsman, J. 2004. Metagenomics: application of genomics to uncultured microorganisms. *Microbiol. Mol. Biol. Rev.* 68:669–685.

Hardin, G. 1960. The competitive exclusion principle. *Science* 131:1292–1297.

Harmsen, H. J. M., A. C. M. Wildeboer, G. C. Raangs, A. A. Wagendorp, N. Klijn, J. G. Bindels, and G. W. Welling. 2000. Analysis of intestinal flora development in breast-fed and formula-fed infants by using molecular identification and detection methods. *J. Pediatr. Gastroenterol. Nutr.* 30:61–67.

Hayashi, H., R. Takahashi, T. Nishi, M. Sakamoto, and Y. Benno. 2005. Molecular analysis of jejunal, ileal, caecal and recto-sigmoidal human colonic microbiota using 16S rRNA gene libraries and terminal restriction fragment length polymorphism. *J. Med. Microbiol.* 54:1093–1101.

Hentges, D. J., and R. Freter. 1962. In vivo and in vitro antagonism of intestinal bacteria against *Shigella flexneri*. I. Correlation between various tests. *J. Infect. Dis.* 110:30–37.

Hooper, L. V., M. H. Wong, A. Thelin, L. Hansson, P. G. Falk, and J. I. Gordon. 2001. Molecular analysis of commensal host-microbial relationships in the intestine. *Science* 291:881–884.

Hooper, L. V., J. Xu, P. G. Falk, T. Midtvedt, and J. I. Gordon. 1999. A molecular sensor that allows a gut commensal to control its nutrient foundation in a competitive ecosystem. *Proc. Natl. Acad. Sci. USA* 96:9833–9838.

Hopkin, J. M. 1997. Mechanisms of enhanced prevalence of asthma and atopy in developed countries. *Curr. Opin. Immunol.* 9:788–792.

Hungate, R. E. 1966. *The Rumen and Its Microbes*. Academic Press, New York, NY.

Kell, D. B., M. Brown, H. M. Davey, W. B. Dunn, I. Spasic, and S. G. Oliver. 2005. Metabolic footprinting and systems biology: the medium is the message. *Nat. Rev.* 3:557–565.

Kimura, K., A. L. McCartney, M. A. McConnell, and G. W. Tannock. 1997. Analysis of fecal populations of bifidobacteria and lactobacilli and investigation of the immunological responses of their human hosts to the predominant strains. *Appl. Environ. Microbiol.* 63:3394–3398.

Konrad, A., Y. Cong, W. Duck, R. Borlaza, and C. O. Elson. 2006. Tight mucosal compartmentation of the murine immune response to antigens of the enteric microbiota. *Gastroenterology* 130:2050–2059.

Lay, C., L. Rigottier-Gois, K. Holmstrom, M. Rajilic, E. E. Vaughan, W. M. de Vos, M. D. Collins, R. Thiel, P. Namsolleck, M. Blaut, and J. Dore. 2005. Colonic microbiota signatures across five northern European countries. *Appl. Environ. Microbiol.* 71:4153–4155.

Lepage, P., P. Seksik, M. Sutren, M.-F. de la Cochetiere, R. Jian, P. Marteau, and J. Dore. 2005. Biodiversity of the mucosa-associated microbiota is stable along the distal digestive tract in healthy individuals and patients with IBD. *Inflamm. Bowel Dis.* 11:473–480.

Lodes, M. J., Y. Cong, C. O. Elson, R. Mohamath, C. J. Landers, S. R. Targan, M. Fort, and R. M. Hershberg. 2004. Bacterial flagellin is a dominant antigen in Crohn disease. *J. Clin. Investig.* 113:1296–1306.

Macdonald, T. T., and G. Monteleone. 2005. Immunity, inflammation, and allergy in the gut. *Science* 307:1920–1925.

McBee, R. H. 1977. Fermentation in the hindgut, p. 185–222. *In* R. T. J. Clarke and T. Bauchop (ed.), *Microbial Ecology of the Gut*. Academic Press, London, United Kingdom.

McCartney, A. L., W. Wenzhi, and G. W. Tannock. 1996. Molecular analysis of the composition of the bifidobacterial and lactobacillus microflora of humans. *Appl. Environ. Microbiol.* 62:4608–4613.

Miller, T. L., and M. J. Wolin. 1983. Stability of *Methanobacter smithii* populations in the microbial flora excreted from the human large bowel. *Appl. Environ. Microbiol.* 45:317–318.

Moore, W. E. C., and L. V. Holdeman. 1974. Special problems associated with the isolation and identification of intestinal bacteria in fecal flora studies. *Am. J. Clin. Nutr.* 27:1450–1455.

Muyzer, G., and K. Smalla. 1998. Application of denaturing gradient gel electrophoresis (DGGE) and temperature gradient gel electrophoresis (TGGE) in microbial ecology. *Antonie van Leeuwenhoek* 73:127–141.

Nicholson, J. K., E. Holmes, J. C. Lindon, and I. D.Wilson. 2004. The challenges of modeling mammalian biocomplexity. *Nat. Biotechnol.* 22:1268–1274.

Norin, K. E., B. E. Gustafsson, B. S. Lindblad, and T. Midtvedt. 1985. The establishment of some microflora associated biochemical characteristics in feces from children during the first years of life. *Acta Paediatr. Scand.* 74:207–212.

Prescott, S. L., C. Macaubus, B. J. Holt, T. B. Smallacombe, R. Loh, P. D. Sly, and P. G. Holt. 1998. Transplacental priming of the human immune system to environmental allergens: universal skewing of initial T cell responses toward the Th2 cytokine profile. *J. Immunol.* 160:4730–4737.

Prindiville, T., M. Cantrell, and K. H. Wilson. 2004. Ribosomal DNA sequence analysis of mucosa-associated bacteria in Crohn's disease. *Inflamm. Bowel Dis.* 10:824–833.

Rawls, J. F., M. A. Mahowald, R. E. Ley, and J. I. Gordon. 2006. Reciprocal gut microbiota transplants from zebrafish and mice to germfree recipients reveal host habitat selection. *Cell* 127:423–433.

Roberton, A. M., and A. P. Corfield. 1999. Mucin degradation and its significance in inflammatory conditions of the gastrointestinal tract, p. 222–261. *In* G. W. Tannock (ed.),

Medical Importance of the Normal Microflora. Kluwer Academic Publishers, Dordrecht, The Netherlands.

Roediger, W. E. 1980. Role of anaerobic bacteria in the metabolic welfare of the colonic mucosa in man. *Gut* **21:**793–798.

Russell, J. B. 2002. *Rumen Microbiology and Its Role in Ruminant Nutrition*. Cornell University, Ithaca, NY.

Russell, J. B., and G. M. Cook. 1995. Energetics of bacterial growth: balance of anabolic and catabolic reactions. *Microbiol. Rev.* **59:**48–62.

Salyers, A. A. 1982. Enzymes involved in degradation of unabsorbed polysaccharides by bacteria of the large bowel, p. 135–138. *In* G. Wallace and L. Bell (ed.), *Fibre in Human and Animal Nutrition*. The Royal Society of New Zealand, Wellington, New Zealand.

Sartor, R. B. 2004. Microbial influences in inflammatory bowel disease: role in pathogenesis and clinical implications, p. 138–162. *In* R. B. Sartor and W. J. Sandborn (ed.), *Kirstner's Inflammatory Bowel Diseases*. Elsevier Publishers, London, United Kingdom.

Schell, M. A., M. Karamirantzou, B. Snel, D. Vilanova, B. Berger, G. Pessi, M. C. Zwahlen, F. Desiere, P. Bork, M. Delby, and R. D. Pridmore. 2002. The genome sequence of *Bifidobacterium longum* reflects its adaptation to the human gastrointestinal tract. *Proc. Natl. Acad. Sci. USA* **99:**14422–14427.

Simon, G. L., and S. L. Gorbach. 1984. Intestinal flora in health and disease. *Gastroenterology* **86:**174–193.

Smith, K. D., E. Andersen-Nissen, F. Hayashi, K. Strobe, M. A. Bergman, S. L. Rassoulian Barrett, B. T. Cookson, and A. Aderem. 2003. Toll-like receptor 5 recognizes a conserved site on flagellin required for protofilament formation and bacterial motility. *Nat. Immunol.* **4:**1247–1253.

Snart, J., R. Bibiloni, T. Grayson, C. Lay, H. Zhang, G. E. Allison, J. K. Laverdiere, F. Temelli, T. Vasanthan, R. Bell, and G. W. Tannock. 2006. Supplementation of the diet with high-viscosity beta-glucan results in enrichment for lactobacilli in the rat cecum. *Appl. Environ. Microbiol.* **72:**1925–1931.

Stappenbeck, T. S., L. V. Hooper, and J. I. Gordon. 2002. Developmental regulation of intestinal angiogenesis by indigenous microbes via Paneth cells. *Proc. Natl. Acad. Sci. USA* **99:**15451–15455.

Suau, A., R. Bonnet, M. Sutren, J.-J. Godon, G. R. Gibson, M. D. Collins, and J. Dore. 1999. Direct analysis of genes encoding 16S rRNA from complex communities reveals many novel molecular species within the human gut. *Appl. Environ. Microbiol.* **65:**4799–4807.

Swidsinski, A., A. Ladhoff, A. Pernthaler, S. Swidsinski, V. Loening-Baucke, M. Ortner, J. Weber, U. Hoffman, S. Schreiber, M. Dietel, and H. Lochs. 2002. Mucosal flora in inflammatory bowel disease. *Gastroenterology* **122:**44–54.

Tannock, G. W. 1984. Control of gastrointestinal pathogens by normal flora, p. 374–382. *In* M. J. Klug and C. A. Reddy (ed.), *Perspectives in Microbial Ecology*. American Society for Microbiology, Washington, DC.

Tannock, G. W. 1992. The lactic microflora of pigs, mice and rats, p. 21–48. *In* J. B. Wood (ed.), *The Lactic Acid Bacteria*, vol. 1. *The Lactic Acid Bacteria in Health and Disease*. Elsevier Applied Science, London, United Kingdom.

Tannock, G. W. 1995. *Normal Microflora. An Introduction to Microbes Inhabiting the Human Body*. Chapman and Hall, London, United Kingdom.

Tannock, G. W. 1997. Influences of the normal microbiota on the animal host, p. 466–497. *In* R. I. Mackie, B. A. White, and R. E. Isaacson (ed.), *Gastrointestinal Microbiology*, vol. 2. *Gastrointestinal Microbes and Host Interactions*. Chapman and Hall, New York, NY.

Tannock, G. W. 2003. The intestinal microflora, p. 1–23. *In* R. Fuller and G. Perdigon (ed.), *Gut Flora. Nutrition, Immunity and Health*. Blackwell Press, Oxford, United Kingdom.

Tannock, G. W. 2004. A special fondness for lactobacilli. *Appl. Environ. Microbiol.* **70:**3189–3194.

Tannock, G. W. 2005. Microbiota of mucosal surfaces in the gut of monogastric animals, p. 163–178. *In* J. P. Nataro, P. S. Cohen, H. L. T. Mobley, and J. N. Weiser (ed.), *Colonization of Mucosal Surfaces*. ASM Press, Washington, DC.

Tannock, G. W., S. Ghazally, J. Walter, D. Loach, H. Brooks, G. Cook, M. Surette, C. Simmers, P. Bremer, F. Dal Bello, and C. Hertel. 2005. Ecological behavior of *Lactobacillus reuteri* 100–23 is affected by mutation of the *luxS* gene. *Appl. Environ. Microbiol.* **71:**8419–8425.

Tannock, G. W., K. Munro, R. Bibiloni, M. A. Simon, P. Hargreaves, P. Gopal, H. Harmsen, and G. Welling. 2004. Impact of consumption of oligosaccharide-containing biscuits on the fecal microbiota of humans. *Appl. Environ. Microbiol.* **70:**2129–2136.

Tannock, G. W., K. Munro, H. J. M. Harmsen, G. W. Welling, J. Smart, and P. K. Gopal. 2000. Analysis of the fecal microflora of human subjects consuming a probiotic product containing *Lactobacillus rhamnosus* DR20. *Appl. Environ. Microbiol.* **66:**2578–2588.

Targan, S. R., C. J. Landers, H. Yang, M. J. Lodes, Y. Cong, K. A. Papadakis, E. Vasiliauskas, C. O. Elson, and R. M. Hershberg. 2005. Antibodies to CBir1 flagellin define a unique response that is associated independently with complicated Crohn's disease. *Gastroenterology* **128:**2020–2028.

Van der Waaij, D., J. M. Berghuis de Vries, and J. E. C. Lekkerkerk. 1971. Colonisation resistance of the digestive tract in conventional and antibiotic-treated mice. *J. Hyg.* **69:**405–411.

Van der Waaij, L., H. J. M. Harmsen, M. Madjipour, F. G. M. Kroese, M. Zwiers, H. M. van Dullemen, N. K. de Boer, G. W. Welling, and P. L. M. Jansen. 2005. Bacterial population analysis of human colon and terminal ileum biopsies with 16S rRNA-based fluorescent probes: commensal bacteria live in suspension and have no direct contact with epithelial cells. *Inflamm. Bowel Dis.* **11:**865–871.

Van der Werf, M. J., R. H. Jellema, and T. Hankemeier. 2005. Microbial metabolomics: replacing trial-and-error by the unbiased selection and ranking of targets. *J. Ind. Microbiol. Biotechnol.* **32:**234–252.

Walter, J., P. Chagnaud, G. W. Tannock, D. M. Loach, F. Dal Bello, H. F. Jenkinson, W. P. Hammes, and C. Hertel. 2005. A high-molecular-mass surface protein (Lsp) and methionine sulfoxide reductase B (MsrB) contribute to the ecological performance of *Lactobacillus reuteri* in the murine gut. *Appl. Environ. Microbiol.* **71:**979–986.

Walter, J., N. C. K. Heng, W. P. Hammes, D. M. Loach, G. W. Tannock, and C. Hertel. 2003. Identification of *Lactobacillus reuteri* genes specifically induced in the mouse gastrointestinal tract. *Appl. Environ. Microbiol.* **69:** 2044–2051.

Walter, J., D. M. Loach, M. Alqumber, C. Rockel, C. Hermann, M. Pfitzenmaier, and G. W. Tannock. 2007. D-alanyl ester depletion of teichoic acids in *Lactobacillus reuteri* 100–23 results in impaired colonization of the mouse gastrointestinal tract. *Environ. Microbiol.* **9:**1750–1760.

Wang, M., S. Ahrne, B. Jeppsson, and G. Molin. 2005. Comparison of bacterial diversity along the human intestinal tract by direct cloning and sequencing of 16S rRNA genes. *FEMS Microbiol. Ecol.* **54:**219–231.

Wilson, M. 2005. *Microbial Inhabitants of Humans: Their Ecology and Role in Health and Disease.* Cambridge University Press, New York, NY.

Xu, J., M. K. Bjursell, J. Himrod, S. Deng, L. K. Carmichael, H. C. Chiang, L. V. Hooper, and J. I. Gordon. 2003. A genomic view of the human-*Bacteroides thetaiotaomicron* symbiosis. *Science* **299:**2074–2076.

Yabuhara, A., C. Macaubas, S. L. Prescott, T. J. Venaille, B. J. Holt, W. Habre, P. D. Sly, and P. G. Holt. 1997. Th2-polarized immunological memory to inhalant allergens in atopics is established during infancy and early childhood. *Clin. Exp. Allergy* **27:**1237–1239.

Yuki, N., T. Shimazaki, A. Kushiro, K. Watanabe, K. Uchida, T. Yuyama, and M. Morotomi. 2000. Colonization of the stratified squamous epithelium of the nonsecreting area of horse stomach by lactobacilli. *Appl. Environ. Microbiol.* **66:**5030–5034.

Zoetendal, E. G., A. D. Akkermans, and W. M. de Vos. 1998. Temperature gradient gel electrophoresis analysis of 16S rRNA from human fecal samples reveals stable and host specific communities of active bacteria. *Appl. Environ. Microbiol.* **64:**3854–3859.

Zoetendal, E. G., A. von Wright, T. Vilpponen-Samela, K. Ben-Amor, A. D. Akkermans, and W. M. De Vos. 2002. Mucosa-associated bacteria in the human gastrointestinal tract are uniformly distributed along the colon and differ from the community recovered from feces. *Appl. Environ. Microbiol.* **68:**3401–3407.

Therapeutic Microbiology: Probiotics and Related Strategies
Edited by J. Versalovic and M. Wilson
© 2008 ASM Press, Washington, DC

2.2. BIOLOGY OF EFFECTOR ORGANISMS FOR PROBIOTIC AND REPLACEMENT THERAPY

Covadonga Barbés

Lactobacilli

3

BRIEF HISTORY

As cited by Hughes and Hillier (1990), Doderlein first isolated gram-positive, catalase-negative, non-spore-forming rods from the vaginas of healthy pregnant women in 1884. "Doderlein bacilli" probably refer to several different genera and species of bacteria. Later, in 1901 M. W. Beijerinck described the genus *Lactobacillus*, and in 1928 Thomas identified the "Doderlein bacilli" as *Lactobacillus acidophilus* by using biochemical methods; this organism is nowadays classified as *Lactobacillus gasseri* (Johnson et al., 1980).

Nowadays, *Lactobacillus* is a well-characterized genus belonging to the phylum *Firmicutes*, class *Bacilli*, order *Lactobacillales*, and family *Lactobacillaceae* together with the genera *Pediococcus* and *Paralactobacillus* (Garrity et al., 2004). They are gram-positive non-spore-forming rods that are catalase and cytochrome negative, usually nonmotile, or motile by peritrichous flagella. Their growth temperature range is 20 to 53°C, with an optimum generally between 30 and 40°C and their pH ranges from 5.5 to 6.2. They are aerotolerant anaerobes, and their growth is enhanced by a microaerophilic atmosphere with 5 to 10% CO_2. They use glucose fermentatively (Kandler and Weiss, 1986), may be either homofermentative or heterofermentative, and have complex nutritional requirements for amino acids, carbohydrates, peptides, nucleic acid derivatives, vitamins, salts, fatty acids, or fatty acid esters.

Lactobacillus comprises 113 recognized species and 16 subspecies, the type species being *Lactobacillus delbrueckii* Leichmann 1896 (Beijerinck, 1901). The genus *Lactobacillus* is very heterogeneous, encompassing species with a large variety of phenotypic, biochemical, and physiological properties. This heterogeneity is reflected in the range of moles percent G+C of the genomic DNA of species included in the genus, this range being 32 to 54%.

Most lactobacilli harbor one or more plasmids, the size of which can vary from 1.2 to 150 kb. On these plasmids have been found genes for lactose metabolism, drug resistance, bacteriocin synthesis, exopolysaccharide production, or DNA restriction-modification. Structurally, plasmids from lactobacilli are closely related to plasmids from other gram-positive bacteria.

Covadonga Barbés, Área de Microbiología, Departamento de Biología Funcional, Facultad de Medicina, Universidad de Oviedo, 33006 Oviedo, Spain.

METABOLISM AND NUTRITIONAL REQUIREMENTS

Lactobacilli possess efficient carbohydrate fermentation pathways coupled to substrate level phosphorylation. A second substrate level phosphorylation site is the conversion of carbamyl phosphate to CO_2 and NH_3, the final step of arginine fermentation. In addition to substrate level phosphorylation, energy may be obtained via the proton motive force generated by lactate efflux (Kandler and Weiss, 1986). Two main sugar fermentation pathways can be distinguished among lactobacilli. The Embden-Meyerhof pathway results almost exclusively in lactic acid as an end product (homolactic fermentation). The 6-phosphogluconate pathway results in significant amounts of other end products such as ethanol, CO_2, acetate, formate, or succinate, in addition to lactic acid (heterolactic fermentation).

Other distinctive metabolic features of lactobacilli are the following: nitrate reduction is highly unusual, gelatine is not liquefied, casein is not digested, and neither indole nor H_2S is produced.

With respect to their nutritional requirements, lactobacilli are extremely fastidious organisms and are adapted to using complex organic substrates. The exact nutritional requirements vary from species to species and are often strain specific. In general, they require carbohydrates as energy and carbon source and also nucleotides, amino acids, and vitamins. Pantothenic acid and nicotinic acid are required by all species, while thiamine is necessary only for the growth of the heterofermentative lactobacilli. The requirements for folic acid, riboflavin, pyridoxal phosphate, and p-aminobenzoic acid vary widely among the various species, riboflavin being the most frequently required, whereas biotin and vitamin B_{12} are required by only a few strains (Kandler and Weiss, 1986).

NATURAL HABITATS

Lactobacilli grow in a variety of habitats wherever high levels of soluble carbohydrates, protein breakdown products, and vitamins occur in conjunction with a low oxygen tension. At the same time, their production of high levels of lactic acid lowers the pH of the environment and suppresses the growth of many other bacteria (Sharpe, 1981). These properties make lactobacilli valuable inhabitants of the intestinal tract of humans and animals and important contributors to food technology. Lactobacilli are widely distributed in nature and have been isolated from various sources. They are part of the indigenous microbiota of the oral cavity, gastrointestinal tract, and vagina in humans and animals, are isolated from plants, and are essential in the manufac-

ture of fermented foods such as dairy products, cured meats, marinated fish, wines, and silages (Morishita et al., 1981).

Humans and Animals

Lactobacilli constitute some of the most common grampositive bacteria in the human microbiota, usually inhabiting various sites as innocuous commensals. The oral cavity and intestinal tract of humans and animals are colonized soon after birth by a diverse microbiota, including lactobacilli. *L. casei*, *L. acidophilus*, and *L. fermentum* are present in the oral cavity in small numbers in dental plaque. Within the gastrointestinal tract, lactobacilli are found at all levels, with quantitative differences depending on the location, being predominant in the ileum and in the large intestine. In general, both qualitative and quantitative variations in this microbiota exist among individuals with respect to individual, ethnic, and nutritional factors (Barbés, 2001). In this organ system, the most frequently encountered lactobacilli belong to the following species: *L. acidophilus* and *L. fermentum* in the stomach; *L. acidophilus*, *L. fermentum*, and *L. salivarius* in the ileum; and *L. fermentum* and *L. salivarius* in the large intestine. Other strains, isolated in lower numbers, are *L. casei*, *L. plantarum*, *L. brevis*, *L. buchneri*, *L. crispatus*, and *L. reuteri* (Lidbeck and Nord, 1993).

Lactobacillus spp. comprise the dominant members of the vaginal microbiota, at 10^7 to 10^8 CFU/g of vaginal fluid in healthy premenopausal women, constituting 61.5% of all microorganisms isolated. Several factors have been found to influence the microbiota of the vagina, such as pregnancy, menstruation, use of oral contraceptives, estrogen replacement therapy, immunosuppression, surgical manipulation of the vagina, and the use of broad-spectrum antibiotics (Fernández et al., 2003). The most frequently isolated species are *L. crispatus*, *L. gasseri*, *L. jensenii*, and *L. iners* (Mehta et al., 1995; Antonio et al., 1999; Vallor et al., 2001; Song et al., 1999; Jin et al., 2007). In addition, lactobacilli have been found on the skin, in nasal and conjunctival secretions, in the ear, in breast milk, and in sperm (Mikelsaar et al., 1998).

With regard to the presence of *Lactobacillus* spp. in other animals, several animals such as pigs, chicken, dogs, mice, rats, and hamsters harbor substantial populations of lactobacilli in their intestines (Mitsuoka, 1992).

Other Habitats

With respect to other habitats, small numbers of lactobacilli are present on intact plant material. *Lactobacillus* spp. are important for both the production and preservation of fermented vegetable foods (e.g., silage, sauerkraut, and mixed pickles). *Lactobacillus* spp. play an important role in the curing process of meat products (e.g., sausages). Lastly, they are also inoculated as a starter or adjunct culture for large-scale commercial milk fermentation processes for making yogurt, cheeses, and sour milks.

TAXONOMY OF RELEVANT ORGANISMS

As mentioned above, the genus *Lactobacillus* was proposed by Beijerinck in 1901. In 1919 Orla-Jensen distinguished three subgenera, *Thermobacterium*, *Streptobacterium*, and *Betabacterium*, on the basis of optimal growth temperature and fermentation end products (Sharpe, 1981). However, the taxonomy of the genus *Lactobacillus* has undergone considerable changes since the time of Orla-Jensen. In 1986 Kandler and Weiss described the following groups. (i) Group I, obligate homofermentative lactobacilli, includes all of the classic representatives of Orla-Jensen's thermobacteria and many other species; the *L. acidophilus* complex composed of six species (*L. acidophilus*, *L. crispatus*, *L. gallinarum*, *L. amylovorus*, *L. gasseri*, and *L. johnsonii*); and other species such as *L. helveticus*, *L. delbrueckii* complex, *L. leichmanii*, *L. salivarius*, and *L. jensenii*. (ii) Group II, facultative heterofermentative lactobacilli, includes Orla-Jensen's streptobacteria and many newly described species, namely, the *L. plantarum* complex, *L. casei* complex, *L. sakei*, *L. curvatus*, and *L. bavaricus*. (iii) Group III contains all the obligate heterofermentative gas-forming lactobacilli of Orla-Jensen's genus *Betabacterium* and other species subsequently described. This group includes *L. fermentum*, *L. cellobiosus*, *L. brevis*, *L. buchneri*, *L. viridescens*, and *L. reuteri*.

In 1991, analyzing 55 species of the genus *Lactobacillus* by reverse transcriptase sequencing of 16s rRNA, Collins et al. demonstrated that the genus *Lactobacillus* is phylogenetically very heterogeneous and the majority of *Lactobacillus* species formed three phylogenetically distinct clusters: Cluster 1 (*L. delbrueckii* group) contains *L. delbrueckii* together with nine other species. Cluster 2 (*L. casei/Pediococcus* group) was the largest and most heterogeneous of the three groups. This cluster comprises 32 *Lactobacillus* species and five pediococcal species. Cluster 3 (designated the *Leuconostoc paramesenteroides* group) contains four *Lactobacillus* species and *L. paramesenteroides*.

The rRNA groups identified by Collins et al. in 1991 do not support the classical division of *Lactobacillus* into the subgenera *Thermobacterium*, *Streptobacterium*, and *Betabacterium* or the three physiological groups described in *Bergey's Manual of Systematic Bacteriology* (Kandler and Weiss, 1986).

In 1995 Schleifer and Ludwig stated that the genus *Lactobacillus* consists of more than 60 described species that are genetically quite diverse. They considered the *L. casei-Pediococcus* group to be heterogeneous and proposed dividing it into the *L. salivarius*, *L. reuteri*, *L. buchneri*, and *L. plantarum* group, as well as renaming the former *L. delbrueckii* group as the *L. acidophilus* group. According to Hammes and Hertel (2003), all former lactobacilli of the *Leuconostoc* group are now reclassified as species of the genus *Leuconostoc* or *Weissella* and all the *Lactobacillus* species listed are members of the former *L. delbrueckii* and *L. casei-Pediococcus* group. Using 16S rRNA sequences, these authors proposed the following phylogenetic groups: *L. buchneri*, *L. casei*, *L. delbrueckii*, *L. plantarum*, *L. reuteri*, *L. sakei*, and *L. salivarius*. On the other hand, *L. brevis* and *L. perolens*, as well as the related species *L. bifermentans* and *L. coryniformis*, are uniquely positioned among the lactobacilli. Finally, according to Dellaglio and Felis (2005), the *L. brevis* group has been included in addition to these and split into two subgroups (*a* and *b*), the *L. buchneri* and *L. plantarum* group and the *L. reuteri* group. Taking these groupings into consideration and according to Euzéby (2007), the genus *Lactobacillus* is composed of 113 species. Phylogenetic groups of the genus *Lactobacillus* are shown in Table 1 with the corresponding species, including their metabolic characteristics and habitats.

Seven species in the genus *Lactobacillus* comprise two subspecies or more: *L. aviarius* (subsp. *araffinosus* and subsp. *aviarius*); *L. coryniformis* (subsp. *coryniformis* and subsp. *torquens*); *L. delbrueckii* (subsp. *bulgaricus*, subsp. *delbrueckii*, subsp. *indicus*, and subsp. *lactis*); *L. kefiranofaciens* (subsp. *kefirgranum* and subsp. *kefiranofaciens*); *L. paracasei* (subsp. *paracasei* and subsp. *tolerans*); *L. plantarum* (subsp. *argentoratensis* and subsp. *plantarum*) and *L. sakei* (subsp. *carnosus* and subsp. *sakei*).

The reclassification of a number of strains and descriptions of several new species have been published recently in the *International Journal of Systematic and Evolutionary Microbiology* (Euzéby, 2007). These are as follows: *L. acidipiscis*, heterotypic synonym of *L. cypricasei*; *L. arizonensis*, heterotypic synonym of *L. plantarum*; *L. durianis*, heterotypic synonym of *L. vaccinostercus*; *L. helveticus*, heterotypic synonym of *L. suntoryeus*; and *L. thermotolerans*, heterotypic synonym of *L. ingluviei*. New species include *L. acidifarinae*, *L. amylotrophicus*, *L. apodemi*, *L. concavus*, *L. hammesii*, *L. harbinensis*, *L. namurensis*, *L. nantensis*, *L. oligofermentans*, *L. plantarum* subsp. *argentoratensis*, *L. rennini*, *L. siliginis*, *L. sobrius*, *L. vini*, and *L. zymae*.

Table 1 Phylogenetic groups of the genus *Lactobacillus*[a]

Full taxon name	Glucose fermentation	Main habitat	Full taxon name	Glucose fermentation	Main habitat
L. brevis group			*L. gallinarum*	O Ho	HA
L. acidifarinae	O He	FF	*L. gasseri*	O Ho	HA
L. brevis	O He	F, FA	*L. hamsteri*	F He	HA
L. hammesii	O He	FF	*L. iners*	O Ho	HA
L. spicheri	F He	FF	*L. intestinalis*	F He	HA
L. zymae	O He	FF	*L. jensenii*	F He	HA
			L. johnsonii	O Ho	HA
L. buchneri group			*L. kalixensis*	O He	HA
L. buchneri a	O He	F, FA	*L. kefiranofaciens* subsp.	O Ho	FF
L. diolivorans a	O He	FF	kefiranofaciens		
L. ferintoshensis a	O He	FF	*L. kefiranofaciens* subsp.	O Ho	FF
L. fructivorans b	O He	FA	kefirgranum		
L. hilgardii a	O He	FA	*L. kitasatonis*	O Ho	HA
L. homohiochii b	F He	FA	*L. psittaci*	O Ho	P
L. kefiri a	O He	FF	*L. sobrius*	O Ho	HA
L. lindneri b	O He	FA	*L. suntoryeus*	O Ho	FF
L. namurensis	O He	FF	*L. ultunensis*	O Ho	HA
L. parabrevis	O He	FA			
L. parabuchneri a	O He	HA	*L. plantarum* group		
L. parakefiri a	O He	FF	*L. alimentarius b*	F He	FF, FA
L. sanfranciscensis b	O He	FF	*L. collinoides a*	O He	FA
			L. farciminis b	O Ho	FF
L. casei group			*L. kimchii b*	F He	FF
L. casei a	F He	HA, FF, FA	*L. mindensis b*	O Ho	FF
L. concavus	O Ho	FF	*L. nantensis*	O Ho	FF
L. manihotivorans b	O Ho	FF	*L. paralimentarius b*	F He	FF
L. pantheris b	O Ho	HA	*L. paraplantarum a*	F He	FA, HA
L. paracasei subsp.	F He	HA, FA, FF	*L. pentosus a*	F He	FF, S
paracasei a			*L. plantarum* subsp.	F He	FF, FA
L. paracasei subsp.	F He	FA	plantarum a		
tolerans a			*L. plantarum* subsp.	F He	FF, FA
L. rhamnosus a	F He	FF	argentoratensis		
L. sharpeae b	O Ho	S	*L. versmoldensis b*	O Ho	FF, FA
L. zeae a	F He	FF			
			L. reuteri group		
L. delbrueckii group			*L. antri a*	O He	HA
L. acetotolerans	F He	FA	*L. coleohominis a*	O He	HA
L. acidophilus	O Ho	HA	*L. fermentum a*	O He	FF, FA
L. amylolyticus	O Ho	FF	*L. frumenti a*	O He	FF
L. amylophilus	O Ho	FF	*L. gastricus a*	O He	HA
L. amylotrophicus	O Ho	FF	*L. ingluviei a*	O He	HA
L. amylovorus	O Ho	FF	*L. mucosae a*	O He	HA, FF
L. crispatus	O Ho	HA	*L. oligofermentans*	O He	FA
L. delbrueckii subsp.	O Ho	FF	*L. oris a*	O He	HA
bulgaricus			*L. panis a*	O He	FF
L. delbrueckii subsp.	O Ho	FF	*L. pontis a*	O He	FF
delbrueckii			*L. reuteri a*	O He	HA, FF
L. delbrueckii subsp.	O Ho	FF	*L. rossiae b*	O He	FF
indicus			*L. suebicus b*	O He	FF
L. delbrueckii subsp.	O Ho	FF	*L. vaccinostercus b*	O He	HA
lactis			*L. vaginalis a*	O He	HA
L. fornicalis	F He	HA			

(*Continued*)

Table 1 (*Continued*)

Full taxon name	Glucose fermentation	Main habitat	Full taxon name	Glucose fermentation	Main habitat
L. sakei group			*L. ruminis*	O Ho	HA
L. curvatus	F He	HA, FF, FA	*L. saerimneri*	O Ho	HA
L. fuchuensis	F He	FA	*L. salivarius*	O Ho	HA
L. graminis	F He	FF	*L. satsumensis*	O Ho	FF
L. sakei subsp. *carnosus*	F He	HA, FF, FA	Unique positions		
L. sakei subsp. *sakei*	FHe	FF, FA	*L. algidus*	F He	FA
L. salivarius group			*L. bifermentans*	F He	FA
L. agilis	F He	S	*L. coryniformis* subsp. *coryniformis*	F He	FF
L. animalis	O Ho	HA			
L. apodemi	O Ho	HA	*L. coryniformis* subsp. *torquens*	F He	FF
L. aviarius subsp. *araffinosus*	O Ho	HA			
			L. harbinensis	F He	FF
L. aviarius subsp. *aviarius*	O Ho	HA	*L. kunkeei*	O He	FA
			L. malefermentans	O He	FA
L. cypricasei	F He	FF	*L. paracollinoides*	O He	FF
L. equi	O Ho	HA	*L. perolens*	F He	FA
L. mali	O Ho	FA	*L. rennini*	O Ho	FA
L. murinus	F He	HA	*L. siliginis*	O He	FF
L. nagelii	O Ho	FA	*L. vini*	O Ho	FF

[a]Abbreviations: O Ho, obligately homofermentative; F He, facultatively heterofermentative; O He, obligately heterofermentative; FA, food associated, usually involved in spoilage; FF, involved in fermentation of food; HA, associated with humans and/or animals; S, sewage; P, opportunistic pathogen; *a* and *b*, subgroups according to Dellaglio and Felis (2005). Adapted from Dellaglio and Felis (2005) and updated in March 2007 (Euzéby, 2007).

IDENTIFICATION OF RELEVANT ORGANISMS

The importance of the genus *Lactobacillus* in both the industrial sphere and human and animal health warrants the extensive development and implementation of strain-typing techniques for this genus. Although phenotypic tests have been used as the primary methods for classifying *Lactobacillus* species, this identification often requires the determination of numerous physiological and biochemical characteristics. As a result, genotypic methods are being increasingly applied in the identification of lactobacilli. Several results (Boyd et al., 2005) suggest that the phenotypic methods most commonly used for the identification of *Lactobacillus* species have poor concordance with genome-based tests. Classical genotypic methods include the determination of DNA base composition (moles percent G+C) and DNA-DNA similarity studies. The G+C content of *Lactobacillus* spp. ranges from 32 to 54 mol%, thereby indicating a high genetic heterogeneity within the genus.

Chemotaxonomic approaches (Kandler and Weiss, 1986; Hammes and Hertel, 2003) have used a variety of characteristics including the following:

- Determination of the isomers of lactic acid produced from glucose

- Presence or absence of meso-diaminopimelic acid in the cell wall
- Determination of the peptidoglycan type
- Determination of the electrophoretic mobility of lactate dehydrogenases in starch gels or polyacrylamide gels
- Use of electrophoretic patterns of peptidoglycan hydrolases with activity against *Micrococcus luteus*
- Comparison of whole-cell protein patterns obtained by standardized sodium dodecyl sulfate polyacrylamide electrophoresis is recognized as a reliable tool for the differentiation of species and subspecies

Genetic methods based on the detection of strain-specific DNA sequences by hybridization or PCR techniques have been developed more recently for the identification and subtyping of strains. Molecular typing methods applicable to *Lactobacillus* include plasmid profiling, restriction enzyme analysis, pulsed-field gel electrophoresis, randomly amplified polymorphic DNA, and ribotyping (Holzapfel et al., 2001). In addition, the application of rRNA technology has become of great importance for bacterial identification. The use of restriction endonucleases is the basis for typing of lactobacilli by using chromosomal DNA (Dykes and von Holy, 1994). Both simple restriction of DNA and modifications of this technique using pulsed-field gel electrophoresis have been used to differentiate strains of lactobacilli. Restriction of PCR-amplified DNA regions has also been applied to this genus. Ribotyping, which is based on patterns generated from the rRNA genes only, has been successfully applied to lactobacilli and represents a rapid and sensitive strain-typing technique.

Molecular methods have been developed for the culture-independent analysis of the diversity of complex microbial communities. Denaturing gradient gel electrophoresis of 16S rRNA gene amplicons has been shown to be both suitable and the fastest tool for the characterization of microbiotas containing *Lactobacillus* spp.

It may thus be concluded that many different genotyping techniques can be applied to the genus *Lactobacillus* as tools for either species identification or differentiation of strains at the clonal level.

MOLECULAR MECHANISMS OF PROBIOTIC ACTION

Lactobacillus spp. are among the most frequent and better characterized microorganisms used as a probiotic. A probiotic may be defined as a preparation of (or a product containing) viable microorganisms of a specific genus and species in sufficient numbers to alter the microbiota (by implantation or colonization) in a compartment of the host and, by so doing, exert beneficial effects in the host (Schrezenmeir and de Vrese, 2001). Important considerations in the choice of a probiotic include safety, functional aspects, and technological aspects (Donohue et al., 1998).

Safety

The genus *Lactobacillus* has a long history of safe use, and most strains are considered commensal microorganisms with no pathogenic potential. New strains must be carefully assessed and tested for the safety and efficacy of their proposed use. Three approaches can be used to assess the safety of potential probiotic strains: (i) studies on the intrinsic properties of the strain such as antibiotic resistance, excessive deconjugation of bile acids, or degradation of mucus; (ii) studies on the pharmacokinetic properties of the strain, determining the efficacy of ingested probiotic bacteria and assessing the effect of massive probiotic doses on the composition of the human microbiota; and (iii) studies investigating the interaction between the strain and the hosts. The last approach consists in verifying that the proposed probiotic does not possess any invasion potential and does not harm the host in any way.

Functional Aspects

Most currently successful strains are reported to be of human origin. Probiotic strains must be able to survive and grow under the physiological conditions of the desired ecological unit. Adherence and colonizing ability are also necessary and are closely related to potential immune effects due to prolonged contact with gut-associated lymphoid tissues. Antimicrobial production including bacteriocins, bacteriocin-like substances, as well as lactic acid and hydrogen peroxide, is often thought to be one means of preventing pathogen growth.

Technological Aspects

Strain viability and the maintenance of desirable characteristics during product manufacture and storage are also a requisite for probiotic strains. Strain survival depends on such factors as the final product pH, the presence of other microorganisms, the storage temperature, and the presence or absence of microbial inhibitors in the substrate. Hardy growth and pleasant aroma and flavor profiles are of importance when developing probiotic functional foods.

The mechanisms via which a probiotic acts include suppression of viruses and pathogenic bacteria, changes in gastrointestinal tract metabolic activity, and enhancement of systemic and local immunity enhancement (Fuller, 1989). With respect to the first of these (also known as competitive exclusion), lactobacilli are believed to interfere with pathogens by a number of mechanisms: (i) adherence to the mucus and coaggregation, thereby forming a barrier which prevents colonization by pathogens or competition for the adhesin receptors of the epithelial cells; and (ii) the production of antimicrobial compounds such as hydrogen peroxide, lactic acid, bacteriocins or bacteriocin-like substances, biosurfactants, and a number of partially purified but unnamed compounds (Fernández et al., 2003).

Adherence of bacteria to epithelial cells has been shown to be an important factor in the colonization of mucous membranes. However, the mechanisms of adhesion are poorly understood. Multiple components of the bacterial cell surface such as glycoproteins, carbohydrates, or lipoteichoic acid appear to participate in the adherence process (Boris et al., 1998). The ability of lactobacilli to coaggregate with intestinal pathogens and uropathogenic bacteria is of special interest, as this feature may constitute a protective mechanism against infection (Boris et al., 1998). Unfortunately, little is known regarding the mechanisms underlying the coaggregation of lactobacilli other than that a variety of surface components are thought to be involved.

Lactobacillus spp. are able to produce biosurfactants such as surlactine (Velraeds et al., 1996). Biosurfactants are surface-active compounds produced by microorganisms that are able to reduce surface and interfacial tensions in both aqueous solutions and hydrocarbon mixtures. The most frequently isolated and most extensively researched biosurfactants are the glycolipids; other groups include lipopeptides and protein-like substances, phospholipids, substituted fatty acids, and lipopolysaccharides. The main physiological role of biosurfactants is to facilitate the uptake of water-immiscible substrates, although they can also exert antimicrobial activity against a variety of microbes. It has also been suggested that biosurfactants could be involved in microbial adhesion (Boris and Barbés, 2000).

With regard to the alteration of microbial and host metabolism, lactobacilli are claimed to affect the cholesterol and bile acid metabolism of the host. On the other hand, the fecal enzymes β-glucuronidase, nitroreductase, and azoreductase were reported to decrease in humans, and these activities remained low as long as the probiotic was being administered. In contrast, ingested lactic acid bacteria (LAB) produce and release hydrolytic enzymes such as β-galactosidase which increase after eating yogurt. Some observations suggest that lactobacilli could also contribute to the digestion of more complex carbohydrates than lactose.

Finally, studies with humans have shown that probiotic lactobacilli can have positive effects on the immune system of their host. It has been suggested by many authors that probiotic bacteria could enhance immunity both locally on the mucosal surfaces and at the systemic level. An increase in antibody levels and macrophage activation have also been reported. Several reports suggest that lactobacilli and other LAB can in fact modulate immunity (Gill, 1998; Perdigon et al., 2001; Seegers, 2002; Maassen et al., 2003).

PROBIOTIC FORMULATIONS (COMMERCIAL PRODUCTS)

Over the last few decades, the field of probiosis has emerged as a new science. Probiotics are being commercially developed for both human and animal consumption, especially in the poultry and aquaculture industries. Their application constitutes alternatives to antibiotics, as well as acting as prophylactics, in particular in the prevention of gastrointestinal infections. Reliability, security, and efficacy are considered fundamental requirements for probiotic products. On the other hand, a daily intake of 10^9 to 10^{10} CFU of viable cells is considered the minimum dose shown to have positive effects on host health (Sanders and Veld, 1999).

Most probiotic formulations usually contain one or several selected strains of generally recognized as safe bacteria, mainly belonging to the genera *Lactobacillus* and *Bifidobacterium*. In addition, other LAB such as *Lactococcus*, *Pediococcus*, *Enterococcus*, and *Streptococcus* and even other bacterial taxa such as *Propionibacterium*, *Bacillus*, and *Escherichia coli* and the yeast *Saccharomyces* have also been used in probiotic products (Huys et al., 2006).

With regard to *Lactobacillus* spp., the following strains are used commercially: *L. acidophilus*, *L. casei*, *L. fermentum*, *L. johnsonii*, *L. paracasei*, *L. plantarum*, *L. reuteri*, *L. rhamnosus*, and *L. salivarius* (Sanders and Veld, 1999; Senok et al., 2005). Concentrates of these bacteria are usually freeze-dried, spray-dried, or microencapsulated and are typically incorporated into dairy products such as fermented milks, yogurts, and cheeses.

A wide variety of novel products containing probiotics has been developed. These can be grouped into three categories: (i) conventional foods such as fermented products with addition of probiotic bacteria, consumed primarily for nutritional purposes; (ii) food supplements or fermented milks with food formulations mostly used as a delivery vehicle for probiotic bacteria; and (iii) dietary supplements in the form of capsules and other formulations conceived to be consumed by healthy individuals (Fasoli et al., 2003).

Numerous commercial probiotic products are currently available on the market all over the world and are gaining popularity. Unfortunately, however, several studies (Yeung et al., 2002; Fasoli et al., 2003) have suggested that improper labeling of probiotic species is common in commercial products. Microbial analyses of probiotic products for human consumption have shown that the identity and number of recovered species do not always correspond to what is stated on the labels. Considering that the beneficial effects of probiotics seem to be strain specific and dose dependent, several findings indicate the need for regulations concerning the labeling of probiotic products. Accurate labeling is essential for their proper use. There is no clear legislation regarding these products in Europe. As mentioned above, several findings suggest the need for clear legislation and adequate control of the manufacturing of probiotic products.

Some commercially probiotic products containing lactobacilli are shown in Table 2.

Table 2   Some commercially probiotic products containing lactobacilli[a]

Lactobacillus species included in probiotic preparations	Type of product
L. acidophilus NCFM	Dairy fermentations, dietary supplement, and toddler formula
L. acidophilus R0052	Pharmaceutical preparation for microbiota replacement
L. acidophilus LB	Pharmaceutical preparation for microbiota replacement
L. casei DN114001	Dairy fermentations
L. casei Shirota	Dairy fermentations
L. fermentum VRI003	Pharmaceutical preparation for microbiota replacement
L. johnsonii Lj-1 (La-1)	Pharmaceutical preparation for microbiota replacement
L. paracasei CRL 431	Dairy fermentations
L. paracasei F19	Pharmaceutical preparation for microbiota replacement
L. plantarum 299V	Fruit juice, dairy fermentations, pharmaceutical preparation for microbiota replacement
L. reuteri RC 14	Pharmaceutical preparation to prevent and treat urogenital infections
L. reuteri SD2112	Pharmaceutical preparation for colicky infants
L. rhamnosus GR-1	Pharmaceutical preparation to prevent and treat urogenital infections
L. rhamnosus R0011	Pharmaceutical preparation for microbiota replacement
L. rhamnosus 271	Dairy fermentations
L. rhamnosus GG	Pharmaceutical preparation for microbiota replacement
L. rhamnosus LB21	Dairy fermentations and fruit juice
L. rhamnosus HN001 (DR 20)	Dairy fermentations and pharmaceutical preparation for microbiota replacement
L. salivarius UCC118	Dairy fermentations

[a]Data from www.usprobiotics.org/.

FOOD APPLICATIONS

Lactobacilli are widespread in nature, and many have been used in food fermentation processes, including milk, meat, and plant material. In addition, a few species of *Lactobacillus* are used as probiotic microorganisms in functional foods. As mentioned above, intense research efforts are under way to develop products incorporating probiotic organisms such as *Lactobacillus*. These probiotic organisms must be prepared in a viable manner on a large scale, remain viable and stable during use and storage, and be able to survive within the intestinal ecosystem. They must also remain metabolically active in the gut and must not produce any biochemical changes such as proteolysis, sugar metabolism, or organic acids in the food products in which they are incorporated (Kaur et al., 2002). These new concepts have led to the introduction of functional foods which comprise a wide range of ingredients and functional aspects (Roberfroid, 1998). The concept of functional foods was first introduced in Japan in the late 1980s, and the term was applied to foods fortified with specific ingredients having certain health benefits (Sanders and Veld, 1999). In recent decades, the market for functional foods has grown at a very fast rate. Probiotic products represent a potential

growth area due to their beneficial effects in promoting gut health as well as their ability to prevent and treat disease. This has consequently raised interest in health-promoting foods.

The benefits derived from a regular intake of probiotic foods are also correlated with their ability to inhibit pathogens and protect humans from gastrointestinal diseases. It is quite likely that certain foods may be superior vehicles for disseminating probiotics. It may also be the case that not all probiotics will be able to colonize the gastrointestinal tract when administered in food, whereas some strains may actually work best when administered in this fashion (Vanderhoof, 2001).

Foods fortified with health-promoting probiotic bacteria are produced at present mainly by using fresh milk or milk derivatives such as yogurt, cheese, ice cream, and desserts, although, more recently, functional food industries have been focusing on new, nondairy foods such as cereals or fruit juices. One approach that is worthy of further research is the combination of probiotics and prebiotics, which can result in an increased number of ingested bacteria reaching the colon in a viable form. Another approach would be to use these probiotics in combination with food enzymes.

At the same time, the antibacterial proteinaceous molecules referred to as bacteriocins produced by LAB may be considered as promising biopreservatives. Among the bacteriocins active against *Listeria* spp. the lantibiotic nisin has been widely studied and is currently used in many countries as a preservative in food products. Another group of antibacterial peptides, a subclass named class IIa bacteriocins, are also used (Ross et al., 2002).

INDUSTRIAL APPLICATIONS

Lactobacillus species are members of the diverse group of gram-positive LAB that are industrially important on account of their long history of use in the fermentation of traditional foods, namely, dairy products (yogurt, butter, cheese, and kefir), meat (salami and sausages), vegetables (sauerkraut, pickled cucumber, and olives), and wine and silage (Geis, 2003). The faster development of LAB and the decrease in pH resulting from acid production lead to microbiologically stable fermented products. Their metabolic activity determines the sensorial and nutritional quality of fermented foods as well as contributing to food preservation.

One of the industrial applications of *Lactobacillus* is as a starter, particularly in dairy products. Since the early 1900s, there has been a notable increase worldwide in the industrial production of cheeses and fermented milks. All this is reflected in enormous demands for starter cultures produced on an industrial scale. Starters are the most important factors determining the final quality and properties of a product, their functions being the following: acid production, proteolytic activity, aroma formation, exopolysaccharide formation, and production of inhibitory compounds such as organic acids, hydrogen peroxide, bacteriocins, bacteriocin-like substances, and biosurfactants. Commercially available forms of starter cultures can be liquid, freeze-dried, concentrated frozen, and concentrated freeze-dried (Mäkinen and Bigret, 1998).

Another application of *Lactobacillus* spp. in industry is as a food preservative. Organic acids and additional metabolites such as bacteriocins produced during fermentation play important roles in the preservation of foods, since these products can inhibit growth of spoilage and pathogenic organisms, thus extending the shelf life of fermented foods. Bacteriocins are defined as bactericidal substances with a narrow inhibitory spectrum centered around homologous species and are essentially composed of a biologically active protein moiety (Tagg et al., 1976). Bacteriogenic strains of lactobacilli have been found among a number of different species, both homo- and heterofermentative. Bacteriocins can be used as biopreservatives in a number of ways in food systems, ranging from the use of the bacteriocin-producing strains directly in food, as starter or protection cultures, to the use of concentrated bacteriocin preparations as food additives.

Lactobacillus spp. also produce heteropolysaccharides. Microbial exopolysaccharides are biothickeners that can be added to a variety of food products, where they serve as viscosifying, stabilizing, emulsifying, and gelling agents. Numerous exopolysaccharides with different composition, size, and structure are synthesized by LAB. Examples of industrially important microbial exopolysaccharides are dextrans, xanthan, gellan, pullulan, and bacterial alginates. Dextrans can also be used in the pharmaceutical and medical industries. There is now renewed interest in heteropolysaccharides, since they play an important role in the reology, texture, and body of fermented milk drinks. For instance, a creamy, smooth texture is one aspect of the quality of yogurt which seems to be improved by the ability of the yogurt bacteria to produce exopolysaccharides. Furthermore, exopolysaccharides from LAB have one of the greatest technical potentials for the development of novel, improved products such as low-milk-solid yogurts, low-fat yogurts, etc. (de Vuyst and Degeest, 1999).

Finally, as mentioned above, metabolites are secreted directly into the fermentation medium. In order to maximize production, commercial strains can be genetically modified to improve inherent properties, to introduce desirable characteristics and novel phenotypes, or to remove unwanted traits. The use of genetic engineering techniques is an effective means of enhancing the industrial applicability of LAB. However, when genetic engineering technology is employed, safety becomes an essential factor for the application of improved LAB to the food industry. The safe use of genetically modified LAB requires the development of food grade cloning systems composed solely of DNA from the homologous host or generally recognized as safe organisms that do not rely on antibiotic markers (Shareck et al., 2004). Plasmids are found in many *Lactobacillus* species. Many of the plasmids that occur in LAB are cryptic, a term used to describe plasmids that do not have any apparent function and have no known effect on the host's phenotype. Research should focus on the further development of food grade selective marker systems that are suitable for large-scale, industrial applications.

MEDICAL APPLICATIONS

Genetically engineered lactobacilli expressing bacterial or viral proteins on the cell surface can potentially be used as oral vaccines. *Lactobacillus* strains have a number of properties that make them attractive candidates as live carriers to deliver protective antigens to the mucosal immune system. These include safety for human consumption, ability to colonize the intestine, gastric acid and bile salts tolerance, and their use in fermentation and preservation of foods for decades. The production of antagonistic substances against pathogenic microorganisms and their ability to adhere to gut epithelium are other important characteristics that make these bacteria useful for oral immunization. Reports indicating that certain *Lactobacillus* spp. can induce a nonspecific immunoadjuvant effect have triggered several studies aimed at determining the capability and feasibility of using these bacteria as safe oral vaccines (Ho et al., 2005). The potential of *Lactobacillus* and other LAB to deliver heterologous antigens to the mucosal immune system offers a number of advantages over traditional parenteral vaccination, such as noninvasiveness and the possibility of eliciting both systemic and mucosal immune responses. In conclusion, *Lactobacillus* spp. are attractive candidates as delivery vehicles for the presentation to the mucosa of compounds with pharmaceutical properties, in particular, vaccines and immunomodulators. These bacteria can induce a specific local and systemic immune response against selected pathogens.

The use of bacteria as biotherapeutic agents started in 1885 when Cantani employed *Bacterium termo* in the treatment of tuberculosis by intrapulmonary instillation. In 1906, Tissier encouraged the use of bifidobacteria for intestinal disorders, and later, in 1907, Mechnikoff demonstrated the beneficial effects of fermented milk in humans. In more recent years, greater attention has been paid to the use of probiotics, and specifically lactobacilli, as an alternative, inexpensive, and natural remedy to restore and maintain health. This approach could, in the future, offer an alternative to antibiotics as a reliable treatment and preventive regimen (Fernández et al., 2003).

L. rhamnosus GG is the most widely studied probiotic agent for adults and children, other strains of *Lactobacillus* used in clinical practice being *L. acidophilus* (La 5, NCFB 1748, and NCFM), *L. casei* (Shirota and DN114001), *L. gasseri* (ADH), *L. johnsonii* (La 1), *L. plantarum* (299v), *L. reuteri* (DSM 20016, SD 2112, and RC-14), *L. rhamnosus* GR-1, and *L. salivarius* (UCC 118). These strains can currently be administered in the form of sachets or capsules or may be added to the food supply. Numerous studies have been conducted to validate the concept of probiotics as a viable therapeutic modality in the treatment of gastrointestinal disease. This refers to diarrhea (antibiotic associated, traveler's, and infectious), prevention of ulcers related to *Helicobacter pylori*, amelioration of lactose maladsorption

symptoms, gastroenteritis, and inflammatory bowel disease (Crohn's disease, ulcerative colitis, and pouchitis) (Limdi et al., 2006). At the same time, some preliminary data are now emerging concerning the usefulness of probiotics in extraintestinal diseases. One of the most promising applications of lactobacilli is as biotherapeutic agents in genital infection (Reid, 2002). These bacteria could be used as a complementary or alternative treatment for these infections.

Finally, although results are inconclusive and often contradictory, an effect has also been suggested for other conditions such as the reduction of serum cholesterol, prevention of caries, treatment of food allergies, reduction of blood pressure in hypertensives, and even respiratory diseases (Dairy Council of California, 2000; Vanderhoof, 2001; Kaur et al., 2002; Marteau, 2002; Brown and Valiere, 2004; Senok et al., 2005).

Gastrointestinal Tract

A great number of studies have been conducted on the use of probiotics for the treatment and prophylaxis of several intestinal disorders over the past 2 decades, and documented clinical data on their effects exist (see Salminen et al., 1998; Gismondo et al., 1999; Marteau, 2002; and Brown and Valiere, 2004, for reviews). Several placebo-controlled studies confirmed the efficacy of *Lactobacillus* in the following clinical situations:

Lactose intolerance. A reduction of symptoms has been observed for lactose intolerance when affected patients replace milk with fermented derivatives in their diet. The greater effect is believed to be due to bacterial β-galactosidase activity, detected in the duodenum after ingesting yogurt containing live microorganisms.

Rotavirus-induced diarrhea. The efficacy of *L. rhamnosus* GG in the treatment of rotavirus-induced children's diarrhea has been demonstrated. Its duration is reduced by half, and a local immune response against the virus is promoted with an increase in immunoglobulin A levels.

Diarrhea consecutive to pelvic radiotherapy. Patients receiving pelvic radiotherapy and fermented milk containing viable *L. acidophilus* NCFB 1748 cells have been found to have a lower incidence of diarrhea.

Antibiotic-associated diarrhea (AAD). Diarrhea occurs frequently in patients who receive antibiotics. *Clostridium difficile* and *Klebsiella oxytoca* contribute to the occurrence of AAD. Several human trials (Gismondo et al., 1999; Gorbach, 2000; Marteau et al., 2001) have shown the efficacy of

L. rhamnosus GG or Lactinex (*L. acidophilus* and *L. bulgaricus*) in decreasing the incidence of diarrhea or preventing recurrence when these strains were coadministered with antibiotics. The evidence to support the routine clinical use of probiotics for prevention or treatment AAD was, however, insufficient.

H. pylori. Colonization of the gastric mucosa by *H. pylori* is strongly associated with gastritis, duodenal and gastric ulcers, gastric carcinoma, or lymphoma. Experimental models and clinical studies have shown antagonistic actions of *Lactobacillus* strains such as *L. gasseri*, *L. johnsonii*, and *L. acidophilus* against *H. pylori* in vitro and reduction of gastric inflammation. However, eradication of *H. pylori* in vivo has not yet been demonstrated. In conclusion, the results obtained so far are confusing, thus limiting the clinical use of this approach (Sakamoto et al., 2001; Penner et al., 2005; Limdi et al., 2006).

Inflammatory bowel disease. This disorder includes Crohn's disease, ulcerative colitis, and pouchitis. Some inconclusive studies exist (Schultz and Sartor, 2000; Gionchetti et al., 2002), but further, controlled studies are required to demonstrate the efficacy of lactobacilli in this clinical situation.

Colon cancer. The *L. casei* Shirota strain has shown inhibiting properties on chemically induced tumors in animals. It has been speculated that butyrate (which reduces the growth of cultured colon cancer cells in vitro) may be a natural antitumor compound, at least partially responsible for probiotic effects (Lidbeck et al., 1992). Other human trials have suggested that the consumption of fermented dairy products containing *Lactobacillus* spp. may have some protective effect against large colon adenoma by decreasing the fecal levels of enzymes, mutagens, and secondary bile salts that may be involved in colon carcinogenesis. This evidence is based on in vitro and animal assays, but not on rigorous human trials (Marteau, 2002).

Genitourinary Tract

Since the first description in 1933 of treatment of vaginitis and vaginosis with replacement of lactobacilli in the United States by Mohler and Brown, the use of probiotics enriched in lactobacilli has been extensively proposed (see Famularo et al., 2001, and Reid and Hammond, 2005, for reviews) as an effective alternative to antibiotics for the treatment of bacterial vaginosis. With regard to the genitourinary tract, depletion of vaginal lactobacilli

has been associated with an increased risk of urogenital infections. Several case reports have presented evidence that lactobacilli might be effective in the the treatment of genitourinary tract infections (Hilton and Rindos, 1995; Sieber and Dietz, 1998; Reid, 2002). Besides the topical application of *L. acidophilus*, *L. rhamnosus* GR-1, *L. fermentum* B-54 or RC-14, and yogurt in the vagina, the ingestion of dairy products fermented by these lactobacilli also seems to have therapeutic effects (Nyirjesy et al., 1997; Reid, 2001; Reid et al., 2001). Moreover, promotion of vaginal colonization with *Lactobacillus* spp. should be assessed as a potential intervention to reduce a woman's risk of acquiring human immunodeficiency virus type 1, gonorrhea, and trichomoniasis (Martin et al., 1999). Dairy products such as yogurt and acidophilus milk, as well as commercially available probiotic products and capsules containing *Lactobacillus* spp., have been used for this purpose as either douching preparations or suppositories.

The idea of treatment of bacterial vaginosis through the colonization of the vagina with exogenous lactobacilli is very attractive and especially interesting for pregnant women and in cases of individuals infected with antibiotic-resistant organisms, but its true efficacy remains controversial despite the numerous efforts that have been made in this respect (see Famularo et al., 2001, and Reid and Hammond, 2005, for reviews).

Other Clinical Applications

More recently, a number of studies have suggested the efficacy of *Lactobacillus* GG and other probiotic strains in reducing the recurrence of early atopic disease or in the curing or prevention of atopic eczema in infants (Kalliomaki et al., 2003; Viljanen et al., 2005). In addition, a few randomized controlled trials (see Marteau, 2002, and Brown and Valiere, 2004, for reviews) have suggested that some probiotics including lactobacilli (*L. reuteri* and *L. gasseri*) may have moderate hypocholesterolemic properties. Furthermore, some preliminary data (Guarino, 1998) reported a significant reduction in the severity of pneumonia in children, the prevention of caries (Caglar et al., 2005), or even the treatment of hypertension (Takano, 1998). Finally, it has been speculated that the inflammation associated with rheumatoid arthritis might be modulated by consuming probiotics such as *Lactobacillus* GG (Malin et al., 1996).

It may be concluded that these other, potential benefits of probiotics remain inconclusive and controversial. Although these bacteria have been used for centuries in the form of fermented dairy products, their potential use as a form of medical nutrition therapy has not received formal recognition. The dose-effect relationship and other pharmacological properties of these strains should be well established, and results need to be confirmed in several different laboratories, while randomized studies as well as a better knowledge of the metabolic properties of the strains used for clinical purposes should be assessed.

Finally, it should be stressed that when lactobacilli are used in humans, it is necessary to take the safety of new strains into consideration, as a few reports have indicated (Rautio et al., 1999; Mackay et al., 1999; Shetty and Woods, 2005; Land et al., 2005) that some species of the genus *Lactobacillus* have been isolated from various types of infection in persons with underlying disease or detrimental conditions. Therefore, assessment of the safety of a probiotic strain involves examination of intrinsic and pharmacokinetic properties and also the interaction between the strain and the host.

SUMMARY AND FUTURE DIRECTIONS

The genus *Lactobacillus* has been studied extensively and is now a well-characterized genus in the LAB group, which is composed of more than 100 recognized species. The genus is of interest for a number of reasons: its long history of safe use in the fermentation and preservation of traditional foods (dairy, meat, and vegetable products) and more recently its incorporation in functional probiotic foods, as well as its ubiquitous presence in human and animal microbiotas, especially in the gastrointestinal and genitourinary tracts (where it dominates the vaginal microbiota). However, the main interest is undoubtedly its role as a probiotic and as a biotherapeutic agent in some clinical situations. Future lines of research should focus on clarifying a number of properties related to its probiotic function and its application as a prophylactic or therapeutic agent in certain human diseases. In this respect, the following topics need elucidating:

- Definition of the active principle
- Carrying out of double-blind placebo-controlled studies to document the individual efficacy of each specific organism for each potential clinical application
- Identification of physiologically relevant biomarkers to assess the parameters of probiotic effectiveness in humans
- Epidemiological and properly controlled human studies to confirm probiotic efficacy
- Pharmacological and pharmacokinetic properties (effective dose for treatment, delivery vehicle, and secondary effects)

- Absence of virulence factors
- Compatibility with indigenous microbiota
- Possibility of use in elderly and immunocompromised patients

The efficacy of probiotics in the treatment of gastrointestinal diseases is well established, as are the potential benefits for other conditions such as genitourinary infections, allergies, and certain bowel disorders. However, a great deal of work is required before credibility can be given to health claims concerning the use of probiotic products in healthy individuals. The ideal approach would be to coordinate efforts and to concentrate on certain topics, such as gastrointestinal and genitourinary disturbances, and not to disperse research in many different directions. It is likely that a mixture of strains will be necessary to obtain success. Accordingly, the relation between strains (antagonism or synergism) needs to be well determined. The markets for functional foods (including essentially *Lactobacillus* spp.) represent a potential growth area. However, internationally standardized regulatory procedures for probiotic products are urgently required.

Finally, another interesting aspect is the fact that *Lactobacillus* spp. constitute attractive candidates as delivery vehicles for the presentation to the mucosa of compounds of pharmaceutical interest, in particular vaccines and immunomodulators. In this respect, a great deal of work is also required to clarify the potential of non-genetically modified or genetically engineered lactobacilli expressing bacterial or viral proteins on the cell surface as oral vaccines.

I acknowledge J. E. Suárez for his useful suggestions.

References

Antonio, M. A. D., S. E. Hawes, and S. L. Hillier. 1999. The identification of vaginal *Lactobacillus* species and the demographic and microbiologic characteristics of women colonized by these species. *J. Infect. Dis.* 180:1950–1956.

Barbés, C. 2001. Microbiota and gastrointestinal system. *Rev. Esp. Enferm. Dig.* 93:328–330.

Beijerinck, M. W. 1901. Anhäufungsversuche mit Ureumbakterien: Ureumspaltung durch Urease und durch Katabolismus. *Zentbl. Bakteriol. Parasitenkd. Infektkrankh. Hyg. Abt. 2* 7:33–61.

Boris, S., J. E. Suárez, F. Vázquez, and C. Barbés. 1998. Adherence of human vaginal lactobacilli to vaginal epithelial cells and interaction with uropathogens. *Infect. Immun.* 66:1985–1989.

Boris, S., and C. Barbés. 2000. Role played by lactobacilli in controlling the population of vaginal pathogens. *Microbes Infect.* 2:543–546.

Boyd, M. A., M. A. D. Antonio, and S. L. Hillier. 2005. Comparison of API 50 CH strips of whole-chromosomal DNA probes for identification of *Lactobacillus* species. *J. Clin. Microbiol.* 43:5309–5311.

Brown, A., C., and A. Valiere. 2004. Probiotics and medical nutrition therapy. *Nutr. Clin. Care* 7:56–58.

Caglar, E., B. Kargul, and I. Tanboga. 2005. Bacteriotherapy and probiotics' role on oral health. *Oral Dis.* 11:131–137.

Collins, M. D., U. Rodrigues, C. Ash, M. Aguirre, J. A. E. Farrow, A. Martinez-Murcia, B. A. Phillips, A. M. Williams, and S. Wallbanks. 1991. Phylogenetic analysis of the Genus *Lactobacillus* and related lactic acid bacteria as determined by reverse transcriptase sequencing of 16S rRNA. *FEMS Microbiol. Lett.* 77:5–12.

Dairy Council of California. 2000. Probiotics—friendly bacteria with a host of benefits. Dairy Council of California, Sacramento, CA. http:www//dairycouncilofca.org/PDFs/probiotics.pdf.

Dellaglio, F., and G. E. Felis. 2005. Taxonomy of lactobacilli and bifidobacteria, p. 25–49. *In* G. W. Tannock (ed.), *Probiotics and Prebiotics: Scientific Aspects.* Academic Press, Norfolk, United Kingdom.

De Vuyst, L., and B. Degeest. 1999. Heteropolysaccharides from lactic acid bacteria. *FEMS Microbiol. Rev.* 23:153–157.

Donohue, D. C., S. Salminen, and P. Marteau. 1998. Safety of probiotic bacteria, p. 369–384. *In* S. Salminen and A. von Wright (ed.), *Lactic Acid Bacteria. Microbiology and Functional Aspects.* Marcel Dekker, Inc., New York, NY.

Dykes, G. A., and A. von Holy. 1994. Strain typing in the genus *Lactobacillus. Lett. Appl. Microbiol.* 19:63–66.

Euzéby, J. P. 2007. List of procaryotic names with standing in nomenclature. http://www.bacterio.cict.fr/twothousand/twothousandsix.htlm.

Famularo, G., M. Pieluigi, R. Coccia, P. Mastroiacovo, and C. De Simone. 2001. Microecology, bacterial vaginosis and probiotics: perspectives for bacteriotherapy. *Med. Hyp.* 56:421–430.

Fasoli, F., M. Marzotto, L. Rizzotti, F. Rossi, F. Dellaglio, and S. Torriani. 2003. Bacterial composition of commercial probiotic products as evaluated by PCR-DGGE analysis. *Int. J. Food Microbiol.* 82:59–70.

Fernández, M. F., S. Boris, and C. Barbés. 2003. Applications of probiotic human lactobacilli, p. 293–301. *In* S. G. Pandalai (ed.), *Recent Research Developments in Infection and Immunity,* vol. 1. Transworld Research Network, Fort P.O. Kerala, India.

Fuller, R. 1989. Probiotics in man and animals. *J. Appl. Bacteriol.* 66:365–378.

Garrity, G. M., J. A. Bell, and T. G. Lilbum. 2004. Taxonomic outline of the Prokaryotes. *Bergey's Manual of Systematic Bacteriology,* 2nd ed. Release 5.0. Springer-Verlag, New York, NY. http://141.150.157.80/bergeysoutline/main.htm.

Geis, A. 2003. Perspectives of genetic engineering of bacteria used in food fermentations, p. 100–118. *In* K. J. Heller (ed.), *Genetically Engineered Food and Methods of Detection.* Wiley-VCH, Weinheim, Germany.

Gill, H. S. 1998. Stimulation of the immune system by lactic cultures. *Int. Dairy J.* 8:535–544.

Gionchetti, P., F. Rizzello, and M. Campieri. 2002. Probiotics in gastroenterology. *Curr. Opin. Gastroenterol.* 17:331–335.

Gismondo, M. R., L. Drago, and A. Lombardi. 1999. Review of probiotics available to modified gastrointestinal flora. *Int. J. Antimicrob. Agents* 12:287–292.

Gorbach, S. L. 2000. Probiotics and gastrointestinal health. *Am. J. Gastroenterol.* 95(Suppl. 1):S2–S4.

Guarino, A. 1998. Effects of probiotics in children with cystic fibrosis. *Gastroenterol. Int.* 11(Suppl.):91.

Hammes, W. P., and C. Hertel. 2003. The genera *Lactobacillus* and *Carnobacterium. In The Prokaryotes: An Evolving Electronic Resource for the Microbiological Community,* 3rd ed. Springer-Verlag. New York, NY. http://link.springer.ny.com/link/service/books/10125/. Accessed 10 April 2007.

Hilton, E., and P. Rindos. 1995. *Lactobacillus* GG vaginal suppositories and vaginitis. *J. Clin. Microbiol.* 33:1433.

Ho, P. S., J. Kwang, and Y. K. Lee. 2005. Intragastric administration of *Lactobacillus casei* expressing transmissible gastroenteritis coronavirus spike glycoprotein induced specific antibody production. *Vaccine* 23:1335–1342.

Holzapfel, W. H., P. Haberer, R. Geisen, J. Björkroth, and U. Schillinger. 2001. Taxonomy and important features of probiotic microorganisms in food and nutrition. *Am. J. Clin. Nutr.* 73(Suppl.):S365–S373.

Hughes, V. L., and S. L. Hillier. 1990. Microbiologic characteristics of *Lactobacillus* products used for colonization of the vagina. *Obstet. Gynecol.* 75:244–248.

Huys, G., M. Vancanneyt, K. D'Haene, V. Vankerckhoven, H. Goossens, and J. Swings. 2006. Accuracy of species identity of commercial bacterial cultures intended for probiotic or nutritional use. *Res. Microbiol.* 157:803–810.

Jin, L., L. Tao, S. I. Pavlova, J. S. So, N. Kiwanuka, Z. Namukwaya, B. A. Saberbein, and M. Wawer. 2007. Species diversity and relative abundance of vaginal lactic acid bacteria from women in Uganda and Korea. *J. Appl. Microbiol.* 102:1107–1115.

Johnson, J. L., C. F. Phelps, C. S. Cummins, J. London, and F. Gasser. 1980. Taxonomy of the *Lactobacillus acidophilus* group. *Int. Syst. Bacteriol.* 30:53–68.

Kalliomaki, M., S. Salminen, T. Poussa, H. Arvilommi, and E. Isolauri. 2003. Probiotics and prevention of atopic disease: a 4 year follow up of a randomised placebo-controlled trial. *Lancet* 361:1869–1871.

Kandler, O., and N. Weiss. 1986. Regular non-sporing Gram-positive rods, p. 1208–1234. *In* P. H. Sneath, N. Mair, M. E. Sharpe, and J. G. Holt (ed.), *Bergey's Manual of Systematic Bacteriology,* vol. 2. William and Wilkins, Baltimore, MD.

Kaur, I. P., K. Chopra, and A. Saini. 2002. Probiotics: potential pharmaceutical applications. *Eur. J. Pharm. Sci.* 15:1–9.

Land, M. H., K. Rouster-Stevens, C. R. Woods, M. L. Cannon, J. Cnota, and A. K. Shetty. 2005. *Lactobacillus* sepsis associated with probiotic therapy. *Pediatrics* 115:178–181.

Lidbeck, A., and C. E. Nord. 1993. Lactobacilli and normal human anaerobic microflora. *Clin. Infect. Dis.* 16:S181–S187.

Lidbeck, A., C. E. Nord, J. A. Gustafsson, and J. Rafter. 1992. Lactobacilli, anticarcinogenic activities and human intestinal microflora. *Eur. J. Cancer Prev.* 1:341–353.

Limdi, J. K., C. O'Neill, and J. McLaughlin. 2006. Do probiotics have a therapeutic role in gastroenterology? *World J. Gastroenterol.* 12:5447–5457.

Maassen, C. B., W. J. Boersma, C. Holten-Neelen, E. Claassen, and J. D. Laman. 2003. Growth phase of orally administered *Lactobacillus* strains differentially affects IgG1/IGg2a ratio for soluble antigens: implications for vaccine development. *Vaccine* **21**:2751–2757.

Mackay, A. D., M. B. Taylor, C. C. Kibbler, and J. M. T. Hamilton-Miller. 1999. *Lactobacillus* endocarditis caused by a probiotic organism. *Clin. Microbiol. Infect.* **5**:290–292.

Mäkinen, A. M., and M. Bigret. 1998. Safety of probiotic bacteria, p. 73-102. *In* S. Salminen and A. von Wright (ed.), *Lactic Acid Bacteria. Microbiology and Functional Aspects.* Marcel Dekker, Inc., New York, NY.

Malin, M., P. Verronen, H. Mykkanen, S. Salminen, and E. Isolauri. 1996. Increased bacterial urease activity in faeces in juvenile chronic arthritis: evidence of altered intestinal microflora. *Br. J. Rheumatol.* **35**:689–694.

Marteau, P. R. 2002. Probiotics in clinical conditions. *Clin. Rev. Allergy. Immunol.* **22**:255–274.

Marteau, P. R., M. de Brese, C. J. Cellier, and J. Schrezenmeir. 2001. Protection from gastrointestinal diseases with the use of probiotics. *Am. J. Clin. Nutr.* **73**(Suppl.):S430–S436.

Martin, H. L., B. A. Richardson, P. M. Nyange, L. Lavreys, S. L. Hillier, B. Chohan, K. Mandaliya, J. O. Ndinya-Achola, J. Bwayo, and J. Kreiss. 1999. Vaginal lactobacilli, microbial flora, and risk of human immunodeficiency virus type 1 and sexually transmitted disease acquisition. *J. Infect. Dis.* **180**:1863–1868.

Mehta, A., J. Talwalkar, C. V. Shetty, and N. D. Motashaw. 1995. Microbial flora of the vagina, p. 1–7. *In* A. B. Onderdonk, P. J. Heidt, and V. C. Rusch (ed.), *Microecology and Therapy*, vol. 23. Institut für Mikroökologie, Herborn-Dill, Germany.

Mikelsaar, M., R. Mändar, and E. Seppo. 1998. Lactic acid microflora in the human microbial ecosystem and its development, p. 279–342. *In* S. Salminen and Atte von Wright (ed.), *Lactic Acid Bacteria: Microbiology and Functional Aspects*, 2nd ed. Marcel Dekker, New York, NY.

Mitsuoka, T. 1992. Intestinal flora and aging. *Nutr. Rev.* **50**:438–446.

Mohler, R. W., and C. P. Brown. 1933. Doderlein's bacillus in the treatment of vaginitis. *Am. J. Obstet. Gynecol.* **25**:718–723.

Morishita, T., Y. Deguchi, M. Yajima, T. Saskurai, and T. Yura. 1981. Multiple nutritional requirements of lactobacilli: genetic lesions affecting amino acid biosynthetic pathways. *J. Bacteriol.* **148**:64–71.

Nyirjesy, P., M. V. Weitz, M. H. T. Grody, and B. Lorber. 1997. Over-the-counter and alternative medicines in the treatment of chronic vaginal symptoms. *Obstet. Gynecol.* **90**:50–53.

Penner, R., R. N. Fedorak, and K. L. Madsen. 2005. Probiotics and nutraceuticals: non-medicinal treatments of gastrointestinal diseases. *Curr. Opin. Pharmacol.* **5**:596–603.

Perdigon, G., R. Fuller, and R. Raya. 2001. Lactic acid bacteria and their effect on the immune system. *Curr. Issues Intest. Microbiol.* **2**:27–42.

Rautio, M., H. Jousimies-Somer, H. Kauma, I. Pietarinen, M. Saxelin, S. Tynkkynen, and M. Koskela. 1999. Liver abscess due to a *Lactobacillus rhamnosus* strain indistinguishable from *L. rhamnosus* strain GG. *Clin. Infect. Dis.* **28**:1160–1161.

Reid, G. 2001. Probiotic agents to protect the urogenital tract against infection. *Am. J. Clin. Nutr.* **73**(Suppl.):S437–S443.

Reid, G. 2002. Probiotics for urogenital health. *Nutr. Clin. Care* **5**:3–8.

Reid, G., A. V. Bruce, N. Fraser, G. H. Heinemann, J. Owen, and B. Henning. 2001. Oral probiotics can resolve urogenital infections. *FEMS Immunol. Med. Microbiol.* **30**:49–52.

Reid, G., and J. A. Hammond. 2005. Probiotics. Some evidence for their effectiveness. *Can. Fam. Phys.* **51**:1487–1493.

Roberfroid, M. B. 1998. Prebiotics and synbiotics: concepts and nutritional properties. *Br. J. Nutr.* **80**:S197–S202.

Ross, R. P., S. Morgan, and C. Hill. 2002. Preservation and fermentation: past, present and future. *Int. J. Food Microbiol.* **79**:3–16.

Sakamoto, I., M. Igarashi, K. Kimura, A. Takagi, T. Miwa, and Y. Koga. 2001. Suppressive effect of *Lactobacillus gasseri* OLL 2716 (LG21) on *Helicobacter pylori* infection in humans. *J. Antimicrob. Chemother.* **47**:709–710.

Salminen, S., M. A. Deighton, Y. Benno, and S. L. Gorbach. 1998. Lactic acid bacteria in health and disease, p. 211–253. *In* S. Salminen and A. von Wright (ed.), *Lactic Acid Bacteria. Microbiology and Functional Aspects.* Marcel Dekker, Inc., New York, NY.

Sanders, M. E., and J. H. Veld. 1999. Bringing a probiotic-containing functional food to the market: microbiological, product regulatory and labelling issues. *Antonie Leeuwenhock* **76**:293–315.

Schleifer, K. H., and W. Ludwig. 1995. Phylogeny of the Genus *Lactobacillus* and related genera. *Syst. Appl. Microbiol.* **18**:461–467.

Schrezenmeir, J., and M. de Vrese. 2001. Probiotics, prebiotics and symbiotics, approaching a definition. *Am. J. Clin. Nutr.* **73**(Suppl.): S361–S364.

Schultz, M., and R. B. Sartor. 2000. Probiotics and inflammatory bowel diseases. *Am. J. Gastroenterol.* **95**(Suppl. 1): S19–S21.

Seegers, J. F. 2002. Lactobacilli as live vaccine delivery vectors: progress and prospects. *Trends Biotechnol.* **20**:508–515.

Senok, A. C., A. Y. Ismaeel, and G. A. Botta. 2005. Probiotics: facts and myths. *Clin. Mirobiol. Infect.* **11**:958–966.

Shareck, J., Y. Choi, B. Lee, and C. B. Miguez. 2004. Cloning vectors based on cryptic plasmids isolated from lactic acid bacteria: their characteristics and potential applications in biotechnology. *Crit. Rev. Biotechnol.* **24**:155–208.

Sharpe, M. E. 1981. The genus *Lactobacillus*, p. 1653–1679. *In* M. P. Starr, H. Stolp, H. G. Trüper, A. Balows, and H. G. Schlegel (ed.), *The Prokaryotes*. Springer-Verlag, Berlin, Germany.

Shetty, A. K., and C. R. Woods. 2005. *Lactobacillus* sepsis associated with probiotic therapy: in reply. *Pediatrics* **116**:517–518.

Sieber, R., and U.-T. Dietz. 1998. *Lactobacillus acidophilus* and yogurt in the prevention and therapy of bacterial vaginosis. *Int. Dairy J.* **8**:599–607.

Song, Y., N. Kato, Y. Matsumiya, C. Liu, H. Kato, and K. Watanabe. 1999. Identification of and hydrogen peroxide production by fecal and vaginal lactobacilli isolated from Japanese women and newborn infants. *J. Clin. Microbiol.* **37**:3062–3064.

Tagg, J. R., A. S. Dajani, and L. W. Watanabe. 1976. Bacteriocins of gram-positive bacteria. *Bacteriol. Rev.* **40**:722–756.

Takano, T. 1998. Milk derived peptides and hypertension reduction. *Int. Dairy J.* **8:**375–378.

Vallor, A. C., M. A. D. Antonio, S. E. Hawes, and S. L. Hillier. 2001. Factors associated with acquisition of, or persistent colonization by, vaginal lactobacilli: role of hydrogen peroxide production. *J. Infect. Dis.* **184:**1431–1436.

Vanderhoof, J. A. 2001. Probiotics: future directions. *Am. J. Clin. Nutr.* **115:**2S–5S.

Velraeds, M., H. Van Der Mei, G. Reid, and H. Busscher. 1996. Inhibition of initial adhesion of uropathogenic *Enterococcus faecalis* by biosurfactants from *Lactobacillus* isolates. *Appl. Environ. Microbiol.* **62:**1958–1963.

Viljanen, M., E. Savilahti, T. Haahtela, K. Juntunen-Backman, R. Korpela, T. Poussa, T. Tuure, and M. Kuitunen. 2005. Probiotics in the treatment of atopic eczema/dermatitis syndrome in infants: a double-blind placebo controlled trial. *Allergy* **60:**494–500.

Yeung, P. S. M., M. E. Sanders, C. L. Kitts, R. Cano, and P. S. Tong. 2002. Species-specific identification of commercial probiotic strains. *J. Dairy Sci.* **85:**1039–1051.

Therapeutic Microbiology: Probiotics and Related Strategies
Edited by J. Versalovic and M. Wilson
© 2008 ASM Press, Washington, DC

Marco Ventura, Francesca Turroni, Angela Ribbera,
Elena Foroni, Douwe van Sinderen

4

Bifidobacteria: the Model Human Gut Commensal

Bifidobacteria are high-C+G gram-positive, non-spore-forming, nonmotile, non-gas-producing, anaerobic, and saccharoclastic microorganisms. Bifidobacteria often occur as Y- or V-shaped rods (Poupard et al., 1973), and under stressful conditions their cell morphology becomes pleomorphic (Fig. 1). It has been shown that the cell shape is also influenced by the abundance of N-acetylglucosamine, alanine, aspartic acid, glutamic acid, and serine in the growth medium. Tissier (1900) was presumably the first to report the isolation of *Bifidobacterium* from the intestine of a child, and he named it *Bacillus bifidus communis*. The genus *Bifidobacterium* was already recognized by Orla-Jensen as a separate taxon in 1924, but it took another 50 years until the genus *Bifidobacterium* was officially established in *Bergey's Manual of Determinative Bacteriology*. Bifidobacteria belong to the *Actinobacteria* phylum, within which they form a distinct order, "*Bifidobacteriales*." This order comprises a single family, *Bifidobacteriaceae*, which in turn consists of four genera, *Bifidobacterium*, *Gardnerella*, *Scardovia*, and *Parascardovia* (Biavati and Mattarelli, 2001; Garrity and Holt, 2001;

Stackebrandt and Schumann, 2000). Except for the *Bifidobacterium* genus, which contains 29 species (Table 1), these genera each contain just a single species.

ECOLOGICAL DISTRIBUTION OF BIFIDOBACTERIA

Bifidobacteria, as mentioned above, were originally isolated from a breast-fed infant (Tissier, 1900). Since then several species have been identified in the gastrointestinal tract (GIT) of mammals and insects. The recognized habitats of bifidobacteria include the human intestine, the human oral cavity, food, the animal (nonhuman) GIT, the insect intestine, and sewage (Table 1), although in the last case fecal contamination may have been the original source of these bifidobacteria. Similarly, *Bifidobacterium animalis* subsp. *lactis*, originally isolated from fermented milk, may also have originated from fecal contamination.

The intestinal microbiota represents a very complex ecosystem whose composition is still far from understood. Host development, genetic background, age, health condition, diet (cultural influences of, for

Marco Ventura, Francesca Turroni, Angela Ribbera, and Elena Foroni, Department of Genetics, Biology of Microorganisms, Anthropology and Evolution, University of Parma, Parma, Italy. **Douwe van Sinderen,** Alimentary, Pharmabiotic Centre and Department of Microbiology, Bioscience Institute, National University of Ireland, Western Road, Cork, Ireland.

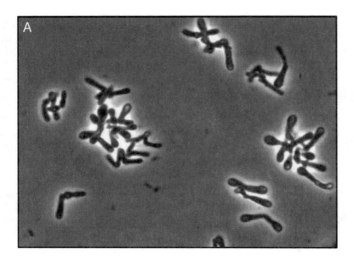

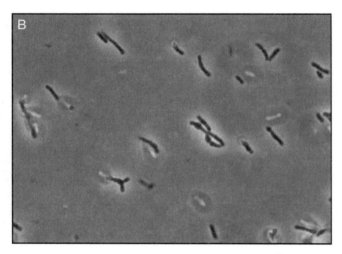

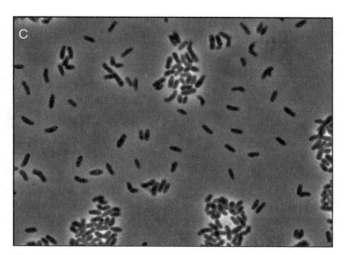

Figure 1 Photomicrographs showing representative bifidobacterial cell shapes. (A) *B. animalis* subsp. *lactis*; (B) *B. longum* biotype longum; (C) *B. pseudolongum*.

example, a more protein- or carbohydrate-based diet), and the adaptability of each bacterial species influence the overall composition of the microbiota in the intestine (Fuller, 1989). The microbiota of infants fed only breast milk becomes dominated by bifidobacteria during the first week, and there is a concomitant decrease in members of the *Enterobacteriaceae* (Yoshioka, 1983; Hopkins et al., 2001). The introduction of solid foods into the diet of breast-fed babies results in a major diversification in the microbiota. Microbial diversity in the human colon is very much affected by aging. The fecal microbiota of children is rather simple, in contrast to that of individuals of an advanced age, which is associated with decreased bifidobacteria and increased *Bacteroides* species diversity (Hopkins et al., 2001, 2002; Langendijk et al., 1995). In the feces of children the most frequently detected bifidobacterial species are *B. longum* biotype longum and *B. longum* biotype infantis followed by *B. breve*, whereas in the feces of adults the most detected species are *B. adolescentis* and *B. catenulatum* (Matsuki et al., 1999). However, a major criticism that could be raised with regard to these studies is that they do not differentiate between the autochthonous bifidobacterial GIT population, which grows in, and has colonized, the human GIT, and the transient bifidobacterial population, which may have been food derived and which cannot survive in the human GIT. Recently, the distribution of autochthonous GIT bifidobacteria has been investigated and it was found that the bifidobacterial microbiota associated with the human colonic mucosa varies with host and/or position in the colon. Such investigations have revealed that species which are widely added to functional foods such as *B. animalis* subsp. *lactis* do not constitute a major component of the GIT autochthonous bifidobacteria, which may raise questions about their efficacy as a probiotic.

Another technical difficulty encountered in determining the ecology of the GIT microbiota is presented by the fact that not all components of the microbiota of the human GIT can be cultivated (Favier et al., 2002; Zoetendal et al., 2004). Thus, all of the enumeration methods which are based on an initial cultivation step followed by selective plating are not reliable approaches for a valid analysis of the GIT microbiota. In recent years, analysis methods using 16S rRNA gene sequences have been widely used in place of conventional culture methods for the analysis of the intestinal microbiota (Amann et al., 1995). In complex mixed populations, 16S rRNA-targeted oligonucleotide probes have been applied to fluorescence in situ hybridization as a culture-independent method (Franks et al., 1998; Langendijk et al., 1995). Fluorescence in situ hybridization involves

Table 1 Bifidobacterial species and their origin

Species	Origin
B. adolescentis	Intestine of adult
B. bifidum	Infant feces
B. angulatum	Human feces
B. breve	Intestine of infant
B. catenulatum	Intestine of adult
B. gallicum	Human feces
B. infantis	Intestine of infant
B. longum	Intestine of adult
B. pseudocatenulatum	Feces of infant
B. dentium	Dental caries
B. lactis	Yogurt
B. animalis	Animal feces
B. boum	Rumen of cattle
B. choerinum	Swine feces
B. cuniculi	Feces of rabbit
B. gallinarum	Chicken cecum
B. suis	Swine feces
B. magnum	Rabbit feces
B. merycicum	Bovine rumen
B. pseudolongum subsp. *globosum*	Bovine rumen
B. pseudolongum subsp. pseudolongum	Swine feces
B. pullorum	Feces of chicken
B. ruminantium	Bovine rumen
B. saeculare	Rabbit feces
B. thermophilum	Swine feces
B. aerophilum	Porcine feces
B. psychraerophilum	Porcine feces
B. thermacidophilum subsp. porcinum	Feces of piglet
B. asteroides	Hindgut of honeybee
B. coryneforme	Hindgut of honeybee
B. indicum	Hindgut of honeybee
B. minimum	Sewage
B. subtile	Sewage
B. thermacidophilum subsp. thermacidophilum	Wastewater

whole-cell hybridization with fluorescent oligonucleotide probes targeted against specific bifidobacterial species. This technique estimates that 4.4% of the adult fecal microbiota consists of bifidobacteria (Lay et al., 2005).

Several proposals have been made concerning the source of initial colonization of a newborn with bifidobacteria. Some early workers reported the isolation of bifidobacteria from the vagina; however, they were not able to successfully demonstrate that bifidobacteria isolated from this environment were similar to those isolated from the infant (Poupard et al., 1973). It was later suggested that the occurrence of bifidobacteria in the stools of adults makes fecal contamination a possible source, either directly at the time of delivery or indirectly from other parts of the mother's body after birth.

GENOMICS AND POSTGENOMICS IN BIFIDOBACTERIAL RESEARCH

Whole-genome sequencing has revolutionized the genetic, biochemical, and molecular biology research on bacteria. Large genome-sequencing efforts have been made to decode the genome sequences of pathogenic bacteria. However, in the last decade a significant emphasis has been placed on whole-genome sequencing of GIT bacteria as well as on food-grade bacteria (Klaenhammer et al., 2005). In this context, the main scientific efforts have focused on the sequencing of members of lactic acid bacteria (LAB), which include strains with industrial interest such as *Streptococcus* and *Lactococcus* strains as well as *Lactobacillus*. In contrast, bifidobacterial genomics is still at a very early stage of development. In fact, of the currently recognized 29 *Bifidobacterium* species, three strains that belong to the *B. longum* phylogenetic group (e.g., *B. longum* biotype longum NCC2705, *B. longum* biotype longum DJO10A, and *B. breve* UCC2003) and two strains harboring the *B. adolescentis* phylogenetic group (*B. adolescentis* ATCC 15703 and *B. dentium* Bd1) have been sequenced to completion or are at various stages of completion (Table 2). Furthermore, genome-sequencing efforts for *B. breve* M-16V, *B. breve* Yakult, *B. animalis* subsp. *lactis*, *B. longum* biotype longum, and *B. longum* biotype infantis (Liu et al., 2005) are under way. All these genomes range in size from 1.9 to 2.9 Mb and generally display architectural features of a typical bacterial chromosome, such as the coorientation of gene transcription and DNA replication (McLean et al., 1998), and a classical origin of replication region, which constitutes (i) a gene constellation composed of *rpmH*, *dnaA*, *dnaN*, and *recF*; (ii) a particular GC nucleotide skew ([G-C]/[G+C]); (iii) the presence of multiple DnaA-boxes; and (iv) AT-rich sequences immediately upstream of the *dnaA* gene (Christensen et al., 1999).

The availability of whole-genome sequences from bifidobacteria is extremely informative for the understanding of the processes underlying speciation and evolution in this genus as well as the adaptation to its specific habitat (e.g., the human intestine). Comparative genomics involving bifidobacterial genomes has revealed a high degree of conservation and synteny across the entire genomes, i.e., *B. longum* biotype longum NCC2705, *B. longum* biotype longum DJO10A, *B. breve* UCC2003, and *B. adolescentis* ATCC15703 (Ventura et al., 2007). However, there are also several breakpoint regions that

Table 2 General features of bifidobacterial genomes[a]

Microorganism	Status	Genome size (bp)	ORF no.	G+C% content	No. of rRNA operons	Reference
B. longum biotype longum NCC2705	C	2,266,000	1730	60	4	Schell et al., 2002
B. longum biotype longum DJO10A	UF	2,375,800	1811	59	4	NCBI source NZ_ AABM00000000
B. adolescentis ATCC15703	UF	2,084,445	1564	59	NA	NCBI source NZ_ BAAD00000000
B. breve UCC2003	UF	2,422,668	1868	58.7	2	Leahy et al., 2005
B. dentium Bd1	UF	~2,600,000	~2270	59.2	NA	NCBI source (project ID: 17583)

[a]C, finished; UF, unfinished; NA, not available; ORF, open reading frame.

seem to represent inversions or DNA insertion/deletion points.

If the use of comparative genomics represents the most reliable route to map differences and similarities among sequenced microorganisms, it nevertheless is still a laborious and highly expensive road. Genomotyping involving DNA microarray technology represents a highly valuable tool for exploring genome variability. The usefulness of such technology has been already demonstrated for the analysis of the interspecific and intraspecific variations in the bacterial genomes of pathogens. These include pathogenic bacteria like *Mycobacterium tuberculosis* (Mahairas et al., 1996), *Vibrio cholerae*, *Staphylococcus aureus* (Fitzgerald, 2001), *Salmonella enterica* (Chan et al., 2003), and *Escherichia coli* (Dobrindt et al., 2003; Peters et al., 2003). Recently, a *B. longum* biotype longum NCC2705-based spotted DNA microarray was employed to compare the genomes of 10 bifidobacterial strains, including other *B. longum* biotype longum strains as well as the closely related *B. longum* biotype infantis and *B. longum* biotype suis taxa (E. Rezzonico, M. Ventura, G. Cuanoud, G. Pessi, G. Giliberti, and F. Arigoni, presented at the Functional Genomics of Gram Positive Microorganisms, Baveno, Italy, 2003). Results showed seven large genome regions of variability, the majority of which encompass DNA with a deviating G+C content. These regions correspond to a prophage remnant, a cluster of genes for enzymes involved in sugar metabolism, such as a β-mannosidase, and a capsular polysaccharide biosynthesis gene cluster, which could play a role in host-bacterium interactions. All of the comparative studies on these bifidobacterial genomes might be useful in identifying strain-specific DNA sequences that may have evolved or been acquired recently and could be responsible for adaptations to their specific habitats. In general, analysis of the microarray hybridization patterns provides an enormous amount of information concerning bacterial genome vari-

ability, strain-specific genes, and bacterial core sequences. Nevertheless, there are some limitations in that the microarray approach is incapable of identifying regions present in the test strains but absent from the strain from which the array was designed. Moreover, genomic comparisons with microarrays do not normally consider synteny of the bacterial genomes. In fact, two genomes could have the same gene content but may be organized differently.

Genome-sequencing efforts have provided a vast reservoir of molecular information that promises to revolutionize our understanding of life. However, genome sequences alone provide only limited insights into the biochemical pathways that drive cell functions. Thus, postgenomic methods such as transcriptomics and proteomics as well as classical molecular biology approaches are necessary for assigning functions to proteins. So far, functional genomic investigations involving bifidobacterial genomes are still in their infancy. Such investigations have so far been limited to the analysis of global transcriptome and proteome profiles of bifidobacterial cells that were submitted to stressful conditions. These analyses revealed a profound modification of gene expression upon cell exposure to bile salts (Sanchez et al., 2005; Savijoki et al., 2005) or high temperatures (Savijoki et al., 2005; Rezzonico et al., 2007). These studies evidenced an increase in the expression of molecular chaperone-encoding genes as well as genes specifying proteins involved in the regulation of transcription and translation. The investigation of genome-wide gene expression in response to such stress stimuli is highly relevant to the industrial application of probiotic strains. In fact, the incorporation of bifidobacteria in health-promoting or probiotic foods requires that they survive industrial food-manufacturing processes, such as starter handling and storage (freeze-drying, freezing, or spray-drying), while remaining viable during storage. The global transcriptome analysis of the heat shock response of

B. longum highlighted an induction of chaperone-encoding genes and the down-regulation of the translation, cell division, and chromosome-partitioning machineries. Furthermore, these postgenomic analyses together with a series of studies directed towards describing the genetic organization and transcriptional regulation of molecular chaperones revealed that bifidobacteria possess the smallest set of chaperone-encoding proteins so far described in the *Actinobacteria* phylum (Ventura et al., 2006b). This may be explained by the fact that bacteria such as bifidobacteria, which live in a more or less isothermal habitat, do not need an elaborate molecular heat stress system responding to temperature fluctuations. In contrast, such bacteria would be expected to possess a more sophisticated system to protect cells against the more frequently occurring environmental stresses such as bile salt, acid, and osmotic stress.

GENOMICS AND THE METABOLIC PROPERTIES OF BIFIDOBACTERIA

The main objective of the postgenomic era is to relate annotated genome sequences to cellular functions (Osterman and Overbeek, 2003). The combination of genomic, physiological, and biochemical information provides the basis for reconstruction of complete metabolic networks. Since bifidobacteria encounter a vast array of substrates in the GIT, information regarding their metabolic properties is crucial to formulate an optimal growth medium. Very rich media (e.g., Rogosa Sharpe Medium or Reinforced Clostridia Medium) are often not able to sustain the growth of many bifidobacterial species. This suggests that the nutritional requirements may change from one strain to another, seemingly due to subtle differences in their metabolic pathways, some of which can be easily identified whereas others may be linked to regulatory differences. The availability of whole-genome sequences will be useful to identify new metabolic pathways or pathways that are incomplete. So far, the only available genome-based information relating to metabolic abilities of bifidobacteria is limited to *B. longum* biotype longum strain NCC2705 (Schell et al., 2002). This strain possesses the genes for the synthesis of at least 19 amino acids from ammonium and major biosynthetic precursors (phosphoenolpyruvate [PEP], oxaloacetate, oxoglutarate, and fumarate). Notably, genes homologous to those encoding asparagine synthetases and asparaginyl-tRNA synthetase are absent, suggesting that *B. longum* biotype longum NCC2705 uses the *gatABC*/asparaginyl-tRNA pathway to produce asparagines from aspartate. Also cysteine biosynthesis and sulfur assimilation are accomplished

by an unusual pathway in this microorganism, which involves homologs of cystathionine γ-synthetase, cystathionine β-synthetase, and cystathionine γ-lyase using succinylhomoserine and an as-yet-unidentified reduced sulfur compound that could be provided through metabolic activity of other GIT commensal bacteria. Moreover, this bifidobacterial strain possesses all the enzymes needed for the biosynthesis of pyrimidine and purine nucleotides for glutamine as well as those necessary for the synthesis of folic acid, thiamine, and nicotinate (Schell et al., 2002). Conversely, the metabolic pathways for the production of riboflavin, biotin, cobalamin, pantothenate, lipoate, and pyridoxine appear to be absent. All of the above-mentioned metabolic capacities indicate that this bacterium seems to be well adapted to growth in an environment which is poor in certain metabolic substrates (e.g., amino acids, vitamins, and nucleotides).

With respect to the carbohydrate fermentative properties of *B. longum* biotype longum NCC2705, the dissection of the genome sequences revealed that this strain possesses all of the required genetic information to channel fructose, galactose, *N*-acetylglucosamine, *N*-acetylgalactosamine, arabinose, xylose, ribose, sucrose, lactose, cellobiose, and melibiose into the fructose-6-phosphate shunt (Schell et al., 2002). Notably, more than 8% of the genes present in the genome of this microorganism encode proteins that are involved in sugar metabolism (e.g., transport and degradation). Such extensive genetic adaptation to carbohydrate metabolism is shared with other bifidobacterial species as well as other enteric bacteria and likely represents an adaptation to living in the GIT (see paragraph below).

Other gene categories that appear to be overrepresented in the bifidobacterial genomes include those involved in cell cycle control and cell division (e.g., Fic, FtsE, FtsK, FtsX, FtsZ, ParA, and Smc). Finally, a large proportion of the *B. longum* biotype longum NCC2705 genome codes for transcriptional regulators, which mainly include negative regulators. Schell et al. (2002) suggested that negative regulation allows a quicker and more stringent response to environmental stimuli, consistent with the need for quick adaptation to the constantly fluctuating substrate availability in the GIT.

PREBIOTICS AND BIFIDOBACTERIA: DEFINITION AND IMPACT ON HUMAN HEALTH

In the industrialized world, diet is an important determinant of the health and lifestyle of a human being. It is generally accepted that a diet rich in fruit and vegetables is associated with a decreased incidence of coronary heart disease and colon cancer. In addition, a lack of physical activity, particularly if associated with over-consumption, increases the risk of the development of nutrition-related chronic diseases such as obesity, hypertension, cardiovascular diseases, osteoporosis, type II diabetes, and several cancers (Bengmark, 2002; Blaut, 2002; Johnson, 2004). It is now well accepted that it is possible to reduce the risk of disease through a healthy lifestyle, which includes a correct and balanced diet. In this context, a new type of food has been recognized that contributes to disease prevention, i.e., functional foods. Functional foods, or functional food ingredients, exert a beneficial effect on host health and/or reduce the risk of chronic disease. The first generation of functional foods was based on deliberate supplementation of foods with minerals (mainly calcium) and vitamins. Only recently the concept has moved towards food additives exerting a positive effect on the gut microbiota, introducing pro-, syn-, and prebiotics (Ziemer and Gibson, 1998).

Prebiotics are food substances which resist digestion in the proximal GIT and reach intact the distal region of the gut, where, besides their direct physiological effect, they also affect the GIT ecosystem by specifically stimulating the growth and activity of the probiotic components of the GIT microbiota (e.g., bifidobacteria), thereby eliciting a beneficial effect on the host's health (Gibson and Roberfroid, 1995). Prebiotics are typically oligosaccharides (Manning and Gibson, 2004) that consist of a mixture of hexose oligomers with a variable extent of polymerization. Oligosaccharides may naturally be present in certain foods, such as fruits and vegetables, or are produced by biosynthesis from natural sugars of polysaccharides and added to food products because of their nutritional properties (Delzenne, 2003). Oligosaccharides present in food differ in their chemical structure, in particular in their degree of polymerization number (ranging from 2 to 20) or in the type of hexose moiety (e.g., glucosyl, fructosyl, galactosyl, and xylosyl). Oligosaccharides that are classified as prebiotics include fructo-oligosaccharides (FOS), trans-galacto-oligosaccharides, gluco-oligosaccharides, inulins, lactulose, lactosucrose, (iso) malto-oligosaccharides, lactilol, pyrodextrins, soybean oligosaccharides, and xylo-oligosaccharides. However, their effect in modulating the intestinal microbiota is highly variable and depends on different factors such as the degree of polymerization as well as the type of polysaccharide. Polysaccharides have not yet been considered as prebiotics. Nevertheless, components of the intestinal microbiota are capable of hydrolyzing polysaccharides to low-molecular-weight oligosaccharides, which are then further degraded and fermented by a wide range of gut bacteria. Among the

prebiotics, inulin possesses the highest molecular weight and consists of a large number of carbohydrate units (plant inulins generally contain between 2 and 140 fructose units) with different degrees of polymerization (Roberfroid, 2005). However, inulin is poorly hydrolyzed by enteric bacteria such as bifidobacteria. It is, therefore, reasonable to assume that an indirect relationship exists between the length of the oligosaccharides and the rate of the fermentative processes. Thus, the lowest-molecular-weight FOS are fermented mainly in the saccharolytic proximal bowel, while long-chain inulins may exert a prebiotic effect in the most distal colonic regions (Gibson, 2004). Many fruits and vegetables contain prebiotic oligosaccharides such as FOS, for example, onion, garlic, banana, asparagus, leek, Jerusalem artichoke, and chicory. However, the level of the prebiotic compound appears to be too low to exert a significant positive effect.

It is necessary to emphasize that not all dietary carbohydrates are classified as prebiotics. In fact, besides their susceptibility to degradation by intestinal bacteria, a prebiotic carbohydrate must fulfill many requisites such as resistance to gastric acidity as well as to hydrolysis by mammalian enzymes and to gastrointestinal absorption (Gibson, 2004; Roberfroid, 2007; Marteau, 2001). Several papers have reported that the bacterial community resident in the human intestinal tract has a major impact on gastrointestinal function and human health (Blaut, 2002; Simmering and Blaut, 2001). The supply of different prebiotics induces a significant modification in the intestinal microbiota, increasing the number of bifidobacteria and LAB (Kruse, 1999; Bouhnik et al., 1996), and hence it directly affects human health. So, it is possible to influence the composition of the intestinal microbiota by the consumption of selected microbes, in particular LAB and/or bifidobacteria, or by the ingestion of nondigestible food components that can act as a prebiotic.

In the last decade, a large number of studies have investigated the health-promoting effects of nondigestible oligosaccharides, which include alleviation of constipation, improvement of mineral absorption, regulation of lipid metabolism, decrease in the risk of colon cancer, treatment of hepatic encephalopathy, influence on glycemia/insulinemia, and modulation of the immune system (Swennen et al., 2006). However, in spite of the above-described positive effects, nondigestible oligosaccharides can also have undesirable effects. Many prebiotic products possess osmotic properties which may cause intestinal discomfort or even function as a laxative if they cause extensive fermentation in the large bowel (at high daily doses) (Conway, 2001; Roberfroid and

Delzenne, 1998). However, both the occurrence and intensity of the above-mentioned effects are clearly dose related, depend on the daily regimen of intake, and may vary significantly from one individual to another (Roberfroid and Delzenne, 1998; Oku, 1996).

PREBIOTICS AND BIFIDOBACTERIA

Genome-sequencing projects of probiotic bacteria have provided an improved understanding of the genetic background of these bacteria and crucial insights into the molecular basis underlying human-bacteria interactions. Within this framework, as mentioned above, the analysis of bifidobacterial genomes provides clear evidence of how the genome content reflects the specific adaptation of these microorganisms to their habitat (e.g., human intestine) (Schell et al., 2002). It has been highlighted that many of the carbohydrate-modifying enzymes, i.e., carbohydrases, present in bifidobacterial genomes are α-galactosidases, β-galactosidases, and enzymes active against gluco-oligosaccharides such as α-glucosidases and sucrose phosphorylases. Another class of enzymes involved in the utilization of prebiotics by bifidobacteria includes the β-galactosidases. These enzymes are essential for bifidobacteria to be able to grow on milk or milk components such as lactose and lactose-derived *trans*-galacto-oligosaccharides. Various β-galactosidase activities have been identified in the genus *Bifidobacterium* (Moller et al., 2001; Hung et al., 2001).

Arabinofuranosyl-containing oligosaccharides derived from plant cell wall constituents such as arabinogalactan, arabinan, and arabinoxylan can be fermented by bifidobacteria through arabinoxylases and arabinofuranohydrolases (van den Broek et al., 2005). However, the rate of degradation of the arabinoxylan and arabinogalactan is rather low and it has been assumed that other bacteria (e.g., *Bacteroides*) are needed for the complete hydrolysis of these polymers. Bifidobacteria are also known to grow rapidly on soy milk substrates that contain large amounts of α-galactosyl oligosaccharides (Garro et al., 1999). Enzymes such as α-galactosidases are responsible for the hydrolysis of such substrates as well as for the utilization of melibiose and galactomannan (Sakai et al., 1987). Apart from oligosaccharides, human milk peptides represent another class of diet-derived compounds, producing bifidogenic effects (Liepke et al., 2002). These are small peptides that are derived from the digestion of milk protein by the gastric protease pepsin and contain a pair of cysteine residues forming a disulfide bond and two small hydrophobic domains located C-terminally to the two cysteines (Liepke et al., 2002). The presence of such peptides has been shown to be 100 times more effective on a molar basis at stimulating the growth of bifidobacteria than certain oligosaccharides, and it has been speculated that the bifidogenic activity of breast milk due to the presence of specific peptides far exceeds that of milk oligosaccharides.

THE BIFIDOBACTERIAL GENOME CONTENTS AND THEIR INTERACTION WITH THE GIT

Genome sequencing provides the blueprint for analyzing the full genetic complement of an organism and provides indications of the genetic determinants that specify the adaptive functions required for the environment in which the microorganism lives. In this context, sugar availability has greatly affected the genome content of the intestinal microbiota. Mammalian biology is partially shaped by the commensal bacteria, including bifidobacteria, that colonize the GIT. Plant-based diets are particularly rich in complex carbohydrates that are not digested by the mammalian enzymes in the upper parts of the GIT and therefore reach the distal compartments of the GIT (e.g., the colon) in an intact form. Most of these sugars are considered prebiotic compounds and include FOS, galacto-oligosaccharides, gluco-oligosaccharides, xylo-oligosaccharides, lactulose, and raffinose (see above and Guarner and Malagelada, 2003). These dietary compounds would have been lost if the distal part of the human GIT had not been colonized by a diverse mixture of anaerobic bacteria, including *Bacteroides*, *Bifidobacterium*, *Clostridium*, and *Enterobacterium* (for a review see Vaughan et al., 2005), which possess the metabolic capacity to degrade many of the above-mentioned oligo- and polysaccharides. In this mutually beneficial relationship, the host gains carbon and energy through adsorption of the short-chain fatty acids that are produced as the end products of bacterial fermentation, whereas bacteria are supplied with a rich buffet of glycans and a protected anoxic environment.

It is interesting that a significant proportion of the genomes of common gut inhabitants such as bifidobacteria is dedicated to sugar metabolism, thus reflecting a critical adaptation to this ecological niche. According to the sequence-based classification of carbohydrate-active enzymes by Coutinho and Henrissat (1999), over 8% of the annotated genes of bifidobacterial genomes are predicted to encode enzymes involved in the metabolism of carbohydrates, including a variety of glycosyl hydrolases that are required for the utilization of diverse, but in most cases not identified, plant-derived dietary fiber or complex carbohydrate structures produced by the host (for a review, see Ventura et al., 2007). Bifidobacteria can also utilize sialic acid-containing complex carbohydrates, which are found in mucin, glycosphingolipids, and human milk (Hoskins et al., 1985). Thus, the mammalian host provides substrates for bifidobacteria, thereby representing a remarkable symbiotic (or altruistic) relationship. Other nutrients that have escaped digestion in the proximal part of the GIT are plant-derived high-molecular-weight carbohydrates like starch and pectin. The capacity to hydrolyze these sugars is not widely distributed among bifidobacteria. Among these, *B. breve* possesses the starch-degrading enzyme amylopullulanase, which may play a crucial role during weaning when nonmilk foods are supplemented to the diet, thus exposing infants for the first time to sugars different from those present in mother's milk (Ryan et al., 2006).

Over 8% of the total bifidobacterial gene content is dedicated to sugar internalization, via ABC transporters, permeases, and proton symporters, rather than PEP-phosphotransferase systems (PEP-PTS) (Schell et al., 2002), although a PEP-PTS has been experimentally demonstrated in *B. breve* to be active for the internalization of glucose (Degnan and Macfarlane, 1993). The PTS acts through the concomitant internalization and phosphorylation of carbohydrates, in which the transfer of phosphate from PEP to the incoming sugar is mediated via a phosphorylation chain involving Enzyme I (EI), histidine-containing protein, and Enzyme II (EII). The *B. longum* biotype longum NCC2705 genome has a single EII-encoding locus, while that of *B. breve* UCC2003 has four (Maze et al., 2007). In the latter organism, one PEP-PTS has been characterized in detail and was shown to transport fructose, although it appears to transport glucose as well (Maze et al., 2007). This difference in the number of PEP-PTS may indicate that *B. breve* more frequently encounters less complex sugars in its preferred habitat, the GIT of infants, than *B. longum* biotype longum encounters in the GIT of adults, where it is prevalent. Thus, the different diets of infants and adults may affect the composition of their GIT microbiome.

Commensal bacteria living in the GIT generally interact with the host through a direct contact between microorganism and the host epithelial cells. The molecular basis of such interactions has been investigated in detail for several GIT pathogens such as *Listeria monocytogenes* and *Salmonella* spp. (Lecuit et al., 2001; Mengaud et al., 1996) or common GIT commensal such as *Bacteroides* (Krinos et al., 2001). Conversely, for commensal bacteria such as bifidobacteria very little is known about the genetic determinants for such bacteria-host interactions. Bifidobacterial genome-sequencing analyses did not reveal clear-cut candidate genes that may play a role in

GIT-bifidobacteria interactions. However, bifidobacteria are predicted to encode cell envelope-associated structures that may play a role in the interactions between host and bacterium. Genome analysis of *B. longum* biotype longum NCC2705 revealed the presence of two regions related to polysaccharide biosynthesis (EPS). The role of EPS produced by nonpathogenic colonic bacteria is poorly understood, but it is likely that these extracellular structures are somehow involved in bacterial adherence to host cells, while they may also endow such colonic bacteria with increased resistance to stomach acids and bile salts (Ruas-Madiedo et al., 2006). Moreover, in the commensal microorganism *Bacteroides thetaiotaomicron*, it has been shown that the presence of different EPS clusters helps the microorganism to escape recognition by the host (Krinos et al., 2001). Interestingly, the *eps* loci of *B. longum* biotype longum NCC2705 are flanked by insertion elements and show a strong divergence in G+C content relative to the remainder of the genome. These appear to be a molecular hallmark of *eps* loci examined thus far and may have an evolutionary implication, allowing inter- and intraspecies transfer of *eps* genes. Recently, a survey of bifidobacteria for evidence of EPS production revealed that those species (e.g., *B. pseudocatenulatum*, *B. longum*, *B. adolescentis*, and *B. animalis*) that are most abundantly present in the intestine of humans and other animals harbored genes related to the synthesis of heteropolysaccharides (Ruas-Madiedo et al., 2006). So one could argue that EPS production is required for adhesion of the bacterial cells to human intestinal mucus and therefore is an interesting property to consider for the selection of probiotic strains.

Another bifidobacterial interaction with its host may be specified by genes that are predicted to encode glyco-protein-binding fimbria-like structures, which have been identified in the genome sequences of both *B. longum* biotype longum NCC2705 and *B. longum* biotype longum DJO10A genomes (Schell et al., 2002). In addition, *B. breve* UCC2003, *B. longum* biotype longum NCC2705, and *B. longum* biotype longum DJO10A appear to encode a serpin-like protease inhibitor that has been demonstrated to contribute to host interactions in the GIT (Ivanov et al., 2006). In fact, bifidobacteria may encounter both pancreatic and neutrophil elastases in their natural environment, and protection against exogenous proteolysis may play an important role in the interaction between these commensal bacteria and their host. It was shown that the *B. longum* biotype longum NCC2705 serpin is an efficient inhibitor of human neutrophil and pancreatic elastases, whose release by activated neutrophils at the sites of intestinal inflammation represents an interesting mechanism of innate immunity (Ivanov et al., 2006).

GENETIC ELEMENTS THAT MAY BE RESPONSIBLE FOR HORIZONTAL GENE TRANSFER IN BIFIDOBACTERIA: PLASMIDS AND BACTERIOPHAGES

Prokaryotes have different mechanisms for genetic adaptation to their environments. These involve different genetic forces that shape the prokaryotic genome such as gene duplication, horizontal gene transfer (HGT), gene loss, and chromosomal rearrangements (Coenye et al., 2005). Among the above-mentioned forces, HGT has been identified as one of the main mechanisms that allow the introduction of novel genes that lead to niche-specific adaptation, which eventually might lead to bacterial diversification and speciation (Ochman et al., 2000; Cohan, 2001). The transmission of novel genes through HGT is generally supported by vectors such as bacteriophages or plasmids which may become integrated into the bacterial chromosome (e.g., integrative plasmids or episome elements). Generally, plasmids are rarely found in bifidobacteria. So far the majority of bifidobacterial plasmids have been identified within different *B. longum* biotype longum strains. These include pMB1 (Rossi et al., 1998), pKJ36 and pKJ50 (Park et al., 1997), pBLO1 (Schell et al., 2002), pNAC1, pNAC2, and pNAC3 (Corneau et al., 2004), pDOJH10S and pDO-JH10L (Lee and O'Sullivan, 2006), pTB6 (Tanaka et al., 2005), pB44 (Gibbs et al., 2006), and pNAL8 (Guglielmetti et al., 2007). In addition, six plasmids from other bifidobacterial species have been sequenced: pVS809 from *Bifidobacterium globosum* (Mattarelli et al., 1994), pCIBb1 from *B. breve* (O'Riordan and Fitzgerald, 1999), pNBb1 from *B. breve* (GenBank accession number E17316), pAP1 from *B. asteroides* (GenBank accession number Y11549), pBC1 from *Bifidobacterium catenulatum* (Alvarez-Martin et al., 2006), and p4M from *Bifidobacterium pseudocatenulatum* (GenBank accession number NC003527). These plasmids do not encode any obvious phenotypic trait, except for the plasmid isolated from *B. bifidum* NCFB 1454 (Yildirim et al., 1999), which was proposed to encode a bacteriocin, bifidocin B. Recently, interest in the characterization of bifidobacterial plasmids has increased significantly because they can be used for the development of molecular tools to genetically manipulate these organisms. In fact, in contrast to the advances achieved in bifidobacterial ecology, the lack of genetic tools has hampered molecular biological investigations of bifidobacteria, certainly when compared to other *Actinobacteria* members such as *Streptomyces* or *Mycobacterium*.

Another vector that may act in the transmission of genes by HGT is represented by bacteriophages. Bifidobacteria have for a long time been considered free from phage infection. However, the identification of three prophage-like elements (Blj1, Bl-1, and Bbr-1) in the genomes of *B. longum* biotype longum NCC2705 and DJO10A and in the genome of *B. breve* UCC2003 has changed this perception (Ventura et al., 2005b). These prophage-like elements display homology to genes of double-stranded DNA phages that infect a broad range of bacteria. Notably, it was shown that the identified prophage-like elements exhibit a close phylogenetic relationship with phages infecting low-G+C gram-positive bacteria, suggesting that these bacteria have shared the same ecological niche during their evolution. This may therefore represent evidence pointing to an ancient exchange of DNA sequences between low- and high-G+C bacteria. The clustering of these prophage-like elements found in bifidobacteria may also be explained by assuming that the forerunner of bifidobacterial phages originally infected the ancestor of high-G+C gram-positive bacteria, which is in agreement with the argument for an evolutionary origin of high-G+C gram-positive bacteria from low-G+C ancestors. Notably, the Blj-1 prophage-like element from *B. longum* biotype longum DJO10A was shown to excise from the genome upon treatment of the bacterium with mitomycin C or hydrogen peroxide (Ventura et al., 2005b). This represents the first reported inducible and molecularly characterized *Bifidobacterium* prophage, presenting possibilities for further studies on the biology of bifidophages. Moreover, all three prophages were shown to be integrated in a $tRNA_{Met}$ gene, which had not previously been shown to act as an *attB* site in gram-positive bacteria (Campbell, 1992). Analysis of the distribution of this integration site in many bifidobacterial taxa, i.e., *B. longum* biotype longum, *B. longum* biotype infantis, *B. longum* biotype suis, *B. breve*, and *B. animalis* subsp. *lactis*, shows that the sequences are well conserved. These conserved sequences might be useful for the construction of an efficient recombination module, analogous to the *Streptomyces* integrating plasmid pSE211 (Brown et al., 1990). This module may represent a valuable source for the construction of vector integration systems that enable the food grade introduction of foreign DNA sequences without disturbing any bacterial function, as was previously described for the genus *Lactococcus* (Martin et al., 2000).

TAXONOMY OF BIFIDOBACTERIA

The availability of several whole-genome sequences has allowed significant progress in the understanding of bacterial evolutionary relationships and thus in the taxonomy of prokaryotes. Nowadays, prokaryotic species are characterized using a polyphasic method that includes genotypic and phenotypic features (Stackebrandt et al., 1997; Vandamme et al., 1996). In particular, significant importance is assigned to the level of genetic relatedness among bacterial species (Coenye et al., 2005) as determined by physicochemical DNA-DNA hybridization methods. Bacteria that exhibit a DNA-DNA hybridization value of more than 70% while displaying less than 5% difference in their melting temperature are considered to belong to the same species. In contrast, strains sharing a level of genomic DNA hybridization that is lower than 50% do not belong to the same species. However, DNA-DNA hybridization methods are time-consuming and sometimes the results achieved are questionable. During the past decades, therefore, the development of molecular biological tools has led to profound modifications with regard to the identification and classification methods of bacteria. In this respect, the use of the 16S rRNA gene as a molecular marker for inferring phylogeny in bacteria has become the preferred tool in bacterial taxonomy. Comparative sequence analysis of the 16S rRNA gene is used to resolve the phylogenetic position of new isolates. In this respect, it has been accepted that isolates depicting a level of 16S rRNA sequence identity greater than 97% are considered to belong to the same taxon. However, according to the recent recommendations of the ad hoc committee for the reevaluation of the definition of the bacterial species, at least one other gene besides the 16S rRNA-encoding gene should be taken into consideration in order to investigate bacterial phylogeny. Among these housekeeping genes, those which encode heat shock proteins such as *groEL-groES* (Ventura et al., 2004b; Jian et al., 2001), *dnaK* (Ventura et al., 2005c), *grpE* (Ventura et al., 2005c), *hrcA* (Ventura et al., 2005a), *clpP* (Ventura et al., 2005d) or *recA* (Kullen et al., 1997; Ventura and Zink, 2003), *tufA* (Ventura and Zink, 2003), and *atpD* (Ventura et al., 2004a) are considered to be valuable molecular markers in bifidobacterial taxonomy. Molecular methods using one or several appropriate genes, i.e., alternative molecular markers, are gaining importance because they provide quick and, in general, reliable results. Alternative molecular markers can be used to correct, corroborate, or fine-tune the rRNA-based system and should fulfill several prerequisites, including wide distribution, functional conservation, genetic stability, and a reasonable number of independently evolving positions or regions. Another desirable prerequisite is that such markers can generate a comprehensive sequence database describing a wide spectrum of phylogenetically diverse bac-

teria. Nevertheless, various studies have raised concerns that phylogenetic investigation based on a single molecular marker may not reflect the "real" phylogeny because of HGT events, incongruous mutational rates, and variable recombination rates. Thus, phylogenetic investigations based on a set of combined alignments of conserved orthologous proteins, also referred to as supertrees, should provide the most reliable image of the phylogenetic relationships existing across bacteria (Brown et al., 2001; Bininda-Emonds, 2004).

Now, as we enter the postgenomics era, the rRNA-based view of microbial phylogeny is subjected to scientific scrutiny. Indeed, the large numbers of microbial genome projects are providing a large database of easily accessible alternative molecular markers in addition to the 16S rRNA gene that can be used to build supertrees. Recently, a phylogenetic study involving all of the currently described bifidobacterial species, using a multigene concatenation approach, demonstrated the increased discriminatory power and robustness of the supertree approach (Ventura et al., 2006a). This phylogenetic analysis displays a subdivision of the genus *Bifidobacterium* in the same phylogenetic groups obtained from the use of 16S rRNA gene-based tree (Fig. 2, part 1). Interestingly, it shows that the projected ancestor of all recognized bifidobacteria groups was most closely related to the current *B. asteroides* species (Fig. 2, part 2).

Although bifidobacteria are classified in the phylum *Actinobacteria*, no clear molecular characteristic was known that was uniquely shared by these bacteria and various other *Actinobacteria*. Nevertheless, a clear evolutionary relationship between bifidobacteria and *Actinobacteria* is now supported by a number of conserved inserts and/or deletions in protein sequences (cytochrome *c* oxidase subunit 1, CTP synthetase, and glutamyl-tRNA synthetase) and the 23S rRNA that are uniquely shared by bifidobacteria and other *Actinobacteria* but are not found in any other bacterial groups (Gao and Gupta, 2005). Comparative analyses of actinobacterial genomes have identified many proteins that are uniquely present in all *Actinobacteria*, homologs of which do not appear to be shared with any other prokaryotic or eukaryotic organism, are specifically present in all currently available bifidobacterial genomes, or are limited to one phylogenetic group of bifidobacteria (e.g., *B. longum* or *B. adolescentis*) (Gao and Gupta, 2006). These studies have highlighted about 90 proteins that are characteristic of the *B. longum* group and an additional 70 proteins that appear to be distinctive of the bifidobacterial genomes sequenced so far. However, for most of the proteins that were earmarked to be specific to either *B. longum* or bifidobacteria, sequence data are

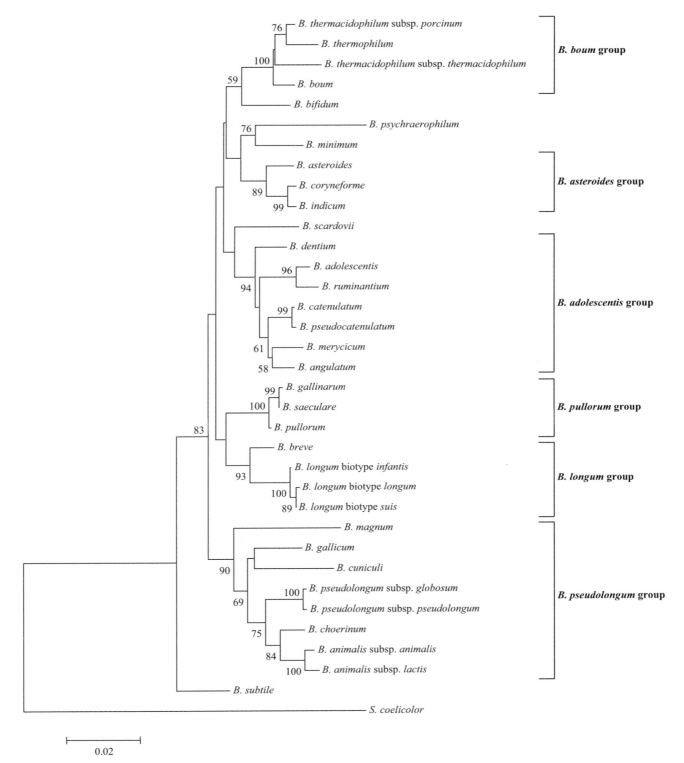

Figure 2 Phylogenetic tree of the genus *Bifidobacterium* based on the 16S rRNA gene sequences (left) and from the concatenation of *clpC*, *dnaB*, *dnaG*, *dnaJ1*, *purF*, *rpoC*, and *xfp* gene sequences (right). The different phylogenetic groups are indicated.

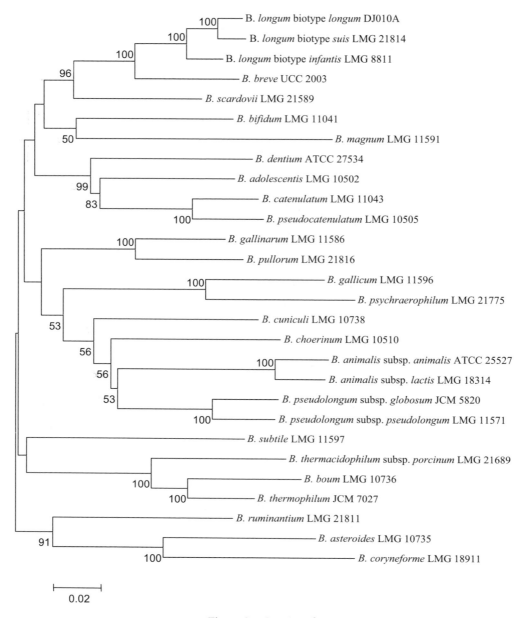

Figure 2 *Continued.*

available only from a restricted number of bifidobacterial species. Thus, it is crucial to gain sequence information for these proteins from other members of this genus. It is likely that, since many of these proteins will be species or strain specific, some may prove to be specific for a subset of bifidobacterial strains or species, revealing their evolutionary relationships and important differences among them. In fact, all bifidobacterial-specific proteins are of unknown function. Therefore,

it is possible to speculate that these proteins may carry out novel functions that make bifidobacteria physiologically distinct from other *Actinobacteria* members. Some of these proteins may also encode probiotic activities of bifidobacterial species in the GIT. Thus, a major task for the future is the understanding of the cellular functions of these bifidobacterium-specific proteins, which may also provide insights into the molecular basis of the probiotic properties of these bacteria.

In phylogenetic trees based on 16S rRNA gene sequences, bifidobacteria form a deep-branching lineage within the *Actinobacteria* phylum (Gao and Gupta, 2005; Stackebrandt and Schumann, 2000). The 29 bifidobacterial species thus far described can be grouped into six different phylogenetic clusters, which include the *B. boum* group, the *B. asteroides* group, the *B. adolescentis* group, the *B. pullorum* group, the *B. longum* group, and the *B. pseudolongum* group (Fig. 2). Taxonomic issues in the genus *Bifidobacterium* were observed for the species *B. longum*, *B. infantis*, and *B. suis*, which have recently been solved by their unification under a single taxon, *B. longum*, being further subdivided into three biotypes, i.e., longum, infantis, and suis (Sakata et al., 2002). Furthermore, another industrially relevant taxonomic topic is represented by the relationship between *B. animalis* and *B. lactis* species, which were reclassified as *B. animalis* subsp. *animalis* and *B. animalis* subsp. *lactis* (Masco et al., 2004). In fact, a polyphasic approach taking into account physiological features (e.g., ability to grow in milk and sugar fermentation profiles) as well as genetic features (e.g., DNA-DNA hybridization and *atpD* and *groEL* gene sequence analysis) demonstrated that representatives of *B. animalis* and *B. lactis* constitute two clear subgroups that have originated from a common ancestor following a recent evolutionary split (Masco et al., 2004; Ventura and Zink, 2002).

CONCLUDING REMARKS

Several issues regarding the sequences of complete bifidobacterial genomes remain unresolved at present. So far only a limited number of completed bifidobacterial genome sequences are available, which, unfortunately, only partially represent the total biodiversity of bifidobacterial communities present in the GIT. It is important that with the accumulation of more bifidobacterial genome sequences, not just representing bifidobacterial isolates of industrial importance, we will be able to obtain molecular insights into the genetic adaptation of bifidobacteria to the human GIT. Moreover, there is a clear scientific incentive to explore how bifidobacteria can coexist with their host while evading the diversity of responses that the host has developed to eliminate pathogenic bacteria. In this context, the understanding of the molecular basis through which the human immune system can discriminate between harmful and beneficial bacteria is an important challenge for the future. Moreover, bifidobacterial activity and bifidobacteria-host interactions in the GIT are still far from fully characterized. Consequently, future postgenomic investigations will be required to provide a molecular knowledge base to help explain the positive health impacts that bifidobacteria have on their mammalian hosts.

This work was financially supported by the Italian Award for Outstanding Young Researcher scheme "Incentivazione alla mobilità di studiosi stranieri e italiani residenti all'estero" to M.V. and by the Science Foundation Ireland Alimentary Pharmabiotic Centre located at University College Cork.

References

Alvarez-Martin, P., A. B. Florez, and B. Mayo. 2006. Screening for plasmids among human bifidobacteria species: sequencing and analysis of pBC1 from *Bifidobacterium catenulatum* L48. *Plasmid* **57:**165–174.

Amann, R. I., W. Ludwig, and K. H. Schleifer. 1995. Phylogenetic identification and in situ detection of individual microbial cells without cultivation. *Microbiol. Rev.* **59:**143–169.

Bengmark, S. 2002. Gut microbial ecology in critical illness: is there a role for prebiotics, probiotics, and synbiotics? *Curr. Opin. Crit. Care* **8:**145–151.

Biavati, B., and P. Mattarelli. 2001. The family *Bifidobacteriaceae. In* M. Dworkin et al. (ed.), *The Prokaryotes: an Evolving Electronic Resource for the Microbiological Community.* http://www.bacterialphylogeny.info/index.html.

Bininda-Emonds, O. R. P. 2004. The evolution of supertrees. *Trends Ecol. Evol.* **19:**315–322.

Blaut, M. 2002. Relationship of prebiotics and food to intestinal microflora. *Eur. J. Nutr.* **41:**I/11–I/16.

Bouhnik, Y., B. Flourie, and M. Riottot. 1996. Effect of fructo-oligosaccharides ingestion on faecal bifidobacteria and selected metabolic index of colon carcinogenesis in healthy humans. *Nutr. Cancer* **26:**21–29.

Brown, D. P., K. B. Idler, and L. Katz. 1990. Characterization of the genetic elements required for site-specific integration of plasmid pSE211 in *Saccharopolyspora erythraea. J. Bacteriol.* **172:**1877–1888.

Brown, J. R., C. J. Douady, M. J. Italia, W. E. Marshall, and M. J. Stanhope. 2001. Universal trees based on large combined protein sequence data sets. *Nat. Genet.* **28:**281–285.

Campbell, A. M. 1992. Chromosomal insertion sites for phages and plasmids. *J. Bacteriol.* **174:**7495–7499.

Chan, K., S. Baker, C. C. Kim, C. S. Detweiler, G. Dougan, and S. Falkow. 2003. Genomic comparison of *Salmonella enterica* serovars and *Salmonella bongori* by use of an *S. enterica* serovar Typhimurium DNA microarray. *J. Bacteriol.* **185:**553–563.

Christensen, B. B., T. Atlung, and F. G. Hansen. 1999. DnaA boxes are important elements in setting the initiation mass of *Escherichia coli. J. Bacteriol.* **181:**2683–2688.

Coenye, T., D. Gevers, Y. Van de Peer, P. Vandamme, and J. Swings. 2005. Towards a prokaryotic genomic taxonomy. *FEMS Microbiol. Rev.* **29:**147–167.

Cohan, F. M. 2001. Bacterial species and speciation. *Syst. Biol.* **50:**513–524.

Conway, P. L. 2001. Prebiotics and human health: the state-of-the-art and future perspectives. *Scand. J. Nutr.* **45:**13–21.

Corneau, N., E. Emond, and G. LaPointe. 2004. Molecular characterization of three plasmids from *Bifidobacterium longum. Plasmid* **51:**87–100.

Coutinho, P. M., and B. Henrissat. 1999. Life with no sugars? *J. Mol. Microbiol. Biotechnol.* 1:307–308.

Degnan, B. A., and G. T. Macfarlane. 1993. Transport and metabolism of glucose and arabinose in *Bifidobacterium breve*. *Arch. Microbiol.* 160:144–151.

Delzenne, N. M. 2003. Oligosaccharides: state of the art. *Proc. Nutr. Soc.* 62:177–182.

Dobrindt, U., F. Agerer, K. Michaelis, A. Janka, C. Buchrieser, M. Samuelson, C. Svanborg, G. Gottschalk, H. Karch, and J. Hacker. 2003. Analysis of genome plasticity in pathogenic and commensal *Escherichia coli* isolates by use of DNA arrays. *J. Bacteriol.* 185:1831–1840.

Favier, C. F., E. E. Vaughan, W. M. De Vos, and A. D. Akkermans. 2002. Molecular monitoring of succession of bacterial communities in human neonates. *Appl. Environ. Microbiol.* 68:219–226.

Fitzgerald, J. R., D. E. Sturdervant, S. M. Mackie, S. R. Gill, and J. M. Musser. 2001. Evolutionary genomics of *Staphylococcus aureus*: insights into the origin of methicillin-resistant strain and the toxic shock syndrome epidemic. *Proc. Natl. Acad. Sci. USA* 98:8821–8826.

Franks, A. H., H. J. Harmsen, G. C. Raangs, G. J. Jansen, F. Schut, and G. W. Welling. 1998. Variations of bacterial populations in human feces measured by fluorescent in situ hybridization with group-specific 16S rRNA-targeted oligonucleotide probes. *Appl. Environ. Microbiol.* 64:3336–3345.

Fuller, R. 1989. Probiotics in man and animals. *J. Appl. Bacteriol.* 66:365–378.

Gao, B., and R. S. Gupta. 2005. Conserved indels in protein sequences that are characteristic of the phylum *Actinobacteria*. *Int. J. Syst. Evol. Microbiol.* 55:2401–2412.

Gao, B., and R. S. Gupta. 2006. Signature proteins that are distinctive characteristics of *Actinobacteria* and their subgroups. *Antonie Leeuwenhoek* 90:69–91.

Garrity, G. M., and J. G. Holt. 2001. The road map to the manual. *In* D. R. Boone and R. W. Castenholz (ed.), *Bergey's Manual of Systematic Bacteriology*. Springer-Verlag, Berlin, Germany.

Garro, M. S., G. F. de Valdez, G. Oliver, and G. S. de Giori. 1999. Hydrolysis of soya milk oligosaccharides by *Bifidobacterium longum* CRL 849. *Z. Lebensm. Unters. Forsch. A* 208:57–59.

Gibbs, M. J., W. Smeianov, J. L. Steel, P. Upcroft, and B. A. Efimov. 2006. Two families of rep-like genes that probably originated by interspecies recombination are represented in viral, plasmid, bacterial, and parasitic protozoan genomes. *Mol. Biol. Evol.* 23:1097–1100.

Gibson, G. R. 2004. Prebiotics. *Best Pract. Res. Clin. Gastroenterol.* 18:287–298.

Gibson, G. R., and M. B. Roberfroid. 1995. Dietary modulation of the human colonic microbiota: introducing the concept of prebiotics. *J. Nutr.* 125:1401–1412.

Guarner, F., and J. R. Malagelada. 2003. Gut flora in health and disease. *Lancet* 361:512–519.

Guglielmetti, S., M. Karp, D. Mora, I. Tamagnini, and C. Parini. 2007. Molecular characterization of *Bifidobacterium longum* biovar longum NAL8 plasmids and construction of a novel replicon screening system. *Appl. Microbiol. Biotechnol.* 74:1053–1061.

Hopkins, M. J., R. Sharp, and G. T. Macfarlane. 2001. Age and disease related changes in intestinal bacterial populations assessed by cell culture, 16S rRNA abundance, and community cellular fatty acid profiles. *Gut* 48:198–205.

Hopkins, M. J., R. Sharp, and G. T. Macfarlane. 2002. Variation in human intestinal microbiota with age. *Dig. Liver Dis.* 34:12–18.

Hoskins, L. C., M. Agustines, W. B. McKee, E. T. Boulding, M. Kriaris, and G. Niedermeyer. 1985. Mucin degradation in human colon ecosystems. Isolation and properties of fecal strains that degrade ABH blood group antigens and oligosaccharides from mucin glycoproteins. *J. Clin. Investig.* 75:944–953.

Hung, M. N., Z. Xia, N. T. Hu, and B. H. Lee. 2001. Molecular and biochemical analysis of two β-galactosidases from *Bifidobacterium infantis* HL96. *Appl. Environ. Microbiol.* 67:4256–4263.

Ivanov, D., C. Emonet, F. Foata, M. Affolter, M. Delley, M. Fisseha, S. Blum-Sperisen, S. Kochhar, and F. Arigoni. 2006. A serpin from the gut bacterium *Bifidobacterium longum* inhibits eukaryotic elastase-like serine proteases. *J. Biol. Chem.* 281:17246–17252.

Jian, W., L. Zhu, and X. Dong. 2001. New approach to phylogenetic analysis of the genus *Bifidobacterium* based on partial HSP60 gene sequences. *Int. J. Syst. Evol. Microbiol.* 51:1633–1638.

Johnson, I. T. 2004. New approaches to the role of diet in the prevention of cancers of the alimentary tract. *Mutat. Res.* 551:9–28.

Klaenhammer, T. R., R. Barrangou, B. L. Buck, M. A. Azcarate-Peril, and E. Altermann. 2005. Genomic features of lactic acid bacteria effecting bioprocessing and health. *FEMS Microbiol. Rev.* 29:393–409.

Krinos, C. M., M. J. Coyne, K. G. Weinacht, A. O. Tzianabos, D. L. Kasper, and L. E. Comstock. 2001. Extensive surface diversity of a commensal microorganism by multiple DNA inversions. *Nature* 414:555–558.

Kruse, H. P., B. Kleessen, and M. Blaut. 1999. Effects of inulin on faecal bifidobacteria in human subjects. *Br. J. Nutr.* 82:375–382.

Kullen, M. J., L. J. Brady, and D. J. O'Sullivan. 1997. Evaluation of using a short region of the *recA* gene for rapid and sensitive speciation of dominant bifidobacteria in the human large intestine. *FEMS Microbiol. Lett.* 154:377–383.

Langendijk, P. S., F. Shut, G. J. Jansen, G. C. Raangs, G. R. Kamphuis, M. H. F. Wilkinson, and G. W. Welling. 1995. Quantitative fluorescence in situ hybridization of *Bifidobacterium* spp. with genus-specific 16S rRNA targeted probes and its application in fecal samples. *Appl. Environ. Microbiol.* 61:3069–3075.

Lay, C., M. Sutren, V. Rochet, K. Saunier, J. Dore, and L. Rigottier-Gois. 2005. Design and validation of 16S rRNA probes to enumerate members of the *Clostridium leptum* subgroup in human faecal microbiota. *Environ. Microbiol.* 7:933–946.

Leahy, S. C., D. G. Higgins, G. F. Fitzgerald, and D. van Sinderen. 2005. Getting better with bifidobacteria. *J. Appl. Microbiol.* 98:1303–1315.

Lecuit, M., S. Vandormael-Pournin, J. Lefort, M. Huerre, P. Gounon, C. Dupuy, C. Babinet, and P. Cossart. 2001. A transgenic model for listeriosis: role of internalin in crossing the intestinal barrier. *Science* 292:1722–1725.

Lee, J. H., and D. J. O'Sullivan. 2006. Sequence analysis of two cryptic plasmids from *Bifidobacterium longum* DJO10A and construction of a shuttle cloning vector. *Appl. Environ. Microbiol.* 72:527–535.

Liepke, C., K. Adermann, M. Raida, H. J. Magert, W. G. Forssmann, and H. D. Zucht. 2002. Human milk provides peptides highly stimulating the growth of bifidobacteria. *Eur. J. Biochem.* 269:712–718.

Liu, M., G. van Enckevort, and R. J. Siezen. 2005. Genome update: lactic acid bacteria genome sequencing is booming. *Microbiology* 151:3811–3814.

Mahairas, G. G., P. J. Sabo, M. J. Hickey, D. C. Singh, and C. K. Stover. 1996. Molecular analysis of genetic differences between *Mycobacterium bovis* BCG and virulent *M. bovis. J. Bacteriol.* 178:1274–1282.

Manning, T. S., and G. R. Gibson. 2004. Microbial-gut interactions in health and disease. Prebiotics. *Best Pract. Res. Clin. Gastroenterol.* 18:287–298.

Marteau, P. 2001. Prebiotics and probiotics for gastrointestinal health. *Clin. Nutr.* 20:41–45.

Martin, M. C., J. C. Alonso, J. E. Suarez, and M. A. Alvarez. 2000. Generation of food-grade recombinant lactic acid bacterium strains by site-specific recombination. *Appl. Environ. Microbiol.* 66:2599–2604.

Masco, L., M. Ventura, R. Zink, G. Huys, and J. Swings. 2004. Polyphasic taxonomic analysis of *Bifidobacterium animalis* and *Bifidobacterium lactis* reveals relatedness at the subspecies level: reclassification of *Bifidobacterium animalis* as *Bifidobacterium animalis* subsp. *animalis* comb. nov. and *Bifidobacterium lactis* as *Bifidobacterium animalis* subsp. *lactis* comb. nov. *Int. J. Syst. Evol. Microbiol.* 54:1137–1143.

Matsuki, T., K. Watanabe, R. Tanaka, M. Fukuda, and H. Oyaizu. 1999. Distribution of bifidobacterial species in human intestinal microflora examined with 16S rRNA-gene-targeted species-specific primers. *Appl. Environ. Microbiol.* 65:4506–4512.

Mattarelli, P., B. Biavati, A. Alessandrini, F. Crociani, and V. Scardovi. 1994. Characterization of the plasmid pVS808 from *Bifidobacterium globosum. New Microbiol.* 17:327–331.

Maze, A., M. O'Connell-Motherway, G. F. Fitzgerald, J. Deutscher, and D. van Sinderen. 2007. Identification and characterization of a fructose phosphotransferase system in *Bifidobacterium breve* UCC2003. *Appl. Environ. Microbiol.* 73:545–553.

McLean, M. J., K. H. Wolfe, and K. M. Devine. 1998. Base composition skews, replication orientation, and gene orientation in 12 prokaryote genomes. *J. Mol. Evol.* 47:691–696.

Mengaud, J., H. Ohayon, P. Gounon, R. M. Mege, and P. Cossart. 1996. E-cadherin is the receptor for internalin, a surface protein required for entry of *L. monocytogenes* into epithelial cells. *Cell* 84:923–932.

Moller, P. L., F. Jorgensen, O. C. Hansen, S. M. Madsen, and P. Stougaard. 2001. Intra- and extracellular β-galactosidases from *Bifidobacterium bifidum* and *B. infantis*. Molecular cloning, heterologous expression, and comparative characterization. *Appl. Environ. Microbiol.* 67:2276–2283.

Ochman, H., J. G. Lawrence, and E. A. Groisman. 2000. Lateral gene transfer and the nature of bacterial innovation. *Nature* 405:299–304.

Oku, T. 1996. Oligosaccharides with beneficial health effects: a Japanese perspective. *Nutr. Rev.* 54(Part 2, Suppl. S): S59–S66.

O'Riordan, K., and G. F. Fitzgerald. 1999. Molecular characterisation of a 5.75-kb cryptic plasmid from *Bifidobacterium breve* NCFB 2258 and determination of mode of replication. *FEMS Microbiol. Lett.* 174:285–294.

Osterman, A., and R. Overbeek. 2003. Missing genes in metabolic pathways: a comparative genomic approach. *Curr. Opin. Chem. Biol.* 7:238–251.

Park, M. S., K. H. Lee, and G. E. Ji. 1997. Isolation and characterization of two plasmids from *Bifidobacterium longum. Lett. Appl. Microbiol.* 25:5–7.

Peters, J. E., T. E. Thate, and N. L. Craig. 2003. Definition of the *Escherichia coli* MC4100 genome by use of a DNA array. *J. Bacteriol.* 185:2017–2021.

Poupard, J. A., I. Husain, and R. F. Norris. 1973. Biology of the bifidobacteria. *Bacteriol. Rev.* 37:136–165.

Rezzonico, E., S. Lariani, C. Barretto, G. Cuanoud, G. Giliberti, M. Delley, F. Arigoni, and G. Pessi. 2007. Global transcriptome analysis of the heat response of *Bifidobacterium longum. FEMS Microbiol. Lett.* 271: 136–145.

Roberfroid, M. 2007. Prebiotics: the concept revisited. *J. Nutr.* 137:830S–837S.

Roberfroid, M. B. 2005. Introducing inulin-type fructans . *Br. J. Nutr.* 93(Suppl. 1):S13–S25.

Roberfroid, M. B., and N. M. Delzenne. 1998. Dietary fructans. *Annu. Rev. Nutr.* 18:117–143.

Rossi, M., P. Brigidi, and D. Matteuzzi. 1998. Improved cloning vectors for *Bifidobacterium* spp. *Lett. Appl. Microbiol.* 26:101–104.

Ruas-Madiedo, P., M. Gueimonde, C. G. de los Reyes-Gavilan, and S. Salminen. 2006. Short communication: effect of exopolysaccharide isolated from "viili" on the adhesion of probiotics and pathogens to intestinal mucus. *J. Dairy Sci.* 89:2355–2358.

Ryan, S. M., G. F. Fitzgerald, and D. van Sinderen. 2006. Screening and identification of starch, amylopectin and pullulan-degrading activities in bifidobacterial strains. *Appl. Environ. Microbiol.* 72:5289–5296.

Sakai, K., T. Tachiki, H. Kumagai, and T. Tochikura. 1987. Hydrolysis of α-D-galactosyl oligosaccharides in soymilk by α-galactosidase of *Bifidobacterium breve. Agric. Biol. Chem.* 51:315–322.

Sakata, S., M. Kitahara, M. Sakamoto, H. Hayashi, M. Fukuyame, and Y. Benno. 2002. Unification of *Bifidobacterium infantis* and *Bifidobacterium suis* as *Bifidobacterium longum. Int. J. Syst. Evol. Microbiol.* 52:1945–1951.

Sanchez, B., M. C. Champomier-Verges, P. Anglade, F. Baraige, C. G. de Los Reyes-Gavilan, A. Margolles, and M. Zagorec. 2005. Proteomic analysis of global changes in protein expression during bile salt exposure of *Bifidobacterium longum* NCIMB 8809. *J. Bacteriol.* **187:**5799–5808.

Savijoki, K., A. Suokko, A. Palva, L. Valmu, N. Kalkkinen, and P. Varmanen. 2005. Effect of heat-shock and bile salts on protein synthesis of *Bifidobacterium longum* revealed by [35S]methionine labelling and two-dimensional gel electrophoresis. *FEMS Microbiol. Lett.* **248:**207–215.

Schell, M. A., M. Karmirantzou, B. Snel, et al. 2002. The genome sequence of *Bifidobacterium longum* reflects its adaptation to the human gastrointestinal tract. *Proc. Natl. Acad. Sci. USA* **99:**14422–14427.

Simmering, R., and M. Blaut. 2001. Pro- and prebiotics—the tasty guardian angels? *Appl. Microbiol. Biotechnol.* **55:**19–28.

Stackebrandt, E., and P. Schumann. 2000. Introduction to the taxonomy of *Actinobacteria. In* M. Dworkin et al. (ed.), *The Prokaryotes: an Evolving Electronic Resource for the Microbiological Community.* http://www.bacterialphylogeny.info/index.html.

Stackebrandt, E., F. A. Rainey, and N. L. WardRainey. 1997. Proposal for a new hierarchic classification system, *Actinobacteria* classis nov. *Int. J. Syst. Bacteriol.* **47:**479–491.

Swennen, K., C. M. Courtin, and J. A. Delcour. 2006. Nondigestible oligosaccharides with prebiotic properties. *Crit. Rev. Food Sci. Nutr.* **46:**459–471.

Tanaka, K., K. Samura, and Y. Kano. 2005. Structural and functional analysis of pTB6 from *Bifidobacterium longum*. *Biosci. Biotechnol. Biochem.* **69:**422–425.

Tissier, H. 1900. Recherches sur la flore intestinale normale et pathologique du nourrisson. Thesis. University of Paris, Paris, France.

Vandamme, P., B. Pot, M. Gillis, P. de Vos, K. Kersters, and J. Swings. 1996. Polyphasic taxonomy, a consensus approach to bacterial systematics. *Microbiol. Rev.* **60:**407–438.

van den Broek, L. A. M., S. W. A. Hinz, G. Beldman, and C. H. L. Doeswijk-Voragen. 2005. Glycosyl hydrolases from *Bifidobacterium adolescentis* DSM20083. *Lait* **85:**125–133.

Vaughan, E. E., H. G. Heilig, K. Ben-Amor, and W. M. de Vos. 2005. Diversity, vitality and activities of intestinal lactic acid bacteria and bifidobacteria assessed by molecular approaches. *FEMS Microbiol. Rev.* **29:**477–490.

Ventura, M., and R. Zink. 2002. Rapid identification, differentiation, and proposed new taxonomic classification of *Bifidobacterium lactis*. *Appl. Environ. Microbiol.* **68:**6429–6434.

Ventura, M., and R. Zink. 2003. Comparative sequence analysis of the *tuf* and *recA* genes and restriction fragment length polymorphism of the internal transcribed spacer region sequences supply additional tools for discriminating *Bifidobacterium lactis* from *Bifidobacterium animalis*. *Appl. Environ. Microbiol.* **69:**7517–7522.

Ventura, M., C. Canchaya, D. van Sinderen, G. F. Fitzgerald, and R. Zink. 2004a. *Bifidobacterium lactis* DSM 10140: identification of the *atp* (*atpBEFHAGDC*) operon and analysis of its genetic structure, characteristics, and phylogeny. *Appl. Environ. Microbiol.* **70:**3110–3121.

Ventura, M., C. Canchaya, R. Zink, G. F. Fitzgerald, and D. van Sinderen. 2004b. Characterization of the *groEL* and *groES* loci in *Bifidobacterium breve* UCC 2003: genetic, transcriptional, and phylogenetic analyses. *Appl. Environ. Microbiol.* **70:**6197–6209.

Ventura, M., C. Canchaya, A. Del Casale, F. Dellaglio, G. F. Fitzgerald, and D. van Sinderen. 2005a. Genetic characterization of the *Bifidobacterium breve* UCC 2003 *hrcA* locus. *Appl. Environ. Microbiol.* **71:**8998–9007.

Ventura, M., J. H. Lee, C. Canchaya, et al. 2005b. Prophage-like elements in bifidobacteria: insights from genomics, transcription, integration, distribution, and phylogenetic analysis. *Appl. Environ. Microbiol.* **71:**8692–8705.

Ventura, M., R. Zink, G. F. Fitzgerald, and D. van Sinderen. 2005c. Gene structure and transcriptional organization of the *dnaK* operon of *Bifidobacterium breve* UCC 2003 and application of the operon in bifidobacterial tracing. *Appl. Environ. Microbiol.* **71:**487–500.

Ventura, M., Z. Zhang, M. Cronin, C. Canchaya, J. G. Kenny, G. F. Fitzgerald, and D. van Sinderen. 2005d. The ClgR protein regulates transcription of the *clpP* operon in *Bifidobacterium breve* UCC 2003. *J. Bacteriol.* **187:**8411–8426.

Ventura, M., C. Canchaya, A. Del Casale, F. Dellaglio, G. F. Fitzgerald, and D. van Sinderen. 2006a. Analysis of bifidobacterial evolution using a multilocus approach. *Int. J. Syst. Evol. Microbiol.* **56:**2783–2792.

Ventura, M., C. Canchaya, Z. Zhang, G. F. Fitzgerald, and D. van Sinderen. 2006b. How high G+C Gram-positive bacteria and in particular bifidobacteria cope with heat stress: protein players and regulators. *FEMS Microbiol. Rev.* **30:**734–759.

Ventura, M., C. Canchaya, G. F. Fitzgerald, R. S. Gupta, and D. van Sinderen. 2007. Genomics as a means to understand bacterial phylogeny and ecological adaptation: the case of bifidobacteria. *Antonie Leeuwenhoek* **91:**351–372.

Yildirim, Z., D. K. Winters, and M. G. Johnson. 1999. Purification, amino acid sequence and mode of action of bifidocin B produced by *Bifidobacterium bifidum* NCFB 1454. *J. Appl. Microbiol.* **86:**45–54.

Yoshioka, H., K. Iseki, and K. Fujita. 1983. Development and differences of intestinal flora in the neonatal period in breast-fed and bottle-fed infants. *Pediatrics* **72:**317–321.

Ziemer, C. J., and G. R. Gibson. 1998. An overview of probiotics, prebiotics and synbiotics in the functional food concept: perspectives and future strategies. *Int. Dairy J.* **8:**473–479.

Zoetendal, E. G., C. T. Collier, S. Koike, R. I. Mackie, and H. R. Gaskins. 2004. Molecular ecological analysis of the gastrointestinal microbiota: a review. *J. Nutr.* **134:**465–472.

Therapeutic Microbiology: Probiotics and Related Strategies
Edited by J. Versalovic and M. Wilson
© 2008 ASM Press, Washington, DC

Xinhua Chen
Ciarán P. Kelly

5

Saccharomyces spp.

HISTORY AND TAXONOMY OF *SACCHAROMYCES* SPECIES

Saccharomyces cerevisiae (baker's yeast or brewer's yeast) has been used for centuries for the production of fermented foods and beverages such as cider, beer, wine, and bread. In addition to those applications, *Saccharomyces* spp. have been tested and used as probiotics to enhance the health and well-being of the human digestive tract. Compared to probiotic bacteria, the natural resistance of yeast to many antimicrobial agents has constituted an advantage for many applications. *Saccharomyces boulardii*, a form of *S. cerevisiae*, has been tested widely in a range of experimental and clinical assays and has shown promising results.

S. *boulardii* is a tropical strain of yeast first isolated in 1923 by the French scientist Henri Boulard, who observed natives of Southeast Asia chewing on the skin of lychee and mangosteen in an attempt to control the symptoms of cholera. Since its introduction to France (Penna et al., 2000), *S. boulardii* has been used widely across Europe to prevent or treat a range of gastrointestinal infectious and inflammatory disorders including infectious diarrhea, antibiotic-associated diarrhea, and idiopathic diarrhea. Currently *S. boulardii* is widely produced commercially in European, African, and South American countries. A lyophilized form for oral administration has been studied in the United States by Biocodex Inc., and the patent strain is held in the American Type Culture Collection (ATCC). *S. boulardii* was initially considered to be a separate species of the hemiascomycete genus *Saccharomyces* (McFarland, 1996). However, there has been controversy as to whether or not *S. boulardii* is a species distinct from *S. cerevisiae*. The claim that *S. boulardii* is a different species from *S. cerevisiae* originated from differentiating assays by multilocus enzyme electrophoresis (McFarland, 1996). Other studies along these lines, including that of Malgoire et al., revealed a genotypic difference between the *S. cerevisiae* and *S. boulardii* strains. By using microsatellite sequence polymorphism as a molecular typing tool, these studies demonstrated a difference between clinical *S. cerevisiae* and *S. boulardii* strains (Malgoire et al., 2005). However, those results have been contradicted by a series of reports from other investigators. Perapoch et al. and McCullough et al. demonstrated, by techniques including randomly amplified polymorphic DNA and restriction

Xinhua Chen and Ciarán P. Kelly, Division of Gastroenterology, Dana 601A, Beth Israel Deaconess Medical Center, Harvard Medical School, 330 Brookline Ave., Boston, MA 02215.

fragment length polymorphism, that *S. cerevisiae* and *S. boulardii* have identical genetic profiles (McCullough et al., 1998; Perapoch et al., 2000). They concluded that the commercial strains of *S. boulardii* are asporogenous subtypes within the circumscription of *S. cerevisiae* and are not representatives of a separate species. Mitterdorfer et al. found that *S. boulardii* strains clustered within the species *S. cerevisiae* by two-dimensional electrophoresis analysis (Mitterdorfer et al., 2001, 2002a, 2002b). Hennequin et al. also demonstrated that *S. cerevisiae* and *S. boulardii* manifest the same profile by microsatellite polymorphism analysis (Hennequin et al., 2001). Thus, a majority of studies, but not all, found that *S. boulardii* and *S. cerevisiae* cannot be distinguished and represent a single species. Perhaps the most comprehensive analysis to date is that of Edwards-Ingram et al. (2004, 2007). Using comparative genomic hybridizations for whole-genome analysis, they concluded that *S. cerevisiae* and *S. boulardii* are members of the same species (Edwards-Ingram et al., 2004). Using a combination of genotypic and physiological characterization, they concluded that *S. boulardii* is a strain of *S. cerevisiae* but has some specific genomic features including a trisomy of chromosome IX and different copy numbers of some genes (Edwards-Ingram et al., 2007). *S. cerevisiae* encompasses a wide range of strains, with various unique characteristics, and whether or not specific genomic differences contribute to the probiotic actions of *S. boulardii* remains to be determined. This review focuses mostly on studies carried out using the commercial strain of *S. boulardii*, as this is the strain of *Saccharomyces* most frequently used in research studies.

MECHANISMS OF ACTION OF *SACCHAROMYCES* SPP. AS PROBIOTIC AGENTS

S. boulardii utilizes multiple mechanisms to exert its beneficial effects. However, like other probiotics, most of these mechanisms have not been studied extensively with many studies, raising questions and opening possibilities rather than providing definitive mechanistic information.

Interference with Bacterial Adhesion

Bacterial attachment is an important colonization requirement and virulence characteristic. Using scanning electron microscopy, Gedek demonstrated that type I fimbrinated *Escherichia coli* cells were strongly bound to the surface of *S. boulardii* cells (Gedek, 1999). Type I pili bind to mannose, and the outer membrane of *S. boulardii* is mannose rich. Once the enteric microbe

has bound to *S. boulardii*, attachment to the brush border is prevented and this leads to the elimination of *E. coli* with the fecal stream. This mechanism may be of importance in the treatment and prophylaxis of many enteric infections and is preferable to the use of antibiotics that are often ineffective, can prolong colonization by certain enteric pathogens, or induce antibiotic-associated diarrhea or *Clostridium difficile* infection (Gedek, 1999).

Inactivation of Bacterial Virulence Factors

A 54-kDa serine protease purified from conditioned medium of *S. boulardii* cultures digests *C. difficile* toxin A and inhibits toxin A binding to enterocyte surface brush border membrane receptors (Castagliuolo et al., 1996; Pothoulakis et al., 1993). Further studies showed that the protease, in addition to cleaving toxin A, also possesses enzymatic activity against *C. difficile* toxin B (Castagliuolo et al., 1999). The protease was effective in protecting against the enterotoxic effects of *C. difficile* toxins both in rat ileal loops and in human colonic mucosa mounted in Ussing chambers. These studies indicate that the protective effects of *S. boulardii* on *C. difficile* toxin-induced intestinal injury are mediated, in part, by proteolytic cleavage of the toxins and possibly their receptors.

It was reported more recently that *S. boulardii* also releases a 63-kDa protein phosphatase that can inhibit the toxicity of *E. coli* surface endotoxins. Compared to purified rat and bovine intestinal alkaline phosphatase, the enzyme from *S. boulardii* showed a greater potency in dephosphorylating lipopolysaccharide (LPS) from *E. coli* 055B5. Furthermore, the dephosphorylated LPS produced much less toxicity in vivo (Buts et al., 2006). Thus, *S. boulardii* secretes enzymes including a protease and a phosphatase that are able to inactivate *C. difficile* toxins and *E. coli* LPS, respectively.

Enhancement of the Mucosal Immune Response

One mechanism whereby *S. boulardii* protects against infection by enteric pathogens is through a stimulation of the host's intestinal mucosal immune response. Buts and colleagues reported that *S. boulardii* significantly increased the secretion of immunoglobulin A (IgA) and secretory component in the rat small intestine. *S. boulardii* caused a twofold increase in IgA levels in small intestine secretions during oral therapy (Buts et al., 1990). *S. boulardii* was also shown to stimulate sIgA production and the phagocytic system of gnotobiotic mice (Rodrigues et al., 2000).

To study the specificity of the secretory IgA response, Qamar and colleagues fed BALB/c mice with *S. boulardii* during oral immunization with inactivated toxoid A from *C. difficile*. The *S. boulardii*-fed mice mounted a specific IgA response to toxin A that was greater than the nonspecific increase in total intestinal IgA concentrations (Qamar et al., 2001). Total small intestinal IgA levels in *S. boulardii*-fed BALB/c mice were 1.8-fold greater than in controls ($P = 0.003$). However, IgA against toxin A was increased 4.4-fold ($P < 0.001$). Thus, *S. boulardii* can act as a mucosal adjuvant to specifically increase intestinal IgA responses to coadministered antigens such as toxin A. An adequate antibody response to toxin A is an important element in asymptomatic carriage of *C. difficile* and in clinical recovery from *C. difficile*-associated diarrhea (Katchar et al., 2007; Kyne et al., 2001; Qamar et al., 2001). Thus, the finding of increased intestinal antitoxin A levels in *S. boulardii*-treated mice may be directly relevant to the protective effects of *S. boulardii* in recurrent *C. difficile* infection. The exact mechanisms underlying the mucosal adjuvant effects of *S. boulardii* are poorly understood. However, stimulation of a more effective host mucosal immune response to prevalent antigens may be a general mechanism for the efficacy of *S. boulardii* in protecting against a wide range of enteric pathogens (Buts et al., 1990; Qamar et al., 2001; Rodrigues et al., 2000).

Modulating Host Signaling Pathways

The activation of intestinal inflammatory and secretory responses is a common characteristic of the many infectious and noninfectious disorders that have been treated using *S. boulardii*. A potential unifying mechanism for these far-reaching effects is that *S. boulardii* can alter critical host cell signaling events that regulate intestinal inflammation, secretion, and barrier function. It has been shown in different cell lines that *S. boulardii* inhibits the production of interleukin-8 (IL-8), a proinflammatory cytokine, induced by IL-1β, tumor necrosis factor alpha, LPS, or *C. difficile* toxin A as well as by whole bacterial pathogens such as enterohemorrhagic *E. coli* (EHEC) (Chen et al., 2006; Dahan et al., 2003; Sougioultzis et al., 2006).

IL-8 gene expression is regulated by several pathways including nuclear factor (NF)-κB and mitogen-activated protein (MAP) kinases. The NF-κB family of transcription factors regulates the expression of many genes associated with immune and inflammatory responses and cell survival (Richmond, 2002; Simeonidis et al., 1999, 2003). NF-κB is also known to be a pivotal mediator of intestinal inflammation in inflammatory bowel disease (IBD) and in infectious enterocolitis (Jobin and Sartor, 2000). NF-κB is tightly regulated by its interaction with inhibitory IκB proteins, and in most resting cells, NF-κB is sequestered in the cytoplasm in an inactive form associated with IκB proteins. Activation signals lead to the degradation of IκB, freeing NF-κB to translocate to the nucleus, where it binds to target gene promoters and up-regulates their transcription (Cohen et al., 1998; Woronicz et al., 1997).

MAP kinases are a family of ubiquitous, highly conserved cell-signaling proteins (Han et al., 1994; Kyriakis et al., 1994; Lee et al., 1994). Key cellular functions that are regulated by MAP kinase signaling include cell proliferation, cell survival, and cytokine production including that of IL-8. Following stimulation by a wide variety of extracellular stimuli and the transmission of signals from the cell surface to the nucleus to regulate gene expression, MAP kinases phosphorylate downstream kinases and/or mediators including transcription factors. Three major groups of MAP kinases have been characterized: the extracellular signal-regulated kinases (ERK), the c-Jun N-terminal kinases, and the p38 MAP kinases (Han et al., 1994; Kyriakis et al., 1994; Lee et al., 1994). These MAP kinase subfamilies form three parallel cascades that can be activated simultaneously or independently.

Preincubation of T84 cells with *S. boulardii* before EHEC infection inhibits phosphorylation and degradation of IκB-α, NF-κB DNA binding activity, and activation of all three MAP kinase classes (Dahan et al., 2003). *S. boulardii* supernatant also prevents IκBα degradation, thereby reducing NF-κB nuclear translocation, DNA binding, and reporter gene transactivation in THP-1 transformed human monocytic cells (Sougioultzis et al., 2006). In T84 cells, *S. boulardii* alters enteropathogenic *E. coli* (EPEC)-induced tyrosine phosphorylation (Czerucka et al., 2000). In another study, *S. boulardii* stimulated PPAR-γ expression and reduced the response of human colon cells to proinflammatory cytokines (Lee et al., 2005).

Studies from our group showed modulation of host signaling events in vivo as well as in vitro. *S. boulardii* conditioned media inhibited IL-1β and toxin A-induced ERK1/2 and c-Jun N-terminal kinase/SAPK but not p38 MAPK activation in human colonocytes (Chen et al., 2006). When *S. boulardii* conditioned medium was inoculated into mouse ileal loops, it again significantly inhibited ERK1/2 activation in response to *C. difficile* toxin A. It also reduced chemokine (KC) production and protected against the histological injury induced by toxin A (Chen et al., 2006). In summary, *S. boulardii* is capable of modulating host signaling events, in response to a wide variety of endogenous and exogenous stimuli including IL-1β (Chen et al., 2006; Sougioultzis et al., 2006), tumor necrosis factor alpha (Sougioultzis et al., 2006), LPS (Sougioultzis et al., 2006), *C. difficile* toxin A (Chen et al., 2006), EHEC (Dahan et al., 2003), and EPEC (Czerucka et al., 2000).

These effects on host signaling may account for the protective and anti-inflammatory effects of S. boulardii in many gastrointestinal disorders. For example, NF-κB is known to play a key role in the pathogenesis of IBD and NF-κB activation in enterocytes following their exposure to microbial factors such as LPS. Furthermore, many commonly used IBD therapies target this critical inflammatory response mediator.

Strengthening of Enterocyte Tight Junctions

One potential mechanism of action of S. boulardii in protecting against diarrheal diseases is through an augmentation of the barrier function of the intestinal epithelium. The ability to maintain epithelial tight-junction integrity and regulate both transcellular and paracellular flux is clearly important in controlling intestinal secretion and absorption (Isolauri, 2001; Keely and Barrett, 2000). Enterocyte and tight-junction integrity may also be of major importance in reducing the exposure of lamina propria antigen-presenting cells and lymphocytes, as well as neuroendocrine cells to bacterial products such as LPS, toxin A, or cholera toxin. Abnormal intestinal permeability may also play a role in the pathogenesis of IBD by facilitating a chronic and inappropriate immune/inflammatory response to luminal microbes and their soluble products.

Castagliuolo et al. and Pothoulakis et al. have reported that S. boulardii augments intestinal epithelial cell barrier function during exposure to C. difficile toxin A (Castagliuolo et al., 1999; Pothoulakis et al., 1993). This effect may result from the actions of the 54-kDa protease factor described above. Studies by Czerucka et al. and Dahan et al. reveal that S. boulardii also maintains the barrier function of EPEC-infected T84 cells through prevention of myosin light chain (MLC) phosphorylation. Serine or threonine phosphorylation of the 20-kDa MLC is an important determinant of contractile tension in cells (de Lanerolle and Paul, 1991; Wilson et al., 1991). EPEC infection leads to MLC phosphorylation, leading to degradation of the tight junctions between intestinal mucosal enterocytes. T84 cell infection by EPEC is characterized by a drop in transepithelial resistance, an increase in permeability, and modification of the distribution of the tight-junction-associated protein ZO-1 (Philpott et al., 1996; Spitz et al., 1995). The phosphorylation of several proteins induced by EPEC in T84 cells is diminished in the presence of S. boulardii, leading to a reduction in mucosal permeability and a resulting decrease in bacterial translocation (Czerucka et al., 2000; Dahan et al., 2003). These data suggest that S. boulardii exerts a preventive effect in EPEC infection by preventing the disruption of tight-junction structure and function, thereby reducing bacterial invasion.

Trophic Effects on Enterocytes

Buts and colleagues have reported that S. boulardii enhances intestinal enzyme expression and exerts trophic effects by the endoluminal release of polyamines (spermine and spermidine) (Buts and De Keyser, 2006; Buts et al., 1994). Polyamines are believed to stimulate the maturation and turnover of small intestinal enterocytes (Dufour et al., 1988; Hosomi et al., 1987). This could lead to improved healing and more rapid recovery from intestinal injury through taking S. boulardii.

Capacity To Affect Immune Cell Redistribution

In a lymphocyte-transferred SCID mouse model of IBD, S. boulardii was reported to induce an accumulation of gamma interferon-producing T-helper 1 cells within the mesenteric lymph nodes correlated with a diminution of CD4+ T-cell number and gamma interferon production by CD4+ T cells within the colon (Dalmasso et al., 2006). An influence of S. boulardii treatment on cell accumulation in mesenteric lymph nodes was also observed in healthy BALB/c mice and involves modifications of lymph node endothelial cell adhesiveness by improving the competence of lymphatic endothelial cells to trap T lymphocytes. Therefore, S. boulardii exerts, in this IBD model, a unique action on inflammation by a specific effect on the migratory behavior of T cells which limits the infiltration of T-helper 1 cells into the inflamed colon (Dalmasso et al., 2006; Fiocchi, 2006).

STUDIES OF *S. BOULARDII* IN ANIMAL DISEASE MODELS

A number of animal disease models have been used to study the mechanisms of action of S. boulardii organisms as well as their potential clinical applications.

Infectious Disease Models

The effects of S. boulardii on C. difficile-associated enteritis and colitis have been studied with animals, including hamsters and gnotobiotic mice, and with mouse ileal loops. When S. boulardii was administered orally to hamsters challenged with C. difficile after clindamycin treatment, the mortality and relapse rates decreased compared to those of controls (Elmer and McFarland, 1987). In gnotobiotic mice, orally administered S. boulardii induced a dose-dependent protection from C. difficile-induced mortality (Elmer and Corthier, 1991). The injurious effects of intraluminal injection of toxin A into mouse ileal loops were also reduced by the coadministration of S. boulardii

(Chen et al., 2006). As discussed above, an enhancement of specific intestinal IgA antitoxin A production, inhibition of Erk1/2 MAP kinase activation, and secretion of a 54-kDa protease are potential mechanisms for the protective effects of *S. boulardii* in *C. difficile* toxin-induced enteritis in animal models (Castagliuolo et al., 1999; Chen et al., 2006; Pothoulakis et al., 1993).

S. boulardii has also demonstrated in vivo protective effects against other intestinal pathogens including *Vibrio cholerae*, *Salmonella enterica* serovar Typhimurium, *Shigella flexneri*, and *Entamoeba histolytica*. Pretreatment with *S. boulardii* for 5 days prevented the small-intestinal morphological damage caused by *V. cholerae* infection in rats (Dias et al., 1995). In both conventional and gnotobiotic mice, *S. boulardii* protected against oral infection with *S. enterica* serovar Typhimurium and *S. flexneri*, resulting in reduced mortality and/or histopathological injury (Rodrigues et al., 1996). Similar results were observed using *S. cerevisiae* strain 905 (Martins et al., 2007). In addition to bacterial pathogens, *S. boulardii* has also been reported to be effective against intestinal parasites such as *E. histolytica*. Treatment with *S. boulardii* reduced mortality in immature rats infected with this protozoan (Rigothier et al., 1990). *S. boulardii* showed no intrinsic amebicidal action in vitro, again suggesting that modulation of host immune and inflammatory responses may be central to its probiotic activities (Rigothier et al., 1994).

Noninfectious-Disease Models

Daily oral intake of *S. boulardii* decreased weight loss, colonic histological injury, and NF-κB activity in a SCID mouse model of IBD induced by intraperitoneal injection of CD4+CD45RBhi T cells from immunocompetent mouse donors. As described above, this protective anti-inflammatory effect of *S. boulardii* was associated with an alteration of the migratory behavior of T cells (Dalmasso et al., 2006). In another mouse IBD model, *S. boulardii* attenuated trinitrobenzene sulfonic acid-induced colitis through a mechanism correlated with the inhibition of NF-κB (G. Dalmasso, G. Alexander, H. Carloson, V. Imbert, P. Lagadec, J. F. Peyron, R. Bomhoff, P. Rampal, and D. Czerucka, presented at the Digestive Disease Week, New Orleans, LA, 15 to 20 May 2004).

CLINICAL STUDIES OF *S. BOULARDII*

S. boulardii has been used for the treatment or prevention of a variety of diarrheal diseases, such as antibiotic-associated diarrhea, acute infectious diarrhea in adults and children, traveler's diarrhea, diarrhea in human immunodeficiency virus-infected patients, *C. difficile*-associated disease, and inflammatory bowel diseases including both Crohn's disease and ulcerative colitis. Below is a description of some clinical trials that have shown the efficacy of *S. boulardii* in different diseases.

AAD

Antibiotic-associated diarrhea (AAD) is a common complication of antibiotic use. AAD usually occurs during, and shortly after, antibiotic exposure as a result of disruption of the intestinal microbiota (McFarland, 1998). Specific therapies for AAD are lacking. Current strategies include discontinuing the inciting antibiotic, restricting the use of high-risk antibiotics, and the use of specific antimicrobial agents if an infectious etiology is known (McFarland, 2006). One of the most frequently recognized etiologic agents of AAD is *C. difficile*, a common source of nosocomial infectious diarrhea in adults. *C. difficile*-associated disease (CDAD) is discussed separately below.

In a randomized, double-blind controlled study, Can et al. investigated the preventive effect of *S. boulardii* on the development of AAD in 151 hospital patients receiving antimicrobial therapy outside the intensive care unit. The prophylactic use of *S. boulardii* was not associated with any serious side effects and reduced the incidence of AAD from 9.0% in controls to 1.4% in those receiving the probiotic ($P < 0.05$) (Can et al., 2006).

In another prospective double-blind controlled study, the effect of *S. boulardii* on AAD in hospitalized patients was again investigated. Over 23 months, 180 patients completed the study. Of the patients receiving a placebo, 22% experienced AAD compared with 9.5% of patients receiving *S. boulardii* ($P = 0.04$). Again, there were no discernible adverse effects of yeast administration (Surawicz et al., 1989).

To determine whether *S. boulardii* prevents AAD in children, Kotowska and colleagues performed a double-blind, randomized placebo-controlled trial in 269 subjects aged 6 months to 14 years treated with broad-spectrum antibiotics. They found that *S. boulardii* (250 mg) effectively reduced the risk of AAD in children from 23 to 8% (relative risk, 0.3; 95% confidence interval, 0.2 to 0.7) (Kotowska et al., 2005).

According to a meta-analysis performed by McFarland (McFarland, 2006), two single probiotic strains showed significant efficacy in protecting against AAD: *S. boulardii* and *Lactobacillus rhamnosus* GG, as well as mixtures composed of two or more different probiotics. Thus, there is good evidence to conclude that cotreatment with *S. boulardii* reduces the risk of AAD in both adults and children receiving broad-spectrum antibiotic therapy.

C. difficile-Associated Disease

C. difficile is the most frequently identified cause of nosocomial infectious diarrhea. CDAD is also the most serious form of AAD, leading, in some cases, to severe pseudomembranous colitis, colectomy, or death (Gerding et al., 1995; Kelly et al., 1994). CDAD is usually treated by discontinuation of the precipitating antibiotic and administration of metronidazole or vancomycin (Kyne and Kelly, 2001). However, one of the main problems associated with the treatment of CDAD is the high incidence (15 to 50%) of recurrent diarrhea following an initial clinical response (Fekety et al., 1997). In a double-blind, randomized, placebo-controlled study involving patients with active CDAD, S. boulardii (500 mg twice daily for 4 weeks) was used in combination with standard antibiotics. A majority of control subjects with a history of recurrent CDAD experienced yet another recurrence (65%), whereas only 35% of those receiving S. boulardii had a recurrence ($P = 0.04$). There was no significant difference in recurrence rates for subjects experiencing their first episode of CDAD (24% versus 19%, $P = 0.86$) (McFarland et al., 1994). However, a subsequent trial by the same investigators showed that, for subjects with a history of recurrent CDAD, a significant decrease in further recurrences occurred only in a group treated with high-dose vancomycin (2 g per day) and S. boulardii (16.7% versus 50% in control; $P = 0.05$) (Surawicz et al., 2000). However, no significant decreases in recurrence rates were seen for other treatment groups.

Thus, there are conflicting data on the efficacy of S. boulardii in preventing CDAD. The best evidence is for patients with a history of recurrent CDAD who are at greatest risk of further recurrences. For those patients, S. boulardii at a dose of 500 mg twice daily for 28 days is safe and may be beneficial. It is worth mentioning that other Saccharomyces preparations including baker's yeast have been used to treat recurrent CDAD, but no controlled study data are available (Chia et al., 1995; Kovacs and Berk, 2000).

Traveler's Diarrhea

Diarrhea is a common disorder among travelers, with a 5 to 50% incidence rate, depending on the destination (McFarland, 2007). Kollaritsch et al. performed a placebo-controlled, double-blind study to evaluate the efficacy of S. boulardii in preventing diarrhea in 3,000 Austrian travelers to several regions of the world. Two dosages of S. boulardii (250 mg or 1,000 mg daily) were tested and administered prophylactically. A significant decrease in the incidence of diarrhea was observed, with success depending directly on compliance with use of the probiotic (Kollaritsch et al., 1993). A meta-analysis by McFarland concluded that among all tested probiotics, S. boulardii and a mixture of Lactobacillus acidophilus and Bifidobacterium bifidum had significant efficacy against traveler's diarrhea with no serious adverse reactions reported in the 12 trials examined (McFarland, 2007). However, the protective effect was relatively small with a pooled relative risk of traveler's diarrhea in subjects taking a probiotic of 0.85 (95% confidence interval, 0.79, 0.91; $P < 0.001$).

Acute Diarrhea

In a randomized placebo-controlled study of acute (presumed infectious) diarrhea in children aged between 3 and 24 months, S. boulardii, when used as an adjuvant to oral rehydration solution, significantly reduced the duration of diarrhea (4.7 days versus 6.2 days in control, $P < 0.05$) (Villarruel et al., 2007). S. boulardii was most effective if administered within 48 h of the onset of diarrhea. A meta-analysis that examined the preventive role of probiotics in different age groups indicates that probiotics reduce the risk of acute diarrhea among adults by 26% (range, 7 to 49%) and by 57% (range, 35 to 71%) among children. In that analysis, the protective effects did not vary significantly between S. boulardii and other probiotic bacterial strains (Sazawal et al., 2006). Therefore, S. boulardii and other probiotics appear to be effective in preventing and in shortening the course of acute infectious diarrheal illnesses both in children and in adults (Szajewska et al., 2007).

Inflammatory Bowel Disease

An open-label, controlled study indicated that S. boulardii may be effective in preventing clinical relapse in Crohn's disease (Guslandi et al., 2000). For 32 patients with Crohn's disease of the ileum or colon, who were in remission for over 3 months, relapse rates of control subjects receiving 6 months of maintenance therapy with 5-ASA (1 g per day) were higher than those of patients receiving 5-ASA plus S. boulardii (1 g per day) (38% versus 6%, respectively) (Guslandi et al., 2000). In an open uncontrolled study of patients with mild to moderate ulcerative colitis, 4 weeks of treatment with S. boulardii was associated with remission in 18 of 25 subjects (71%) (Guslandi et al., 2003). These studies suggest that S. boulardii may have some efficacy in treating IBD. However, larger randomized controlled studies are needed to confirm these preliminary findings.

S. boulardii has also demonstrated efficacy in treating AIDS-related diarrhea (Saint-Marc et al., 1991). However, caution has been advocated when using S. boulardii in immunocompromised patients because of the potential for serious complications as discussed below.

ADVERSE EFFECTS OF *SACCHAROMYCES* PROBIOTIC USE

In light of the duration and extent of its use, *S. boulardii* has been shown to be a remarkably safe biotherapeutic agent for the majority of recipients. However, a number of cases of fungemia due to *S. cerevisiae* or *S. boulardii* have been reported. Riquelme et al. reported two cases of fungemia caused by *S. cerevisiae* occurring in immunosuppressed patients treated orally with *S. boulardii*. Molecular typing confirmed clonality in the strains isolated from the patients and the *S. boulardii* capsule (Riquelme et al., 2003). In another case series, Munoz et al. demonstrated that the *Saccharomyces* strains were identical in three patients with fungemia. Moreover, the isolated strains were identical to the strain given orally as Ultralevura to these patients before the onset of fungemia (Munoz et al., 2005). Besides translocation from the digestive tract, the fungemia may also have originated from contamination of central venous catheter lines from the hands of health care workers after the probiotic capsules had been opened to allow for nasogastric administration (Hennequin et al., 2000). In a review, Herbrecht and Nivoix concluded that the use of *Saccharomyces* as a probiotic is an important risk factor for *S. cerevisiae* fungemia. This finding led them to question the risk-benefit ratio of using *S. boulardii* in critically ill or immunocompromised patients who are at risk of developing infection from exposure to high doses of an organism with low intrinsic virulence (Herbrecht and Nivoix, 2005).

FUTURE DIRECTIONS

Currently, *S. boulardii* remains the primary yeast to be used commercially as a probiotic in humans. Some authors have suggested the use of other yeast species or genera. However, these proposals are based on in vitro data or the results of very limited clinical trials (Kovacs and Berk, 2000; Kumura et al., 2004; Martins et al., 2007). Clinical reports describing the use of *S. cerevisiae* (baker's yeast) in recurrent CDAD (Chia et al., 1995; Kovacs and Berk, 2000) and its in vitro effects against *S. enterica* (Martins et al., 2007) and the claims of genomic similarity or identity with *S. boulardii* (McCullough et al., 1998; Mitterdorfer et al., 2002a, 2002b) certainly opened possibilities for further studies using other *S. cerevisiae* strains, with the goal of identifying additional yeast strains with protective and therapeutic effects.

The anti-inflammatory effects of *S. boulardii* make it a promising agent for use in IBD. To date, clinical trials in IBD have been extremely limited. Additional, larger controlled clinical trials of *Saccharomyces* in various IBD populations are expected in the future.

A high priority in *S. boulardii* research, as in other probiotic studies, is to define specific mechanisms of action and to characterize active moieties responsible for the probiotic effects. This should facilitate optimization and standardization of the beneficial clinical effects. To date, however, most mechanistic studies in the field of probiotics have been limited by a lack of knowledge regarding the active compounds responsible for the observed effects. In the case of CDAD, for example, multiple effects of *S. boulardii* have been described including protease activity, activation of the immune response, and anti-inflammatory effects. It seems likely, therefore, that the effects of *S. boulardii* on intestinal physiology in health and in disease do not reside in a single chemical or receptor but instead rely on a complex and interacting network of yeast factors and host responses.

References

Buts, J. P., P. Bernasconi, J. P. Vaerman, and C. Dive. 1990. Stimulation of secretory IgA and secretory component of immunoglobulins in small intestine of rats treated with *Saccharomyces boulardii*. *Dig. Dis. Sci.* 35:251–256.

Buts, J. P., and N. De Keyser. 2006. Effects of *Saccharomyces boulardii* on intestinal mucosa. *Dig. Dis. Sci.* 51:1485–1492.

Buts, J. P., N. De Keyser, and L. De Raedemaeker. 1994. *Saccharomyces boulardii* enhances rat intestinal enzyme expression by endoluminal release of polyamines. *Pediatr. Res.* 36:522–527.

Buts, J. P., N. Dekeyser, C. Stilmant, E. Delem, F. Smets, and E. Sokal. 2006. *Saccharomyces boulardii* produces in rat small intestine a novel protein phosphatase that inhibits *Escherichia coli* endotoxin by dephosphorylation. *Pediatr. Res.* 60:24–29.

Can, M., B. A. Besirbellioglu, I. Y. Avci, C. M. Beker, and A. Pahsa. 2006. Prophylactic *Saccharomyces boulardii* in the prevention of antibiotic-associated diarrhea: a prospective study. *Med. Sci. Monit.* 12:PI19–PI22.

Castagliuolo, I., J. T. LaMont, S. T. Nikulasson, and C. Pothoulakis. 1996. *Saccharomyces boulardii* protease inhibits *Clostridium difficile* toxin A effects in the rat ileum. *Infect. Immun.* 64:5225–5232.

Castagliuolo, I., M. F. Riegler, L. Valenick, J. T. LaMont, and C. Pothoulakis. 1999. *Saccharomyces boulardii* protease inhibits the effects of *Clostridium difficile* toxins A and B in human colonic mucosa. *Infect. Immun.* 67:302–307.

Chen, X., E. G. Kokkotou, N. Mustafa, K. R. Bhaskar, S. Sougioultzis, M. O'Brien, C. Pothoulakis, and C. P. Kelly. 2006. *Saccharomyces boulardii* inhibits ERK1/2 mitogen-activated protein kinase activation both in vitro and in vivo and protects against *Clostridium difficile* toxin A-induced enteritis. *J. Biol. Chem.* 281:24449–24454.

Chia, J. K., S. M. Chan, and H. Goldstein. 1995. Baker's yeast as adjunctive therapy for relapses of *Clostridium difficile* diarrhea. *Clin. Infect. Dis.* 20:1581.

Cohen, L., W. J. Henzel, and P. A. Baeuerle. 1998. IKAP is a scaffold protein of the IkappaB kinase complex. *Nature* 395:292–296.

Czerucka, D., S. Dahan, B. Mograbi, B. Rossi, and P. Rampal. 2000. *Saccharomyces boulardii* preserves the barrier function and modulates the signal transduction pathway induced in enteropathogenic *Escherichia coli*-infected T84 cells. *Infect. Immun.* **68**:5998–6004.

Dahan, S., G. Dalmasso, V. Imbert, J. F. Peyron, P. Rampal, and D. Czerucka. 2003. *Saccharomyces boulardii* interferes with enterohemorrhagic *Escherichia coli*-induced signaling pathways in T84 cells. *Infect. Immun.* **71**:766–773.

Dalmasso, G., F. Cottrez, V. Imbert, P. Lagadec, J. F. Peyron, P. Rampal, D. Czerucka, H. Groux, A. Foussat, and V. Brun. 2006. *Saccharomyces boulardii* inhibits inflammatory bowel disease by trapping T cells in mesenteric lymph nodes. *Gastroenterology***131**:1812–1825.

de Lanerolle, P., and R. J. Paul. 1991. Myosin phosphorylation/dephosphorylation and regulation of airway smooth muscle contractility. *Am. J. Physiol.* **261**:L1–L14.

Dias, R. S., E. A. Bambirra, M. E. Silva, and J. R. Nicoli. 1995. Protective effect of *Saccharomyces boulardii* against the cholera toxin in rats. *Braz. J. Med. Biol. Res.* **28**:323–325.

Dufour, C., G. Dandrifosse, P. Forget, F. Vermesse, N. Romain, and P. Lepoint. 1988. Spermine and spermidine induce intestinal maturation in the rat. *Gastroenterology* **95**:112–116.

Edwards-Ingram, L., P. Gitsham, N. Burton, G. Warhurst, I. Clarke, D. Hoyle, S. G. Oliver, and L. Stateva. 2007. Genotypic and physiological characterization of *Saccharomyces boulardii*, the probiotic strain of *Saccharomyces cerevisiae*. *Appl. Environ. Microbiol.* **73**:2458–2467.

Edwards-Ingram, L. C., M. E. Gent, D. C. Hoyle, A. Hayes, L. I. Stateva, and S. G. Oliver. 2004. Comparative genomic hybridization provides new insights into the molecular taxonomy of the *Saccharomyces* sensu stricto complex. *Genome Res.* **14**:1043–1051.

Elmer, G. W., and G. Corthier. 1991. Modulation of *Clostridium difficile* induced mortality as a function of the dose and the viability of the *Saccharomyces boulardii* used as a preventative agent in gnotobiotic mice. *Can. J. Microbiol.* **37**:315–317.

Elmer, G. W., and L. V. McFarland. 1987. Suppression by *Saccharomyces boulardii* of toxigenic *Clostridium difficile* overgrowth after vancomycin treatment in hamsters. *Antimicrob. Agents Chemother.* **31**:129–131.

Fekety, R., et al. 1997. Guidelines for the diagnosis and management of *Clostridium difficile*-associated diarrhea and colitis. *Am. J. Gastroenterol.* **92**:739–750.

Fiocchi, C. 2006. Probiotics in inflammatory bowel disease: yet another mechanism of action? *Gastroenterology* **131**:2009–2012.

Gedek, B. R. 1999. Adherence of *Escherichia coli* serogroup O 157 and the *Salmonella typhimurium* mutant DT 104 to the surface of *Saccharomyces boulardii*. *Mycoses* **42**:261–264.

Gerding, D. N., S. Johnson, L. R. Peterson, M. E. Mulligan, and J. Silva, Jr. 1995. *Clostridium difficile*-associated diarrhea and colitis. *Infect. Control. Hosp. Epidemiol.* **16**:459–477.

Guslandi, M., P. Giollo, and P. A. Testoni. 2003. A pilot trial of *Saccharomyces boulardii* in ulcerative colitis. *Eur. J. Gastroenterol. Hepatol.* **15**:697–698.

Guslandi, M., G. Mezzi, M. Sorghi, and P. A. Testoni. 2000. *Saccharomyces boulardii* in maintenance treatment of Crohn's disease. *Dig. Dis. Sci.* **45**:1462–1464.

Han, J., J. D. Lee, L. Bibbs, and R. J. Ulevitch. 1994. A MAP kinase targeted by endotoxin and hyperosmolarity in mammalian cells. *Science* **265**:808–811.

Hennequin, C., C. Kauffmann-Lacroix, A. Jobert, J. P. Viard, C. Ricour, J. L. Jacquemin, and P. Berche. 2000. Possible role of catheters in *Saccharomyces boulardii* fungemia. *Eur. J. Clin. Microbiol. Infect. Dis.* **19**:16–20.

Hennequin, C., A. Thierry, G. F. Richard, G. Lecointre, H. V. Nguyen, C. Gaillardin, and B. Dujon. 2001. Microsatellite typing as a new tool for identification of *Saccharomyces cerevisiae* strains. *J. Clin. Microbiol.* **39**:551–559.

Herbrecht, R., and Y. Nivoix. 2005. *Saccharomyces cerevisiae* fungemia: an adverse effect of *Saccharomyces boulardii* probiotic administration. *Clin. Infect. Dis.* **40**:1635–1637.

Hosomi, M., N. H. Stace, F. Lirussi, S. M. Smith, G. M. Murphy, and R. H. Dowling. 1987. Role of polyamines in intestinal adaptation in the rat. *Eur. J. Clin. Investig.* **17**:375–385.

Isolauri, E. 2001. Probiotics in human disease. *Am. J. Clin. Nutr.* **73**:1142S–1146S.

Jobin, C., and R. B. Sartor. 2000. The I kappa B/NF-kappa B system: a key determinant of mucosal inflammation and protection. *Am. J. Physiol. Cell Physiol.* **278**:C451–C462.

Katchar, K., C. P. Taylor, S. Tummala, X. Chen, J. Sheikh, and C. P. Kelly. 2007. Association between IgG2 and IgG3 subclass responses to toxin A and recurrent *Clostridium difficile*-associated disease. *Clin. Gastroenterol. Hepatol.* **5**:707–713.

Keely, S. J., and K. E. Barrett. 2000. Regulation of chloride secretion. Novel pathways and messengers. *Ann. N. Y. Acad. Sci.* **915**:67–76.

Kelly, C. P., C. Pothoulakis, and J. T. LaMont. 1994. *Clostridium difficile* colitis. *N. Engl. J. Med.* **330**:257–262.

Kollaritsch, H., H. Holst, P. Grobara, and G. Wiedermann. 1993. [Prevention of traveler's diarrhea with *Saccharomyces boulardii*. Results of a placebo controlled double-blind study]. *Fortschr. Med.* **111**:152–156.

Kotowska, M., P. Albrecht, and H. Szajewska. 2005. *Saccharomyces boulardii* in the prevention of antibiotic-associated diarrhea in children: a randomized double-blind placebo-controlled trial. *Aliment. Pharmacol. Ther.* **21**:583–590.

Kovacs, D. J., and T. Berk. 2000. Recurrent *Clostridium difficile*-associated diarrhea and colitis treated with *Saccharomyces cerevisiae* (baker's yeast) in combination with antibiotic therapy: a case report. *J. Am. Board Fam. Pract.* **13**:138–140.

Kumura, H., Y. Tanoue, M. Tsukahara, T. Tanaka, and K. Shimazaki. 2004. Screening of dairy yeast strains for probiotic applications. *J. Dairy Sci.* **87**:4050–4056.

Kyne, L., and C. P. Kelly. 2001. Recurrent *Clostridium difficile* diarrhoea. *Gut* **49**:152–153.

Kyne, L., M. Warny, A. Qamar, and C. P. Kelly. 2001. Association between antibody response to toxin A and protection against recurrent *Clostridium difficile* diarrhoea. *Lancet* **357**:189–193.

Kyriakis, J. M., P. Banerjee, E. Nikolakaki, T. Dai, E. A. Rubie, M. F. Ahmad, J. Avruch, and J. R. Woodgett. 1994. The stress-activated protein kinase subfamily of c-Jun kinases. *Nature* **369**:156–160.

Lee, J. C., J. T. Laydon, P. C. McDonnell, T. F. Gallagher, S. Kumar, D. Green, D. McNulty, M. J. Blumenthal, J. R. Heys,

S. W. Landvatter, et al. 1994. A protein kinase involved in the regulation of inflammatory cytokine biosynthesis. *Nature* 372:739–746.

Lee, S. K., H. J. Kim, S. G. Chi, J. Y. Jang, K. D. Nam, N. H. Kim, K. R. Joo, S. H. Dong, B. H. Kim, Y. W. Chang, J. I. Lee, and R. Chang. 2005. [*Saccharomyces boulardii* activates expression of peroxisome proliferator-activated receptor-gamma in HT-29 cells]. *Korean J. Gastroenterol.* 45:328–334.

Malgoire, J. Y., S. Bertout, F. Renaud, J. M. Bastide, and M. Mallie. 2005. Typing of *Saccharomyces cerevisiae* clinical strains by using microsatellite sequence polymorphism. *J. Clin. Microbiol.* 43:1133–1137.

Martins, F. S., A. C. Rodrigues, F. C. Tiago, F. J. Penna, C. A. Rosa, R. M. Arantes, R. M. Nardi, M. J. Neves, and J. R. Nicoli. 2007. *Saccharomyces cerevisiae* strain 905 reduces the translocation of *Salmonella enterica* serotype Typhimurium and stimulates the immune system in gnotobiotic and conventional mice. *J. Med. Microbiol.* 56:352–359.

McCullough, M. J., K. V. Clemons, J. H. McCusker, and D. A. Stevens. 1998. Species identification and virulence attributes of *Saccharomyces boulardii* (nom. inval.). *J. Clin. Microbiol.* 36:2613–2617.

McFarland, L. V. 1998. Epidemiology, risk factors and treatments for antibiotic-associated diarrhea. *Dig. Dis.* 16:292–307.

McFarland, L. V. 2006. Meta-analysis of probiotics for the prevention of antibiotic associated diarrhea and the treatment of *Clostridium difficile* disease. *Am. J. Gastroenterol.* 101:812–822.

McFarland, L. V. 2007. Meta-analysis of probiotics for the prevention of traveler's diarrhea. *Travel Med. Infect. Dis.* 5:97–105.

McFarland, L. V. 1996. *Saccharomyces boulardii* is not *Saccharomyces cerevisiae*. *Clin. Infect. Dis.* 22:200–201.

McFarland, L. V., C. M. Surawicz, R. N. Greenberg, R. Fekety, G. W. Elmer, K. A. Moyer, S. A. Melcher, K. E. Bowen, J. L. Cox, Z. Noorani, et al. 1994. A randomized placebo-controlled trial of *Saccharomyces boulardii* in combination with standard antibiotics for *Clostridium difficile* disease. *JAMA* 271:1913–1918.

Mitterdorfer, G., W. Kneifel, and H. Viernstein. 2001. Utilization of prebiotic carbohydrates by yeasts of therapeutic relevance. *Lett. Appl. Microbiol.* 33:251–255.

Mitterdorfer, G., H. K. Mayer, W. Kneifel, and H. Viernstein. 2002a. Clustering of *Saccharomyces boulardii* strains within the species *S. cerevisiae* using molecular typing techniques. *J. Appl. Microbiol.* 93:521–530.

Mitterdorfer, G., H. K. Mayer, W. Kneifel, and H. Viernstein. 2002b. Protein fingerprinting of *Saccharomyces* isolates with therapeutic relevance using one- and two-dimensional electrophoresis. *Proteomics* 2:1532–1538.

Munoz, P., E. Bouza, M. Cuenca-Estrella, J. M. Eiros, M. J. Perez, M. Sanchez-Somolinos, C. Rincon, J. Hortal, and T. Pelaez. 2005. *Saccharomyces cerevisiae* fungemia: an emerging infectious disease. *Clin. Infect. Dis.* 40:1625–1634.

Penna, F. J., L. A. Filho, A. C. Calcado, H. R. Junior, and J. R. Nicolli. 2000. [Up-to-date clinical and experimental basis for the use of probiotics]. *J. Pediatr.* (Rio de Janeiro) 76(Suppl. 1):S209–S217. (In Portuguese.)

Perapoch, J., A. M. Planes, A. Querol, V. Lopez, I. Martinez-Bendayan, R. Tormo, F. Fernandez, G. Peguero, and S. Salcedo. 2000. Fungemia with *Saccharomyces cerevisiae* in two newborns, only one of whom had been treated with ultra-levura. *Eur. J. Clin. Microbiol. Infect. Dis.* 19:468–470.

Philpott, D. J., D. M. McKay, P. M. Sherman, and M. H. Perdue. 1996. Infection of T84 cells with enteropathogenic *Escherichia coli* alters barrier and transport functions. *Am. J. Physiol.* 270:G634–G645.

Pothoulakis, C., C. P. Kelly, M. A. Joshi, N. Gao, C. J. O'Keane, I. Castagliuolo, and J. T. Lamont. 1993. *Saccharomyces boulardii* inhibits *Clostridium difficile* toxin A binding and enterotoxicity in rat ileum. *Gastroenterology* 104:1108–1115.

Qamar, A., S. Aboudola, M. Warny, P. Michetti, C. Pothoulakis, J. T. LaMont, and C. P. Kelly. 2001. *Saccharomyces boulardii* stimulates intestinal immunoglobulin A immune response to *Clostridium difficile* toxin A in mice. *Infect. Immun.* 69:2762–2765.

Richmond, A. 2002. Nf-kappa B, chemokine gene transcription and tumour growth. *Nat. Rev. Immunol.* 2:664–674.

Rigothier, M. C., J. Maccario, and P. Gayral. 1994. Inhibitory activity of saccharomyces yeasts on the adhesion of *Entamoeba histolytica* trophozoites to human erythrocytes in vitro. *Parasitol. Res.* 80:10–15.

Rigothier, M. C., J. Maccario, P. N. Vuong, and P. Gayral. 1990. [Effects of *Saccharomyces boulardii* yeast on trophozoites of *Entamoeba histolytica* in vitro and in cecal amebiasis in young rats]. *Ann. Parasitol. Hum. Comp.* 65:51–60. (In French.)

Riquelme, A. J., M. A. Calvo, A. M. Guzman, M. S. Depix, P. Garcia, C. Perez, M. Arrese, and J. A. Labarca. 2003. *Saccharomyces cerevisiae* fungemia after *Saccharomyces boulardii* treatment in immunocompromised patients. *J. Clin. Gastroenterol.* 36:41–43.

Rodrigues, A. C., D. C. Cara, S. H. Fretez, F. Q. Cunha, E. C. Vieira, J. R. Nicoli, and L. Q. Vieira. 2000. *Saccharomyces boulardii* stimulates sIgA production and the phagocytic system of gnotobiotic mice. *J. Appl. Microbiol.* 89:404–414.

Rodrigues, A. C. P., R. M. Nardi, E. A. Bambirra, E. C. Vieira, and J. R. Nicoli. 1996. Effect of *Saccharomyces boulardii* against experimental oral infection with *Salmonella typhimurium* and *Shigella flexneri* in conventional and gnotobiotic mice. *J. Appl. Bacteriol.* 81:251–256.

Saint-Marc, T., L. Rossello-Prats, and J. L. Touraine. 1991. [Efficacy of *Saccharomyces boulardii* in the treatment of diarrhea in AIDS]. *Ann. Med. Interne* (Paris) 142:64–65.

Sazawal, S., G. Hiremath, U. Dhingra, P. Malik, S. Deb, and R. E. Black. 2006. Efficacy of probiotics in prevention of acute diarrhoea: a meta-analysis of masked, randomised, placebo-controlled trials. *Lancet Infect. Dis.* 6:374–382.

Simeonidis, S., I. Castagliuolo, A. Pan, J. Liu, C. C. Wang, A. Mykoniatis, A. Pasha, L. Valenick, S. Sougioultzis, D. Zhao, and C. Pothoulakis. 2003. Regulation of the NK-1 receptor gene expression in human macrophage cells via an NF-kappa B site on its promoter. *Proc. Natl. Acad. Sci. USA* 100:2957–2962.

Simeonidis, S., D. Stauber, G. Chen, W. A. Hendrickson, and D. Thanos. 1999. Mechanisms by which IkappaB proteins control NF-kappaB activity. *Proc. Natl. Acad. Sci. USA* 96:49–54.

Sougioultzis, S., S. Simeonidis, K. R. Bhaskar, X. Chen, P. M. Anton, S. Keates, C. Pothoulakis, and C. P. Kelly. 2006. *Saccharomyces boulardii* produces a soluble anti-inflammatory factor that inhibits NF-kappaB-mediated IL-8 gene expression. *Biochem. Biophys. Res. Commun.* **343:**69–76.

Spitz, J., R. Yuhan, A. Koutsouris, C. Blatt, J. Alverdy, and G. Hecht. 1995. Enteropathogenic *Escherichia coli* adherence to intestinal epithelial monolayers diminishes barrier function. *Am. J. Physiol.* **268:**G374–G379.

Surawicz, C. M., G. W. Elmer, P. Speelman, L. V. McFarland, J. Chinn, and G. van Belle. 1989. Prevention of antibiotic-associated diarrhea by *Saccharomyces boulardii*: a prospective study. *Gastroenterology* **96:**981–988.

Surawicz, C. M., L. V. McFarland, R. N. Greenberg, M. Rubin, R. Fekety, M. E. Mulligan, R. J. Garcia, S. Brandmarker, K. Bowen, D. Borjal, and G. W. Elmer. 2000. The search for a better treatment for recurrent *Clostridium difficile* disease: use of high-dose vancomycin combined with *Saccharomyces boulardii*. *Clin. Infect. Dis.* **31:**1012–1017.

Szajewska, H., A. Skorka, and M. Dylag. 2007. Meta-analysis: *Saccharomyces boulardii* for treating acute diarrhoea in children. *Aliment. Pharmacol. Ther.* **25:**257–264.

Villarruel, G., D. M. Rubio, F. Lopez, J. Cintioni, R. Gurevech, G. Romero, and Y. Vandenplas. 2007. *Saccharomyces boulardii* in acute childhood diarrhoea: a randomized, placebo-controlled study. *Acta Paediatr.* **96:**538–541.

Wilson, A. K., G. Gorgas, W. D. Claypool, and P. de Lanerolle. 1991. An increase or a decrease in myosin II phosphorylation inhibits macrophage motility. *J. Cell Biol.* **114:**277–283.

Woronicz, J. D., X. Gao, Z. Cao, M. Rothe, and D. V. Goeddel. 1997. IkappaB kinase-beta: NF-kappaB activation and complex formation with IkappaB kinase-alpha and NIK. *Science* **278:**866–869.

Therapeutic Microbiology: Probiotics and Related Strategies
Edited by J. Versalovic and M. Wilson
© 2008 ASM Press, Washington, DC

John R. Tagg, Jeremy P. Burton,
Philip A. Wescombe, Chris N. Chilcott

6

Streptococci as Effector Organisms for Probiotic and Replacement Therapy

The struggle among microorganisms to survive and to establish an ecological niche in the human body has fascinated medical scientists almost as much as the struggle between a specific infectious agent and its human host (Wannamaker, 1980).

HISTORICAL PERSPECTIVE

Following our birth, a generally predictable and orderly succession of microorganisms establishes residence upon all of the accessible surfaces of our body, ultimately forming site-specific climax communities: highly resilient microbial menageries, many members of which appear uniquely adapted to the exigencies of life in just this particular microhabitat. The affiliates of this normal microflora (or indigenous microbiota) have a keen interest in our well-being, since our healthy tissues constitute their preferred homeland. For humans, there has been only a relatively recent realization that our body cells are substantially outnumbered by our microbial symbionts and that this situation is both inevitable and desirable.

The individual members of our indigenous microbiota are under continuous territorial siege by competing microbes, both endogenous and extrinsic, some of which have pathogenic potential for the host should they be allowed to grow unchecked. Aggressively virulent space-invading microbes are sometimes able to supplant the incumbents and especially so if the tissue landscape is damaged or our innate and specific immune defenses are compromised. Broad-spectrum antibiotics indiscriminately kill a wide variety of natives within the host's normal microbiota, resulting in the formation of ecological instabilities and encouraging the proliferation of antibiotic resistance and superinfection by the more robust and opportunistic members of the surviving home guard. Humans have made a variety of attempts, generally ad hoc, to intervene in these bacterial skirmishes and civil wars. The practice of ingesting probiotic bacteria, particularly intestinal lactobacilli and bifidobacteria, has evolved from its folk medicine origins to current widespread public popularity and increased scientific scrutiny as a relatively uncomplicated self-help way of achieving tangible health benefits. Recent advancements and applications of genomic and proteomic technologies have increased our understanding of the ecology of the human indigenous microbiota, and with the benefit of

John R. Tagg, Department of Microbiology and Immunology, University of Otago, PO Box 56, Dunedin, New Zealand. **Jeremy P. Burton, Philip A. Wescombe,** and **Chris N. Chilcott,** BLIS Technologies Ltd, Centre for Innovation, University of Otago, PO Box 56, Dunedin, New Zealand.

this knowledge a more scientifically informed basis can now be adopted for the selection (or construction) of probiotic mercenaries, equipped with targeted antibiotic weaponry, to bolster the frontline defenses of the normal human microbiota.

It was Pasteur who first introduced the notion of bacteriotherapy: the utilization of "harmless" bacteria to displace pathogenic organisms as a means of treating infection (Pasteur and Joubert, 1877). Throughout the early 1900s physicians continued to pit bacterium against bacterium in both test tubes and infected patients, because there was no other treatment option available to them (Florey, 1946). However, with the advent of the antibiotic era there now was an alternative—or at least for a time. Indeed, in the mid-1940s scientists dealt two "trump cards" having the potential to indiscriminately decimate microbes and mankind—penicillin and the atomic bomb, respectively. The practice of bacteriotherapy and bacterioprophylaxis was largely discontinued as both physicians and the public at large appeared to develop an almost smug complacency about the level of risk posed by our potential microbial adversaries. Humans clearly now had the upper hand. However, in the face of their persistent exposure to antibiotic-laced ecosystems the microbes have fought back and countless variants now flourish with apparent impunity despite even our most potent designer antimicrobials. The medical community now faces the specter of microbial clones capable of defying all of our conventional chemical weapons of microbe destruction. This dilemma has encouraged many researchers to reconsider the Pasteurian creed—that bacteria themselves could prove to be our most effective allies—as we continue to confront that relatively small but resilient band of miscreant microbes that are capable of causing infections of humans and other animals (Huovinen, 2001).

The whole concept of either deliberately ingesting or otherwise seeding our tissues with microbes is anathema to many humans. After all, the only good germ is a dead germ—at least that is the message imprinted upon us by the media from an early age. We are urged, are we not, to rid our homes of all germs and to douse every accessible body crevice with antibiotics, antiseptics, and assorted antimicrobials in a heroic attempt to achieve a germfree environment. This then is the antimicrobial gospel, and let's face it—most microbes have overwhelmingly had bad press.

However, with increased knowledge has come a greater awareness that our sanitized cuisine and habitat may have impacted negatively upon both our immunological and our microbial defenses. By minimizing our contact with nonpathogenic microbes, we may have reduced important antigenic stimulation and increased the risk of developing unbalanced populations of bacteria on our various body surfaces.

In recent years researchers have started to apply strains of a wider variety of bacterial species, some not principally adapted to an intestinal lifestyle, as new-age probiotics to modulate and mobilize our microbial and immunological defenses in various of the far-flung outposts of the human indigenous microbiota. Some of these strains do their work by competing with potential pathogens for resources and space. Others excrete metabolic by-products or antibiotics that are toxic to disease-causing microbes but harmless to people or that trigger the host's immune system. The present chapter examines the involvement of members of the genus *Streptococcus* in some of these new developments.

STREPTOCOCCI AS PROBIOTICS OR AS CANDIDATES FOR REPLACEMENT THERAPY

The principal natural habitat for streptococci in their associations with humans is the oral cavity and, to a lesser extent, the nasopharynx. Until recently, probiotic principles have not been widely applied to the specific protection of oral and nasopharyngeal surfaces against bacterial infection. Although the conventional lactobacillus and bifidobacterial probiotics do not naturally colonize these tissues, randomized controlled trials have shown that ingestion of certain strains may be correlated with reduced nasal colonization by some potentially pathogenic bacteria including *Streptococcus pneumoniae*, *Staphylococcus aureus*, and beta-hemolytic streptococci (Gluck and Gebbers, 2003) and also with reduced oral levels of candida (Hatakka et al., 2007) and the dental caries pathogen, *Streptococcus mutans* (Caglar et al., 2005, 2006; Meurman 2005).

Some researchers have turned to the development of replacement therapy strategies using relatively harmless indigenous streptococci as oral and nasopharyngeal probiotics, since (it is reasoned) these should have greater colonization potential than lactobacilli and bifidobacteria for these target tissues. The objective of replacement therapy is to achieve the implantation and persistence within the normal microbiota of relatively innocuous "effector" bacteria that are somehow able to competitively exclude, or limit the outgrowth of, potential disease-causing bacteria, without significantly disturbing the balance of the existing microbial ecosystem. This process of microbe-based competitive exclusion of other microbes is sometimes termed microbial (or bacterial) interference (Brook, 1999). Streptococcal strains derived from the indigenous microbiota have been used in preliminary attempts to afford protection against the bacterial consortia diseases otitis media (Roos et al., 2001), dental caries (Hillman and Socransky, 1987), and halitosis (Burton et al., 2006a, 2006b) or against specific infection by *Streptococcus pyogenes* (Roos et al., 1996; Tagg, 2004), and further details of these trials are provided later in this chapter.

Sometimes, the mechanisms operating in situ to confer host protection in documented studies of replacement therapy are not known, such as with the proposed anti-*S. mutans* action of *Streptococcus salivarius* strain TOVE-R (Kurasz et al., 1986). Nevertheless, it is generally considered that the principal mechanisms contributing to microbial interference (or preemptive niche occupancy) may typically include either the greater ability of the effector bacterium to compete with others for limited attachment sites and essential nutrients or the superior capability of that bacterium to produce, and to be resistant to, anticompetitor molecules, some of which may be rather nonspecific in their targeting (e.g., acids, hydrogen peroxide, and ammonia), while others (e.g., bacteriocins, bacteriocin-like inhibitory substances [BLIS], and bacteriophages) appear generally to be more specifically targeted against some of those bacteria that are relatively similar to the effector strain (Tagg et al., 1976). Table 1 gives representative examples of phenotypic characteristics of streptococci especially relevant to their application as oral probiotics.

In the past, most probiotic candidates have been naturally occurring, generally regarded as safe strains of dairy industry origins that have had a long history of safe use and acceptance by humans. Many of these bacteria, which include lactobacilli, bifidobacteria, and *Streptococcus thermophilus*, have not been directly sourced from humans and are thus unlikely to be efficacious colonizers or to be directly competitive with pathogenic bacteria for the same niche in human tissues. As such, their role in bacterial interference appears more likely to be in the initiation of short-term immunological responses in the host tissues (Corthesy et al., 2007), rather than in effecting direct competition with pathogens by occupancy of common attachment sites or through bacteriocin-mediated inhibition.

Streptococcal probiotics are generally considered most likely to confer health benefits to sites other than the intestines, since their numbers within the adult human gut microbiota, either in health or in disease, are relatively small. *S. thermophilus* (Hols et al., 2005), however, is a nominated component of some "intestinal" probiotic mixes, and since large numbers of its cells are often consumed in yogurts, this species could potentially

contribute to systemic or local immune stimulation in the intestines as well as conferring health benefits for subjects either exhibiting lactose intolerance (due to its high content of beta-galactosidase) (Rizkalla et al., 2000) or having inflammatory bowel disease (part of the VSL-3 probiotic mix) (Chapman et al., 2007). Indeed, the potential importance of *S. thermophilus*, in spite of its perhaps somewhat fleeting interactions with human tissues, should not be underestimated, given that this species has very close genetic linkages to the numerically predominant oral commensal, *S. salivarius* (Bentley et al., 1991; Farrow and Collins, 1984; Innings et al., 2005; Mora et al., 2003; Poyart et al., 1998).

S. salivarius, although best known as a foundation member of the adult oral microbiota, is also a significant early contributor to the intestinal microbiota of infants (Park et al., 2005). *S. salivarius* probiotics, ingested with the intention of achieving oral colonization, bolster the indigenous *S. salivarius* populations that are regularly shed from the oral mucosae, and these cells (whether dead or alive) and perhaps especially their dispersed cell surface teichoic acid fragments may exhibit immunoreactivity, either in the oral cavity or during the course of their transit through the gastrointestinal tract (Cosseau et al., 2007).

The conventional concept of replacement therapy is the use of "good" bacteria to compete with, or antagonize, "bad" bacteria in order to prevent and treat infections. From an optimistic perspective, replacement therapy offers the possibility of achieving relatively extended protection for the human host against a variety of microbial infections or maladies: an intrinsically simple and inexpensive solution to the serious problem of escalating levels of resistance to conventional therapeutic antibiotics. Streptococci have considerable appeal as "effector" organisms for replacement therapy in the oral cavity, since some species (e.g., the phylogenetically closely related *S. salivarius* and *Streptococcus vestibularis*) (Delorme et al., 2007) are low-virulence commensals, well suited to competitively exclude undesirable family members such as *S. mutans*, *S. pyogenes*, and *S. pneumoniae*, which are incriminated in a number of diseases of this region. Indeed, several relatively innocuous streptococcal species have a numerically significant presence in the oral cavity and nasopharyngeal microbial consortia, and within these multicellular communities they have become evolutionarily highly adapted to interact, coexist, and compete with other streptococci.

For the purposes of replacement therapy, one option is to use a naturally occurring isolate of a low-virulence species that will either (i) competitively occupy a particular habitat or niche required by the target pathogen or (ii) seed into the saliva diffusible agent(s) capable of

Table 1 Characteristics of streptococci having potential relevance to their use as oral probiotics

Characteristic	Species	Potential role in situ or in vitro	Reference(s)
Lactate dehydrogenase deficiency	S. mutans (genetically modified)	No production of cariogenic lactic acid by S. mutans in biofilm Lactic acid nonproducers for use in anti-MS bacterial interference studies	Anderson and Shi, 2006; Hillman, 2002
Urease production	Various oral streptococci especially S. salivarius	Increase in pH may reduce acid-mediated damage by acid producers such as S. mutans and lactobacilli	Schaumann and Tagg, 1991
Biofilm modulation	S. thermophilus	Incorporated into plaque, reduces its cariogenicity	Comelli et al., 2002
	S. salivarius	Dextranase degradation of certain extracellular polysaccharides in plaque	Lawman and Bleiweis, 1991; Ohnishi et al., 1995
	Streptococcus gordonii, S. mutans, and various other oral bacteria	Competence-stimulating factor influences biofilm production and S. mutans	Kuramitsu and Wang, 2006; Li et al., 2001a, 2001b
Bacteriocin production	Streptococci, enterococci, and staphylococci	Target MS	Balakrishnan et al., 2001
	Streptococci and actinomyces	Inhibit S. mutans regrowth in animal studies	van der Hoeven and Schaeken, 1995
	S. mutans and S. sanguinis	Interfere with carriage of staphylococci	Tzannetis et al., 1991
	Streptococcus species	Compete with lactobacilli and staphylococci in mouse studies	Marcotte et al., 1995
	S. salivarius and alpha-hemolytic streptococci	Compete with S. pyogenes, S. aureus, and organisms implicated in halitosis	Brook, 2005; Burton et al., 2006a; Fujimori et al., 1995, 1997; Hyink et al., 2007; Roos et al., 2001; Tagg, 2004; Tagg and Dierksen, 2003
	S. gordonii	Inhibits bacteriocin production by MS	Wang and Kuramitsu, 2005
	S. equi subsp. zooepidemicus	Targets S. mutans	Simmonds et al., 1997
Hydrogen peroxide production	Viridans group streptococci	Inhibit methicillin-resistant S. aureus	Uehara et al., 2001
	S. sanguinis	Competes with S. mutans in biofilms	Kreth et al., 2005
Adhesion	S. thermophilus	Adheres to saliva-coated hydroxyapatite beads	Comelli et al., 2002
Host epithelium homeostasis	S. salivarius	Induction of homeostasis-related genes	Cosseau et al., 2007
Local immune modulation	S. salivarius	Increased salivary gamma interferon production	Chilcott et al., 2005[a], Cosseau et al., 2007
Unknown antagonism or competitive action	Alpha-hemolytic streptococci	Inhibit S. pyogenes and S. aureus	Fujimori et al., 1995
	S. salivarius	Inhibits S. mutans	Tanzer et al., 1985
	Streptococcus oligofermentans	Inhibits S. mutans	Tong et al., 2006

[a]Chilcott, C. N., L. Crowley, V. Kulkarni, R. W. Jack, A. D. McLellan, and J. R. Tagg, 2005. Presented at the Joint Meeting of New Zealand Microbiological Society and New Zealand Biochemistry and Molecular Biology, Dunedin, New Zealand.

controlling the numbers or metabolism of the target pathogen located at some other oral cavity site which is infiltrated by this saliva. An alternative option for replacement therapy is for the effector strain to be a "genetically crippled" virulence-enfeebled variant of the pathogenic species. These specifically engineered avirulent variants must, however, in order to be successful, have a strong competitive edge over any disease-causing native members of that same species in the battle for niche dominance. This gene manipulation approach to replacement therapy, actively pursued by Jeffrey Hillman and his associates in relation to dental caries control (Hillman et al., 2007), is discussed in some detail later.

INTERBACTERIAL COMPETITIVE ATTRIBUTES OF STREPTOCOCCI USED AS PROBIOTICS AND IN REPLACEMENT THERAPY

Bacteriocins, the activity of which is typically most strongly directed against species closely related to the producer cell, are produced ubiquitously by bacterial isolates from natural ecosystems and appear likely to be the prime effectors of interbacterial competition (Riley and Gordon, 1999). Bacteriocin-producing bacteria potentially offer (at least theoretically) a relatively targeted approach to pathogen control. In contrast to conventional therapeutic antibiotics, they effect relatively little collateral killing of unrelated bacteria, since they deliver low concentrations of narrow-spectrum antimicrobials principally to their immediate vicinity.

The bacteriocins of gram-positive bacteria are a heterogeneous array of antibiotics (Jack et al., 1995; Tagg et al., 1976), recently classified into four clusters (Heng et al., 2007b). Examples of each cluster known to be produced by streptococci are shown in Fig. 1. As a group, the bacteriocins are apparently united only by their ribosomally synthesized proteinaceous composition and

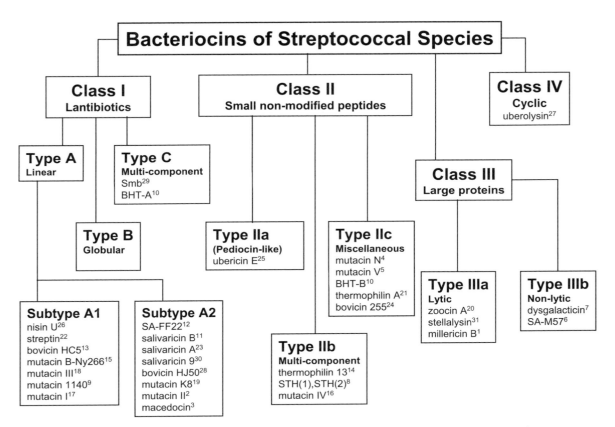

Figure 1 Illustration of the four classes of bacteriocins produced by gram-positive bacteria with examples currently known to be produced by streptococci. Footnotes: 1, Beukes et al., 2000; 2, Chikindas et al., 1995; 3, Georgalaki et al., 2002; 4, Hale et al., 2004; 5, Hale et al., 2005a, 2005b; 6, Heng et al., 2004; 7, Heng et al., 2006a; 8, Heng et al., 2007a; 9, Hillman et al., 1998; Smith et al., 2003; 10, Hyink et al., 2005; 11, Hyink et al., 2007; 12, Jack et al., 1994a, 1994b; 13, Mantovani et al., 2002; 14, Marciset et al., 1997; 15, Mota-Meira et al., 1997; 16, Qi et al., 2001; 17, Qi et al., 2000; 18, Qi et al., 1999; 19, Robson et al., 2007; 20, Simmonds et al., 1996; 21, Ward and Somkuti, 1995; 22, Wescombe and Tagg, 2003; 23, Wescombe et al., 2006b; Ross et al., 1993; 24, Whitford et al., 2001; 25, R. E. Wirawan, N. C. K. Heng, R. W. Jack, and J. R. Tagg, abstr. B14, 7th ASM Conference on Streptococcal Genetics, St. Malo, France, 2006; 26, Wirawan et al., 2006; 27, Wirawan et al., 2007; 28, Xiao et al., 2004; 29, Yonezawa and Kuramitsu, 2005; 30, Wescombe et al., unpublished (GenBank accession no. DQ889747); 31, Heng et al., 2006b.

by their targeted killing of bacteria closely related to the producer bacterium. There are very few reports of bacteriocins also exhibiting toxicity for eukaryotic cells, although in some instances the genetic loci for bacteriocins may be closely linked, either chromosomally or on plasmids, to bacterial virulence determinants (Wescombe et al., 2005).

Bacteriocins are the most abundant of the antimicrobial compounds facultatively produced by bacteria, and they are found in all major bacterial lineages (Riley and Wertz, 2002a, 2002b). It is supposed that they can influence the composition of heterogeneous bacterial populations, such as those found in naturally occurring biofilms, by mechanisms that include molecular signaling (quorum sensing) and antibiosis (Quadri, 2002). Our own research interests are focused upon the commensal and pathogenic oral streptococci, and these have been shown to produce a particularly wide variety of bacteriocins (Heng et al., 2007b; Nes et al., 2007). The lethal activity of bacteriocins is often (but not always) largely directed against closely related members of the same genus as the producer, implying that they have a major role in niche competition. Due to the high diversity of bacteriocin production, the potential possibly exists for the development of novel bacteriocin-producing probiotic strains that will specifically target just certain bacterial species.

The producer bacterium and its progeny are protected from the toxic action of their bacteriocins by the activity of dedicated immunity gene products (generally also encoded by the bacteriocin locus) that specifically exclude or deactivate the bacteriocins (Baba and Schneewind, 1998; Cotter et al., 2005; Fimland et al., 2005). There are significant metabolic and genetic costs associated with the maintenance of bacteriocin production and immunity: resources must be diverted from other cellular functions, or (for some gram-negative bacteria) the release of bacteriocins requires cell lysis (Riley and Wertz, 2002a, 2002b). The metabolic costs associated with the expression of bacteriocin immunity are thought to be a critical element in accounting for the observed coexistence between bacteriocin-sensitive and bacteriocin-insensitive strains in heterogeneous microbial ecosystems such as in dental plaque and on oral mucosae (Czaran et al., 2002).

Whereas bacteria have traditionally been studied as populations of cells that act independently, it is now clear that there is extensive interaction and communication between similar (and sometimes surprisingly different) cells cohabiting complex natural communities such as the biofilms on oral surfaces (Jenkinson and Lamont, 2005). Bacteria can produce an impressive repertoire

of secondary metabolites and, in turn, can respond to a wide variety of chemical stimuli in their environment. Some of these secondary metabolites have vital roles in the cell-density-dependent regulation of gene expression (Keller and Surette, 2006). The signaling molecules bind to receptors on or in the bacterial cell, and at some threshold concentration this effects changes in the expression of particular genes. Both intra- and interspecific signaling activities have been described, and these are thought to provide a mechanism for the coordinated regulation of bacterial population behavior. Although a number of different classes of molecules have been implicated in bacterial signaling, in streptococci this function appears largely to be effected by oligopeptides, some of which also function as anticompetitor molecules (or bacteriocins) (Cvitkovitch et al., 2003; Quadri, 2002).

The coexpression of specific bacteriocin immunity is necessary to avoid suicide in the killer (bacteriocin-producing) phenotype. The genes encoding bacteriocin production and immunity to the homologous bacteriocin are typically contiguous and frequently are plasmid-borne. Variant cells that have lost the capability of expressing the bacteriocin structural gene while maintaining bacteriocin immunity (bac$^-$ immune$^+$) may (by avoiding the metabolic cost of bacteriocin production) constitute a relatively efficient and therefore favored phenotype in an ecosystem in which some exposure to that homologous bacteriocin occurs. However, once these bac$^-$ immune$^+$ populations come to predominate within the ecosystem, bacteriocin-sensitive (bac$^-$ immune$^-$) variants of these cells, since they do not even have to bear the cost of immunity expression, will now have the chance to proliferate—at least until reentry of fully fledged bacteriocin producers (bac$^+$ immune$^+$) into the ecosystem. This killer-immune-sensitive cell system has been described as a cycle of competitive dominance and has been likened to the childhood game of "rock-scissors-paper" (Czaran et al., 2002). Killers are dominant over sensitives, but immunes outcompete killers and sensitives replace the immunes due to their more efficient competition for limited resources (Riley and Gordon, 1999).

Recent studies have shown that the production by *S. pyogenes* of SalY, the immunity protein for the lantibiotic salivaricin A, is important for the intracellular survival of this bacterium (Phelps and Neely, 2007). The suggestion is that SalY may function as a virulence factor for *S. pyogenes*, presumably conferring cross-protection against the killing action of eukaryotic cationic peptides. Although in *S. pyogenes* some components of the salivaricin A locus (including *salY*) are present in the vast majority of strains tested, only isolates of serotype M4 appear to express the biologically active bacteriocin

(Johnson et al., 1979; Simpson et al., 1995; Upton et al., 2001). The implication is that, at least in *S. pyogenes*, the bac⁻ immune⁺ phenotype has been evolutionarily advantageous and is overwhelmingly conserved. Interestingly, our own (unpublished) studies have shown that SalY is also expressed by some indigenous *S. salivarius* strains in the absence of expression of the bioactive salivaricin A. In the case of *S. salivarius*, however, it appears more likely that the expression of SalY in the absence of the homologous bacteriocin is to confer a survival advantage to the host (bac⁻ immune⁺) strain in the face of niche competition from salivaricin A-producing *S. salivarius*, since more than 10% of natural isolates of *S. salivarius* are capable of expressing salivaricin A (Tagg et al., 1983). Nevertheless, in view of the demonstrated contribution of SalY to *S. pyogenes* intracellular survival, it will be of interest to determine whether SalY expression confers a similar phenotypic capability upon *S. salivarius*.

Some attributes other than the production of bacteriocins have been proposed to increase the competitiveness of streptococcal strains within the oral cavity. These include the depletion or competitive inhibition of uptake of an essential substance (e.g., substrate or vitamin), alteration of the microenvironment (e.g., change in pH), or production of nonprotein antagonistic substances. More than 25 years ago Sanders and Sanders (1982) showed that the low-molecular-weight pantothenic acid antagonist enocin produced by *S. salivarius* may have a role in the competitive exclusion of *S. pyogenes*. No follow-up of these landmark investigations has been reported.

The production of bioactive metabolites such as hydrogen peroxide may also be a mechanism by which the oral or nasopharyngeal microbiota can be altered (Kreth et al., 2005; Tano et al., 2003). Several oral streptococci, lactobacilli, and related bacteria appear to be capable of producing excess hydrogen peroxide, and *S. aureus* organisms located in the nasopharyngeal cavity appear to be particularly susceptible to hydrogen peroxide-mediated inhibition (Regev-Yochay et al., 2006; Uehara et al., 2001). Unlike the case with bacteriocins, this is a relatively nonspecific action that probably relies upon the close association of bacteria in order to be effective. However, at other sites in the human body, such as the vagina, hydrogen peroxide-producing bacteria such as the lactobacilli appear to play a key role in the maintenance of homeostasis (Vallor et al., 2001).

The individual members of consortia may act either as individuals or in groups to promote or suppress the proliferation of other microbes, either directly contiguous to them or within range of their diffusible bioactive products. Promotion of the growth of others may occur via the production of metabolic end products directly utilizable by other microbes and by homotypic or heterotypic coaggregation. Inhibition of other bacteria may be through competitive binding to adhesion receptors on host or other microbe surfaces as well as through the production of antibiotics or metabolic end products antagonistic to the growth of others. The emphasis of the present review is largely on current knowledge of the contribution of dedicated interbacterial inhibitors, the bacteriocins and BLIS, to the efficacy of streptococci as potential probiotics. The acronym BLIS is applied as a convenient preliminary descriptor for interbacterial inhibitory effects observed in vitro, prior to the complete chemical and genetic characterization of the specific bioactive agent(s) (Ragland and Tagg, 1990). The practical value of the use of this term with reference to streptococci is highlighted by our findings that (i) these bacteria typically produce a variety of nonproteinaceous inhibitors such as lactic acid and hydrogen peroxide and (ii) many streptococci produce multiple bacteriocins (and also bacteriolytic enzymes and bacteriophages) that can contribute to the total activity spectrum of the bacteria during the initial phases of their in vitro screening for inhibitory activity.

FACTORS INFLUENCING THE EFFICACY OF STREPTOCOCCAL PREPARATIONS FOR PROBIOTIC OR REPLACEMENT THERAPY APPLICATIONS

Desirable properties for effector strains proposed for application as probiotics or in replacement therapy include (i) low pathogenic potential; (ii) pathogen-specific targeting; (iii) ease of propagation in vitro and of delivery in a viable format to the human host; (iv) reliable integration within the host indigenous microbiota; (v) ease of elimination, if required, from the human host (e.g., with antibiotic dosing); (vi) genetic stability; and (vii) persistence at effective levels within a chosen habitat. Some of the practical factors that may need to be taken into consideration when evaluating oral streptococcal probiotics are listed in Table 2.

Safety

Since most probiotics are marketed as foods or dietary supplements, the consideration of safety is of utmost importance. The safety of conventional probiotics that have been traditionally used (e.g., *Lactobacillus*, *Bifidobacterium*, *Leuconostoc*, *Lactococcus*, and *S. thermophilus*) has been established through long periods of use. However, the introduction of new probiotic species requires rigorous investigation of their safety

Table 2 Major considerations when developing a new probiotic

Consideration	Issues to be considered
Safety	Virulence
	Antibiotic resistance profile
	Toxicological data
	Enzyme profile
	Genetic stability
	Human and animal trials
Stability	Shelf life
Formulation	Product format
	Supplementary ingredients
	Consumer acceptance
	Organoleptic properties
Colonization efficacy	Pretreatment requirements
	Adhesion to host cells
	Indigenous microflora competition
Health benefits	Immune stimulation
	Exclusion of specific pathogens
	Postantibiotic microbiota replenishment

(Donohue, 2006; von Wright, 2005) and epidemiological surveillance of subjects for strain retention or horizontal acquisition of newly introduced probiotics.

Stability

Probiotics, by definition, must be viable when administered, even though some research has shown that killed cells can also exert a beneficial effect, especially in regard to immune stimulation. However, if the effectiveness of the probiotic relies upon achieving colonization for the production of antimicrobial substances, then the use of live cells is critical.

Formulation

A variety of different delivery formats have been devised for the convenience of the consumer (chewing gum, lozenges, drinks, yogurt, and drinking straws). The ingredients should provide stability and desirable organoleptic (taste and texture) profiles for the product. The addition of prebiotics, which aid the growth of the probiotic organisms, may increase colonization efficacy and provide additional health benefits.

Colonization Efficacy

Probiotics to be used in oral replacement therapy are required to colonize either a mucosal or enamel surface. These surfaces are already populated by existing endogenous populations, and therefore, the introduction of a new strain first requires the exposure of adhesion sites to allow it to achieve initial attachment. A reduction in the existing population can be achieved using antibiotics

or other antimicrobial substances such as chlorhexidine or chlorine dioxide. A 0.2% chlorhexidine mouthwash or 400-ppm chlorine dioxide mouthwash can effect at least a 10-fold temporary reduction in the total bacterial counts of saliva, and in the case of chlorhexidine, these lowered counts will persist for 3 to 4 h (Burton et al., 2006a).

The adhesion characteristics of probiotic cells have been shown to be influenced by the culture conditions, the number of seed culture transfers, and the type of lyoprotectants used in freeze-drying. The condition of the cells is important, and many probiotics in current use have inadequate quality controls in place. Other factors potentially influencing colonization efficacy include (i) the number of doses delivered and viable cell counts of the preparations, (ii) the production by the indigenous microbiota of BLIS activity directed against the probiotic strain, (iii) secretory antibody blocking adhesion of the probiotic strain, and (iv) the presence of indigenous populations expressing specific immunity to the bacteriocin(s) of the probiotic bacterium—these bac$^-$ immune$^+$ strains outcompeting the probiotic strain because of the relative energetic advantage they derive from not expressing the homologous bacteriocin(s). On the other hand, bac$^+$ immune$^+$ probiotics may supplant indigenous bac$^-$ immune$^-$ cells of the same species competing for the same niche, but only if the probiotic strain, following its adhesion, produces levels of bacteriocin that are bactericidal for its bac$^-$ immune$^-$ competitors.

Health Benefits

Some of the established and potential health benefits attributed to the consumption of traditional intestinal probiotics include (i) enhanced gut function and stability, (ii) increased protection against infectious and noninfectious diseases, (iii) immune system modulation, (iv) alleviation of lactose intolerance, (v) improved digestion and nutrient absorption, (vi) reduced blood cholesterol, (vii) reduced allergy risk, and (viii) reduced risk of urinary tract infections.

There is a tendency to generalize health claims for probiotics based on the assumption that the research on specific probiotic strains can then be extrapolated to any marketed strain of that same species. Health effects should be scientifically determined for each specific probiotic strain with information provided about the efficacious dose and formulations tested. Positive results from well-conducted clinical studies will expand and increase the acceptance of probiotics for the prevention/treatment of specific diseases. Some probiotics may exert effects locally or during transit through the gastrointestinal system. It is generally considered that at least 10^7 viable cells per day need to be ingested to achieve health benefits (Sanders, 2000). Ideally these health benefits should be scientifically established by clinical studies with humans performed by several independent research groups and published in peer-reviewed journals. Acid resistance and adhesion to intestinal mucosa are desirable characteristics for traditional probiotics. For streptococcal probiotics targeting the oral cavity, acid tolerance is not a critical factor.

INTERACTIONS OF SOME STREPTOCOCCAL FRIENDS AND FIENDS IN THE HUMAN ORAL CAVITY

The oral cavity is a complex ecosystem and presents a wide variety of niches influenced by a range of pH values, nutrient limitations, and exposed surfaces (shedding and nonshedding). In addition, it is bathed regularly by salivary and crevicular fluids and is periodically inundated by heterogeneous gluts of nutrients. The major oral habitats include the buccal mucosa, tongue dorsum, tooth surfaces (supra- and subgingival), crevicular epithelium, gingival crevice, and (sometimes) prosthodontic and orthodontic appliances. The tongue dorsum is highly papillated and provides a heavily colonized microbial refuge with a sufficiently low redox potential for anaerobes to flourish. The various oral microbial communities consist of metabolically interdependent microbes having their base camps rooted in biofilms on the exposed surfaces of the mouth, but also having a significant (if ephemeral) planktonic presence in the saliva, especially at night when, under the influence of our programmed circadian biorhythms, the rate of salivation is markedly reduced (Dawes, 1972). As one side effect of this relative salivary stasis, it can be predicted that for most humans the salivary levels of bacteriocins will peak, as will the corresponding carnage of susceptible bacteria, during the night hours.

So-called "viridans" group streptococci are among the pioneer colonizers in the oral cavity and are especially abundant in the first days of life (Kononen et al., 2002). One of the first streptococcal species to establish residence in the mouth of the newborn child is *S. salivarius* (Pearce et al., 1995). The number of distinctive *S. salivarius* strains is at first relatively large, but within a few days the predominant clonal types in a baby's mouth often come to more closely resemble those of the mother (Tagg et al., 1983). Although mostly considered a professional resident of the human oral cavity, *S. salivarius* can also be found in the normal microbiota of the nasopharynx (Kononen et al., 2002) and intestinal tract (Park et al., 2005), especially in the early years of life. Large populations persist throughout our lives on healthy oral epithelia, especially the papillary surface of

the tongue (Sklavounou and Germaine, 1980). When *S. salivarius* numbers are depleted, unbalanced overgrowth of *Candida* or of anaerobes can occur, resulting in maladies such as oral thrush (Liljemark and Gibbons, 1973), halitosis (Kazor et al., 2003), and Sjogren's syndrome (MacFarlane, 1984).

Due to its strategic location and predominant numbers, *S. salivarius* is particularly well placed to perform a population surveillance and management (i.e., "sentinel") role within the oral microbiota. We consider that anticompetitor molecules such as bacteriocins are central to this function. For example, (i) when a salivaricin A-producing *S. salivarius* population is present, some other oral bacterial species show increased levels of specific resistance to this bacteriocin (Tompkins and Tagg, 1989); (ii) children carrying dominant salivaricin A-producing *S. salivarius* acquire *S. pyogenes* less frequently (Dierksen et al., 2000); (iii) the absence of *S. salivarius* has been linked to the occurrence of halitosis, and administration of the oral probiotic *S. salivarius* strain K12 (which produces both salivaricin A and salivaricin B) alleviates the symptoms (Burton et al., 2006a); (iv) the expression of salivaricin A by *S. salivarius* is up-regulated (induced) by exposure of the producer cells to either the homologous salivaricin A peptide or to any of a number of salivaricin A variant peptides produced by different oral streptococcal species (Wescombe et al., 2006b). A practical consequence of this is that when the salivaricin A peptide is taken into the oral cavity, the production of the homologous bacteriocin by indigenous salivaricin A-positive *S. salivarius* is stimulated, and this in turn can lead to expansion of the relative numbers of salivaricin A-positive clones within the oral microbiota (Dierksen et al., 2007); (v) very large plasmids (megaplasmids) encode the production of salivaricin A, salivaricin B, and other, as-yet-uncharacterized bacteriocins in *S. salivarius* K12 and other BLIS-positive *S. salivarius* (Wescombe et al., 2006a). Furthermore in some strains, including K12, the loci for fimbria formation and for a putative nonribosomal peptide synthetase of currently unknown function are also located on these megaplasmids (unpublished data); and (vi) demonstration that megaplasmids can transfer in vivo to other *S. salivarius* isolates leads us to speculate that the genetic flexibility conferred by these plasmids may enable strains such as *S. salivarius* K12 to have a major role in regulating population dynamics and to function as a "genetic clearing house," i.e., to act as both an intra- and interspecies recipient (and expresser) and donor of genetic material within the oral cavity (Fig. 2).

Other consistent contributors to the normal microbiota of the oral cavity prior to the eruption of the dentition, and indeed then throughout life, are *S. vestibularis* and

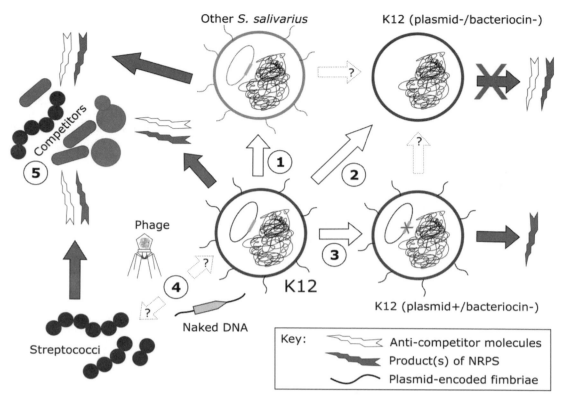

Figure 2 Overview of the proposed role of *S. salivarius* in regulating population dynamics in the oral cavity. 1, megaplasmid transfer to other *S. salivarius*; 2, complete loss of megaplasmid and related function(s); 3, mutation(s) in specific loci resulting in loss of certain function(s); 4, acquisition and/or transfer of ecologically relevant loci between *S. salivarius* K12 and other streptococci; 5, potential superinfecting microbes. Filled arrows indicate expression of ecologically relevant loci; complete arrows (filled and unfilled) indicate observed phenotypic changes; dashed, unfilled arrows (containing question marks) indicate hypothetical processes. (Courtesy of R.W. Jack.)

Streptococcus oralis. These may also be good oral probiotic candidates, since they have low virulence and widespread oral cavity distribution in humans, although they may not exhibit the same high frequencies of BLIS production that are found for *S. salivarius* (Dierksen and Tagg, 2000). With the appearance of the primary dentition and the availability of nonshedding enamel surfaces, the opportunity arises for formation of dental plaque and with it an appropriate habitat for some additional streptococcal species (e.g., the mutans streptococci and *Streptococcus sanguinis*) to establish a presence within the oral microbiota. These dental plaque-adapted streptococci, shrouded in situ by water-insoluble dextran polymers, provide a more formidable challenge for probiotic control. Although the mutans streptococci are prolific producers of bacteriocins having powerful killing activity against other mutans streptococci, they appear themselves to be uncommonly resistant to the

BLIS activities of most other oral streptococci (Balakrishnan et al., 2001).

Chronic multispecies bacterial infections of the oral cavity (e.g., dental caries, periodontal disease, and halitosis) are endemic, expensive to treat, and recalcitrant to conventional preventative protocols. These infections appear typically to be caused by the collective actions of more than one organism—the microbial community producing damage that individual microorganisms are probably incapable of inflicting (Jenkinson and Lamont, 2005). The majority of adults have either gum disease or tooth decay. Cavities are the single most common chronic disease of childhood. About one-third of the general population suffers from halitosis. In healthy mouths the "good" bacteria exert control. If conditions change, the "bad guys" can take control of surfaces, with cavities, bleeding gums, and bad breath as possible consequences (Pennisi, 2005).

The oral cavity is lined by various surfaces, including different types of soft tissues, some relatively permeable and capable of becoming much more permeable to bacterial translocation when influenced by inflammation and disease. Other intrinsic factors that can affect microbial growth and population balance include the flow of nutrients, host molecules such as tissue proteins and immune molecules, microbial extracellular products or cellular components, differences in redox potentials, and the complex infrastructure of the oral biofilms. Saliva not only provides a critical source of microbial nutrients and cofactors, it also has important roles as a biological buffer and as the conduit for intraoral translocation of biologically active molecules, microbes, and nutrients.

DENTAL CARIES

Dental caries is the localized destruction of tooth tissues by acid accumulation from the bacterial fermentation of dietary carbohydrates. Lesion formation results when enamel demineralization exceeds remineralization. The mainstay for treatment of dental caries has long been the surgical "drill and fill" approach, and preventative measures have been either behavior based (attempting to motivate individuals to improve their oral hygiene and diet) or chemical based (applying fluoride, chlorhexidine, povidone iodine, etc.). In spite of many years of endeavor, efforts to introduce measures to control dental caries by immunization have been uniformly unsuccessful (Russell et al., 2004).

On the basis of several decades of epidemiological observations and laboratory-based research, S. mutans and, to a lesser extent, Streptococcus sobrinus are generally considered to be the principal etiological agents of dental caries in humans. This tenet, primarily implicating the so-called mutans streptococcus (MS) species in dental caries, stemmed from the pioneering work of Loesche as a cornerstone example of his "specific plaque hypothesis" for the etiology of dental diseases (Loesche, 1979). More recently, however, sophisticated tools to enable molecular evaluation of the total plaque microbiota have facilitated reconsiderations of the pathogenic potential of the entire plaque community in dental caries as well as in other diseases of the oral tissues (Jenkinson and Lamont, 2005; Marsh, 2006; Munson et al., 2004).

Two attributes of the MS that are particularly relevant to their proposed key involvement in dental caries are their production of large quantities of acid from dietary carbohydrate and their formation from sucrose of highly branched extracellular polysaccharides (glucans) that help trap acidic metabolites within the plaque matrix.

According to the acidogenic theory of dental caries, it is the products of bacterial fermentation, particularly lactic acid, that mediate the caries process, reducing the pH of the microenvironment of the tooth surface below the critical threshold at which dissolution of the mineral phase of enamel and dentine is initiated, the weakened surface eventually cavitating to form a clinically evident lesion.

Attempts to devise a microbial interference-based strategy to prevent dental caries have sometimes logically first focused on identifying relatively nonpathogenic oral commensals capable of inhibiting the growth of MS (James and Tagg, 1991). However, with the notable exception of certain enterococci (Jett and Gilmore, 1990), S. salivarius (Kurasz et al., 1986), and Streptococcus equi subsp. zooepidemicus (Simmonds et al., 1997), the strongest producers of anti-MS activity appear to be other strains of MS. Zoocin A, a muralytic bacteriocin from S. equi subsp. zooepidemicus strain 4881, when tested in a triple-species plaque biofilm system, resulted in a specific 2-log reduction of the S. mutans component of the biofilm for up to 20 h posttreatment (Simmonds et al., 1995).

The potential for traditional probiotics of intestinal origin to contribute to dental caries management has recently been explored (Anderson and Shi, 2006). Ingestion of lactobacilli-containing probiotics was linked to reduction in MS counts in some trials, even though the lactobacilli themselves did not show any oral cavity persistence. In other studies, Comelli and associates (Comelli et al., 2002) showed that S. thermophilus bound in vitro to saliva-coated hydroxyapatite to the same degree as S. sobrinus, even though this may bear little relationship to reality since S. thermophilus has never been found to contribute significantly to the oral indigenous microbiota of humans.

Building upon the premise that most human tooth decay is initiated by S. mutans, Hillman has taken the replacement therapy control of dental caries to a new level of sophistication (Hillman, 2002). It was inferred that dental plaque might be more readily colonized by a naturally occurring or genetically engineered MS effector strain that was not only relatively avirulent (i.e., only weakly cariogenic) but also highly competitive due to its production of potent anti-MS BLIS activity. These researchers propose to utilize an S. mutans effector strain genetically crippled by deletion of the lactate dehydrogenase (LDH) gene such that it is no longer strongly acidogenic but still retains its powerful anti-MS activity. This strain is equipped to compete aggressively with wild-type S. mutans for its favored ecological niche in human dental plaque by virtue of production of the epidermin-like lantibiotic mutacin 1140 (Smith et al., 2003). The effector strain appears to be capable of killing all other tested strains of *S. mutans*, a feature possibly attributable in part to its production of an especially large number of different mutacins. Indeed, in our screening of MS, this strain has the widest variety of mutacin loci (mutacin 1140, mutacin IV, mutacin K8, and mutacin Smb) of all those tested (Robson et al., 2007).

Early attempts at replacement therapy for dental caries control had demonstrated that it is generally difficult to achieve persistent colonization of plaque with laboratory strains of MS (Svanberg and Loesche, 1978), particularly in subjects already harboring indigenous MS. Indeed, horizontal transfer of MS, even between close contacts, is a rare event other than for a period of several months following the onset of tooth eruption, when children tend to acquire MS strains from their primary caregiver (Caufield et al., 1993). This "window of infectivity" period is the preferred time to attempt implantation of MS effector strains.

S. mutans JH1000 was the original effector strain chosen by Hillman for further development (Hillman et al., 1985a, 1985b). A variant of this strain, named JH1140, was found to produce elevated levels of BLIS, and this strain was tested in human subjects to demonstrate that colonization efficacy and persistence correlated directly with BLIS production (Hillman et al., 1985b). Although good colonization was demonstrated, the problem of these strains themselves being highly acidogenic MS clearly precluded their application in replacement therapy. Parallel studies explored techniques for reducing the cariogenicity of the potential effector strains. Mutants exhibiting defects in glucan synthesis have reduced cariogenicity in animal models but are unlikely to compete successfully with glucan-synthesizing strains for prime plaque locations (Tanzer et al., 1985). Thus, attention became focused on the introduction of mutations affecting acid production (Hillman et al., 2000). Inactivation of the LDH gene was a lethal mutation in *S. mutans*, but compensatory introduction of a *Zygomonas mobilis* alcohol dehydrogenase gene helped to overcome the LDH deficiency. This produced a strain (BCS3-L1) that combined the traits of low acidogenicity and strong mutacin production. This is the candidate replacement therapy strain that the company Oragenics hopes to test for efficacy in human trials.

Some issues remain to be addressed. (i) The modified strain forms more plaque when grown in vitro in the presence of sucrose than does the wild-type strain (Hillman et al., 2000). (ii) The potential (although minimal) exists for reversion to LDH production (resulting in a strongly competitive cariogenic strain). (iii) Though

similar structurally to nisin, the toxicity of mutacin 1140 has not yet been directly tested, nor has the toxicity of the other mutacins putatively produced by this strain been evaluated. (iv) The potent mutacin output and the different fermentation profile of the effector strain could potentially modulate plaque ecology and result in the proliferation of other organisms having pathogenic potential.

OTITIS MEDIA

Acute otitis media (AOM) is perhaps the most common bacterial infection in young children (peak age, 1 to 2 years), with *S. pneumoniae*, *Haemophilus influenzae*, and, less often, *Moraxella catarrhalis* and *S. pyogenes* most commonly implicated. The infecting bacteria typically translocate via the eustachian tube from their base camp in the nasopharynx to the middle ear (Faden et al., 1997). Many children seem especially predisposed to develop recurrent otitis media, and the principal strategies currently used to provide them some protection against repeat infections are antibiotic prophylaxis and the fitting of tympanostomy tubes. However, the steadily increasing number of antibiotic-resistant otitis media pathogens raises questions about the net benefits of antibiotic prophylaxis. Moreover, antibiotic exposure inevitably impacts on the balance of the normal nasopharyngeal microbiota, facilitating colonization with additional antibiotic-resistant pathogens. Indeed, antibiotic treatment can increase the risk of recurrent OM (Roos et al., 2001). The placement of tympanostomy tubes can be effective, but this is expensive and involves the recognized risks of general anesthesia and surgery.

The normal bacterial population of the upper airways provides an important barrier to invading pathogens. Several studies have reported higher levels of alpha streptococci in the nasopharyngeal microbiota of healthy children than in those of children who are prone to AOM (Bernstein et al., 1993; Brook, 1999, 2005; Fujimori et al., 1996). Moreover, the alpha streptococci recovered from the openings of their eustachian tubes appear more likely to have interfering activity against AOM pathogens than those isolated from the adenoid tissue (Tano et al., 1999). Roos and associates showed how commensal alpha streptococci can be used to replace the normal nasopharyngeal microbiota in children with recurrent otitis media, a strategy based on a similar approach that these researchers had previously used to prevent recurrent streptococcal tonsillitis (Roos et al., 1996). A nasal spray containing five alpha streptococci (two strains of *S. sanguinis*, two strains of *Streptococcus mitis*, and one strain of *S. oralis*) showing in vitro inhibitory activity against AOM pathogens when tested in a double-blind, randomized, placebo-controlled study significantly reduced the recurrence rate of AOM and the frequency of secretory OM (Roos et al., 2001). At 3 months post-treatment, 42% of children given the streptococcal spray were healthy compared with 22% of the controls—and the need for new courses of antimicrobials decreased. Significantly, the children enrolled in this study had been given antibiotic therapy for 10 days prior to use of either the streptococcal or the placebo spray. By contrast, in a similar study, but with no prior use of antibiotics, there was no significant decrease in the levels of AOM pathogens or protection against repeat episodes of AOM for children treated with the alpha-streptococcal spray (Tano et al., 2002a). This highlights the importance of using probiotics hand-in-hand with conventional therapies in the oropharynx, where there may be colonization resistance to the probiotic strains because of the interfering activities of established biofilm populations. To date, the nature of the interfering activities of the alpha streptococci against the AOM pathogens has not been established (Tano et al., 2002b). In future studies it would also be beneficial to document the levels of long-term persistence of each of the colonizing strains in the mixture.

A more recent preliminary study of the contribution of known streptococcal bacteriocins to the inhibitory activities of the nasopharyngeal streptococcal populations of 20 OM-prone and 15 control children found that two of the controls, but none of the OM subjects, had *S. salivarius* producing two lantibiotics (salivaricin A and salivaricin B) present in their nasopharygeal specimens (Walls et al., 2003). Interestingly, tongue swabbings of these two subjects failed to detect the double-lantibiotic-producing *S. salivarius*, indicating perhaps that these strongly inhibitory strains may have a relative trophism for the nasopharynx. Although there is no clear evidence that these organisms protect against AOM, their low pathogenicity and strong in vitro lantibiotic production capability indicate that they should be incorporated in future trials of bacteriotherapy for recurrent AOM. Although *S. salivarius* is not generally considered a predominant member of the nasopharyngeal microbiota of adults (Rasmussen et al., 2000), in children under age 2, however, it is the second most common streptococcus (after *S. mitis*).

STREPTOCOCCAL PHARYNGITIS

S. pyogenes infections cause a variety of pathologies and are especially prevalent in children. The sequelae to these infections (especially rheumatic fever) are a major public health concern. Worldwide, rheumatic fever currently affects at least 12 million people, and some 400,000 die annually as a consequence of rheumatic heart disease (Carapetis et al., 2005). At present, the only effective means of protecting children against the possible complications of *S. pyogenes* infection is the prompt administration of a high and persisting (10-day) dose of an antibiotic such as penicillin. Unfortunately, this happens only if symptoms of acute infection have caused the child to be taken to a doctor, which does not happen in most countries. The World Health Organization has recently noted the need to develop novel strategies for the primary prevention of rheumatic fever and other streptococcal diseases (Carapetis, 2004). Vaccines are being developed but are likely to be at least a decade away, and even then cost and logistical constraints mean that they will not be available for the populations most in need for many years to come.

The investigation of inhibitory interactions between streptococci and other bacteria in the throat by Sanders and collaborators showed that children who became colonized with *S. pyogenes* had a lower percentage of throat cultures containing bacteria inhibitory or bactericidal for *S. pyogenes* than those who did not become colonized with *S. pyogenes* (Crowe et al., 1973). They also found that interfering bacteria were more often recovered during the months with highest prevalence of *S. pyogenes* infection and that the occurrence of bactericidal organisms increased with age, possibly contributing to the relative resistance of adults to *S. pyogenes* infection. The most inhibitory bacteria were alpha- or nonhemolytic streptococci and neisseriae (Sanders et al., 1977). Eradication of alpha-hemolytic streptococci can result in overgrowth of gram-negative enteric bacilli (Sprunt et al., 1971).

Implementation of anti-*S. pyogenes* replacement therapy appears to offer an ecologically sound alternative for streptococcal control. Since commensal streptococci are numerically predominant in the oral cavity, they are likely to be central to any naturally occurring anti-*S. pyogenes* activity. Several groups have investigated the *S. pyogenes*-interfering activities of the streptococcal residents of the oral microbiota. Children who develop *S. pyogenes* pharyngitis have a lower proportion of throat cultures containing bacteria inhibitory or bacteriocidal for *S. pyogenes* than those who do not become infected (Grahn and Holm, 1983; Sanders, 1969; Tagg and Dierksen, 2003). The pantothenic acid antagonist enocin, produced by some *S. salivarius* strains, was speculated to contribute to protection against *S. pyogenes* infections (Sanders and Sanders, 1982). Of all the bacterial species known to regularly inhabit the human oral microbiota in large numbers, *S. salivarius* is perhaps the most innocuous. There are no reports of this species causing infections in the oral cavity, and the rare instances of its association with bacteremia or meningitis have occurred in immunologically compromised patients or following trauma to the patient's tissues (Burton et al., 2006b; Carley, 1992). Since *S. salivarius* is common, not only on the dorsum of the tongue but also on the oropharyngeal mucosa (Frandsen et al., 1991), it is well positioned to directly repel invasion by *S. pyogenes*. Approximately 45% of *S. salivarius* strains inhibited the growth of one or more members of a set of nine indicator strains used to detect streptococcal BLIS (Dempster and Tagg, 1982). In a longitudinal study of the distribution of hemolytic streptococci in schoolchildren, it was observed that carriage or acquisition of *S. pyogenes* was not randomly distributed. Many of the rarely infected children were found to harbor large populations of *S. salivarius* producing anti-*S. pyogenes* BLIS activity (Tagg et al., 1990). Children naturally harboring populations of these bacteriocin-producing *S. salivarius* organisms were significantly less likely to acquire *S. pyogenes*. This led to the hypothesis that the presence in the oral cavity of certain BLIS-producing *S. salivarius* strains could afford protection against *S. pyogenes*.

A follow-up study of 780 Dunedin school children found two major types of BLIS activities produced by their *S. salivarius* strains, the corresponding P-type patterns being referred to as 226 (11% of children positive) and 677 (9% positive) (Dierksen and Tagg, 2000). A further 20% of the children had *S. salivarius* organisms of various other P-type designations, including some isolates producing particularly strong (P-type 777) BLIS activity. The P-type 777 prototype strain K12 produces two lantibiotics, salivaricin A2 (a variant of salivaricin A) and salivaricin B, each having strong anti-*S. pyogenes* inhibitory activity (Hyink et al., 2007; Ross et al., 1993; Upton et al., 2001). Strain K12 has subsequently been utilized by the company BLIS Technologies Ltd (www.blis.co.nz) in a series of probiotic products intended to (i) help maintain oral health (K12 Throat Guard), (ii) replenish the oral and intestinal microbiota following antibiotic usage (BLIS BioRestore), (iii) treat halitosis (BLIS K12 Fresh Breath Kit), or (iv) support the throat's natural immune defense (BLIS K12 Travel Guard). The major objectives in relationship to *S. pyogenes* is to provide a simple, inexpensive, and specific means of preventing acute pharyngeal infections and also potentially to serve as an alternative to antibiotic prophylaxis for prevention of rheumatic fever recurrences. The potential for achieving considerable reductions in

morbidity and mortality associated with streptococcal pharyngitis and its complications, coupled with the savings in health care dollars provide compelling incentives for implementation of replacement therapy strategies to control the proliferation of *S. pyogenes*.

HALITOSIS

Oral malodor afflicts up to one-half of the adult human population to varying degrees. Although not considered a major medical concern, halitosis can nevertheless be a debilitating condition for some individuals and is of major concern to many others. The most common oral malodor compounds are the by-products of metabolism of bacteria, especially anaerobes, located on the tongue dorsum. People having halitosis originating in this region appear to have decreased levels of *S. salivarius* when compared to normal controls (Kazor et al., 2003). Restoration of *S. salivarius* population levels following the use of a bacteriocin-producing *S. salivarius* strain can positively influence malodor parameters such as the volatile sulfur compound levels (Burton et al., 2006a). In vitro testing showed that *S. salivarius* K12 can suppress the growth of black-pigmented bacteria in saliva samples and also of pure cultures of various reference strains of other bacteria commonly implicated in halitosis (Burton et al., 2006a).

OTHER ORAL DISEASES POTENTIALLY AMENABLE TO STREPTOCOCCAL PROBIOTIC CONTROL

Observations that certain streptococcal species may be more commonly present in plaque specimens from healthy individuals than from those affected by periodontitis (Hillman et al., 1985) have encouraged Oragenics to develop a probiotic mixture containing strains of *Streptococcus uberis* and *S. oralis* for potential application to the control of periodontitis.

Candida albicans is the most frequently isolated fungal pathogen in humans, commonly causing oral candidosis in immunocompromised individuals or those having antibiotic therapy. In a preliminary study, *S. salivarius*, *Escherichia coli*, and *Porphyromonas gingivalis* were all found to significantly suppress adhesion of *C. albicans* to human buccal epithelial cells (Nair and Samaranayake, 1996). In other studies, *S. salivarius* caused some weak suppression of germ tube formation by *C. albicans*, while other oral species such as *P. gingivalis*, *Lactobacillus casei*, and *Prevotella intermedia* elicited significant enhancement of their formation (Nair et al., 2001).

BENEFITS OF REPLACEMENT THERAPY

A strong motivator for application of replacement therapy is the increased desire of consumers to make their own informed decisions about the application of natural methods for health maintenance. Broad-spectrum therapeutic antibiotics indiscriminately kill many members of the host microbiota, resulting in the formation of an ecological vacuum and encouraging superinfection and resistance development. By contrast, BLIS-producing bacteria potentially offer a more targeted solution to runaway pathogen control. Carefully selected BLIS producers would effect relatively little collateral killing of unrelated bacteria, since they deliver narrow-spectrum antimicrobial activity in concentrations that are probably inhibitory only to target bacteria in their immediate vicinity. Modulation of the microbiota composition by specific introduction of strains of "naturally occurring" species that are capable of excluding colonization/infection by target pathogens could be viewed as the controlled manipulation of a process that otherwise occurs only haphazardly in nature. Directed implantation of relatively harmless effector bacteria known to be strongly competitive with potential pathogens offers (even on a relatively short-term basis) a cost-effective means of achieving protection for the host against specific bacterial infections. It may also foster increased herd protection through natural transmission of the effector strain to the close contacts of the host.

DIFFICULTIES AND POTENTIAL RISKS

Although the outcomes have been reported to be promising, none of the pilot studies involving streptococcal probiotics has yet resulted in routine widespread acceptance and application as a preventative regimen. One mitigating factor may be the ethical consideration that even reputedly low-virulence colonizing strains may sometimes cause infections in compromised individuals. The normal microbiota in healthy humans is remarkably stable, a reflection of it being a finely tuned climax community that is normally well equipped to limit invasion by any foreign microbe or to prevent overgrowth by a minority member of the population. However, the status quo equilibrium is regularly upset by some events, most dramatically by exposure to broad-spectrum antibiotics or antiseptics, but also possibly following substantial nutritional, hormonal, or physical changes to the microenvironment. Any significant reductions in the numbers of individual components of the climax community could potentially result in overgrowth (superinfection) by previously suppressed minority members. Similarly, the high intrinsic stability of the indigenous microbiota can present a major obstacle to probiotic colonization. Success is unlikely unless the effector strain is very strongly competitive. Alternatively, the effector strain could be administered either prior to establishment of the microbial climax community (in the perinatal period) or upon creation of an appropriate niche following disruption of the microbiota by exposure to antimicrobials. Long-term retention of antibiotic-producing effector strains may not be easily achieved. The additional energy and nutritional demands of bacteriocin production may be sufficiently disadvantageous to organisms in some ecosystems that this will counterbalance any competitive benefit conferred by antibiosis. Under such circumstances, the bacteriocin-producing strain will gradually be replaced within the population, first by bacteriocin-nonproducing but immune cells, and then, when the levels of bacteriocin in that habitat have dropped below a critical threshold, the favored derivative of the original probiotic strain will be phenotypically negative for both bacteriocin production and bacteriocin immunity. The selection of pathogens resistant to the effector strain remains one tangible potential problem, particularly if the microbial interference is largely mediated by antibiosis. Typically, however, once an antibiotic selective pressure is removed, resistant variants tend to be disadvantaged and are lost to the population. Also, the effector strain, no matter how generally harmless, may potentially initiate disease under unusual circumstances such as immunosuppression, immunodeficiency, burns, drugs, stress, and climatic variation. Since not all risks can be predicted, new opportunistic infections could conceivably be initiated. However, it seems that the risks of this occurring would be minimized by the application of naturally occurring strains commonly isolated from balanced ecosystems in healthy individuals.

OUTLOOK FOR FUTURE USE

Intestinal probiotics are widely accepted for microbial population replacement and recolonization of the gastrointestinal tract, and a variety of beneficial strains are now inexpensively provided for the consumer. By contrast, the development and application of bacterial replacement therapy for the prevention of infections of the oral cavity and other tissue surfaces are not very advanced. Changes are now under way, and an increasingly prominent role for bacterial replacement therapy can be anticipated as an ecologically sound strategy for the prevention and control of a whole variety of topical bacterial infections of humans and other animals. More research is needed to identify (and possibly to genetically modify) the most appropriate effector strains and to optimize the conditions for their in vitro propagation and preservation, for enhancing their colonization efficiency, and for favoring their prolonged retention within the normal microbiota.

References

Anderson, M. H., and W. Shi. 2006. A probiotic approach to caries management. *Pediatr. Dent.* **28**:151–153, 192–198.

Baba, T., and O. Schneewind. 1998. Instruments of microbial warfare: bacteriocin synthesis, toxicity and immunity. *Trends Microbiol.* **6**:66–71.

Balakrishnan, M., R. S. Simmonds, and J. R. Tagg. 2001. Diverse activity spectra of bacteriocin-like inhibitory substances having activity against mutans streptococci. *Caries Res.* **35**:75–80.

Bentley, R. W., J. A. Leigh, and M. D. Collins. 1991. Intrageneric structure of *Streptococcus* based on comparative analysis of small-subunit rRNA sequences. *Int. J. Syst. Bacteriol.* **41**:487–494.

Bernstein, J. M., H. F. Faden, D. M. Dryja, and J. Wactawski-Wende. 1993. Micro-ecology of the nasopharyngeal bacterial flora in otitis-prone and non-otitis-prone children. *Acta Otolaryngol.* **113**:88–92.

Beukes, M., G. Bierbaum, H. G. Sahl, and J. W. Hastings. 2000. Purification and partial characterization of a murein hydrolase, millericin B, produced by *Streptococcus milleri* NMSCC 061. *Appl. Environ. Microbiol.* **66**:23–28.

Brook, I. 1999. Bacterial interference. *Crit. Rev. Microbiol.* **25**:155–172.

Brook, I. 2005. The role of bacterial interference in otitis, sinusitis and tonsillitis. *Otolaryngol. Head Neck Surg.* **133**:139–146.

Burton, J. P., C. N. Chilcott, C. J. Moore, G. Speiser, and J. R. Tagg. 2006a. A preliminary study of the effect of probiotic *Streptococcus salivarius* K12 on oral malodour parameters. *J. Appl. Microbiol.* **100**:754–764.

Burton, J. P., P. A. Wescombe, C. J. Moore, C. N. Chilcott, and J. R. Tagg. 2006b. Safety assessment of the oral cavity probiotic *Streptococcus salivarius* K12. *Appl. Environ. Microbiol.* **72**:3050–3053.

Caglar, E., S. K. Cildir, S. Ergeneli, N. Sandalli, and S. Twetman. 2006. Salivary mutans streptococci and lactobacilli levels after ingestion of the probiotic bacterium *Lactobacillus reuteri* ATCC 55730 by straws or tablets. *Acta Odontol. Scand.* **64**:314–318.

Caglar, E., N. Sandalli, S. Twetman, S. Kavaloglu, S. Ergeneli, and S. Selvi. 2005. Effect of yogurt with *Bifidobacterium* DN-173 010 on salivary mutans streptococci and lactobacilli in young adults. *Acta Odontol. Scand.* **63**:317–320.

Carapetis, J. R. 2004. Group A streptococcal vaccine development: current status and issues of relevance to less developed countries. WHO/FCH/CAH/05.09. World Health Organization, Switzerland. Geneva, http://www.who.int/child-adolescent-health/New_Publications/CHILD_HEALTH/DP/WHO_FCH_CAH_05.09.pdf.

Carapetis, J. R., A. C. Steer, E. K. Mulholland, and M. Weber. 2005. The global burden of group A streptococcal diseases. *Lancet Infect. Dis.* **5**:685–694.

Carley, N. H. 1992. *Streptococcus salivarius* bacteremia and meningitis following upper gastrointestinal endoscopy and cauterization for gastric bleeding. *Clin. Infect. Dis.* **14**:947–948.

Caufield, P. W., G. R. Cutter, and A. P. Dasanayake. 1993. Initial acquisition of mutans streptococci by infants: evidence for a discrete window of infectivity. *J. Dent. Res.* **72**:37–45.

Chapman, T. M., G. L. Plosker, and D. P. Figgitt. 2007. Spotlight on VSL#3 probiotic mixture in chronic inflammatory bowel diseases. *BioDrugs* **21**:61–63.

Chikindas, M. L., J. Novak, A. J. Driessen, W. N. Konings, K. M. Schilling, and P. W. Caufield. 1995. Mutacin II, a bactericidal antibiotic from *Streptococcus mutans*. *Antimicrob. Agents Chemother.* **39**:2656–2660.

Comelli, E. M., B. Guggenheim, F. Stingele, and J. R. Neeser. 2002. Selection of dairy bacterial strains as probiotics for oral health. *Eur. J. Oral Sci.* **110**:218–224.

Corthesy, B., H. R. Gaskins, and A. Mercenier. 2007. Crosstalk between probiotic bacteria and the host immune system. *J. Nutr.* **137**:781S–790S.

Cosseau, C., D. Devine, E. Dullaghan, R. Falsafi, I. Yu, J. Tagg, and R. Hancock. 2007. Mechanisms underlying the commensal and probiotic properties of *Streptococcus salivarius*, abstr. 0146. *I ADR/AADR/CADR 85th General Session and Exhibition*, New Orleans, LA.

Cotter, P. D., C. Hill, and R. P. Ross. 2005. Bacteriocins: developing innate immunity for food. *Nat. Rev. Microbiol.* **3**:777–788.

Crowe, C. C., W. E. Sanders, Jr., and S. Longley. 1973. Bacterial interference. II. Role of the normal throat flora in prevention of colonization by group A streptococcus. *J. Infect. Dis.* **128**:527–532.

Cvitkovich, D. G., Y. H. Li, and R. P. Ellen. 2003. Quorum sensing and biofilm formation in streptococcal infections. *J. Clin. Investig.* **112**:1626–1632.

Czaran, T. L., R. F. Hoekstra, and L. Pagie. 2002. Chemical warfare between microbes promotes biodiversity. *Proc. Natl. Acad. Sci. USA* **99**:786–790.

Dawes, C. 1972. Circadian rhythms in human salivary flow rate and composition. *J. Physiol.* **220**:529–545.

Delorme, C., C. Poyart, S. D. Ehrlich, and P. Renault. 2007. Extent of horizontal gene transfer in evolution of streptococci of the salivarius group. *J. Bacteriol.* **189**:1330–1341.

Dempster, R. P., and J. R. Tagg. 1982. The production of bacteriocin-like substances by the oral bacterium *Streptococcus salivarius*. *Arch. Oral Biol.* **27**:151–157.

Dierksen, K. P., M. Inglis, and J. R. Tagg. 2000. High pharyngeal carriage rates of *Streptococcus pyogenes* in Dunedin school children with a low incidence of rheumatic fever. *N. Z. Med. J.* **113**:496–499.

Dierksen, K. P., C. J. Moore, M. Inglis, P. A. Wescombe, and J. R. Tagg. 2007. The effect of ingestion of milk supplemented with salivaricin A-producing *Streptococcus salivarius* on the bacteriocin-like inhibitory activity of streptococcal populations on the tongue. *FEMS Microbiol. Ecol.* **59**:584–591.

Dierksen, K. P., and J. Tagg. 2000. Distribution of bacteriocin-producing *Streptococcus salivarius* within primary school populations in Dunedin, New Zealand and their influence on acquisition or carriage of *Streptococcus pyogenes*, p. 81–85. *In* D. R. Martin and J. Tagg (ed.), *Streptococci and Streptococcal Diseases Entering the New Millennium.* Securacopy, Auckland, New Zealand.

Donohue, D. C. 2006. Safety of probiotics. *Asia Pac. J. Clin. Nutr.* **15**:563–569.

Faden, H., L. Duffy, R. Wasielewski, J. Wolf, D. Krystofik, and Y. Tung. 1997. Relationship between nasopharyngeal colonization and the development of otitis media in children. *J. Infect. Dis.* **175**:1440–1445.

Farrow, J. A., and M. D. Collins. 1984. DNA base composition, DNA-DNA homology and long-chain fatty acid studies on *Streptococcus thermophilus* and *Streptococcus salivarius. J. Gen. Microbiol.* **130**:357–362.

Fimland, G., L. Johnsen, B. Dalhus, and J. Nissen-Meyer. 2005. Pediocin-like antimicrobial peptides (class IIa bacteriocins) and their immunity proteins: biosynthesis, structure, and mode of action. *J. Pept. Sci.* **11**:688–696.

Florey, H. W. 1946. The use of micro-organisms for therapeutic purposes. *Yale J. Biol. Med.* **19**:101–117.

Frandsen, E. V., V. Pedrazzoli, and M. Kilian. 1991. Ecology of viridans streptococci in the oral cavity and pharynx. *Oral Microbiol. Immunol.* **6**:129–133.

Fujimori, I., R. Goto, K. Kikushima, K. Hisamatsu, Y. Murakami, and T. Yamada. 1995. Investigation of oral alpha-streptococcus showing inhibitory activity against pathogens in children with tonsillitis. *Int. J. Pediatr. Otorhinolaryngol.* **33**:249–255.

Fujimori, I., K. Hisamatsu, K. Kikushima, R. Goto, Y. Murakami, and T. Yamada. 1996. The nasopharyngeal bacterial flora in children with otitis media with effusion. *Eur. Arch. Otorhinolaryngol.* **253**:260–263.

Fujimori, I., K. Kikushima, K. Hisamatsu, I. Nozawa, R. Goto, and Y. Murakami. 1997. Interaction between oral alpha-streptococci and group A streptococci in patients with tonsillitis. *Ann. Otol. Rhinol. Laryngol.* **106**:571–574.

Georgalaki, M. D., E. Van Den Berghe, D. Kritikos, B. Devreese, J. Van Beeumen, G. Kalantzopoulos, L. De Vuyst, and E. Tsakalidou. 2002. Macedocin, a food-grade lantibiotic produced by *Streptococcus macedonicus* ACA-DC 198. *Appl. Environ. Microbiol.* **68**:5891–5903.

Gluck, U., and J. O. Gebbers. 2003. Ingested probiotics reduce nasal colonization with pathogenic bacteria (*Staphylococcus aureus, Streptococcus pneumoniae,* and beta-hemolytic streptococci). *Am. J. Clin. Nutr.* **77**:517–520.

Grahn, E., and S. E. Holm. 1983. Bacterial interference in the throat flora during a streptococcal tonsillitis outbreak in an apartment house area. *Zentbl. Bakteriol. Mikrobiol. Hyg. A* **256**:72–79.

Hale, J. D., B. Balakrishnan, and J. R. Tagg. 2004. Genetic basis for mutacin N and of its relationship to mutacin I. *Indian J. Med. Res.* **119**(Suppl.):247–251.

Hale, J. D., N. C. Heng, R. W. Jack, and J. R. Tagg. 2005a. Identification of *nlmTE*, the locus encoding the ABC transport system required for export of nonlantibiotic mutacins in *Streptococcus mutans. J. Bacteriol.* **187**:5036–5039.

Hale, J. D., Y. T. Ting, R. W. Jack, J. R. Tagg, and N. C. Heng. 2005b. Bacteriocin (mutacin) production by *Streptococcus mutans* genome sequence reference strain UA159: elucidation of the antimicrobial repertoire by genetic dissection. *Appl. Env iron. Microbiol.* **71**:7613–7617.

Hatakka, K., A. J. Ahola, H. Yli-Knuuttila, M. Richardson, T. Poussa, J. H. Meurman, and R. Korpela. 2007. Probiotics

reduce the prevalence of oral candida in the elderly—a randomized controlled trial. *J. Dent. Res.* **86**:125–130.

Heng, N. C., G. A. Burtenshaw, R. W. Jack, and J. R. Tagg. 2004. Sequence analysis of pDN571, a plasmid encoding novel bacteriocin production in M-type 57 *Streptococcus pyogenes. Plasmid* **52**:225–229.

Heng, N. C., N. L. Ragland, P. M. Swe, H. J. Baird, M. A. Inglis, J. R. Tagg, and R. W. Jack. 2006a. Dysgalacticin: a novel, plasmid-encoded antimicrobial protein (bacteriocin) produced by *Streptococcus dysgalactiae* subsp. *equisimilis. Microbiology* **152**:1991–2001.

Heng, N. C. K., P. M. Swe, Y.-T. Ting, M. Dufour, H. J. Baird, N. L. Ragland, G. A. Burtenshaw, R. W. Jack, and J. R. Tagg. 2006b. The large antimicrobial proteins (bacteriocins) of streptococci, p. 351–354. *In* K.S. Sriprakash et al. (ed.), *International Congress Series #1289: Conference Proceedings of the 16th Lancefield International Symposium on Streptococci and Streptococcal Diseases.* Elsevier, Amsterdam, The Netherlands.

Heng, N. C., J. R. Tagg, and G. R. Tompkins. 2007a. Competence-dependent bacteriocin production by *Streptococcus gordonii* DL1 (Challis). *J. Bacteriol.* **189**:1468–1472.

Heng, N. C. K., P. A. Wescombe, J. P. Burton, R. W. Jack, and J. R. Tagg. 2007b. The diversity of bacteriocins in grampositive bacteria, p. 45–92. *In* M. A. Riley and M. A. Chavan (ed.), *Bacteriocins: Ecology and Evolution.* Springer-Verlag, Berlin, Germany.

Hillman, J. D. 2002. Genetically modified *Streptococcus mutans* for the prevention of dental caries. *Antonie Leeuwenhoek* **82**:361–366.

Hillman, J. D., T. A. Brooks, S. M. Michalek, C. C. Harmon, J. L. Snoep, and C. C. van Der Weijden. 2000. Construction and characterization of an effector strain of *Streptococcus mutans* for replacement therapy of dental caries. *Infect. Immun.* **68**:543–549.

Hillman, J. D., J. Mo, E. McDonell, D. Cvitkovitch, and C. H. Hillman. 2007. Modification of an effector strain for replacement therapy of dental caries to enable clinical safety trials. *J. Appl. Microbiol.* **102**:1209–1219.

Hillman, J. D., J. Novak, E. Sagura, J. A. Gutierrez, T. A. Brooks, P. J. Crowley, M. Hess, A. Azizi, K. Leung, D. Cvitkovitch, and A. S. Bleiweis. 1998. Genetic and biochemical analysis of mutacin 1140, a lantibiotic from *Streptococcus mutans. Infect. Immun.* **66**:2743–2749.

Hillman, J. D., and S. S. Socransky. 1987. Replacement therapy of the prevention of dental disease. *Adv. Dent. Res.* **1**:119–125.

Hillman, J. D., S. S. Socransky, and M. Shivers. 1985a. The relationships between streptococcal species and periodontopathic bacteria in human dental plaque. *Arch. Oral Biol.* **30**:791–795.

Hillman, J. D., B. I. Yaphe, and K. P. Johnson. 1985b. Colonization of the human oral cavity by a strain of *Streptococcus mutans. J. Dent. Res.* **64**:1272–1274.

Hols, P., F. Hancy, L. Fontaine, B. Grossiord, D. Prozzi, N. Leblond-Bourget, B. Decaris, A. Bolotin, C. Delorme, S. Dusko Ehrlich, E. Guedon, V. Monnet, P. Renault, and M. Kleerebezem. 2005. New insights in the molecular biology and physiology of *Streptococcus thermophilus* revealed by comparative genomics. *FEMS Microbiol. Rev.* **29**:435–463.

Huovinen, P. 2001. Bacteriotherapy: the time has come. *BMJ* **323:**353–354.

Hyink, O., M. Balakrishnan, and J. R. Tagg. 2005. *Streptococcus rattus* strain BHT produces both a class I two-component lantibiotic and a class II bacteriocin. *FEMS Microbiol. Lett.* **252:**235–241.

Hyink, O., P. A. Wescombe, M. Upton, N. Ragland, J. P. Burton, and J. R. Tagg. 2007. Salivaricin A2 and the novel lantibiotic salivaricin B are encoded at adjacent loci on a 190-kilobase transmissible megaplasmid in the oral probiotic strain *Streptococcus salivarius* K12. *Appl. Environ. Microbiol.* **73:**1107–1113.

Innings, A., M. Krabbe, M. Ullberg, and B. Herrmann. 2005. Identification of 43 *Streptococcus* species by pyrosequencing analysis of the *rnpB* gene. *J. Clin. Microbiol.* **43:**5983–5991.

Jack, R., R. Benz, J. Tagg, and H. G. Sahl. 1994a. The mode of action of SA-FF22, a lantibiotic isolated from *Streptococcus pyogenes* strain FF22. *Eur. J. Biochem.* **219:**699–705.

Jack, R. W., A. Carne, J. Metzger, S. Stefanovic, H. G. Sahl, G. Jung, and J. Tagg. 1994b. Elucidation of the structure of SA-FF22, a lanthionine-containing antibacterial peptide produced by *Streptococcus pyogenes* strain FF22. *Eur. J. Biochem.* **220:**455–462.

Jack, R. W., J. R. Tagg, and B. Ray. 1995. Bacteriocins of gram-positive bacteria. *Microbiol. Rev.* **59:**171–200.

James, S. M., and J. R. Tagg. 1991. The prevention of dental caries by BLIS-mediated inhibition of mutans streptococci. *N. Z. Dent. J.* **87:**80–83.

Jenkinson, H. F., and R. J. Lamont. 2005. Oral microbial communities in sickness and in health. *Trends Microbiol.* **13:**589–595.

Jett, B. D., and M. S. Gilmore. 1990. The growth-inhibitory effect of the *Enterococcus faecalis* bacteriocin encoded by pAD1 extends to the oral streptococci. *J. Dent. Res.* **69:**1640–1645.

Johnson, D. W., J. R. Tagg, and L. W. Wannamaker. 1979. Production of a bacteriocine-like substance by group-A streptococci of M-type 4 and T-pattern 4. *J. Med. Microbiol.* **12:**413–427.

Kazor, C. E., P. M. Mitchell, A. M. Lee, L. N. Stokes, W. J. Loesche, F. E. Dewhirst, and B. J. Paster. 2003. Diversity of bacterial populations on the tongue dorsa of patients with halitosis and healthy patients. *J. Clin. Microbiol.* **41:**558–563.

Keller, L., and M. G. Surette. 2006. Communication in bacteria: an ecological and evolutionary perspective. *Nat. Rev. Microbiol.* **4:**249–258.

Kononen, E., H. Jousimies-Somer, A. Bryk, T. Kilp, and M. Kilian. 2002. Establishment of streptococci in the upper respiratory tract: longitudinal changes in the mouth and nasopharynx up to 2 years of age. *J. Med. Microbiol.* **51:**723–730.

Kreth, J., J. Merritt, W. Shi, and F. Qi. 2005. Competition and coexistence between *Streptococcus mutans* and *Streptococcus sanguinis* in the dental biofilm. *J. Bacteriol.* **187:**7193–7203.

Kuramitsu, H. K., and B. Y. Wang. 2006. Virulence properties of cariogenic bacteria. *BMC Oral Health* **6**(Suppl. 1):S11.

Kurasz, A. B., J. M. Tanzer, L. Bazer, and E. Savoldi. 1986. In vitro studies of growth and competition between

S. salivarius TOVE-R and mutans streptococci. *J. Dent. Res.* **65:**1149–1153.

Lawman, P., and A. S. Bleiweis. 1991. Molecular cloning of the extracellular endodextranase of *Streptococcus salivarius*. *J. Bacteriol.* **173:**7423–7428.

Li, Y. H., M. N. Hanna, G. Svensater, R. P. Ellen, and D. G. Cvitkovitch. 2001a. Cell density modulates acid adaptation in *Streptococcus mutans*: implications for survival in biofilms. *J. Bacteriol.* **183:**6875–6884.

Li, Y. H., P. C. Lau, J. H. Lee, R. P. Ellen, and D. G. Cvitkovitch. 2001b. Natural genetic transformation of *Streptococcus mutans* growing in biofilms. *J. Bacteriol.* **183:**897–908.

Liljemark, W. F., and R. J. Gibbons. 1973. Suppression of *Candida albicans* by human oral streptococci in gnotobiotic mice. *Infect. Immun.* **8:**846–849.

Loesche, W. J. 1979. Clinical and microbiological aspects of chemotherapeutic agents used according to the specific plaque hypothesis. *J. Dent. Res.* **58:**2404–2412.

MacFarlane, T. W. 1984. The oral ecology of patients with severe Sjogren's syndrome. *Microbios* **41:**99–106.

Mantovani, H. C., H. Hu, R. W. Worobo, and J. B. Russell. 2002. Bovicin HC5, a bacteriocin from *Streptococcus bovis* HC5. *Microbiology* **148:**3347–3352.

Marciset, O., M. C. Jeronimus-Stratingh, B. Mollet, and B. Poolman. 1997. Thermophilin 13, a nontypical antilisterial poration complex bacteriocin, that functions without a receptor. *J. Biol. Chem.* **272:**14277–14284.

Marcotte, H., L. Rodrigue, C. Coulombe, N. Goyette, and M. C. Lavoie. 1995. Colonization of the oral cavity of mice by an unidentified streptococcus. *Oral Microbiol. Immunol.* **10:**168–174.

Marsh, P. D. 2006. Dental plaque as a biofilm and a microbial community—implications for health and disease. *BMC Oral Health* **6**(Suppl. 1):S14.

Meurman, J. H. 2005. Probiotics: do they have a role in oral medicine and dentistry? *Eur. J. Oral Sci.* **113:**188–196.

Mora, D., G. Ricci, S. Guglielmetti, D. Daffonchio, and M. G. Fortina. 2003. 16S-23S rRNA intergenic spacer region sequence variation in *Streptococcus thermophilus* and related dairy streptococci and development of a multiplex ITS-SSCP analysis for their identification. *Microbiology* **149:**807–813.

Mota-Meira, M., C. Lacroix, G. LaPointe, and M. C. Lavoie. 1997. Purification and structure of mutacin B-Ny266: a new lantibiotic produced by *Streptococcus mutans*. *FEBS Lett.* **410:**275–279.

Munson, M. A., A. Banerjee, T. F. Watson, and W. G. Wade. 2004. Molecular analysis of the microflora associated with dental caries. *J. Clin. Microbiol.* **42:**3023–3029.

Nair, R. G., S. Anil, and L. P. Samaranayake. 2001. The effect of oral bacteria on *Candida albicans* germ-tube formation. *APMIS* **109:**147–154.

Nair, R. G., and L. P. Samaranayake. 1996. The effect of oral commensal bacteria on candidal adhesion to human buccal epithelial cells *in vitro*. *J. Med. Microbiol.* **45:**179–185.

Nes, I. F., D. B. Diep, and H. Holo. 2007. Bacteriocin diversity in *Streptococcus* and *Enterococcus*. *J. Bacteriol.* **189:**1189–1198.

Ohnishi, Y., S. Kubo, Y. Ono, M. Nozaki, Y. Gonda, H. Okano, T. Matsuya, A. Matsushiro, and T. Morita. 1995.

Cloning and sequencing of the gene coding for dextranase from *Streptococcus salivarius*. *Gene* **156**:93–96.

Park, H. K., S. S. Shim, S. Y. Kim, J. H. Park, S. E. Park, H. J. Kim, B. C. Kang, and C. M. Kim. 2005. Molecular analysis of colonized bacteria in a human newborn infant gut. *J. Microbiol.* **43**:345–353.

Pasteur, L., and J. F. Joubert. 1877. Charbon et septicémie. *C. R. Soc. Biol.* (Paris) **85**:101–115.

Pearce, C., G. H. Bowden, M. Evans, S. P. Fitzsimmons, J. Johnson, M. J. Sheridan, R. Wientzen, and M. F. Cole. 1995. Identification of pioneer viridans streptococci in the oral cavity of human neonates. *J. Med. Microbiol.* **42**:67–72.

Pennisi, E. 2005. A mouthful of microbes. *Science* **307**:1899–1901.

Phelps, H. A., and M. N. Neely. 2007. SalY of the *Streptococcus pyogenes* lantibiotic locus is required for full virulence and intracellular survival in macrophages. *Infect. Immun.* **75**:4541–4551.

Poyart, C., G. Quesne, S. Coulon, P. Berche, and P. Trieu-Cuot. 1998. Identification of streptococci to species level by sequencing the gene encoding the manganese-dependent superoxide dismutase. *J. Clin. Microbiol.* **36**:41–47.

Qi, F., P. Chen, and P. W. Caufield. 2001. The group I strain of *Streptococcus mutans*, UA140, produces both the lantibiotic mutacin I and a nonlantibiotic bacteriocin, mutacin IV. *Appl. Environ. Microbiol.* **67**:15–21.

Qi, F., P. Chen, and P. W. Caufield. 2000. Purification and biochemical characterization of mutacin I from the group I strain of *Streptococcus mutans*, CH43, and genetic analysis of mutacin I biosynthesis genes. *Appl. Environ. Microbiol.* **66**:3221–3229.

Qi, F., P. Chen, and P. W. Caufield. 1999. Purification of mutacin III from group III *Streptococcus mutans* UA787 and genetic analyses of mutacin III biosynthesis genes. *Appl. Environ. Microbiol.* **65**:3880–3887.

Quadri, L. E. 2002. Regulation of antimicrobial peptide production by autoinducer-mediated quorum sensing in lactic acid bacteria. *Antonie Leeuwenhoek* **82**:133–145.

Ragland, N., and J. Tagg. 1990. Applications of bacteriocin-like inhibitory substance (BLIS) typing in a longitudinal study of the oral carriage of beta-haemolytic streptococci by a group of Dunedin schoolchildren. *Zentbl. Bakteriol.* **274**:100–108.

Rasmussen, T. T., L. P. Kirkeby, K. Poulsen, J. Reinholdt, and M. Kilian. 2000. Resident aerobic microbiota of the adult human nasal cavity. *APMIS* **108**:663–675.

Regev-Yochay, G., K. Trzcinski, C. M. Thompson, R. Malley, and M. Lipsitch. 2006. Interference between *Streptococcus pneumoniae* and *Staphylococcus aureus*: in vitro hydrogen peroxide-mediated killing by *Streptococcus pneumoniae*. *J. Bacteriol.* **188**:4996–5001.

Riley, M. A., and D. M. Gordon. 1999. The ecological role of bacteriocins in bacterial competition. *Trends Microbiol.* **7**:129–133.

Riley, M. A., and J. E. Wertz. 2002a. Bacteriocin diversity: ecological and evolutionary perspectives. *Biochimie* **84**:357–364.

Riley, M. A., and J. E. Wertz. 2002b. Bacteriocins: evolution, ecology, and application. *Annu. Rev. Microbiol.* **56**:117–137.

Rizkalla, S. W., J. Luo, M. Kabir, A. Chevalier, N. Pacher, and G. Slama. 2000. Chronic consumption of fresh but not heated yogurt improves breath-hydrogen status and short-chain fatty acid profiles: a controlled study in healthy men with or without lactose maldigestion. *Am. J. Clin. Nutr.* **72**:1474–1479.

Robson, C. L., P. A. Wescombe, N. A. Klesse, and J. R. Tagg. 2007. Isolation and partial characterization of the *Streptococcus mutans* type AII lantibiotic mutacin K8. *Microbiology* **153**:1631–1641.

Roos, K., E. G. Hakansson, and S. Holm. 2001. Effect of recolonisation with "interfering" alpha streptococci on recurrences of acute and secretory otitis media in children: randomized placebo controlled trial. *BMJ* **322**:210–212.

Roos, K., S. E. Holm, E. Grahn-Hakansson, and L. Lagergren. 1996. Recolonization with selected alpha-streptococci for prophylaxis of recurrent streptococcal pharyngotonsillitis—a randomized placebo-controlled multicentre study. *Scand. J. Infect. Dis.* **28**:459–462.

Ross, K. F., C. W. Ronson, and J. R. Tagg. 1993. Isolation and characterization of the lantibiotic salivaricin A and its structural gene *salA* from *Streptococcus salivarius* 20P3. *Appl. Environ. Microbiol.* **59**:2014–2021.

Russell, M. W., N. K. Childers, S. M. Michalek, D. J. Smith, and M. A. Taubman. 2004. A caries vaccine? The state of the science of immunization against dental caries. *Caries Res.* **38**:230–235.

Sanders, C. C., G. E. Nelson, and W. E. Sanders, Jr. 1977. Bacterial interference. IV. Epidemiological determinants of the antagonistic activity of the normal throat flora against group A streptococci. *Infect. Immun.* **16**:599–603.

Sanders, C. C., and W. E. Sanders, Jr. 1982. Enocin: an antibiotic produced by *Streptococcus salivarius* that may contribute to protection against infections due to group A streptococci. *J. Infect. Dis.* **146**:683–690.

Sanders, E. 1969. Bacterial interference. I. Its occurrence among the respiratory tract flora and characterization of inhibition of group A streptococci by viridans streptococci. *J. Infect. Dis.* **120**:698–707.

Sanders, M. E. 2000. Considerations for use of probiotic bacteria to modulate human health. *J. Nutr.* **130**:384S–390S.

Schaumann, J. B., and J. R. Tagg. 1991. Development and application of a simple filter paper imprinting technique for the detection and enumeration of colonies of ureolytic micro-organisms. *Lett. Appl. Microbiol.* **12**:117–120.

Simmonds, R. S., J. Naidoo, C. L. Jones, and J. R. Tagg. 1995. The streptococcal bacteriocin-like inhibitory substance, zoocin A, reduces the proportion of *Streptococcus mutans* in an artificial plaque. *Microb. Ecol. Health Dis.* **8**:281–292.

Simmonds, R. S., L. Pearson, R. C. Kennedy, and J. R. Tagg. 1996. Mode of action of a lysostaphin-like bacteriolytic agent produced by *Streptococcus zooepidemicus* 4881. *Appl. Environ. Microbiol.* **62**:4536–4541.

Simmonds, R. S., W. J. Simpson, and J. R. Tagg. 1997. Cloning and sequence analysis of zooA, a *Streptococcus zooepidemicus* gene encoding a bacteriocin-like inhibitory substance having a domain structure similar to that of lysostaphin. *Gene* **189**:255–261.

Simpson, W. J., N. L. Ragland, C. W. Ronson, and J. R. Tagg. 1995. A lantibiotic gene family widely distributed in *Streptococcus salivarius* and *Streptococcus pyogenes*, p. 639–643. In J. J. E. A. Ferretti (ed.), *Genetics of Streptococci, Enterococci and Lactococci*, vol. 85. Karger, Basel, Switzerland.

Sklavounou, A., and G. R. Germaine. 1980. Adherence of oral streptococci to keratinized and nonkeratinized human oral epithelial cells. *Infect. Immun.* 27:686–689.

Smith, L., C. Zachariah, R. Thirumoorthy, J. Rocca, J. Novak, J. D. Hillman, and A. S. Edison. 2003. Structure and dynamics of the lantibiotic mutacin 1140. *Biochemistry* 42:10372–10384.

Sprunt, K., G. A. Leidy, and W. Redman. 1971. Prevention of bacterial overgrowth. *J. Infect. Dis.* 123:1–10.

Svanberg, M. L., and W. J. Loesche. 1978. Implantation of *Streptococcus mutans* on tooth surfaces in man. *Arch. Oral Biol.* 23:551–556.

Tagg, J. R. 2004. Prevention of streptococcal pharyngitis by anti- *Streptococcus pyogenes* bacteriocin-like inhibitory substances (BLIS) produced by *Streptococcus salivarius*. *Indian J. Med. Res.* 119(Suppl.):13–16.

Tagg, J. R., A. S. Dajani, and L. W. Wannamaker. 1976. Bacteriocins of gram-positive bacteria. *Bacteriol. Rev.* 40:722–756.

Tagg, J. R., and K. P. Dierksen. 2003. Bacterial replacement therapy: adapting "germ warfare" to infection prevention. *Trends Biotechnol.* 21:217–223.

Tagg, J. R., V. Pybus, L. V. Phillips, and T. M. Fiddes. 1983. Application of inhibitor typing in a study of the transmission and retention in the human mouth of the bacterium *Streptococcus salivarius*. *Arch. Oral Biol.* 28:911–915.

Tagg, J. R., N. L. Ragland, and N. P. Dickson. 1990. A longitudinal study of Lancefield group A streptococcus acquisitions by a group of young Dunedin schoolchildren. *N. Z. Med. J.* 103:429–431.

Tano, K., E. Grahn Hakansson, S. E. Holm, and S. Hellstrom. 2002a. A nasal spray with alpha-haemolytic streptococci as long term prophylaxis against recurrent otitis media. *Int. J. Pediatr. Otorhinolaryngol.* 62:17–23.

Tano, K., E. Grahn Hakansson, P. Wallbrandt, D. Ronnqvist, S. E. Holm, and S. Hellstrom. 2003. Is hydrogen peroxide responsible for the inhibitory activity of alpha-haemolytic streptococci sampled from the nasopharynx? *Acta Otolaryngol.* 123:724–729.

Tano, K., E. G. Hakansson, S. E. Holm, and S. Hellstrom. 2002b. Bacterial interference between pathogens in otitis media and alpha-haemolytic streptococci analyzed in an in vitro model. *Acta Otolaryngol.* 122:78–85.

Tano, K., C. Olofsson, E. Grahn-Hakansson, and S. E. Holm. 1999. In vitro inhibition of *S. pneumoniae*, nontypable *H. influenzae* and *M. catharralis* by alpha-hemolytic streptococci from healthy children. *Int. J. Pediatr. Otorhinolaryngol.* 47:49–56.

Tanzer, J. M., A. B. Kurasz, and J. Clive. 1985. Competitive displacement of mutans streptococci and inhibition of tooth decay by *Streptococcus salivarius* TOVE-R. *Infect. Immun.* 48:44–50.

Tompkins, G. R., and J. R. Tagg. 1989. The ecology of bacteriocin-producing strains of *Streptococcus salivarius*. *Microb. Ecol. Health Dis.* 2:19–28.

Tong, H., B. Zhu, W. Chen, F. Qi, W. Shi, and X. Dong. 2006. Establishing a genetic system for ecological studies of *Streptococcus oligofermentans*. *FEMS Microbiol. Lett.* 264:213–219.

Tzannetis, S. E., A. Bigis, N. Konidaris, H. Ioannidis, V. Genimatas, and J. Papavassiliou. 1991. In-vitro bacteriocin-mediated antagonism by oral streptococci against human carrier strains of staphylococci. *J. Appl. Bacteriol.* 70:294–301.

Uehara, Y., K. Kikuchi, T. Nakamura, H. Nakama, K. Agematsu, Y. Kawakami, N. Maruchi, and K. Totsuka. 2001. H_2O_2 produced by viridans group streptococci may contribute to inhibition of methicillin-resistant *Staphylococcus aureus* colonization of oral cavities in newborns. *Clin. Infect. Dis.* 32:1408–1413.

Upton, M., J. R. Tagg, P. Wescombe, and H. F. Jenkinson. 2001. Intra- and interspecies signaling between *Streptococcus salivarius* and *Streptococcus pyogenes* mediated by SalA and SalA1 lantibiotic peptides. *J. Bacteriol.* 183:3931–3938.

Vallor, A. C., M. A. Antonio, S. E. Hawes, and S. L. Hillier. 2001. Factors associated with acquisition of, or persistent colonization by, vaginal lactobacilli: role of hydrogen peroxide production. *J. Infect. Dis.* 184:1431–1436.

van der Hoeven, J. S., and M. J. Schaeken. 1995. Streptococci and actinomyces inhibit regrowth of *Streptococcus mutans* on gnotobiotic rat molar teeth after chlorhexidine varnish treatment. *Caries Res.* 29:159–162.

von Wright, A. 2005. Regulating the safety of probiotics—the European approach. *Curr. Pharm. Des.* 11:17–23.

Walls, T., D. Power, and J. Tagg. 2003. Bacteriocin-like inhibitory substance (BLIS) production by the normal flora of the nasopharynx: potential to protect against otitis media? *J. Med. Microbiol.* 52:829–833.

Wang, B. Y., and H. K. Kuramitsu. 2005. Interactions between oral bacteria: inhibition of *Streptococcus mutans* bacteriocin production by *Streptococcus gordonii*. *Appl. Environ. Microbiol.* 71:354–362.

Wannamaker, L. W. 1980. Bacterial interference and competition. *Scand. J. Infect. Dis.* Suppl. 24:82–85.

Ward, D. J., and G. A. Somkuti. 1995. Characterization of a bacteriocin produced by *Streptococcus thermophilus* ST134. *Appl. Microbiol. Biotechnol.* 43:330–335.

Wescombe, P. A., J. P. Burton, P. A. Cadieux, N. A. Klesse, O. Hyink, N. C. Heng, C. N. Chilcott, G. Reid, and J. R. Tagg. 2006a. Megaplasmids encode differing combinations of lantibiotics in *Streptococcus salivarius*. *Antonie Leeuwenhoek* 90:269–280.

Wescombe, P. A., N. C. K. Heng, R. W. Jack, and J. R. Tagg. 2005. Bacteriocins associated with cytotoxicity for eukaryotic cells, p. 399–448. In T. Proft (ed.), *Microbial Toxins: Molecular and Cellular Biology*. Horizon Bioscience, Wymondham, United Kingdom.

Wescombe, P. A., and J. R. Tagg. 2003. Purification and characterization of streptin, a type A1 lantibiotic produced by *Streptococcus pyogenes*. *Appl. Environ. Microbiol.* 69:2737–2747.

Wescombe, P. A., M. Upton, K. P. Dierksen, N. L. Ragland, S. Sivabalan, R. E. Wirawan, M. A. Inglis, C. J. Moore, G. V. Walker, C. N. Chilcott, H. F. Jenkinson, and J. R. Tagg. 2006b. Production of the lantibiotic salivaricin A and its variants by oral streptococci and use of a specific induction assay to detect their presence in human saliva. *Appl. Environ. Microbiol.* **72:**1459–1466.

Whitford, M. F., M. A. McPherson, R. J. Forster, and R. M. Teather. 2001. Identification of bacteriocin-like inhibitors from rumen *Streptococcus* spp. and isolation and characterization of bovicin 255. *Appl. Environ. Microbiol.* **67:**569–574.

Wirawan, R. E., N. A. Klesse, R. W. Jack, and J. R. Tagg. 2006. Molecular and genetic characterization of a novel nisin variant produced by *Streptococcus uberis. Appl. Environ. Microbiol.* **72:**1148–1156.

Wirawan, R. E., K. M. Swanson, T. Kleffmann, R. W. Jack, and J. R. Tagg. 2007. Uberolysin: a novel cyclic bacteriocin produced by *Streptococcus uberis. Microbiology* **153:**1619–1630.

Xiao, H., X. Chen, M. Chen, S. Tang, X. Zhao, and L. Huan. 2004. Bovicin HJ50, a novel lantibiotic produced by *Streptococcus bovis* HJ50. *Microbiology* **150:**103–108.

Yonezawa, H., and H. K. Kuramitsu. 2005. Genetic analysis of a unique bacteriocin, Smb, produced by *Streptococcus mutans* GS5. *Antimicrob. Agents Chemother.* **49:**541–548.

Therapeutic Microbiology: Probiotics and Related Strategies
Edited by J. Versalovic and M. Wilson
© 2008 ASM Press, Washington, DC

Michael Schultz

7

Escherichia coli

It is generally accepted that the probiotic era started with the notations of the Russian Nobel Prize laureate Elias Metchnikoff regarding the effects of certain lactobacilli on the longevity of Bulgarian peasants (Metchnikoff and Chalmers, 1907). Metchnikoff did not pursue this idea any further and was later awarded the Nobel Prize for his work on phagocytosis. Shortly before, in 1885, at a time when Robert Koch revolutionized modern microbiology with his new scientific theories and working methods, Theodor Escherich, a newly appointed lecturer at the Medical University of Munich, demonstrated that the human meconium is sterile but bacterial colonization of the intestine occurs from the infants' surroundings within 3 to 24 h after birth (Escherich, 1885). The International Committee for Bacteriological Nomenclature in 1958 named this "Bacterium coli commune" *Escherichia coli* in his honor. His discovery sparked research into the human intestinal microbiota, work that is sustained to this date. In 1916, Alfred Nissle, then superintendent of the Baden Medical Examination Centre for Infectious Diseases in Freiburg, Germany, performed what can now be regarded as pioneering experiments demonstrating the probiotic properties of intestinal

E. coli. He was engaged in analyzing the antagonism of various *E. coli* strains against pathogenic intestinal bacteria. When students were growing petri dish cultures in bacteriological courses, he had observed that mixing human stool samples with typhus pathogens had resulted in the bacteria growing at very different rates. In some cases *E. coli* colonies were dominant, in others typhus colonies. It was in 1917, during World War I, that Nissle managed to isolate a particular high-grade *E. coli* strain from the feces of an officer, who, unlike his comrades, had not suffered from any of the intestinal disorders then rampant in southeastern Europe. Self-experiments convinced him of the complete harmlessness of his method, and in 1916, he began to place bacteria, grown on agar plates, in gelatin capsules sealed with wax or paraffin (Nissle, 1916). At the end of this year, the Mutaflor trademark was registered with the Imperial Patents Office in Berlin. This was the start of a large number of publications by Nissle describing how *E. coli* Nissle 1917/Mutaflor (EcN; DSM 6601 [German Collection for Microorganisms]) can be used therapeutically (Nissle, 1918) (Fig. 1).

While EcN is by far the most studied probiotic *E. coli* strain, the probiotic effects of several other *E. coli* strains

Michael Schultz, Department of Medical and Surgical Sciences, Medicine Section, University of Otago Medical School, PO Box 913, Dunedin, New Zealand.

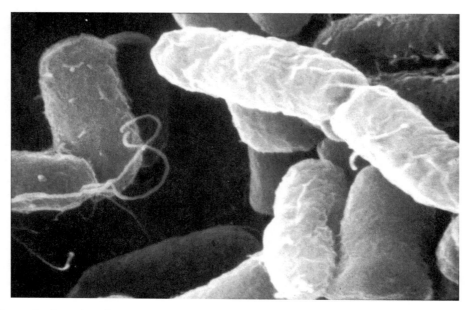

Figure 1 Scanning electron microscopic image (magnification, 20, ×000) of *E. coli* Nissle 1917, kindly provided by H. J. Jacob, Ruhr University, Bochum, Germany.

have also been reported. In the early 1960s, *E. coli* M-17 was demonstrated in open-label trials with children and adults, initially in Russia and later in Israel, to be effective in treating various intestinal infections. This strain has shown a possible effect in patients with irritable bowel syndrome (IBS) and is now marketed in the United States. *E. coli* H22, a nonpathogenic isolate from the feces of Amazonian rubber tree tappers and Indians (Nascimento et al., 1999), a population that has had little to no contact with civilization and therefore with antibiotic therapy, was recently shown to exhibit antagonistic effects towards a range of intestinal pathogens, suggesting potential use as a probiotic for livestock and humans (Cursino et al., 2006; Smarda et al., 2007). Duval-Iflah et al. have achieved some success in reducing the number of antibiotic-resistant *E. coli* organisms in infant feces by postpartum intestinal inoculation of newborn children with a plasmid-free human *E. coli* strain, EM0 (Duval-Iflah et al., 1982).

In this chapter on probiotic *E. coli* we focus on the properties, underlying mechanisms, and clinical uses of *Escherichia coli* strain Nissle 1917 as this is the most widely used and studied strain. However, we also refer to important work that has been done using other *E. coli* strains.

ISOLATION AND IDENTIFICATION

E. coli, a gram-negative bacterium, belongs to the *Enterobacteriaceae* family and is one of the first bacterial species to colonize infants' intestines. *E. coli* can thrive

only in the intestines of humans or animals, and by day 3 after birth approximately 45% of vaginally delivered babies are positive for *E. coli*, which was most likely passed on from mother to child, while only about 12% of babies delivered by cesarean section are positive for *E. coli* (Nowrouzian et al., 2003). This is in contrast to almost 70% of children who were colonized by *E. coli* during their first week of life in the 1970s. Nowrouzian et al. reported results from the late 1990s indicating that colonization of close to 100% took at least 6 months or more and this is probably due to reduced spreading of fecal bacteria because of increased hygiene in hospitals and families (Nowrouzian et al., 2003). It is noteworthy that some *E. coli* strains, but also other microorganisms that are acquired at a very young age (Schultz et al., 2004a), persist in the intestinal microbiota of an individual for months or years while others disappear within a few weeks (Adlerberth et al., 1998).

Approximately 50,000 different *E. coli* strains occur naturally. *E. coli* strains are classified and identified according to their O and H serogroups: O antigens are carbohydrates and are part of the lipopolysaccharide (LPS). For many years, the O serogroup was used to distinguish between pathogenic and commensal *E. coli*. To date, close to 200 different O serotypes have been described, with the O6 serogroup being very common (Wolf, 1997). Certain O serotypes are considered clearly pathogenic, while the *E. coli* O6 serogroup is very heterogeneous, including nonpathogenic commensal and pathogenic (diarrheagenic and uropathogenic) variants

(Blum et al., 1995). The H serogroup is determined by the flagellar antigen, long known to be the major antigen of *Salmonella* and *E. coli* strains. Recently it has been discovered that flagellin, a major subunit of bacterial flagella, serves as a potent activator of the innate immune system via stimulation of Toll-like receptor 5 (TLR-5), which triggers a massive induction of host gene expression (Gewirtz, 2007; van Aubel et al., 2007).

E. coli strain Nissle 1917 (O6:K5:H1) is a typical example of a nonpathogenic, commensal fecal *E. coli* isolate. Comparison of the genome structure of *E. coli* Nissle 1917 with other O6 strains, especially uropathogenic strains, has revealed striking structural similarities at the genomic level. It seems that the lack of defined virulence factors (e.g., *E. coli* alpha-hemolysin and P-fimbrial adhesins) combined with the expression of additional fitness factors (e.g., microcins, different iron uptake systems, adhesins, and proteases) supports its survival and successful colonization of the human gut and most likely contributes to the probiotic nature of this strain (Grozdanov et al., 2004).

Although *E. coli* does not represent a major group of bacteria of the intestinal microbiota, it is a normal and important inhabitant of the human gut. Isolation of a particular strain can therefore become a challenge. EcN has been fully characterized (Grozdanov et al., 2004; Sun et al., 2005) and has been identified by the use of different methods. Although conventional biochemical microbiological methods are reliable (G. W. Tannock, personal communication), they require several days to complete. Furthermore, it is presumed that the therapeutic effect of EcN is linked to the presence of the strain in the region of interest. It remains difficult, however, to follow the orally administered strain on its passage through the complex microbial environment of the intestine in vivo. We have transformed EcN, without alteration of strain-specific characteristics, with a plasmid carrying a *gfp* gene (pUC-gfp) to obtain EcN-GFP in order to enable in vivo detection. Following oral administration of a single dose containing 5×10^{10} CFU of EcN-GFP per ml to an animal model, green fluorescent colonies were readily detectable by fluorescence microscopy in luminal samples and also by immunohistochemistry in histological sections (Fig. 2). By this method, EcN-GFP was identified in fecal samples for initially 14 days and following direct selection by the administration of ampicillin until day 45. A limitation of the use of EcN-GFP is the instability of the marker in vivo, possibly due to the lack of applied selection pressure, while obvious ethical concerns do not allow its use in humans (Schultz et al., 2005). Because of this, and the variability of commensal *E. coli* strains that lack specific virulence factors, a PCR assay has been developed by Blum-Oehler et al. that allows accurate identification of this strain not only from pure cultures but also from fecal samples after its oral application in the presence of other *E. coli* strains (Blum-Oehler et al., 2003). Initially five PCR assays were developed which were based on the small cryptic plasmids or major fimbrial subunits, while the most specific results

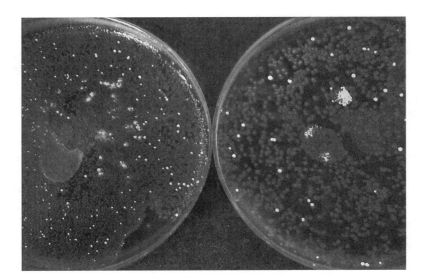

Figure 2 Fecal sample from a mouse following oral administration of green fluorescent protein expressing *E. coli* Nissle 1917 cultured on MacConkey agar plates and photographed under UV light. In this black and white image, colonies of fluorescent *E. coli* Nissle 1917 appear white in contrast to the gray colonies of the other organisms.

were obtained with primers based on DNA sequences from plasmid pMUT2. This plasmid is without any obvious function other than coding for a mobilization function. This plasmid-based PCR assay can be used to detect EcN directly from fecal samples without prior cultivation (Blum-Oehler et al., 2003) with a detection limit of 10^3 to 10^4 CFU of EcN per ml.

MECHANISMS OF PROBIOTIC ACTION

Perhaps the most appropriate definition for probiotics was published by an Expert Consultation at a meeting convened by the FAO/WHO in October, 2001: "Probiotics are live microorganisms which when administered in adequate amounts confer a health benefit on the host" (Sanders, 2003). Although the body of evidence for significant clinical benefits of probiotic therapy is growing, the underlying pathways that are utilized to mediate these effects remain largely unclear. In order to reach the lower gastrointestinal tract and to, at least temporarily, colonize, probiotic bacteria have to be equipped with a number of so-called fitness factors. EcN displays several properties that eventually allow the exertion of probiotic effects. Besides the obvious modulation of the host's intestinal microbiota, EcN is thought to either directly, or indirectly via mediators, influence the immune response and to have a profound effect on gut barrier function. These pathways are most likely the result of a complex interaction of host and bacterial characteristics which we are only just beginning to understand (Marco et al., 2006; Reid et al., 2006; Saavedra, 2007). In this context, the beneficial effect of probiotics, mainly lactobacilli but also EcN, in the prevention of allergies can be discussed (Rasche et al., 2007).

E. coli strain Nissle 1917 (O6:K5:H1) is a bacterium of the *Enterobacteriaceae* family, and certain strains of this serotype are capable of uropathogenicity. The uniqueness of EcN has been studied intensively, and it is evident that this strain exhibits a specific pattern of fitness factors to guarantee superior survival in a hostile environment but lacks prominent virulence factors (Grozdanov et al., 2004). This unique combination constitutes, most likely, the basis for the probiotic properties that we observe.

FITNESS FACTORS OF PROBIOTIC *E. COLI*

Early studies indicated a pronounced antagonism of EcN towards other *E. coli* strains and enterobacteria. In a letter to *Nature* in 1959, J. Papavassiliou announced the discovery of a new, very powerful antibiotic substance, colicin X, produced by EcN as the basis of this antagonism (Papavassiliou, 1959). Further characterization of colicin X indicated strong activity against 74 strains of *E. coli* but limited effect towards other intestinal pathogens like *Salmonella*, *Proteus*, and *Pseudomonas* (Papavassiliou, 1961). Later work showed that colicin X consists of the microcins H47 and M (Patzer et al., 2003). However, powerful antibacterial capabilities cannot by themselves guarantee survival of an organism in a highly competitive environment such as the intestinal microbiota; other fitness factors are also required. In bacteria, iron is an indispensable component in the generation of the energy source ATP. EcN produces at least six different iron uptake systems (enterobactin, salmochelin, aerobactin, yersiniabactin, ChuA, and EfeU), which is rare for a nonpathogenic strain but found more often in uropathogenic strains (Grosse et al., 2006; Valdebenito et al., 2006). Uropathogenic microorganisms of the O6:K5:H1 clone produce (with a few exceptions) alpha-hemolysin, CNF1, and P fimbriae. Also, these variants are all resistant to the bactericidal effects of the serum complement system. LPS are a key component of the outer membrane of *E. coli* and other gram-negative bacteria and are believed to play a significant role in serum resistance and other features of the cell surface. In contrast to uropathogenic strains, EcN displays an increased serum sensitivity (this is also in contrast to probiotic lactobacilli) and therefore decreased virulence. This has been attributed by Grozdanov et al. to a single nucleotide exchange resulting in an incomplete O antigen that is responsible for the semirough O6 LPS phenotype of EcN as indicated by the special smooth-and-rough colonial appearance on agar plates (Grozdanov et al., 2002). Further analysis of the genome structure and comparison of EcN to five other *E. coli* strains revealed that EcN carries no genes for alpha-hemolysin, CNF1, or P-fimbrial adhesins (mannose-resistant) but expresses type 1 and F1C fimbriae (Blum et al., 1995; Grozdanov et al., 2004). The exact links between these findings and their physiological consequences need to be studied further but certainly contribute to the efficient colonization of this strain (Nagy et al., 2005; Sun et al., 2005).

Antagonistic, antibacterial effects of *E. coli* M-17 were discovered in the early 1960s by Russian scientists and were, unfortunately, published only in Russian (Tamarin Iu, 1965; Iukhimenko et al., 1968; Grabovskaia, 1969). The first clinical observations on the relationship between *E. coli* M-17 and other *E. coli* strains were recorded in the 1970s in healthy children (Bila et al., 1971). The probiotic, antibacterial effect was partly attributed to a substance, produced by *E. coli* M-17, that inhibited the production of hemolysins active against sheep erythrocytes in mice (Stanislavsky et al., 1977).

PROBIOTIC EFFECTS OF *E. COLI* IN VITRO AND IN VIVO

The intestinal epithelial barrier in humans and animals separates the inside from the outside world. This separation is sophisticated as it allows nutrients and a controlled amount of bacteria and other antigens, etc., to enter the body while most bacteria and other microorganisms are confined to the lumen. The epithelial barrier function is the result of a complex interaction of luminal factors (e.g., microbiota), physical properties (e.g., mucus, epithelial cell layer, etc.), and the intestinal immune system. A breakdown of this tightly regulated homeostasis is seen in enteric infections but also in chronic diseases such as ulcerative colitis (UC) and Crohn's disease (CD), commonly referred to as inflammatory bowel diseases (IBD) (Schölmerich, 2006). Unique fitness factors make EcN a superior colonizer in the gastrointestinal ecosystem. Besides the already discussed antimicrobial properties of EcN leading to a modulation of the composition of the intestinal microbiota, other mechanisms have been elucidated affecting the host's immune system as well as gut barrier function. The observation that EcN protects gnotobiotic piglets against invasion by *Salmonella* (Mandel et al., 1995) led to further studies of the antagonistic effects of EcN. Gnotobiotic rats were challenged with *Candida albicans*. Prior monoassociation with EcN followed by *C. albicans* reduced the proliferation rate of the yeast, whereas EcN inoculation following *C. albicans* association had limited effects (Lorenz and Schulze, 1996). Altenhoefer et al. demonstrated in vitro in the INT407 cell line that EcN not only inhibited invasion by *Salmonella* but also by *Yersinia enterocolitica*, *Shigella flexneri*, *Listeria pneumophila*, and *Listeria monocytogenes* (Altenhoefer et al., 2004). This effect appeared to be independent of the production of microcins or physical contact of EcN with the INT407 cell line (Altenhoefer et al., 2004). Boudeau et al. confirmed the inhibitory effect on adhesion and invasion of EcN on adherent-invasive *E. coli* (Boudeau et al., 2003). This antagonism was then again put to the test in vivo based on a suggestion by Nissle that colonization of newborns with EcN might be of potential benefit (Nissle, 1916). Lodinova-Zadnikova et al. administered EcN orally to full-term and premature infants and demonstrated increased anti-SK22 antibodies of immunoglobulin A (IgA) and IgM isotypes in stool filtrates and in sera of colonized infants compared to controls (Lodinova-Zadnikova et al., 1992). This was later confirmed, and the authors concluded that EcN significantly stimulates specific humoral and cellular responses and simultaneously induces nonspecific natural immunity (Cukrowska et al., 2002). Further detailed analysis of the influence of EcN on the immune system was provided by Sturm et al., aiming to investigate the effect of EcN on peripheral and mucosal T-cell function (Sturm et al., 2005). While proliferation of peripheral blood T cells in response to antigen stimulation is necessary to mount a significant immune response, which may itself contribute to disease, this has been shown to be effectively downregulated by EcN while apoptosis was not increased, as seen in the treatment with anti-tumor necrosis factor alpha antibody (Lugering et al., 2001). The effect of EcN on lamina propria T cells (LPT) is quite different. LPT are important factors in maintaining the tightly regulated immunological homeostasis between the inside of the body and the lumen. Cell cycling on mucosal T cells was not suppressed by EcN. This differential effect on distinct T-cell populations might be the basis for immunoregulatory properties of EcN allowing a potent but limited inflammatory response possibly on the mucosal level without the possibility to recruit more T cells from the peripheral pool. This inflammatory cascade is regulated by cytokine signaling. Stimulation of peripheral blood T cells, LPT, or cell lines with live EcN or cell debris resulted in reduced interleukin-2 (IL-2), gamma interferon, and tumor necrosis factor alpha secretion and an upregulation of the secretion of regulatory IL-10, IL-8, and IL-1β (Otte and Podolsky, 2004; Sturm et al., 2005; Helwig et al., 2006). It was further shown that these effects were mediated by TLR-2 signaling, expressed on activated T cells (Sturm et al., 2005). TLRs have been recently shown to recognize microbes in order to initiate an appropriate immune response. Different TLRs are selectively activated by different microbial components (Takeda et al., 2003). This concept of recognition of EcN by TLRs was tested in TLR-2 and TLR-4 knockout mice. While EcN significantly ameliorated dextran sodium sulfate (DSS)-induced colitis and secretion of proinflammatory cytokines in wild-type animals, no effect was seen in either knockout (Grabig et al., 2006). Ukena et al. have chosen the broad approach of measuring gene expression in vitro on Caco-2 cells upon stimulation with EcN. The result was astounding in that EcN largely led to an up-regulation of proinflammatory genes and the secretion of MCP-1 protein, which is usually up-regulated in infection and inflammation. While the authors regarded this result as unexpected, they see a role of MCP-1 in protection of the host from bacterial infection (Ukena et al., 2005).

It has furthermore been demonstrated that EcN also strengthens the intestinal epithelial barrier. The family of defensins consists of human antimicrobial peptides, produced by the intestinal epithelium in order to limit access of enteric bacteria. Wehkamp et al. demonstrated that EcN induces human β-defensin-2 in intestinal epithelial cells via nuclear factor κB and AP-1 (Wehkamp et al., 2004). Important in this context is the finding that human β-defensin-2 is normally expressed only in cases of inflammation such as UC and, to a lesser degree, in CD (Wehkamp et al., 2003), possibly explaining the successful use of EcN in UC (Rembacken et al., 1999). This finding was not restricted to EcN and was observed with other probiotic strains as well (Wehkamp et al., 2004). Calprotectin, a calcium- and zinc-binding protein of the S100 family, is produced by neutrophils in response to stimulation with bacterial LPS and exerts antimicrobial effects. High levels of calprotectin are regarded as useful markers of IBD (Roseth, 2003). EcN has been shown to significantly increase the secretion of calprotectin in monoassociated piglets within 24 h of colonization (Splichal et al., 2005). Furthermore, EcN seems to directly influence properties of the paracellular pathway. Incubation of T84 cells with enteropathogenic *E. coli* leads to a disruption of tight junctions, while coincubation with EcN leads to an increase of zonula occludens-2 expression, its redistribution towards cell boundaries, and silencing of PKC isotypes, resulting in tight junction and epithelial barrier repair (Zyrek et al., 2007). However, Otte and Podolsky could not demonstrate an effect of EcN on barrier function including mucin production, modulation of resistance, etc., in HT-29 cells in contrast to the probiotic mixture VSL#3 (Otte and Podolsky, 2004). This tightening of the mucosal barrier was also seen in acute secretory diarrhea in a pig model of intestinal infection. Treatment with EcN prior to infection with the porcine enterotoxigenic *E. coli* Abbotstown (EcA) resulted in the absence of clinical signs and no overshooting secretory response upon stimulation with forskolin. In this model no histological inflammation was seen (Schroeder et al., 2006).

Further work regarding the probiotic effects of *E. coli* M-17 has been published. Shelkovaia et al. described the phenomenon of "selective destructive adsorption" of rotaviruses by *E. coli* M-17 as an important biological mechanism responsible for the protection of the body from rotavirus infection (Shelkovaia et al., 1991). These pronounced antimicrobial effects have led to interesting suggestions regarding the possible probiotic use of *E. coli* M-17. Klymniuk and Smirnov have assessed the effects of *E. coli* M-17 against the aerobic microbiota of the human skin and recommended *E. coli* M-17 for clinical testing for the correction of skin microbiocenoses and for preventing the development of pyoseptic complications of skin (Klymniuk and Smirnov, 1997).

PRECLINICAL IN VIVO DATA

Some of the preclinical data have been obtained using highly specialized animal models as discussed above. The potential clinical relevance has also been evaluated in several animal models for intestinal inflammation based on Nissle's initial observation of protection against gastrointestinal infection (Nissle, 1916). However, not all animal models have shown equal benefit, and acute colitis (commonly induced by various concentrations [1 to 5%] of DSS in the drinking water) was more resistant to treatment than chronic colitis. Using 5% DSS to induce colitis, we and others observed a significant reduction in the secretion of proinflammatory cytokines and other markers of intestinal inflammation, but no effect on the histological severity was seen (Schultz et al., 2004b; Kokesova et al., 2006). Using only 1.3% DSS to induce colitis, histological amelioration of the intestinal inflammation was also observed. In contrast, chronic colitis was more amenable to treatment. In a transfer model of chronic colitis (transfer of CD4$^+$ CD62L$^+$ T-lymphocytes from BALB/c mice in SCID mice) as well as in IL-10$^{-/-}$ mice, proinflammatory cytokine secretion was reduced and clinical markers of intestinal inflammation as well as histological findings improved (Schultz et al., 2004b; Kamada et al., 2005). EcN has also been investigated in an animal model with increased postinfectious visceral hyperalgesia resembling the features of human IBS. Inflammation was initiated in rats with colorectal instillation of TNBS, and the visceromotor reflex of abdominal wall muscles was determined by electromyographia. Control rats demonstrated an elevated level of the visceromotor reflex, while treatment with EcN abolished this finding, suggesting a possible role of EcN in patients with IBS (Liebregts et al., 2005).

In contrast to the effects of the probiotic EcN in vitro and in vivo using animal models of intestinal inflammation or infection, Duncker et al. assessed the effects of EcN in healthy young pigs with regard to the number and distribution of intestinal immune cells and the mucosal mRNA expression of cytokines and antimicrobial peptides. This particular animal model was used because of the anatomical and immunological similarity of its gastrointestinal tract to humans. As expected, EcN did not induce any toxicity, and furthermore, the authors concluded that EcN, apart from increasing the number of CD8$^+$ cells in the mucosa of the ascending colon, had only minor effects on the immune system in healthy individuals (Duncker et al., 2006).

E. coli M-17 has also been assessed in animal models for intestinal inflammation. Oral administration of 6 × 10^8 CFU of *E. coli* M-17 in a mouse model with chronic

DSS-induced colitis improved the disease activity index as well as reducing IFN-γ and IL-1β levels (Fitzpatrick et al., 2006). These effects were partly attributed to the inhibition of NF-κB and the subsequent secretion of proinflammatory cytokines. Interestingly, in comparison to VSL#3, live *E. coli* M-17 isolates were necessary to mediate this effect (Fitzpatrick et al., 2007).

CLINICAL USE OF PROBIOTIC *E. COLI*

Safety and Efficacy

Different probiotic bacteria of the species *E. coli* have been widely used in patients for a variety of mainly gastrointestinal disorders (Table 1). EcN was isolated in 1917 and has been available on the German market since then. In postmarketing surveillance studies, data from close to 4,500 patients were gathered prospectively and analyzed for indication, efficacy, and side effects (Krammer et al., 2006; Rohrenbach et al., 2007). Because it has few side effects, EcN is used widely for infants and children. Rohrenbach et al. analyzed prospective treatment data of 668 children aged up to 11 years (Rohrenbach et al., 2007). The dosage ranged from 10^8 CFU of EcN for babies and infants (<23 months) to 10×10^9 CFU of EcN for children (>23 months to <11 years) for a maximum of 12 weeks. In 86.7% of the patients ($n = 579$), EcN was used in the treatment of gastrointestinal disorders (acute and chronic diarrhea, constipation, etc.). Other indications ($n = 89$) included extraintestinal disorders such as eczema and an elevated susceptibility to infections. Overall, good efficacy and significant improvement of symptoms were scored by physicians for 84.4% of the children and by parents for 81.2% of the children. Different forms of diarrhea responded well to treatment with a significant reduction of stool frequency, while in the case of chronic constipation the stool frequency significantly increased. All in all, 20 cases of suspected side effects were noted (2.9%). These included flatulence, bloating, diarrhea, abdominal pain, nausea, and vomiting.

Krammer et al. analyzed prospective treatment data from 3,807 patients (163 infants, 505 children, 132 teenagers, and 3,007 adults gathered in 446 centers in Germany and Austria) (Krammer et al., 2006). The dosage ranged from up to 50×10^9 CFU of EcN for adults to 10×10^9 CFU of EcN for children and 10^8 CFU of EcN for toddlers and babies and was administered for up to 12 weeks. Again, EcN was mainly used in the treatment of gastrointestinal disorders ($n = 3,511$, 92.2%; mainly diarrhea and IBS). Other indications included infectious diseases, eczema, and urinary tract infections ($n = 296$,

7.8%). Overall, good efficacy and significant improvement of symptoms were scored by physicians for 81.4% of individuals and by parents for 77.8%. Again, treatment with EcN achieved a significant reduction in stool frequency in patients with chronic diarrhea and an increase in stool frequency in patients with chronic constipation. Of interest are the results concerning patients with IBS ($n = 679$). For these, significant improvement of abdominal pain, flatulence, bloating, and stool consistency was observed. Side effects as a result of treatment with EcN were recorded for 2.8% of patients ($n = 109$), of which almost all were confined to the gastrointestinal tract (bloating, flatulence, abdominal pain, nausea, and vomiting). Two patients developed erythema and pruritus.

Inflammatory Bowel Disease

Besides these large, open-label, postmarketing observations, EcN has been used in a number of clinical trials performed according to good clinical practice. Two trials demonstrated statistical equivalence of standard mesalazine treatment (1.5 g/day) and EcN (50×10^9 CFU) in the maintenance of remission of UC (Kruis et al., 1997, 2004). The observation period of the 2004 study spanned 1 year, and, also in 2004, the guidelines for diagnosis and treatment of UC as issued by the German Society of Gastroenterology and Digestive Diseases recommended EcN as an alternative to standard mesalazine treatment to maintain remission (Hoffmann et al., 2004). A smaller trial ($n = 60$/group) indicated the successful use of EcN in acute and remissive UC compared to 2.4 g of mesalazine per day (Rembacken et al., 1999). However, interpretation of the results is rather difficult because patients with exacerbation of mild to severe colitis were randomized and besides EcN or mesalazine, concomitant medication ranged from hydrocortisone acetate enemas to oral prednisone (30 to 60 mg/day). All patients received a 1-week course of gentamicin prior to treatment with EcN (Rembacken et al., 1999). In addition, a combination of EcN with mesalazine seems possible, since even high doses of the aminosalicylate do not harm EcN in vivo (T. Nguyen-Xuan, G. Blum-Oehler, et al., MON-G-241, presented at the 14th United European Gastroenterology week, Berlin, Germany, 2006). While EcN seems to confer significant benefits in the treatment of UC, only one small double-blind, placebo-controlled trial was initiated in active CD predominantly affecting the colon (Malchow, 1997). EcN was combined with steroid treatment, and emphasis was placed on the relapse rate after remission was reached and possible steroid-sparing effects. Because of the small number of patients, positive results did not reach statistical significance.

Table 1 Clinical trials and observations with *E. coli* Nissle 1917

Diagnosis or analysis[a]	Study design	No. of patients	Duration	Aim of study	Outcome	Reference
IBD						
Active and inactive CD predominantly in the colon (CDAI, >150)	Double-blind, randomized, placebo controlled	Group 1 (n = 16): prednisolone + EcN Group 2 (n = 12): prednisolone + placebo	1 yr	Steroid sparing effect Maintenance of remission	Improved maintenance of remission and steroid sparing effect (nonsignificant finding)	Malchow, 1997
Active and inactive UC	Double-blind, randomized, placebo controlled	Group 1 (n = 59): mesalazine (2.4 g/day) Group 2 (n = 57): EcN	1 yr	Time to relapse, rate of relapse, steroid sparing effect	EcN is as effective as mesalazine in maintaining remission	Rembacken et al., 1999
Inactive UC (CAI, ≤ 4)	Double-blind, randomized, placebo controlled	Group 1 (n = 50): EcN Group 2 (n = 53): mesalazine (1.5 g/day)	12 wks	Equivalence of EcN and mesalazine	No significant difference between EcN and mesalazine	Kruis et al., 1997
Inactive UC (CAI, ≤ 4)	Double-blind, randomized, placebo controlled	Group 1 (n = 162): EcN Group 2 (n = 165): mesalazine (1.5 g/day)	1 yr	Equivalence of EcN and mesalazine	EcN is as effective as mesalazine in maintaining remission (significant equivalence)	Kruis et al., 2004
Active pouchitis (PDAI, 13–15)	Case report	n = 2	315 days and 56 days, respectively	Induction and maintenance of remission	Significant reduction in PDAI score to 6 and 3, respectively	Kuzela et al., 2001
Diverticular disease						
Symptomatic uncomplicated diverticulosis	Open label	1st flare-up (n = 15): antibiotic + absorbent therapy for 1 wk 2nd flare-up (n = 15): see 1st flare-up followed by EcN for 5.2 wks	Up to 40 months follow-up	Maintenance of remission of diverticulosis	EcN increased remission periods and decreased symptoms	Fric and Zavoral, 2003
Diarrhea						
Acute diarrhea in infants and toddlers	Double-blind, randomized, placebo controlled	Group 1 (n = 58): EcN Group 2 (n = 55): placebo	Until response (10 days at maximum)	Time to response Effect on symptoms	EcN shortened the duration of symptoms	Henker et al., 2007
Prolonged diarrhea in infants and toddlers	Double-blind, randomized, placebo controlled	Group 1 (n = 75): EcN Group 2 (n = 76): placebo	21 days	Lasting reduction of symptoms	EcN was significantly superior to placebo	Henker et al., 2006

Modulation of Colonization in Full-Term and Premature Newborns

Indication	Study design	Study population	Duration	Parameter investigated	Results	Reference
Preventive colonization in full-term newborns	Double-blind, randomized, placebo controlled	Group 1 (n = 27): EcN Group 2 (n = 27): placebo	5 days treatment with 6 mo follow-up	Prevention of colonization with pathogenic and potentially pathogenic bacteria	Colonization with EcN in 90% for 6 mo; Significant reduction of pathogenic and potentially pathogenic bacteria	Lodinova-Zadnikova and Sonnenborn, 1997
Preventive colonization in full-term newborns	Open label	EcN: n = 23 Controls: n = 20 (historic sample)	5 days treatment with 6–12 mo follow-up	Development of the aerobic intestinal flora	Reduction of pathogenic and potentially pathogenic bacteria; Colonization in 10/16 children	Schroeder, 1992
Preventive colonization in full-term and premature newborns	Controlled	Group 1 (n = 22, full-term): EcN Group 2 (n = 9, preterm): placebo Group 3 (n = 9, preterm): untreated	5 days treatment with 3 wks follow-up	Immunological status	Increase of IgA and IgM isotypes in stools of both full-term and preterm infants	Lodinova-Zadnikova et al, 1992
Preventive colonization in premature newborns	Blind, randomized, placebo controlled	Group 1 (n = 34): EcN Group 2 (n = 27): placebo	5 days treatment with 3 wks follow-up	Immunological status	Proliferation of blood cells, increase of EcN-specific IgA and unspecific IgM	Cukrowska et al., 2002
Collagenous colitis						
Symptomatic collagenous colitis	Open label	EcN (n = 14)	4 wks	Effect on stool consistency and frequency	Significant clinical benefit	Tromm et al., 2004
Halitosis						
Gut-caused halitosis	Case report	n = 1	3 mo		Normalization of breath gas analysis	Henker et al., 2001
Postmarketing analysis						
Safety and efficacy for children	Prospective study	n = 668	Maximum, 12 wks	Analysis of indication, efficacy, and safety	Mainly gastrointestinal indications (86.7%); Side effects in 2.9%; Clinical benefit in 81.2 to 84.4%	Rohrenbach et al., 2007
Safety and efficacy for adults and children	Prospective study	n = 3,807	Maximum, 12 wks	Analysis of indication, efficacy, and safety	Mainly gastrointestinal indications (92.2%); Side effects in 2.8%; Clinical benefit in 81.4%	Krammer et al., 2006

[a]CDAI, Crohn's disease activity index; CAI, colitis activity index; PDAI, pediatric disease activity index.

Table 2 Clinical trials and observations with other probiotic *E. coli* preparations

Diagnosis	Strain used	Study design	No. of patients	Duration	Aim of study	Outcome	Reference
Small bowel inflammation	*E. coli* M-17	Open label	*n* = 20	1 mo	Healing of mucosal lesions as assessed by capsule endoscopy	Possible effect on mucosal healing	Adler, 2006

Preventive Colonization of Full-Term and Premature Newborns

Based on Nissle's initial observations (Nissle, 1916, 1918), EcN has been used to prevent colonization of the newborn's intestinal tract by potentially pathogenic microorganisms (Lodinova-Zadnikova and Sonnenborn, 1997). Oral administration of EcN (10^8 CFU) from day 1 to day 5 after birth significantly reduced the concentration of a range of pathogenic and potentially pathogenic microorganisms, and colonization with EcN was demonstrated in 94% of children of up to 6 months. Also in premature infants, similar treatment with EcN had important effects on immunological parameters such as blood cell proliferation and the secretion of IgA and IgM antibodies (Lodinova-Zadnikova et al., 1992; Cukrowska et al., 2002).

Acute and Prolonged Diarrhea in Infants and Toddlers

In 113 children with acute unspecific diarrhea (maximum duration, 3 days), EcN (1×10^8 to 3×10^8 CFU, depending on the age of the children), in comparison to a placebo, significantly improved symptoms in more patients (94.5% versus 67.2%) and shortened the time to response to treatment (2.5 versus 4.8 days) (Henker et al., 2007). Children (*n* = 151) with prolonged unspecific diarrhea (duration, between 4 and 14 days) also benefited from a similar EcN therapy plus initial rehydration. In comparison with a placebo, the response rates were significantly higher on days 14 (93.3% versus 65.8%) and 21 (98.7% versus 71.1%) (Henker et al., 2006).

Other Gastrointestinal Indications

Several other smaller or open-label trials have suggested that EcN is beneficial in other gastrointestinal disorders. While the exact etiology of pouchitis is unknown, an association with dysbiosis has been suggested (Lim et al., 2006). Effective use of EcN in this setting seems logical and has been tried (Kuzela et al., 2001) and also

suggested for other probiotic preparations (Gionchetti et al., 2003).

A small open-label trial investigated the use of EcN in symptomatic but uncomplicated diverticulosis and demonstrated increased remission periods and a decrease in symptoms (Fric and Zavoral, 2003). However, due to the design of trials used in assessing its usefulness for symptomatic collagenous colitis (Tromm et al., 2004), gut-caused halitosis (Henker et al., 2001), and IBS, the results of larger studies will have to be awaited before treatment recommendations can be given.

Extraintestinal Indications

There is mounting evidence in favor of the use of probiotic bacteria in the prevention and treatment of urinary tract infections (Falagas et al., 2006). This is based on the fact that uropathogenic bacteria, most commonly *E. coli*, originate from the bowel microbiota. In the early 1920s, EcN was an accepted treatment modality for recurrent urinary tract infections (Roerig, 1919, 1921). However, evidence was based on individual observations only and larger studies did not demonstrate the desired effect (unpublished data). Lately, lactobacillus-based preparations have seemed to be the preferred treatment alternative in urinary tract infections. As evidenced by large postmarketing analyses, EcN is also used for eczema and elevated susceptibility to infections (Krammer et al., 2006; Rohrenbach et al., 2007), but no robust data exist for these indications.

FUTURE PERSPECTIVES

EcN is a clinically relevant, well-characterized, and safe probiotic microorganism that temporarily colonizes the human (and animal) intestinal tract. It is effective in UC maintenance treatment. Besides the obvious areas of interest such as IBS, pouchitis, collagenous colitis, and even urinary tract infections, for which clinical observations and open-label trials have indicated its use to be beneficial and the results of larger trials are awaited, other possible uses are also being explored. Steidler et al. used a probiotic *Lactococcus lactis* strain to produce and locally secrete high levels of human IL-10 in the inflamed intestine (Steidler et al., 2000), and a phase I trial has been completed (Braat et al., 2006). However, a major disadvantage might be the short-lived persistence of *L. lactis* in the intestine, possibly requiring continuous administration. Westendorf et al. successfully tested EcN as a carrier of therapeutic molecules in a mouse model (Westendorf et al., 2005). The possible clinical relevance of this approach was suggested by Stritzker et al., who demonstrated in a mouse model of mammary cancer that EcN administered by tail vein injection specifically targeted tumor tissue. Colonization was found to be long lasting, as demonstrated by the use of an in vitro L-arabinose induction system to track EcN (Stritzker et al., 2007). The fact that EcN as a human fecal isolate is able to temporarily colonize the human intestinal tract makes the use of this strain also very attractive for other future developments. Hamer et al. used EcN and *Lactobacillus jensenii* 1153 following genetical engineering to successfully block in vitro infection of T cells and macrophages by human immunodeficiency virus primary isolates. In vivo, following colonization with EcN, approximately 50% of primates, challenged by a pathogenic human immunodeficiency virus strain, were protected from infection (Rao et al., 2005; Hamer et al., 2006).

CONCLUSION

The enterobacterium *E. coli* can be extraintestinally pathogenic (e.g., uropathogenic), intestinally pathogenic (e.g., enteropathogenic or enterohemorrhagic), and non-pathogenic or commensal (e.g., probiotic). The probiotic *E. coli* strain Nissle 1917 was isolated in 1917 from a soldier who appeared to be protected from gastrointestinal infections causing severe diarrhea in many of his comrades. Since that time, EcN has been studied intensively, not only with a focus on its apparent clinical use but also with a view to understanding how it counteracts the pathogenic mechanisms underlying a number of diseases. Its uniqueness, not only among other *E. coli* strains but also among other probiotic microorganisms, is evident. While being the subject of research for many other indications, this strain seems to be particularly relevant as an alternative to mesalazine in the maintenance of remission of UC and has potential for the treatment of IBS.

The cited work by M. Schultz was funded through a grant by the Deutsche Morbus Crohn/Colitis ulzerosa Vereinigung e. V. (German Crohn's and Colitis Foundation), the ReForM program by the University of Regensburg, Germany, and Ardeypharm GmbH, Herdecke, Germany.

References

Adlerberth, I., F. Jalil, B. Carlsson, L. Mellander, A. L. Hanson, P. Larsson, K. Khalil, and A. Wold. 1998. High turnover rate of *Escherichia coli* strains in the intestinal flora of infants in Pakistan. *Epidemiol. Infect.* **121:**587–598.

Altenhoefer, A., S. Oswald, U. Sonnenborn, C. Enders, J. Schulze, J. Hacker, and T. A. Oelschlaeger. 2004. The probiotic *Escherichia coli* strain Nissle 1917 interferes with invasion of human intestinal epithelial cells by different enteroinvasive bacterial pathogens. *FEMS Immunol. Med. Microbiol.* **40:**223–229.

Bila, S. O., I. A. Shulichenko, and A. A. Sutulova. 1971. The relationship between *Escherichia coli* from the intestines of healthy children and strain M-17-a producing colibacterine. *Mikrobiol. Zh.* **33:**787–788.

Blum, G., R. Marre, and J. Hacker. 1995. Properties of *Escherichia coli* strains of serotype O6. *Infection* **23:**234–236.

Blum-Oehler, G., S. Oswald, K. Eiteljorge, U. Sonnenborn, J. Schulze, W. Kruis, and J. Hacker. 2003. Development of strain-specific PCR reactions for the detection of the probiotic *Escherichia coli* strain Nissle 1917 in fecal samples. *Res. Microbiol.* **154:**59–66.

Boudeau, J., L. A. Glasser, S. Julien, J. F. Colombel, and A. Darfeuille-Michaud. 2003. Inhibitory effect of probiotic *Escherichia coli* strain Nissle 1917 on adhesion to and invasion of intestinal epithelial cells by adherent-invasive *E. coli* strains isolated from patients with Crohn's disease. *Aliment. Pharmacol. Ther.* **18:**45–56.

Braat, H., P. Rottiers, W. D. Hommes, N. Huyghebaert, E. Remaut, P. J. Remon, S. J. van Deventer, S. Neirynck, P. M. Peppelenbosch, and L. Steidler. 2006. A phase I trial with transgenic bacteria expressing interleukin-10 in Crohn's disease. *Clin. Gastroenterol. Hepatol.* **4:**754–759.

Cukrowska, B., R. Lodinova-Zadnikova, C. Enders, U. Sonnenborn, J. Schulze, and H. Tlaskalova-Hogenova. 2002. Specific proliferative and antibody responses of premature infants to intestinal colonization with nonpathogenic probiotic *E. coli* strain Nissle 1917. *Scand. J. Immunol.* **55:**204–209.

Cursino, L., D. Smajs, J. Smarda, R. M. Nardi, J. R. Nicoli, E. Chartone-Souza, and A. M. Nascimento. 2006. Exoproducts of the *Escherichia coli* strain H22 inhibiting some enteric pathogens both in vitro and in vivo. *J. Appl. Microbiol.* **100:**821–829.

Duncker, S. C., A. Lorentz, B. Schroeder, G. Breves, and S. C. Bischoff. 2006. Effect of orally administered probiotic *E. coli* strain Nissle 1917 on intestinal mucosal immune cells of healthy young pigs. *Vet. Immunol. Immunopathol.* **111:**239–250.

Duval-Iflah, Y., M. F. Ouriet, C. Moreau, N. Daniel, J. C. Gabilan, and P. Raibaud. 1982. Implantation of a strain of "*Escherichia coli*" in the digestive tract of human new-borns: barrier effect against antibioresistant "*E. coli*" (author's translation). *Ann. Microbiol.* (Paris) **133:**393–408. (In French.)

Escherich, T. 1885. Die Darmbakterien des Neugeborenen und Saeuglings. *Fortschr. Med.* **16:**512–522.

Falagas, E. M., I. G. Betsi, T. Tokas, and S. Athanasiou. 2006. Probiotics for prevention of recurrent urinary tract infections in women: a review of the evidence from microbiological and clinical studies. *Drugs* 66:1253–1261.

Fitzpatrick, L. R., J. Small, E. Bostwick, R. Hoerr, and W. A. Koltun. 2006. Effects of the probiotic *E. coli* strain M-17 on chronic dextran sulfate sodium-induced colitis in mice. *Gastroenterology* 130:A313.

Fitzpatrick, L. R., J. Small, E. Bostwick, R. Hoerr, L. W. Maines, and A. W. Koltun. 2007. In vitro effects of the probiotic *Escherichia coli* strain M-17: inhibition of nuclear factor-kappa B and pro-inflammatory cytokines. *Gastroenterology* 112:A400.

Fric, P., and M. Zavoral. 2003. The effect of non-pathogenic *Escherichia coli* in symptomatic uncomplicated diverticular disease of the colon. *Eur. J. Gastroenterol. Hepatol.* 15:313–315.

Gewirtz, A. T. 2007. TLRs in the gut. III. Immune responses to flagellin in Crohn's disease: good, bad, or irrelevant? *Am. J. Physiol. Gastrointest. Liver Physiol.* 292:G706–G710.

Gionchetti, P., F. Rizzello, U. Helwig, A. Venturi, M. K. Lammers, P. Brigidi, B. Vitali, G. Poggioli, M. Miglioli, and M. Campieri. 2003. Prophylaxis of pouchitis onset with probiotic therapy: a double-blind placebo controlled trial. *Gastroenterology* 124:12–22.

Grabig, A., D. Paclik, C. Guzy, A. Dankof, D. C. Baumgart, J. Erckenbrecht, B. Raupach, U. Sonnenborn, J. Eckert, R. R. Schumann, B. Wiedenmann, A. U. Dignass, and A. Sturm. 2006. *Escherichia coli* strain Nissle 1917 ameliorates experimental colitis via toll-like receptor 2- and toll-like receptor 4-dependent pathways. *Infect. Immun.* 74:4075–4082.

Grabovskaia, B. K. 1969. The antagonistic activity of *Escherichia coli* strain M-17-P. *Zh. Mikrobiol. Epidemiol. Immunobiol.* 46:104–107.

Grosse, C., J. Scherer, D. Koch, M. Otto, N. Taudte, and G. Grass. 2006. A new ferrous iron-uptake transporter, EfeU (YcdN), from *Escherichia coli*. *Mol. Microbiol.* 62:120–131.

Grozdanov, L., U. Zahringer, G. Blum-Oehler, L. Brade, A. Henne, A. Y. Knirel, U. Schombel, J. Schulze, U. Sonnenborn, G. Gottschalk, J. Hacker, T. E. Rietschel, and U. Dobrindt. 2002. A single nucleotide exchange in the *wzy* gene is responsible for the semirough O6 lipopolysaccharide phenotype and serum sensitivity of *Escherichia coli* strain Nissle 1917. *J. Bacteriol.* 184:5912–5925.

Grozdanov, L., C. Raasch, J. Schulze, U. Sonnenborn, G. Gottschalk, J. Hacker, and U. Dobrindt. 2004. Analysis of the genome structure of the nonpathogenic probiotic *Escherichia coli* strain Nissle 1917. *J. Bacteriol.* 186:5432–5441.

Hamer, D., L. McHugh, M. McKinney, C. Richards, K. Schully, L. Lagenaur, and S. Rao. 2006. Live microbial microbicides for HIV. *Retrovirology* 3(Suppl. 1):S50.

Helwig, U., K. M. Lammers, F. Rizzello, P. Brigidi, V. Rohleder, E. Caramelli, P. Gionchetti, J. Schrezenmeir, U. R. Foelsch, S. Schreiber, and M. Campieri. 2006. Lactobacilli, bifidobacteria and *E. coli* Nissle induce pro- and anti-inflammatory cytokines in peripheral blood mononuclear cells. *World J. Gastroenterol.* 12:5978–5986.

Henker, J., B. Blokhin, J. Bolbot, V. Maydannik, L. Joeres, C. Wolff, and J. Schulze. 2006. Successful therapy of unspecific prolonged diarrhea in infants and toddlers with the probiotic *E. coli* Nissle 1917. *Gastroenterology* 130:A315.

Henker, J., M. Laass, B. M. Blokhin, Y. K. Bolbot, V. G. Maydannik, M. Elze, C. Wolff, and J. Schulze. 2007. The probiotic *Escherichia coli* strain Nissle 1917 (EcN) stops acute diarrhoea in infants and toddlers. *Eur. J. Pediatr.* 166:311–318.

Henker, J., F. Schuster, and K. Nissler. 2001. Successful treatment of gut-caused halitosis with a suspension of living non-pathogenic *Escherichia coli* bacteria—a case report. *Eur. J. Pediatr.* 160:592–594.

Hoffmann, J. C., M. Zeitz, C. S. Bischoff, J. H. Brambs, P. H. Bruch, H. J. Buhr, A. Dignass, I. Fischer, W. Fleig, R. U. Folsch, K. Herrlinger, W. Hohne, G. Jantschek, B. Kaltz, M. K. Keller, U. Knebel, J. A. Kroesen, W. Kruis, H. Matthes, G. Moser, S. Mundt, C. Pox, M. Reinshagen, A. Reissmann, J. Riemann, G. Rogler, W. Schmiegel, J. Scholmerich, S. Schreiber, O. Schwandner, K. H. Selbmann, E. F. Stange, M. Utzig, and C. Wittekind. 2004. Diagnosis and therapy of ulcerative colitis: results of an evidence based consensus conference by the German Society of Digestive and Metabolic Diseases and the competence network on inflammatory bowel disease. *Z. Gastroenterol.* 42:979–983.

Iukhimenko, N. L., I. P. Emel'ianov, S. M. Lenkina, E. I. Tron, and M. L. Tishina. 1968. The spectrum of activity of a polycolicinogenic strain of *E. coli* M-17 with regard to enterobacteria. *Zh. Mikrobiol. Epidemiol. Immunobiol.* 45:11–14.

Kamada, N., N. Inoue, T. Hisamatsu, S. Okamoto, K. Matsuoka, T. Sato, H. Chinen, K. S. Hong, T. Yamada, Y. Suzuki, T. Suzuki, N. Watanabe, K. Tsuchimoto, and T. Hibi. 2005. Nonpathogenic *Escherichia coli* strain Nissle 1917 prevents murine acute and chronic colitis. *Inflamm. Bowel. Dis.* 11:455–463.

Klymniuk, I. S., and V. V. Smirnov. 1997. The action of bacterial antagonists on the aerobic microflora of human skin. *Mikrobiol. Z.* 59:53–60.

Kokesova, A., L. Frolova, M. Kverka, D. Sokol, P. Rossmann, J. Bartova, and H. Tlaskalova-Hogenova. 2006. Oral administration of probiotic bacteria (*E. coli* Nissle, *E. coli* O83, *Lactobacillus casei*) influences the severity of dextran sodium sulfate-induced colitis in BALB/c mice. *Folia Microbiol.* 51:478–484.

Krammer, H. J., H. Kamper, R. von Bunau, E. Zieseniss, C. Stange, F. Schlieger, I. Clever, and J. Schulze. 2006. Probiotic drug therapy with *E. coli* strain Nissle 1917 (EcN): results of a prospective study of the records of 3,807 patients. *Z. Gastroenterol.* 44:651–656.

Kruis, W., P. Fric, J. Pokrotnieks, B. Fixa, M. Kascak, A. M. Kamm, J. Weismueller, C. Beglinger, M. Stolte, C. Wolff, and J. Schulze. 2004. Maintaining remission of ulcerative colitis with the probiotic *Escherichia coli* Nissle 1917 is as effective as with standard mesalazine. *Gut* 53:1617–1623.

Kruis, W., E. Schutz, P. Fric, B. Fixa, G. Judmaier, and M. Stolte. 1997. Double-blind comparison of an oral *Escherichia coli* preparation and mesalazine in maintaining remission of ulcerative colitis. *Aliment. Pharmacol. Ther.* 11:853–858.

Kuzela, L., M. Kascak, and A. Vavrecka. 2001. Induction and maintenance of remission with nonpathogenic *Escherichia coli* in patients with pouchitis. *Am. J. Gastroenterol.* 96:3218–3219.

Liebregts, T., B. Adam, A. Bertel, S. Jones, J. Schulze, C. Enders, U. Sonnenborn, K. Lackner, and G. Holtmann. 2005. Effect of *E. coli* Nissle 1917 on post-inflammatory visceral sensory function in a rat model. *Neurogastroenterol. Motil.* 17:410–414.

Lim, M., P. Sagar, P. Finan, D. Burke, and H. Schuster. 2006. Dysbiosis and pouchitis. *Br. J. Surg.* 93:1325–1334.

Lodinova-Zadnikova, R., and U. Sonnenborn. 1997. Effect of preventive administration of a nonpathogenic *Escherichia coli* strain on the colonization of the intestine with microbial pathogens in newborn infants. *Biol. Neonate.* 71:224–232.

Lodinova-Zadnikova, R., H. Tlaskalova-Hogenova, and U. Sonnenborn. 1992. Local and serum antibody response in full-term and premature infants after artificial colonization of the intestine with *E. coli* strain Nissle 1917 (Mutaflor©). *Pediatr. Allergy Immunol.* 3:43–48.

Lorenz, A., and J. Schulze. 1996. Establishment of *E. coli* Nissle 1917 and its interaction with *Candida albicans* in gnotobiotic rats. *Microecol. Ther.* 24:45–51.

Lugering, A., M. Schmidt, N. Lugering, G. H. Pauels, W. Domschke, and T. Kucharzik. 2001. Infliximab induces apoptosis in monocytes from patients with chronic active Crohn's disease by using a caspase-dependent pathway. *Gastroenterology* 121:1145–1157.

Malchow, H. A. 1997 Crohn's disease and *Escherichia coli*. A new approach in therapy to maintain remission of colonic Crohn's disease? *J. Clin. Gastroenterol.* 25:653–658.

Mandel, L., I. Trebichavsky, I. Splichal, and J. Schulze. 1995. Stimulation of intestinal immune cells by *E. coli* in gnotobiotic piglets, p. 463–464. *In* J. Mestecky (ed.), *Advances in Mucosal Immunology.* Plenum Press, New York, NY.

Marco, M. L., S. Pavan, and M. Kleerebezem. 2006. Towards understanding molecular modes of probiotic action. *Curr. Opin. Biotechnol.* 17:204–210.

Metchnikoff, E., and E. Chalmers. 1907. *The Prolongation of Life: Optimistic Studies*, p. 161. Heinemann, London, United Kingdom.

Nagy, G., U. Dobrindt, L. Grozdanov, J. Hacker, and L. Emody. 2005. Transcriptional regulation through RfaH contributes to intestinal colonization by *Escherichia coli*. *FEMS Microbiol. Lett.* 244:173–180.

Nascimento, A. M., C. E. Campos, E. P. Campos, J. L. Azevedo, and E. Chartone-Souza. 1999. Re-evaluation of antibiotic and mercury resistance in *Escherichia coli* populations isolated in 1978 from Amazonian rubber tree tappers and Indians. *Res. Microbiol.* 150:407–411.

Nissle, A. 1916. Ueber die Grundlagen einer neuen ursaechlichen Bekaempfung der pathologischen Darmflora (On the fundamentals for new causal control of pathological intestinal microflora). *Dtsch. Med. Wochenschr.* 42:1181–1184.

Nissle, A. 1918. Die antagonistische Behandlung chronischer Darmstoerungen mit Colibakterien (The antagonistical therapy of chronic intestinal disturbances). *Med. Klinik* 1918:29–30.

Nowrouzian, F., B. Hesselmar, R. Saalman, I. L. Strannegard, N. Aberg, A. E. Wold, and I. Adlerberth. 2003. *Escherichia coli* in infants' intestinal microflora: colonization rate, strain turnover, and virulence gene carriage. *Pediatr. Res.* 54:8–14.

Otte, J. M., and D. K. Podolsky. 2004. Functional modulation of enterocytes by gram-positive and gram-negative microorganisms. *Am. J. Physiol. Gastrointest. Liver Physiol.* 286:G613–G626.

Papavassiliou, J. 1959. Production of colicines in Simmons's citrate agar. *Nature* 184:1339–1340.

Papavassiliou, J. 1961. Biological characteristics of colicine X. *Nature* 190:110.

Patzer, S. I., M. R. Baquero, D. Bravo, F. Moreno, and K. Hantke. 2003. The colicin G, H and X determinants encode microcins M and H47, which might utilize the catecholate siderophore receptors FepA, Cir, Fiu and IroN. *Microbiology* 149:2557–2570.

Rao, S., S. Hu, L. McHugh, K. Lueders, K. Henry, Q. Zhao, R. A. Fekete, S. Kar, S. Adhya, and D. H. Hamer. 2005. Toward a live microbial microbicide for HIV: commensal bacteria secreting an HIV fusion inhibitor peptide. *Proc. Natl. Acad. Sci. USA* 102:11993–11998.

Rasche, C., C. Wolfram, M. Wahls, and M. Worm. 2007. Differential immunomodulating effects of inactivated probiotic bacteria on the allergic immune response. *Acta Derm. Venereol* 87:305–311.

Reid, G., S. O. Kim, and G. K. Kohler. 2006. Selecting, testing and understanding probiotic microorganisms. *FEMS Immunol. Med. Microbiol.* 46:149–157.

Rembacken, B. J., A. M. Snelling, P. M. Hawkey, D. M. Chalmers, and A. T. Axon. 1999. Non-pathogenic *Escherichia coli* versus mesalazine for the treatment of ulcerative colitis: a randomised trial. *Lancet* 354:635.

Roerig, F. 1919. Behandlung der Koliinfection der Harnwege mit Mutaflor (Treatment of *E. coli* associated urinary tract infections with Mutaflor). *Munch. Med. Wochenschr.* 50:1442–1443.

Roerig, F. 1921. Weiteres ueber Mutaflor bei Koliinfection der Harnwege. *Munch. Med. Wochenschr.* 31:480–481.

Rohrenbach, J., A. Matthess, R. Maier, R. von Bunau, E. Zieseniss, C. Stange, and J. Schulze. 2007. *Escherichia coli* Stamm Nissle 1917 (EcN) bei Kindern (*E. coli* Nissle 1917 in children). *Kinder- und Jugendarzt* 38:1–5.

Roseth, G. A. 2003. Determination of faecal calprotectin, a novel marker of organic gastrointestinal disorders. *Dig. Liver Dis.* 35:607–609.

Saavedra, J. M. 2007. Use of probiotics in pediatrics: rationale, mechanisms of action, and practical aspects. *Nutr. Clin. Pract.* 22:351–365.

Sanders, M. E. 2003. Probiotics: considerations for human health. *Nutr. Rev.* 61:91–99.

Schölmerich, J. 2006. Inflammatory bowel disease: Pandora's box, present and future. *Ann. N. Y. Acad. Sci.* 1072:365–378.

Schroeder, B., S. Duncker, S. Barth, R. Bauerfeind, A. D. Gruber, S. Deppenmeier, and G. Breves. 2006. Preventive effects of the probiotic *Escherichia coli* strain Nissle 1917 on acute secretory diarrhea in a pig model of intestinal infection. *Dig. Dis. Sci.* 51:724–731.

Schultz, M., C. Gottl, R. J. Young, P. Iwen, and J. A. Vanderhoof. 2004a. Administration of oral probiotic bacteria to pregnant women causes temporary infantile colonization. *J. Pediatr. Gastroenterol. Nutr.* 38:293–297.

Schultz, M., U. G. Strauch, H. J. Linde, S. Watzl, F. Obermeier, C. Gottl, N. Dunger, N. Grunwald, J. Scholmerich, and H. C. Rath. 2004b. Preventive effects of *Escherichia coli* strain Nissle 1917 on acute and chronic intestinal inflammation in two different murine models of colitis. *Clin. Diagn. Lab. Immunol.* **11**:372–378.

Schultz, M., S. Watzl, T. A. Oelschlaeger, H. Rath, C. Goettl, N. Lehn, J. Schoelmerich, and H. J. Linde. 2005. Green fluorescent protein for detection of the probiotic microorganism *Escherichia coli* strain Nissle (EcN) in vivo. *J. Microbiol. Methods* **61**:389–398.

Shelkovaia, N. G., L. G. Kupchinskii, V. A. Znamenskii, and V. M. Bondarenko. 1991. [An electron microscopic study of the interaction of bacterial intestinal microflora and rotavirus virions]. *Zh. Mikrobiol. Epidemiol. Immunobiol.* **1991**:18–21. (In Russian.)

Smarda, J., D. Smajs, H. Lhotova, and D. Dedicova. 2007. Occurrence of strains producing specific antibacterial inhibitory agents in five genera of *Enterobacteriaceae*. *Curr. Microbiol.* **54**:113-118.

Splichal, I., M. K. Fagerhol, I. Trebichavsky, A. Splichalova, and J. Schulze. 2005. The effect of intestinal colonization of germ-free pigs with *Escherichia coli* on calprotectin levels in plasma, intestinal and bronchoalveolar lavages. *Immunobiology* **209**:681–687.

Stanislavsky, S. E., V. V. Bogdanova, D. I. Kirpatovsky, and M. ZhvanetskayaI. 1977. Isolation and immunochemical characteristics of the immunodepressive substance from *Escherichia coli*. *J. Hyg. Epidemiol. Microbiol. Immunol.* **21**:84–94.

Steidler, L., W. Hans, L. Schotte, S. Neirynck, F. Obermeier, W. Falk, W. Fiers, and E. Remaut. 2000. Treatment of murine colitis by *Lactococcus lactis* secreting interleukin-10. *Science* **289**:1352–1355.

Stritzker, J., S. Weibel, P. J. Hill, T. A. Oelschlaeger, W. Goebel, and A. A. Szalay. 2007. Tumor-specific colonization, tissue distribution, and gene induction by probiotic *Escherichia coli* Nissle 1917 in live mice. *Int. J. Med. Microbiol.* **297**:151–162.

Sturm, A., K. Rilling, D. C. Baumgart, K. Gargas, T. Abou-Ghazale, B. Raupach, J. Eckert, R. R. Schumann, C. Enders, U. Sonnenborn, B. Wiedenmann, and A. U. Dignass. 2005. *Escherichia coli* Nissle 1917 distinctively modulates T cell cycling and expansion via toll-like receptor 2 signaling. *Infect. Immun.* **73**:1452–1465.

Sun, J., F. Gunzer, A. M. Westendorf, J. Buer, M. Scharfe, M. Jarek, F. Goessling, H. Bloecker, and A. P. Zeng. 2005. Genomic peculiarity of coding sequences and metabolic potential of probiotic *Escherichia coli* strain Nissle 1917 inferred from raw genome data. *J. Biotechnol.* **117**: 147–161.

Takeda, K., T. Kaisho, and S. Akira. 2003. Toll-like receptors. *Annu. Rev. Immunol.* **21**:335–376.

Tamarin Iu, A. 1965. [Antagonistic activity of *E. coli* M-17 on solid media containing different amounts of sodium chloride]. *Zh. Mikrobiol. Epidemiol. Immunobiol.* **42**:143–144. (In Russian.)

Tromm, A., U. Niewerth, M. Khoury, E. Baestlein, G. Wilhelms, J. Schulze, and M. Stolte. 2004. The probiotic *E. coli* strain Nissle 1917 for the treatment of collagenous colitis: first results of an open-label trial. *Z. Gastroenterol.* **42**:365–369.

Ukena, S. N., A. M. Westendorf, W. Hansen, M. Rohde, R. Geffers, S. Coldewey, S. Suerbaum, J. Buer, and F. Gunzer. 2005. The host response to the probiotic *Escherichia coli* strain Nissle 1917: specific up-regulation of the proinflammatory chemokine MCP-1. *BMC Med. Genet.* **6**:43.

Valdebenito, M., A. L. Crumbliss, G. Winkelmann, and K. Hantke. 2006. Environmental factors influence the production of enterobactin, salmochelin, aerobactin, and yersiniabactin in *Escherichia coli* strain Nissle 1917. *Int. J. Med. Microbiol.* **296**:513–520.

van Aubel, R. A., A. M. Keestra, D. J. Krooshoop, W. van Eden, and J. P. van Putten. 2007. Ligand-induced differential cross-regulation of Toll-like receptors 2, 4 and 5 in intestinal epithelial cells. *Mol. Immunol.* **44**:3702–3714.

Wehkamp, J., J. Harder, K. Wehkamp, B. Wehkamp-von Meissner, M. Schlee, C. Enders, U. Sonnenborn, S. Nuding, S. Bengmark, K. Fellermann, J. M. Schroeder, and E. F. Stange. 2004. NF-kappaB- and AP-1-mediated induction of human beta defensin-2 in intestinal epithelial cells by *Escherichia coli* Nissle 1917: a novel effect of a probiotic bacterium. *Infect. Immun.* **72**:5750–5758.

Wehkamp, J., J. Harder, M. Weichenthal, O. Mueller, K. R. Herrlinger, K. Fellermann, J. M. Schroeder, and E. F. Stange. 2003. Inducible and constitutive beta-defensins are differentially expressed in Crohn's disease and ulcerative colitis. *Inflamm. Bowel Dis.* **9**:215–223.

Westendorf, A. M., F. Gunzer, S. Deppenmeier, D. Tapadar, J. K. Hunger, M. A. Schmidt, J. Buer, and D. Bruder. 2005. Intestinal immunity of *Escherichia coli* Nissle 1917: a safe carrier for therapeutic molecules. *FEMS Immunol. Med. Microbiol.* **43**:373–384.

Wolf, M. K. 1997. Occurrence, distribution, and associations of O and H serogroups, colonization factor antigens, and toxins of enterotoxigenic *Escherichia coli*. *Clin. Microbiol. Rev.* **10**:569–584.

Zyrek, A. A., C. Cichon, S. Helms, C. Enders, U. Sonnenborn, and M. A. Schmidt. 2007. Molecular mechanisms underlying the probiotic effects of *Escherichia coli* Nissle 1917 involve ZO-2 and PKCzeta redistribution resulting in tight junction and epithelial barrier repair. *Cell. Microbiol.* **9**:804–816.

Therapeutic Microbiology: Probiotics and Related Strategies
Edited by J. Versalovic and M. Wilson
© 2008 ASM Press, Washington, DC

Kasipathy Kailasapathy

8

Formulation, Administration, and Delivery of Probiotics

Modern consumers are increasingly interested in their personal health and expect the food they eat to be healthy or even capable of preventing illness. Foods are no longer considered by consumers solely in terms of taste and immediate nutritional needs, but also in terms of their ability to provide specific benefits above and beyond their basic nutritional value. Functional foods targeted towards gut health currently provide the largest segment of the functional food market in Europe, Japan, and Australia (Hilliam and Young, 2000; Heasman and Mellentin, 2001). The recognition of cultured dairy products with probiotic bacteria as functional foods that provide health benefits beyond basic nutrition and the emerging clinical evidence of their potential in preventing certain diseases have boosted their consumption (Playne et al., 2003; Boylston et al., 2004). There is growing scientific evidence to suggest that the maintenance of a healthy gut microbiota may provide protection against gastrointestinal (GI) disorders including infections and inflammatory bowel diseases.

The emergence of antibiotic-resistant bacteria and natural ways of suppressing the growth of pathogens has contributed to the growth of probiotic foods and nutraceuticals. Probiotic bacteria not only compete and suppress "unhealthy fermentation" in the human intestine but also produce a number of beneficial health effects of their own (Goldin, 1998).

The reported therapeutic potential and health benefits of probiotic bacteria are enhancement of immunity against intestinal infections, immune enhancement, prevention of diarrheal diseases, prevention of colon cancer, prevention of hypercholesterolemia, improvement in lactose utilization, prevention of upper GI tract diseases, and stabilization of the gut mucosal barrier (Kailasapathy and Chin, 2000).

Tissier (1906) originally proposed the concept of beneficial bacteria. He advocated the administration of *Bifidobacterium* to infants with diarrhea, based on the concept that the beneficial bifidobacteria will replace the "bad bacteria" responsible for causing the intestinal disturbance. Metchnikoff (1907) recommended the consumption of yogurt containing *Lactobacillus* spp. The consumed bacteria were to replace toxin-producing bacteria present in the intestines. He suggested that the long life of Bulgarian peasants resulted from the consumption of fermented milk products. The term probiotic,

Kasipathy Kailasapathy, Probiotics and Encapsulated Functional Foods Research Unit, School of Natural Sciences, Centre for Plant and Food Science, University of Western Sydney, Locked Bag 1797, South Penrith DC, NSW 1797, Australia.

meaning "for life," was first coined in the 1960s in order to describe "substances secreted by one microorganism that stimulate the growth of another" (Lilly and Stillwell, 1965). Parker (1974) referred to the term probiotics with reference to animal feed supplements. However, the role of these beneficial bacteria in promoting positive health benefits upon the host has been fully recognized only in the last 2 decades. Fuller (1989) redefined the word probiotics as "viable micro-organisms that contribute to intestinal microbial balance and have the potential to improve the health of their human host." Recently, probiotics have been defined as "live micro-organisms which, when administered in adequate amounts, confer a health benefit on the host" (Reid et al., 2003).

Probiotics are live microbial feed supplements that have been used for many years in the animal feed industry. However, probiotics are now widely used in the manufacturing of fermented dairy products. Probiotic bacteria have been increasingly incorporated into fermented dairy products, including yogurts, soft-semihard cheeses, ice cream, and frozen fermented dairy desserts (Anal and Singh, 2007).

Many different organisms are used as probiotics; however, *Lactobacillus acidophilus*, *Lactobacillus casei*, *Bifidobacterium bifidum*, *Bifidobacterium longum*, and *Saccharomyces boulardii* are most frequently used as probiotics in products for human consumption (Playne, 1994). Generally *Lactobacillus* and *Bifidobacterium* strains are used in the development of probiotic products intended for human consumption due to the belief that these bacteria are members of the intestinal microbiota and are also considered "generally safe" (Berg, 1998; Klein et al., 1998).

A probiotic must have good technological properties so that it can be manufactured and incorporated into food products without losing viability and functionality or creating unpleasant flavors or textures in the product. Food and Agriculture Organization (FAO) and World Health Organization (WHO) guidelines (FAO/WHO, 2001, 2002) suggest that probiotic bacteria incorporated into food products must demonstrate their tolerance to gastric juices and bile in order to survive during their transit through the gut. Additionally, probiotic bacteria must be capable of colonizing the GI tract, and they must be safe and have the potential to maintain their efficiency during the shelf life of the product. Several aspects, including safety, functional, and technological characteristics, must be taken into consideration in the selection process for probiotic microorganisms. Potential probiotic bacteria should have some or all of the following functional properties: (i) tolerance to gastric acid and intestinal bile, enzyme, and oxygen (incorporated during processing); (ii) ability to adhere to host epithelial cells;

(iii) ability to colonize the GI tract; (iv) pathogen exclusion; (v) production of antimicrobial substances toward pathogens; (vi) nonpathogenicity and noncarcinogenicity; and (vii) characteristics favoring a well-balanced microbial gut ecosystem (Kailasapathy and Rybka, 1997). Careful screening of probiotic bacteria for their technological suitability can also allow the selection of strains with the best manufacturing and food technology characteristics. However, even the most robust probiotic strains are currently limited in the range of food applications to which they can be applied. Additionally, bacteria with exceptional functional health properties are often ruled out due to technological limitations. New process and formulation technologies need to be developed that will enable both the expansion of the range of probiotic products and the use of efficacious strains that currently cannot be incorporated into food fermentations or stored using existing technologies.

The viability of probiotics has been both a marketing and a technological challenge for many processing industries. The standard for any food sold with health claims derived from the addition of probiotics is that it must contain per gram at least 10^6 to 10^7 CFU of viable probiotic bacteria (FAO/WHO, 2001). Viability during the shelf life of the product and survival in the GI tract to populate the human gut are two important issues in health benefit provision by probiotics. Additionally, factors related to the technological and sensory aspects of probiotic food production are of importance since only by satisfying the demands of consumers can the food industry succeed in promoting the consumption of functional probiotic products in the future.

GI TRACT AND GUT MICROBIOTA

The GI tract of humans consists of a diverse microbiota with between 300 and 500 bacterial species. The microbiota of the GI tract of an adult consists of 99% of obligate anaerobes; gastric secretions and rapid mobility in the upper small intestine restrict the microbiota to approximately 10^3 organisms per ml of luminal fluids at this site and between 10^{11} and 10^{12} organisms per g or ml of colon contents (Xu and Gordon, 2003; Backhead et al., 2005). The bacterial composition of the microbiota in different regions of the GI tract differs due to the anatomical properties of the sites and other conditions such as pH, oxygen availability, and transit time of the food contents. Bacterial species belonging to the genera *Bacteroides*, *Bifidobacterium*, *Fusobacterium*, *Butyrivibrio*, *Clostridium*, *Eubacterium*, *Enterobacter*, *Peptococcus*, and *Lactobacillus* are common members of the resident microbiota of the GI tract (Benno and Mitsuoka, 1986).

Bifidobacteria and lactobacilli represent 90% of the bacterial population, whereas less than 0.01% consists of a diversified bacterial population which may include potential pathogens (Tournut, 1993). The microbiota alters throughout the GI tract and also changes as a person ages. The pH, the presence of bile salts, and the availability of oxygen are the predominant factors determining which species of bacteria reside in the different regions of the GI tract (Hoier, 1992; Goldin, 1996).

The stomach, with a pH of 2.3 and substantial level of gastric juices, is inhabited by a few, hardy gram-positive bacteria and some yeasts. Further down the GI tract as bile salt levels decrease and pH increases, more bacterial species are present in higher numbers. The small intestine is a zone of transition, with gram-negative bacteria and anaerobes becoming predominant (Richardson, 1996). The number of aerobic bacteria decreases towards the colon, where 95% of the bacterial population are strict anaerobes. The ileocecal sphincter acts as a doorway to the enormous bacterial concentrations found in the colon (Goldin, 1996). In the small intestine, the limiting factors for the intestinal microbiota are the presence of gastric juices and contents movement, whereas in the large intestine, the limiting factors are microbiologically produced antimicrobial substances and competition for food (Richardson, 1996). As the intestinal contents pass through the colon, nutrients are depleted by microbial activity until very little remains in the distal or descending colon (Cummings and MacFarlane, 1991). There is a more neutral pH and less metabolite production in the descending colon (Gibson and Roberfroid, 1995). Although bacteria are distributed throughout the GI tract, the major concentrations of microbes and metabolic activity are to be found in the large intestine.

Microbial colonization of the intestines begins immediately after birth (Benno and Mitsuoka, 1986). The microbes derived from the mother have a strong stimulatory effect for both the normal development of the microbiota and the maturation of the gut-associated lymphoid tissue. These effects are less apparent in cesarean-born infants (Gronlund et al., 1999). Initial colonization is by Enterobacteriaceae and streptococci. These species are followed by those of Bacteroides, Bifidobacterium, and Clostridium, with Bifidobacterium spp. becoming predominant approximately 1 week after birth. As children are weaned from breast milk, the number of bifidobacteria decreases while those of Bacteroides, Eubacterium, and Peptococcus increase. Diet can have a major effect on the gut microbial activities. Breast-fed infants have a natural predominance of bifidobacteria, and also specific strains of these. Children fed with infant formula have lower levels of bifidobacteria and a microbiota that is more complex and similar to that of adults (Ishibashi and Shimamura, 1993). In the elderly, the number of bifidobacteria decreases, whereas the number of clostridia and lactobacilli increases (Mitsuoka, 1996).

The intestinal bacteria live in symbiotic or antagonistic relationships with their host. The indigenous bacteria may be grouped either as potentially pathogenic or as health promoting (Salminen et al., 1998). Strains with beneficial properties include, among others, bifidobacteria and lactobacilli, which are also among the predominant culturable microbes in healthy infants (He et al., 2001). Normalization of the indigenous microbiota by specific strains of the healthy gut microbiota forms the basis of probiotic therapy (Salminen et al., 1998). The targets for probiotic interventions include clinical conditions with impaired mucosal barrier function, particularly manifested by infections and inflammatory diseases (Saarela et al., 2002).

PROBIOTIC FOODS AND NUTRACEUTICALS

Probiotic Foods

Probiotic foods can be made in two ways: (i) fermentation of raw ingredients by probiotic bacteria, with or without starter culture strains; and (ii) addition of suitable concentrations of probiotics to the finished product (O'Sullivan et al., 1992; Svensson, 1999). Probiotic fermentation of raw ingredients allows the bacteria to multiply and impart distinctive flavors, organoleptic flavors, and organoleptic changes to the food. The probiotic strains selected for each different food system affect the qualities of the final product, depending on the type and amount of acids and other metabolites that are produced. Hetero- and homofermentative lactobacilli impart different flavors during fermentation. Homofermenters produce an "acid-sour" flavor from lactic acid, and heterofermenters yield an "acid-sharp" flavor from the acetic acid (Marshall and Tamime, 1997). The composition of the food determines which probiotic strain is more suited to good growth and survival. When probiotic bacteria are added to the final product without fermentation, bacterial survival, rather than growth, is the important factor (Svensson, 1999). Bacteria must be added at a suitable cell concentration to remain above 10^6 CFU/g of food during the shelf life of the product. However, any bacterial growth during this period may produce undesirable changes such as postacidification, resulting in a less acceptable product.

Whether probiotics are used in the manufacture of the food product or are added postproduction, the important factor is the ability of the product to convey the desired health benefits. Strain selection, food composition, and the use of prebiotics and food-processing parameters such as pH and temperature determine the successful survival of the bacteria (Hull et al., 1992). Product taste, composition, and marketing determine the success of the product in the marketplace (Saxelin et al., 1999). The majority of foods containing probiotic bacteria are dairy foods due to the traditional association of lactic acid bacteria (LAB) with fermented milks (Sanders, 1998). Probiotics have been incorporated into fermented milks, yogurts, soft and semihard cheeses, ice cream, frozen dairy desserts, quark cheese, and cottage cheese as well as fermented cereals, infant formulas, beverages, salami, sausages, and bread (Varnam and Sutherland, 1994; Lee at al., 1999). Over 70 products all over the world including sour cream, buttermilk, yogurt, powdered milk, and frozen desserts contain bifidobacteria and lactobacilli (Shah, 2000).

Nutraceuticals

Probiotic-containing nutraceuticals are produced by specialized manufacturers who typically carry out fermentation in vats, recover and concentrate the cells by centrifugation or filtration, dry the concentrate, and market it in the form of a powder, caplets, or chewable tablets. Legislation, particularly in the United States, allows probiotic supplements under the Dietary Supplement Health and Education Act of 1994. Probiotic supplements are available in different forms, the two most popular being capsules or caplets and freeze-dried powders. Probiotic strains of L. acidophilus 50 ME are sold by Institut Rosell/Lallemand, The Americas, Montreal, Canada (www.lallemand.com). Probiocap TM (L. acidophilus in a hydrophobic matrix) is marketed with claims to have increased tolerance to gastric juices, improved survival during tableting, enhanced temperature resistance during food processing, and extended shelf life at room temperatures. Cerebios-Pharma (www.cerbios.ch) markets Cernivet LBC ME 10 as a pelletable microbial feed additive for the stabilization of the intestinal microbiota. Other examples include Probio-Tec capsules for innovative probiotic product solutions for dietary supplements and infant formulas marketed by Chr Hansen (www.chbiosystems.com). Geneflora manufactured and sold by Americas Bio-Plus Corporation (www.yeastbuster.com) claims to be a robust friendly intestinal microbiota classified by the U.S. Department of Agriculture as a probiotic. Bio-Three tablets are marketed by the Japanese TOA Pharmaceutical Co. Ltd. These tablets contain a mixture of three probiotic organisms: Enterococcus T-110, Clostridium butyricum TO-A, and Bacillus mesentericus

TO-A. It is claimed that a symbiosis of these three bacteria strongly inhibits harmful bacteria in the intestine, facilitates proliferation of bifidobacteria, and normalizes the intestinal microbiota (Kailasapathy, 2002).

VIABILITY, SURVIVAL, AND REGULATORY ASPECTS OF PROBIOTIC BACTERIA

Viability Issues

Although there are instances where nonviable probiotics can still exert their biological effects (Ouwehand and Salminen, 1998; Tabrizi et al., 2004; Stanton et al., 2005), it is widely believed that products which contain viable probiotics are the most desirable. The viability of probiotic cultures in functional foods is therefore a critical issue of their functionality. The viability and metabolic activity of probiotic bacteria are important considerations because the bacteria must survive in the food or nutraceutical during its shelf life and during transit through the acidic conditions of the stomach and must resist any degradation by hydrolytic enzymes and bile salts in the small intestine. It is essential that products sold with any health claims meet the recommended criterion of a minimum of 10^6 to 10^7 CFU of viable probiotic bacteria per g (FAO/WHO, 2001).

Analysis of probiotic products in many different countries has confirmed that probiotic strains exhibit poor survival in food such as yogurts and fermented milks, with cell numbers being much lower than the recommended levels at the expiry date (Kailasapathy and Rybka, 1997; Shah, 2000; Lourens-Hattingh and Viljoen, 2001). Rybka and Fleet (1997) found that the viable population of L. acidophilus and Bifidobacterium spp. exceeded 10^6 CFU/g only in 24 and 15%, respectively, of the 50 commercial yogurts tested. Shah et al. (2000) observed that counts of both L. acidophilus and Bifidobacterium spp. decreased to less than the recommended 10^6 CFU/g by the expiry date in most of the Australian yogurts in their study. Similar results have been reported in the United Kingdom and in North America. Eight commercial yogurt samples sold in London, which claimed to contain viable bifidobacteria were enumerated for the presence of this organism. Only five of the eight yogurts tested contained viable bifidobacteria at $>10^6$ CFU/ml, while the remaining three did not contain any bifidobacteria (Iwana et al., 1993). Modler and Villa-Garcia (1993) reported that bifidobacteria do not survive in several yogurt products in North America, due to highly acidic conditions.

Probiotic preparations such as tablets, powders, etc., may contain lower viable counts. Among 15 feed supplements supposedly containing L. acidophilus, the viable counts were found to vary greatly, with 3 products containing no lactobacilli at all (Gilliland, 1981).

Regulatory Issues

The efficiency of added probiotic bacteria depends on the dose level, their viability must be maintained throughout the product's shelf life, and they must survive the gut environment (Kailasapathy and Chin, 2000). The introduction of various standards for probiotic dairy foods has required that yogurt manufacturers ensure the presence of viable lactobacilli and bifidobacteria in their products throughout the shelf life (International Dairy Federation, 1992; Lourens-Hattingh and Viljoen, 2001; Shah, 2000). These high numbers (10^8 CFU/g of product) have been suggested to compensate for the possible reduction in the numbers of probiotic organisms during passage through the stomach and intestine. The International Dairy Federation requires 10^7 CFU of *L. acidophilus* per g in products such as acidophilus milk and 10^6 CFU of bifidobacteria per g in fermented milks containing bifidobacteria at the time of sale (International Dairy Federation, 1992). The Swiss Food Regulation and the MERCOSOR regulations (Argentina, Paraguay, Brazil, and Uruguay) require a minimum of 10^6 CFU of viable bifidobacteria per g in similar products (Bibiloni et al., 2001). The Fermented Milk and Lactic Acid Beverages Association of Japan has specified that there be at least 10^7 CFU of viable bifidobacteria per g in fermented milk drinks (Lourens-Hattingh and Viljoen, 2001). In the United States, the National Yogurt Association specifies that in order to use the National Yogurt Association's "Live and Active Culture" logo on the container, a product should contain 10^8 CFU of lactic acid bacteria per g at the time of manufacture (Lourens-Hattingh and Viljoen, 2001). According to the Australian and New Zealand Food Standards Code (ANZFA), the microorganisms used in the manufacture of fermented milk products should remain viable in the product and the combined total of the viable lactic acid cultures used for yogurt fermentation should be at least 10^6 CFU/g (ANZFA, 2001).

Factors Affecting the Survival of Probiotic Bacteria

The ability of microorganisms to survive and multiply in the host strongly influences their probiotic benefits. The bacteria should be metabolically stable and active in the product, survive passage through the upper digestive tract in large numbers, and confer beneficial effects when in the intestine of the host (Kailasapathy and Chin, 2000; Shah, 2000). *L. acidophilus* and *Bifidobacterium* spp. are considered to be sensitive in a yogurt environment. Bifidobacteria are not as acid tolerant as *L. acidophilus* and

have been reported to exhibit weak growth in milk and require an anaerobic environment (Lourens-Hattingh and Viljoen, 2001). Kneifel et al. (1993) reported that factors such as the acidity of yogurt, its chemical and microbiological composition, the availability of nutrients, and growth promoters and inhibitors affect probiotic survival. Various other factors such as acid and hydrogen peroxide produced by yogurt bacteria, the concentrations of lactic and acetic acids, interaction of the probiotic species with the yogurt starters, buffering capacity, whey proteins, sugars, incubation temperature, fermentation time, and the fat content of the yogurt can affect the survival of *L. acidophilus* and *Bifidobacterium* spp. in yogurt (Kailasapathy and Supriadi, 1996; Lourens-Hattingh and Viljoen, 2001; Micanel et al., 1997; Shah, 2000; Vinderola et al., 2002). Vinderola et al. (2000) observed that full-fat yogurt was more inhibitory for *B. bifidum* than reduced-fat yogurt. Dave and Shah (1997) suggested that variations in the inoculum levels of commercial probiotic yogurt cultures and their incubation temperature could affect the viability of probiotic microorganisms as observed in their study. The influences of incubation temperature, fermentation time, and storage temperature on bacterial viability have been reported by Kneifel et al. (1993), Sultana et al. (2000), and Godward et al. (2000).

The bacterial strains selected as probiotics must also be able to survive gastric acidity (pH 1 to 4), bile salts, enzymes such as lysozyme present in the intestines, toxic metabolites including phenols produced during digestion, bacteriophages, antibiotics, and anaerobic conditions (Hoier, 1992; Lankaputhra and Shah, 1995; Tejada-Simon et al., 1999; Wang et al., 1999; Kailasapathy and Chin, 2000). The human GI tract and stomach have the highest acidity; the probiotic bacteria not only must survive these conditions but also are required to colonize the gut. Therefore, probiotic strain selection is very important, as many strains of *L. acidophilus* and *Bifidobacterium* spp. cannot survive these conditions.

Ways To Improve the Viability of Probiotic Bacteria

A number of methods have been reported in the literature to improve the viability of probiotic bacteria during manufacture and storage of fermented dairy products and also during gastric transit.

1. Lowering the storage temperature to less than 3 to 4°C increases *L. acidophilus* and bifidobacterial survival (Sakai et al., 1987).
2. Lowering the incubation temperature to 37°C favors growth of bifidobacteria and increases

incubation time (M. Costello, presented at the Food Industry Conference, International Food Processing Machinery and Technology Exhibition and Conference, Sydney, Australia, 12 to 14 July 1993).

3. Enrichment of yogurt mix with whey protein concentrate increases the buffering capacity of yogurt, retards decrease in pH, and prevents pH change during storage of yogurt (Supriadi et al., 1994).

4. Terminating yogurt fermentation at a higher pH (>5) allows better survival of LAB (Varnam and Sutherland, 1994).

5. Heat shock (58°C for 5 min) of the yogurt prevents excess acid production, and the acidity remains constant during storage (Marshall, 1992).

6. Application of hydrostatic pressure (200 to 300 MPa for 10 min at room temperature) to yogurt prevents after-acidification and hence maintains the initial number of viable LAB (Tanaka and Hatanake, 1992).

7. Addition of cysteine and other nutrients, e.g., baker's yeast, tomato juice, papaya pulp, acetate, and oligosaccharides (Ahmed and Mittal, 1990; Babu et al., 1992; Marshall, 1991; Saxena et al., 1994; Shah, 2000; Shimamura, 1982).

8. Other approaches that increase the resistance of these sensitive microorganisms to adverse conditions have been proposed, including appropriate selection of acid- and bile-resistant strains, the use of oxygen-impermeable containers, two-step fermentation, stress adaptation, and the incorporation of micronutrients such as peptides (Gismondo et al., 1999).

IMMOBILIZATION AND MICROENCAPSULATION TECHNOLOGIES FOR PROBIOTICS

Incorporating probiotic bacteria into functional food presents many challenges, particularly with respect to the stability of probiotic bacterial cells during processing and storage and the need to prevent undesirable interactions with the carrier food matrix. Therefore, there is a need to protect the bacterial cells against adverse processing and storage conditions as well as during GI transit. Providing probiotic living cells with a physical barrier against adverse external conditions is an approach currently receiving considerable interest in the food industry (Kailasapathy, 2002). Clearly, obtaining a health benefit requires the viability of the bacterial cells in the GI tract and their controlled release in the target areas of the GI

tract. Microencapsulation (ME) could be useful for this purpose.

In the past, microorganisms were immobilized or entrapped in polymer matrices for use in food and biotechnological applications. The physical retention of cells in the matrix facilitates the separation of the cells from their metabolites. As the technique of immobilization or entrapment became refined, the immobilized cell technology has evolved into encapsulation of cells. Encapsulation tends to stabilize cells, potentially enhancing their viability and stability in the production, storage, and handling of lactic cultures. An immobilized environment also conferred additional protection to lactobacillus and bifidobacterial cells during rehydration and lyophilization (Kim et al., 1996).

ME is an inclusion technique for confining a bioactive substance into a polymeric matrix coated by one or more semipermeable polymers by virtue of which the encapsulated compound becomes more stable and protected than its isolated or free form. Encapsulation of food bioactives can provide the final product with better technological and nutritional properties and, in addition, controlled release of encapsulated compounds under specific conditions. A microcapsule consists of a semipermeable, spherical, thin, and strong membrane surrounding a solid/liquid core with a diameter varying from a few micrometers to 1 mm (Anal and Singh, 2007). ME can be used for many applications in the food and nutraceutical industries, including stabilizing the core material, controlling the oxidative reactions, providing sustained or controlled release (both temporal and time-controlled release), masking flavors, colors, or odors, extending the shelf life, and protecting components against nutritional losses. There are numerous methods of ME. ME of probiotics presents two challenges: the size of the cell (typically 1 to 5 μm in diameter) and the need to keep the cell alive, with little or no stress imposed on it during the ME process and during the encapsulated shelf life. The latter aspect has been considered crucial in selecting the appropriate ME technology. Encapsulation occurs naturally when bacterial cells grow and produce exopolysaccharides. The microbial cells are entrapped within their own secretions, which act as a protective structure or a capsule, reducing the permeability of material through the capsules, and therefore, they are less exposed to adverse environmental factors. Many LAB synthesize exopolysaccharides, but they produce insufficient amounts of these to enable full encapsulation (N. Shah, presented at the Symposium on New Developments in Technology of Fermented Milks, International Dairy Federation, Cornwell Scanticon, Kolding, Denmark, 3 June 2002).

ME helps to separate a core material from its environment until it is released. It protects the unstable core from its environment, thereby improving its stability, extends the core's shelf life, and provides a sustained and controlled release (Fig. 1). The structure formed by the microencapsulation agent around the core substance is known as the wall. The properties of the wall system are designed to protect the core and to release it at controlled rates under specific conditions while allowing small molecules to pass in and out of the membrane (Franjione and Vasishtha, 1995; Gibbs et al., 1999). The capsules may range from submicrometers to several millimeters in size and can be of different shapes (Shahidi and Han, 1993; Franjione and Vasishtha, 1995).

Compared to immobilization/entrapment techniques, ME has many advantages. The microcapsule is composed of a semipermeable, spherical, thin, and strong membranous wall. Therefore, the bacterial cells are retained within the microcapsules (Jankowski et al., 1997). Moreover, compared to an entrapment matrix, there is no solid or gelled core in the microcapsule and its small diameter helps to reduce mass transfer limitations. Nutrients and metabolites can diffuse through the semipermeable membrane easily. The membrane serves as a barrier to cell release and minimizes contamination. The encapsulated core material is released by several mechanisms such as mechanical rupture of the cell wall, dissolution of the wall, melting of the wall, and diffusion through the wall (Franjione and Vasishtha, 1995).

ME Technologies for Probiotics

There are several methods of ME. However, technologies applied to probiotics are generally limited to gelling, spray-drying, spray-cooling, extrusion, and emulsions (Kailasapathy, 2002; Anal and Singh, 2007; Champagne and Fustier, 2007).

ME Using Polymer Hydrogelling Technologies

In hydrogelling, polymers are used in the presence of monovalent or divalent cations to microentrap probiotic bacterial cells in hydrogel beads. The polymerization is induced by the interaction of cations with the hydropolymers, resulting in the production of solid matrices which contain the cells. Food grade polymers such as alginate, chitosan, carboxymethylcellulose, carrageenan, gelatin, starch, and pectin are mainly employed, using various ME techniques (Table 1). In some cases a filler polymer is used which does not get involved in the cation-induced gelling but helps to strengthen the solid matrix of the gel beads. For example, Hi-Maize starch (a cross-

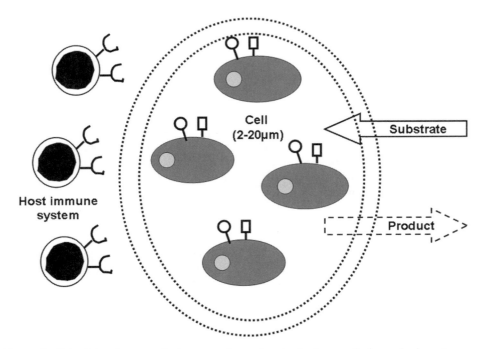

Figure 1 Principle of encapsulation: membrane barrier isolates cells from the host immune system while allowing transport of metabolites and extracellular nutrients. Membrane with size-selective pores (30 to 70 kDa) (Kailasapathy, 2002).

Table 1 Encapsulation of lactic acid and probiotic bacteria[a]

Capsule material	Special treatment	Bacteria	Application	Reference
Extrusion method				
A	N	L, S	Yogurt	Prevost et al., 1985
A	N	S	Cheese	Prevost and Davies, 1987
A	N	S	Phage protection	Steenson et al., 1987
A	N	S	Yogurt	Prevost and Davies, 1988
A	Chitosan	L	Biomass production	Zhou et al., 1998
A	Glycerol	L	Biomass production	Kearney et al., 1990
A	N	L, S	Biomass production	Champagne et al., 1993
A	Starch	L	Biomass production	Jankowski et al., 1997
A	N	L, B	Biomass production	Lee and Heo, 2000
A	N	L, B	Yogurt	Talwalkar and Kailasapathy, 2003
A	N	L, B	Biomass production	Anjani et al., 2004
A	N	L	Yogurt/Biomass production	Krasaekoopt et al., 2003
Emulsion technique				
Ca	Soy oil	S, L	Yogurt	Audet et al., 1998
CAP	Paraffin	S		Rao et al., 1989
A	Vegetable oil	L	Ice cream	Sheu and Marshall, 1991
Ca	Vegetable oil	L	Biomass production	Arnaud et al., 1992
Ch	Mineral oil	L	Biomass production	Groboillot et al., 1993
A	Vegetable oil	L	Frozen ice milk	Sheu et al., 1993
A	Canola oil	L	Biomass production	Larisch et al., 1994
A	Corn oil	B	Ice milk	Kebary et al., 1998
A	Vegetable oil	L, B	Yogurt	Sultana et al., 2000
A	Vegetable oil	B	Yogurt	Adhikari et al., 2003

[a]A, alginate; Ca, carrageenan; CAP, cellulose acetate phthalate; Ch, chitosan; L, *Lactobacillus* spp.; S, *Streptococcus* spp.; B, *Bifidobacterium* spp.; N, no treatment. Modified from Iyer, 2005.

linked resistant starch) is used as a filler in the calcium-induced alginate (encapsulant) hydrogelling to entrap probiotic bacteria (Sultana et al., 2000). Entrapment of probiotic cells in an alginate matrix is the most popular system of immobilization reported (Champagne et al., 1994). Probiotic bacteria (1 to 3 µm in diameter) are well retained in the alginate hydrogel matrix, which is estimated to have a pore size of less than 17 nm (Klein et al., 1983).

Encapsulation of Probiotics in Polymer-Cation Systems

Polymerization induced by cation has several advantages: easy handling of gel beads, control of dosage (in CFU per gram), facilitation of incorporation of cryoprotectants and application of surface coatings for extra protection, desirable dissolution properties, controlled release, desirable adhesion properties, and enhanced sensorial properties (Anal and Singh, 2007). The most

popular cation-ME system is the alginate extraction process in a calcium chloride solution. On addition of sodium alginate solution to a calcium chloride solution, interfacial polymerization is instantaneous, with precipitation of calcium alginate followed by a more gradual gelation of the interior as calcium ions permeate through the alginate systems. In some cases, filler material such as resistant starch (Sultana et al., 2000; Muthukumaraswamy et al., 2006), pectin, and whey proteins (Guerin et al., 2003) have been blended with alginate to improve the matrix for subsequent applications. Encapsulated probiotic bacteria (*L. acidophilus* and *Bifidobacterium infantis*) in a calcium-alginate-Hi-Maize starch (a resistant starch and a prebiotic) matrix produced are shown in Fig. 2. This ME method has been reported to protect probiotic bacteria from harsh acidic conditions of gastric fluid and to increase survival of encapsulated bacteria under acidic and alkaline conditions (Chandramouli et al., 2004).

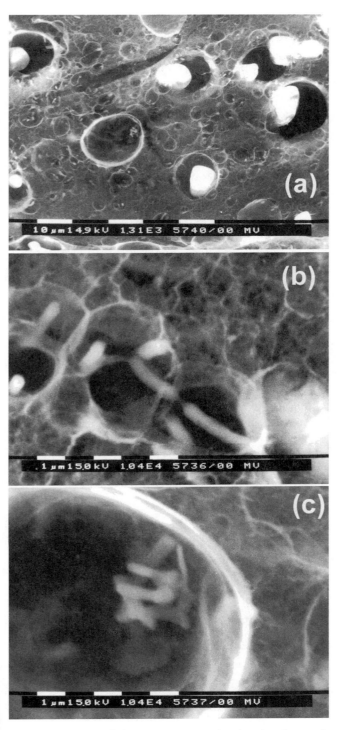

Figure 2 Section of alginate microcapsules showing the starch granules in the cavities (a), *L. acidophilus* (b), and *B. infantis* (c) (Kailasapathy, 2002).

There are various scale-up methods as well as industrial suppliers of extrusion bead-forming equipment (Champagne, 2006; Heinzen, 2002), and production can be on an industrial scale. Coating of the alginate beads can also be accomplished to improve their protective properties. The alginate hydrogel beads are simply dipped in a solution containing a cationic polymer, such as chitosan, gelatin, or poly-L-lysine (Krasaekoopt et al., 2004; Groboillot et al., 1993). Chen et al. (2005) reported using fructo-oligosaccharides or isomalto-oligosaccharides, a growth promoter (peptide), and sodium alginate as coating materials to microencapsulate different probiotics such as *L. acidophilus*, *L. casei*, *B. bifidum*, and *B. longum*.

Chan and Zhang (2002) developed an enteric coating encapsulation method for an industrially sourced strain of *L. acidophilus*, to protect the bacterial cells as they pass through the GI tract. The coating material used was a mixture of sodium alginate and hydroxypropylcellulose. Some protein-based ME techniques are also carried out by ionic gellification. Limited data suggest that alginate gels offer better protection to probiotics than other carbohydrate-based or protein-based gels (Muthukumaraswamy et al., 2006; Kailasapathy and Sureeta, 2004), but more data are needed on the effect of the gelling matrix. Cui et al. (2001) reported the preparation of poly-L-lysine-cross-linked alginate microparticles loaded with bifidobacteria and demonstrated the increased survival of bifidobacteria even in the lower-pH media during storage at 4°C in a refrigerator compared with free cultures.

Rao et al. (1989) reported the encapsulation of *Bifidobacterium pseudolongum* in cellulose acetate phthalate by using an emulsion technique and reported that microencapsulated bacteria survived in larger numbers (10^9 CFU/ml) in an acidic environment than nonencapsulated organisms, which did not retain any viability when exposed to a simulated gastric environment for 1 h. Gelatin is useful as a thermally reversible gelling agent for encapsulation. Hyndman et al. (1993) used high concentrations of gelatin (24%, wt/vol) to encapsulate *Lactobacillus lactis* by cross-linking with toluene-2-4-diisocyanate for industrial biomass production.

Mixed hydrogel polymerization to encapsulate *Bifidobacterium* cells comprising alginate, pectin, and whey proteins has been reported (Guerin et al., 2003). The additional membrane formed by the conjugation of whey protein and pectin provided protection to the probiotic bacterial cells against acidic and bile conditions. The biopolymer chitosan, the *N*-deacetylated product of the polysaccharide chitin, is increasingly being used in the ME of probiotic bacterial cells. Krasaekoopt et al. (2003, 2004) evaluated the survival of probiotics encapsulated in chitosan-coated alginate beads in yogurt and in ultrahigh-temperature-treated and conventionally treated milk during storage. They reported that the survival of the encapsulated bacteria was higher than that of the free cells by approximately 1 log. The number of bacterial cells was maintained above the recommended therapeutic minimum (10^7 CFU/g) throughout storage for the lactobacilli but not for the bifidobacteria. ME of *Lactobacillus bulgaricus* KFR1763 in chitosan-coated alginate beads protected the bacteria in gastric fluid (pH 2.0) and is therefore an effective means of delivering viable cells to the GI tract (Lee et al., 2004).

Bacteria have been observed to adhere to starch granules (Anderson and Salyers, 1989), and this property has been specifically utilized for ME of probiotics in maize (corn), potato, oat, or barley (Crittenden et al., 2001; Myllarinen et al., 2000; Myllarinen, 2002). The starch could be used as a filler material, and the growing cells can adhere to the granules or grow inside the gel matrix. These probiotic-containing starch granules could constitute carriers for probiotics in the development of functional foods. Resistant starch (not digested by pancreatic amylases in the small intestine so that it reaches the colon, where it can be fermented by the resident microbiota) can be used in ME to ensure the viability of probiotic organisms in food and in the GI system. Resistant starch also offers an ideal surface for adherence of the probiotics to the starch granule during processing, storage, and transit through the upper GI tract, providing robustness and resilience to environmental stresses. Mattila-Sandholm et al. (2002) reported using enzymically treated large potato starch granules as a probiotic carrier. They found that starch-encapsulated LAB survived at least 6 months at room temperature under normal atmospheric humidity and at least 18 months when frozen. The incorporation of Hi-Maize starch improved the encapsulation of viable bacteria compared with encapsulation without starch (Sultana et al., 2000). Talwalkar and Kailasapathy (2003) reported that ME of *L. acidophilus* and *B. lactis* in calcium-induced alginate-starch hydrogel beads prevented cell death from oxygen toxicity. The ME restricted the diffusion of oxygen through the gel, creating anoxic regions in the center of the beads.

Gibson and Roberfroid (1995) reported that prebiotics selectively stimulated probiotic strains. Some authors (Fooks et al., 1999; Roberfroid, 2000) suggest that prebiotics may improve the survival of bacteria traversing the upper part of the GI tract, thereby enhancing their effects on the large bowel. Iyer and Kailasapathy (2005) introduced the concept of coencapsulation which includes ME of probiotic bacteria (*L. acidophilus* CSCC 2400 and CSCC 2409) and complementary prebiotic substances (Hi-Maize starch, Raftiline, and Raftiolse) as filler materials in calcium-induced alginate microcapsules coated with alginate, poly-L-lysine, or chitosan polymers. They reported that Hi-Maize starch capsules provided enhanced protection to the bacterial cells in acidic conditions (pH 2 up to 3 h) compared to Raftiline and Raftilose. It was also observed that addition of Hi-Maize (1%, wt/vol) to capsules containing *Lactobacillus* spp. and further coating with chitosan significantly increased ($P < 0.05$) the survival of encapsulated bacteria under in vitro acidic and bile salt conditions and also in stored yogurt compared with alginate encapsulated cells.

Extrusion and Emulsion Technologies

ME by extrusion involves projecting an emulsion core and coating material through a nozzle at high pressure. Extrusion of polymer solutions through nozzles to produce capsules has been reported on a laboratory scale but can also be scaled up. If droplet formation occurs in a controlled manner (in contrast to spraying), the technique is known as prilling (Heinzen, 2002). Mass production of beads is achieved by either multinozzle systems, rotating-disk atomizers, or jet-cutting techniques. Centrifugal systems using either a multinozzle system or a rotating disk have also been developed for the mass production of microcapsules (Heinzen, 2002). The emulsion technique involves the dispersion of an aqueous phase containing the bacterial cells and polymer suspension into an organic phase such as oil, resulting in a water-in-oil emulsion. The dispersed aqueous droplets are hardened by cooling or by the addition of a gelling agent or a cross-linking agent. Following gelation, the beads are partitioned into water and washed to remove oil. However, the residual oil and emulsifiers such as Tween 20 in the microcapsules may be detrimental to the viability of probiotic bacteria, particularly if remaining within the capsules with the bacteria during extended storage periods. Extrusion and emulsion techniques are not easily applied to probiotics because of their "large" particle size (Champagne and Fustier, 2007).

Spray-Drying, Spray-Coating, and Spray-Chilling Technologies

Spray-drying has traditionally had limited industrial use for probiotics, as most probiotic bacteria do not survive well during the temperature and osmotic extremes to which they are exposed during the spray-drying process (Selmer-Olsen et al., 1999). The spray-dried cells lose their activity after a few weeks of storage at room temperature due to stress-induced damage to cell membranes and associated proteins. Additions of thermoprotectants, such as trehalose (Conrad et al., 2000) and granular starch (Crittenden et al., 2006), have been shown to improve culture viability during drying and storage. In spray-coating, the partially dried core material is kept in motion in a specially designed vessel, either by injection of air at the bottom or by a rotary action (Champagne and Fustier, 2007). This is followed by a spray of a coating material which solidifies and forms a layer over the dried core material. In food applications, the coating is mostly lipid based, but a wide group of compounds such as proteins, gluten, casein, cellulose and its derivatives, carrageenan, and alginate can be used (Ubbink et al., 2003). Spray-coating is useful for coats having multiple layers. For example, the first coating may confer a protective property and the second coating could be used to facilitate the suspension of microcapsules containing the probiotic bacteria, which may be useful for probiotic beverage development. Spray-chilling involves atomizing a molten matrix with a low melting point (32 to 42°C) containing the probiotic bacteria (Champagne and Fustier, 2007). It is similar to spray-drying but is based on the injection of cold air into the chamber to enable solidification of the gel particle, rather than the hot air which dries the droplet into a fine powder particle in the case of spray-drying.

ME Technologies for Probiotic Nutraceuticals

Probiotic-containing nutraceuticals are produced by harvesting cells from large-scale biomass industrial fermentation, microencapsulating the concentrated cell mass, and drying the products. They are then marketed in the form of a powder, caplets, or chewable tablets. Currently, the encapsulation process is carried out by spray-coating. Examples include the STAR and Probiocap technologies (Goulet and Wozniak, 2002). Fat-based polymers are used to spray-coat fine particles of probiotic cultures to enhance the survival rate against the gastric contents (Goulet and Wozniak, 2002). Probiotic strains of *L. acidophilus* 50 ME are sold in a microencapsulated form by Institut Rosell/Lallemand The Americas, Montreal, Canada (www.lallemand.com). Probiocap (microencapsulated *L. acidophilus* 50 ME in a hydrophobic matrix) claims to have increased tolerance to gastric juices, improved survival during tableting, enhanced temperature resistance during processing, and extended shelf life at room temperatures (Kailasapathy, 2002).

ME is beneficial in probiotic tablet manufacture. When spray-coated particles containing probiotics were exposed to compression into tablets, the survival rate was higher than with uncoated particles (Goulet and Wozniak, 2002). It was also observed that when free cells and compression-generated tablets were exposed

to simulated gastric fluid (SGF), much higher survival was recorded with the cells in the tablet, but only in very acidic environments (between pH 1.2 and 2.0) (Chan and Zhang, 2005). In the compression-ME system, the formation of a hydrogel surrounding the cell was thought to be the basis for cell protection (Chan and Zhang, 2005). However, only 50% of the tablet was hydrated after 2 h of exposure to the SGF, suggesting that there is limited entry of the acidic solution into the tablet. These observations are useful to ascertain the value of encapsulation when the tablet is taken as a whole. However, further studies are needed to examine the usefulness of the technique when the tablet is chewed and broken down to small particles. It can be expected that the "limitation of mass transfer of SGF" type of protection offered by encapsulation would be lower in that instance. The encapsulated powders with enteric coating may protect the probiotic bacteria from gastric acidity and deliver large numbers of bacteria to the small intestine.

DELIVERY OF PROBIOTIC BACTERIA: CONTROLLED RELEASE

The viability of probiotic bacteria is an important consideration because they must survive in the food or beverage during processing and shelf life and during transit through the acidic and alkaline conditions in the GI tract. They should also resist any degradation by hydrolytic enzymes and bile salts in the small intestine. Controlled release of bacteria is a critical benefit of ME. While ME provides protection to probiotic bacteria and prevents cell death due to acid, alkali, and degenerative enzymes in the GI tract, there is no guarantee that bacteria are released from capsules at the target site in the required numbers. It is beneficial for encapsulated probiotic bacteria to be released in the small intestine, where Peyer's patches exist, to activate the immune system. Therefore, the polymers used for ME should be able to protect the bacteria in the acidic stomach and release the bacteria under the alkaline conditions in the small intestine. Many reports show that ME in alginate or pectin-based beads can be used for controlled release of bioactive substances. In vitro studies with calcium alginate or pectinate beads have shown that they maintain their integrity in the simulated upper GI tract but subsequently release the bioactive substances (Mandal et al., 2006).

To evaluate the release profiles of encapsulated bacteria from calcium alginate and chitosan-coated-alginate-starch (CCAS) capsules, two different experiments have been carried out (ex vivo and in vivo) (Iyer et al., 2004, 2005). In the first experiment, the release profiles of two different bacteria, *L. casei* strain Shirota (LCS) and green fluorescent protein (GFP)-tagged *Escherichia coli* K-12 (*E. coli* GFP[+] K-12), from CCAS capsules were investigated in porcine GI contents by using an ex vivo method. In a second experiment, calcium alginate and CCAS capsules containing LCS were fed to mice and bacterial release at different sites in the GI tract was monitored for up to 24 h. In the latter experiment, LCS was used as a model probiotic strain because of the availability of specific selective media that allowed differentiation of the inoculated bacteria from food and from the GI tract microbiota. The microcapsules were prepared aseptically using an InoTech Encapsulator with a 300-μm nozzle as described by Iyer et al. (2004). The contents of different sections of the GI tract (stomach, duodenum, anterior small intestine, posterior small intestine, and colon) were collected from three different pigs. Encapsulated bacteria (0.1 g; approximately 10[8] CFU) were incubated in different intestinal contents (10 ml) anaerobically at 37°C for 12 h. Samples were removed at different time intervals, and the *E. coli* GFP[+] bacterial release was evaluated using a fluorescent microscope. For the enumeration of

LCS, spread plates of lactitol-lactobacillus-vancomycin (LLV) agar (Yuki et al., 1999) were used. Six BALB/c mice (6 weeks old) were force-fed 0.1 g of encapsulated bacteria (approximately 10[8] CFU). The force-fed animals were euthanized at different time intervals. The total contents of the stomach, small intestine, and colon were immediately collected after slaughtering, weighed, and diluted in sterile water. The release of encapsulated LCS was determined using LLV agar. The colonies from LLV agar plates were randomly picked and further confirmed for identification by amplification with a species-specific primer and then subjection to denaturation gradient gel electrophoresis (Walter et al., 2000) (Fig. 3). The release of calcium alginate encapsulated *E. coli* GFP[+] in porcine intestinal contents is shown in Fig. 4. There was essentially no release of encapsulated bacteria from the capsules in the gastric contents. In contrast, there was a complete release of *E. coli* within 1 h of incubation in the small intestinal contents (pH 6.5 to 6.8) at 37°C, while it took 8 h to nearly completely release the *E. coli* in the colon contents (pH 6.9) under similar conditions. The

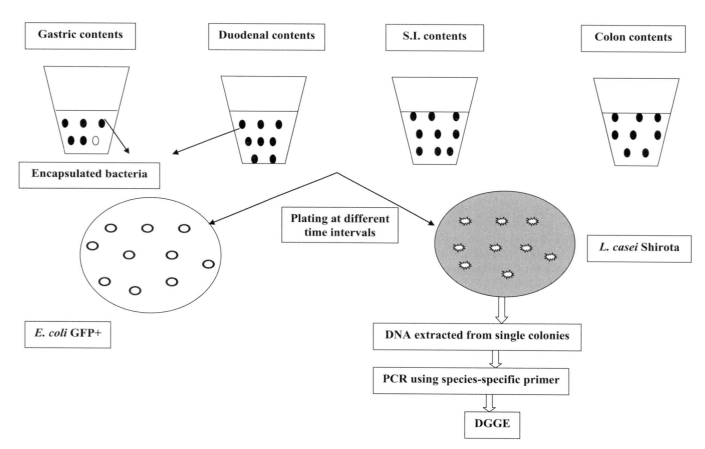

Figure 3   Release of encapsulated bacteria in ex vivo GI contents (Iyer, 2005).

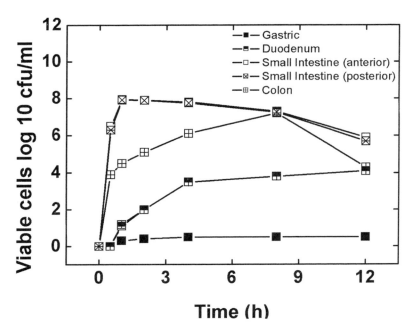

Figure 4 Release of encapsulated bacteria (*E. coli* GFP⁺ K-12 strain) in porcine intestinal contents (Iyer et al., 2004).

release profile of LCS from CCAS capsules in different sections of porcine GI contents is shown in Fig. 5. The release of LCS from capsules was different in different GI contents. There was no significant release of LCS in gastric porcine contents (pH 2.5) even after 24 h of incubation. There was a complete release of LCS in the ileal contents (pH 6.8) after 8 h of incubation. As in the ileum, there was a complete release of LCS from capsules in colon contents, but it took nearly 12 h. While there was a complete release of *E. coli* GFP⁺ from calcium

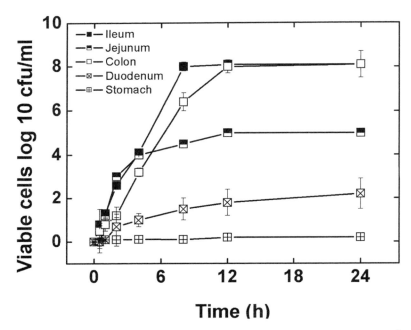

Figure 5 Release of encapsulated bacteria (*L. casei* Shirota) in porcine intestinal contents (Iyer et al., 2005).

alginate capsules within 1 h in porcine ileal contents ex vivo, it took nearly 8 h to completely release LCS from CCAS capsules. The difference between the release of *E. coli* and LCS could be due to the chitosan coating of the capsules. *E. coli* GFP$^+$ was encapsulated with alginates while alginate capsules containing LCS were coated with chitosan polymer. Chitosan, a positively charged polyamine, forms a semipermeable membrane around a negatively charged polymer such as alginate. This membrane provides a barrier to cell release.

The results of these porcine ex vivo experiments demonstrated that the most likely site of bacterial release from the capsule will be the small intestine. Both *E. coli* and LCS were released in large numbers more quickly in the ileal contents of the porcine GI tract than in other GI tract contents. These results are very encouraging because, first, the encapsulated bacteria are not released in the acidic stomach, hence protecting them from gastric acidity, and second, they are released in the segments of the GI tract where are found Peyer's patches and other mucosa-associated lymphatic tissues that are thought to play a critical role in immunostimulation (Rescigno et al., 2001). Therefore, it could be said that ME in alginates with or without coating effectively minimizes the bactericidal effects of the gastric pH and maximizes the number of organisms reaching the ileum and, subsequently, the colon.

The release of LCS from CCAS capsules in different regions of the murine GI tract is shown in Table 2. There was no release of LCS from capsules in the gastric and duodenal contents up to 24 h. There was very low release of LCS from capsules in the jejunal contents (circa 10^3 CFU/g), whereas there was greater but incomplete release of LCS (2.4×10^5 CFU/g) from capsules in the colon contents after 24 h of feeding. There was a complete release of LCS from CCAS capsules in the ileal regions after 12 h, whereas there was only a partial release of encapsulated bacteria in the duodenal, jejunal, and colon contents.

The release profiles of probiotic bacteria from alginate and CCAS capsules ex vivo and in vivo porcine and murine gastrointestinal contents have been reported. In summary, this study has shown that it is possible to release completely the viable probiotic bacteria in the ileum and colon regions (ex vivo and in vivo studies) from microcapsules over a 24-h period. The results of this study indicate that encapsulation efficiently minimizes the bactericidal effects of the gastric pH and maximizes the number of organisms reaching the ileum and, subsequently, the colon.

APPLICATION IN FUNCTIONAL FOODS

Processing of probiotic foods involves heat treatment (pasteurization), pumping, homogenizing and stirring (incorporation of air), freezing (frozen dairy products), addition of ingredients which can be antimicrobial (e.g., salt), drying (powdered milk products), packaging (oxygen ingress through packaging during storage), unfavorable storage conditions (e.g., postacidification in yogurt), heat shock (in cold chain products), and the possible development of antimicrobial compounds secreted by the starter cultures during fermentation. Culture companies select probiotic strains to withstand these adverse technological considerations; however, the recent trend has been for these companies to focus the selection of strains on the basis of health-enhancing and therapeutic effects, and therefore the latest probiotic strains may have lost their ability to withstand unfavorable processing and storage conditions. Hence, the viability of probiotic bacteria is of paramount importance in the marketability of probiotic-based products. ME offers the necessary protection to enhance the survival of probiotics in food and nutraceutical products. It has been reported that ME using calcium-induced alginate-starch polymers (Godward and Kailasapathy, 2003a, 2003b; Sultana et al., 2000), potassium-induced kappa-carrageenan polymers (Adhikari et al., 2000,

Table 2 Release profile of *L. casei* strain Shirota from chitosan-coated alginate-starch capsules in mouse GI tract at different time intervals[a]

Region	Time (h)				
	2	4	8	12	24
Stomach	ND	ND	ND	ND	ND
Duodenum	$4.2 \times 10^1 \pm 0.2 \times 10^1$	$2.6 \times 10^1 \pm 0.2 \times 10^1$	ND	ND	ND
Jejunum	ND	$2.1 \times 10^1 \pm 0.6 \times 10^1$	$7.3 \times 10^3 \pm 0.1 \times 10^3$	$4.1 \times 10^3 \pm 0.6 \times 10^3$	$3.3 \times 10^3 \pm 0.1 \times 10^3$
Ileum	ND	$4.1 \times 10^2 \pm 1.04 \times 10^2$	$3.0 \times 10^5 \pm 0.1 \times 10^5$	$1.2 \times 10^7 \pm 0.5 \times 10^7$	$3.1 \times 10^7 \pm 1.1 \times 10^7$
Colon	ND	ND	$5.4 \times 10^5 \pm 0.9 \times 10^5$	$3.8 \times 10^5 \pm 0.3 \times 10^5$	$1.0 \times 10^5 \pm 1.0 \times 10^5$

[a]Results expressed as $\log_{10}$ CFU/g of tissue samples (mean $\pm$ SE) ($n = 7$) (Iyer, 2005). ND, not detectable.

2003), and whey protein polymers (Picot and Lacroix, 2004) has increased the survival and viability of probiotic bacteria in yogurts during storage. Kailasapathy (2006) reported that incorporation of calcium-induced alginate starch microcapsules containing probiotic bacteria (*L. acidophilus* and *B. lactis*) did not substantially alter the overall sensory characteristics of yogurts. ME also appears to provide anoxic regions inside the capsules, thus reducing oxygen trapped inside the capsules, which prevented the viability losses of oxygen-sensitive strains (Talwalkar and Kailasapathy, 2003, 2004) in addition to protecting the cells against the detrimental effect of the acid environment in the yogurt. McMaster et al. (2005) also showed increased oxygen tolerance by bifidobacteria in gel beads. The efficiency of ME in protecting the probiotic bacteria, however, depends on the oxygen sensitivity of the bacteria and the dissolved oxygen levels in the product. The addition of starch as a filler material to the alginate core (Sultana et al., 2000), coencapsulated with prebiotic substances (Iyer and Kailasapathy, 2005), or coating of the bead with chitosan (Krasaekoopt et al., 2006) appears to improve the viability of the cultures.

Compared to most of the traditional dairy probiotic foods, Cheddar cheese has a markedly higher pH (4.8 to 5.6) than fermented milks and yogurt (pH 3.7 to 4.3) and can thus help in providing a more stable medium to support the long-term survival of acid-sensitive probiotic bacteria (Stanton et al., 1998). The metabolism of various LAB in Cheddar cheese results in an anaerobic environment within a few weeks of ripening, favoring the survival of probiotic bacteria (Van den Tempel et al., 2002). Furthermore, the matrix of Cheddar cheese and its relatively high fat content offer protection to probiotic bacteria during passage through the GI tract (Vinderola et al., 2002). Thus, it appears that ME may not be beneficial in protecting probiotic bacteria in Cheddar cheese. However, compared to yogurt, Cheddar cheese has a longer ripening, storage, and shelf life during which the pH decreases, making the cheese acidic in nature during ripening. The combination of long maturation periods and acidic conditions could make it difficult for probiotic bacteria to survive during the 6- to 12-month ripening period. Additionally, unlike yogurts, Cheddar cheese also contains starter and nonstarter LAB, which may affect the survival of probiotic bacteria. Dinakar and Mistry (1994) reported improved survival of *B. bifidum* in Cheddar cheese over a 6-month ripening period. Gardiner et al. (2002) reported improved survival, as well as an increased survival and increased growth rate, of *Lactobacillus paracasei* in Cheddar cheese after 3 months of ripening. Similar results have been reported by McBrearty et al. (2001), Godward and Kailasapathy (2003c), and Darukaradhya (2005).

Numerous studies have reported that probiotics entrapped in alginate or carrageenan beads have greater viability following freezing in dairy desserts (Kebary et al., 1998; Sheu et al., 1993; Godward and Kailasapathy, 2003a, 2003b, 2003c; Shah and Ravula, 2000). The high fat content of ice cream and the neutral pH of dairy desserts may be the main factors responsible for the additional protection provided to probiotic bacteria. However, the addition of cryoprotectants such as glycerol (Sheu et al., 1993; Sultana et al., 2000) seems to improve the viability of probiotic bacteria during freezing of the dairy desserts. The milk fat in ice cream formulations may also act as an encapsulant material for probiotic bacteria during the homogenization of the ice cream mix. The high total solids in ice cream mix, including the fat (emulsion), may provide protection for the bacteria (Kailasapathy and Sultana, 2003).

In unfermented probiotic milk products, the probiotic cultures are added after the milk is pasteurized and cooled. Addition of cultures after pasteurization may cause contamination. The effect of ME in microgel particles on the survival of cultures during pasteurization has been determined, and it was found that some protection was offered by ME when the cultures were pasteurized at 62°C for 30 min. However, viability losses were found to be high when pasteurization was carried out at 70°C for 1 min (Kushal et al., 2005). Even if the milk provides some protection to the cells during heating, it appears that ME in alginate beads is inadequate to provide protection to the bacterial cells.

In powdered milk products, the challenge is to protect the probiotics from the excessive heat and osmotic dehydration during spray-drying. The addition of a thermoprotectant such as trehalose (Conrad et al., 2000) may help to improve viability during drying and storage. Some studies have examined the stability of encapsulated probiotics in dried milk. Freeze-dried microencapsulated hydrogel beads seem to be more stable during incubation at room temperature (Kailasapathy and Sureeta, 2004; Capela et al., 2006). Spray-coating of a freeze-dried culture seems to be more effective for additional protection (Siuta-Cruce and Goulet, 2001). When a lipid coating is used, it may form a barrier to moisture and oxygen entry into the microcapsules. The nature of the packaging materials including their oxygen scavenging capacity, together with the addition of antioxidants, desiccants, etc., may need to be considered for effective protection of probiotic cells during storage (Hsiao et al., 2004; Miller et al., 2003). Spray-drying of starch-encapsulated bifidobacteria did not result in good survival of the organism during storage at 19 to 24°C (Crittenden et al., 2006). Hence, improvements in ME technology are described in order to enhance the viability of cells during storage of dairy products. ME is also being studied to protect probiotic bacteria in meat systems. In contrast to the dairy products, there are few reported data available on encapsulation of meat products (Saucier and Champagne, 2005).

With regard to plant-based products, probiotics are most frequently incorporated into soy products (Wang et al., 2002), although interest is increasing in the use of fermented cereals (Charalampopoulos et al., 2003; Laine et al., 2003) and vegetables (Savard et al., 2003). In a traditional African fermented maize product, ME in gellan/xanthan beads was found to improve the stability of bifidobacteria during storage (McMaster et al., 2005). ME improved the survival of *Lactobacillus rhamnosus* subjected to freezing in a cranberry juice concentrate and during storage of the frozen product (Reid et al., 2007). ME can be of benefit to the stability of probiotic cultures; however, the way the bacteria are grown, harvested, and dried for subsequent industrial use can be as important in promoting the viability of the cultures in food systems as the ME itself. Although the probiotic bacteria show good stability in products having a low water activity such as peanut butter (water activity, 0.24), when *L. rhamnosus* was spray-coated and incorporated into peanut butter (incubated at 21°C), there was decreased viability of cells (J. Belvis, T. A. Tompkins, T. A. Wallace, L. Casavant, C. Fortin, and C. Carson, presented at the CIFIST Meeting, Montreal, Canada, 30 May 2006). ME by spray-coating did not improve the survival and stability of lactobacilli during bread-making (Belvis et al., presented). However, ME in a whey-based protein particle was reported to be effective at enhancing the survival of probiotic lactobacilli during the heat treatment applied during biscuit manufacture (Reid et al., 2007).

A vegetarian product by definition must be free from detectable dairy- and animal-derived proteins including allergens. From an ethical viewpoint, probiotic vegetarian products must not have used animal-derived ingredients during manufacture. Vegetarian probiotic products, inoculated with cells grown and preserved in animal- or milk-derived ingredients, have problems with carryover of undesirable constituents. Growth media containing no animal-derived ingredients have been developed for culturing probiotic organisms to cell concentrations equal to those of standard laboratory media, and a vegetarian product incorporating *L. acidophilus* MJLA1 has been prepared. This product had excellent sensory appeal and better storage characteristics than the uninoculated control (Heenan, 2001). When bifidobacteria were microentrapped into alginate beads and added to mayonnaise, the stability of the cells during storage was greater than with free cells (Khalil and Mansour, 1998).

FUTURE TRENDS

The therapeutic effect of probiotic bacteria and their use in preventive medicine are increasingly being reported. As clinical evidence of the beneficial effects of probiotics accumulates, the food, nutraceutical, and pharmaceutical industries will formulate new and innovative probiotic-based therapeutic products. Culture companies will invest large sums of money to develop more efficacious probiotic strains that can provide significantly enhanced health benefits and withstand the rigors of processing and storage. Innovative ways of administering, delivering, and effecting controlled releasing of probiotics will be developed in the near future. Yogurt and fermented milks have spearheaded the development of probiotic functional foods. The tendency is for other fermented products such as cheese, dairy-vegetable blended spreads, frozen desserts, and meat and vegetable products to follow. Some of these products are already in the development stages. Personal products, sports and health products, and cosmetics containing specific strains of probiotics are currently being either developed or planned, and more innovative products will be developed in the future. Designer probiotic products delivering specific therapeutic strains will be the next phase of development. This will include food, pharmaceutical, and nutraceutical products. These products may take the form of tablets, pills, reconstitutable single-serve sachet products, or convenient packs with instructions on how to prepare and administer them. Some food companies have already developed formulations to prepare probiotic yogurts in the kitchen at home by using a yogurt maker.

An important question in the development of functional foods is the functionality of bioactive cultures. It has been demonstrated that the food matrix has a significant effect on the survival of the cells in the upper regions of the GI tract (Saarela et al., 2006). Therefore, a therapeutic effect noted with a nutraceutical probiotic product cannot be directly transposed to a food product (Champagne and Fustier, 2007). In some cases, functional foods might prove to be better than nutraceuticals as consumers are becoming increasingly health conscious and looking for foods that prevent diseases.

The viability of probiotic bacteria is important for their efficacy, and a large number of reports have shown that many probiotic-based food products do not have the recommended number of viable cells. Thus, ME is a valuable means of protecting and improving the viability of probiotic bacteria. ME will also be important in nutraceutical development. It has been shown that non-protected cells consumed in a dried form have lower recovery levels in stools than those consumed in milk or cheese (Saxelin et al., 2003). The high viability losses that occur when free cells in a powder enter the stomach explain why ME is beneficial for the functionality of probiotics in nutraceuticals (Champagne and Fustier, 2007). ME or enteric-coated probiotic nutraceuticals may deliver the recommended number of viable cells. ME offers the potential to reduce the adverse effects on probiotic viability of the food and GI tract environment as well as during food or nutraceutical processing, storage, and consumption. A number of efficient shell materials and controlled-release trigger mechanisms have been developed in ME, and this trend will continue, particularly with reference to food grade materials and the controlled and targeted release of probiotic bacteria in the GI tract. Probiotic bacteria are already being considered as de novo vaccines (Kailasapathy and Chin, 2000) with the ability to modulate immune responses to a higher level of competence, thereby arming the immune system to better cope with incoming pathogens. The ability of probiotic bacteria to modulate immunity and to improve the composition of the entire microbiota offers the consumer a more effective alternative to better health than the consumption of therapeutic drugs.

The biological activity of probiotic bacteria is due in part to their ability to attach to enterocytes and thereby prevent binding of pathogens. The attachment of probiotic bacteria to receptors on the cell surface of intestinal epithelial cells can activate signaling processes leading to the synthesis of cytokines that affect the function of mucosal lymphocytes. Many of these receptors, such as glycosphingolipids, mannosylated glycoproteins, and TOLL, are already utilized by pathogens. This could be used to develop designer probiotic bacteria by coating with the selected receptor compound and targeting and directing the probiotic bacteria to areas in the GI tract, such as Peyer's patches (small intestine) for maximum activation of the immune system. Further selection of suitable receptor polymers and ME can also help to direct the probiotic bacteria to access areas of medical interest such as tumors in the colon. More research is needed to study the adhesion properties of probiotic bacteria and the selection of polymers that can trigger successful adhesion to targeted intestinal cells and to design these polymers as capsular wall materials or coatings. This could achieve targeted delivery of probiotic bacteria to various sites within the GI tract.

In addition to efficacious capsular wall materials or coatings, cell loading of the capsules is an important challenge. Capsules greater than 20 to 50 μm in diameter may influence the texture of the food products and hence the overall sensory characteristics. However, the microbial cell has a larger size (typically 2 to 5 μm) and therefore could limit the cell loading within the capsules. Another challenge is to improve the heat resistance of these probiotic cells. There appears to be no commercial probiotic product available that is stable at higher temperatures. Discovering or manipulating strains that are heat stable or that have been genetically modified and developing new heat-insulating-encapsulating systems are two of the major challenges in this area of functional food development.

ME can also serve to coentrap prebiotics which could pave the way to designer capsules for gut health. Adding fructo-oligosaccharides or isomalto-oligosaccharides into alginate beads has helped to improve the stability of bifidobacteria during storage in unfermented milk as well as in simulated gastric solutions (Chen et al., 2005). The concept of coencapsulation offers the potential for increased efficiency of functional foods by exploiting the synergy between probiotic and prebiotic ingredients. Addition of Hi-Maize starch as a coencapsulant appears to improve the survival of encapsulated probiotic bacteria in yogurts.

The sensory aspects of foods are critical in the acceptance of new products. Food scientists have generally tried to prevent sensory changes related to the addition of probiotics (Champagne et al., 2005), but in many instances there are no major changes in texture or organoleptic quality that significantly affect the sensorial properties of food (Kailasapathy, 2006). An emerging marketing strategy is to develop food products that clearly show the microcapsules (possibly colored) distributed within the product. Thus, ME could become a future marketing tool for the food and nutraceutical industry.

References

Adhikari, K., A. Mustapha, I. U. Grun, and L. Fernando. 2000. Viability of microencapsulated bifidobacteria in set yoghurt during refrigerated storage *J. Dairy Sci.* **83:**1946–951.

Adhikari, K., A. Mustapha, and I. U. Grun. 2003. Survival and metabolic activity of microencapsulated *Bifidobacterium longum* in stirred yoghurt. *J. Food Sci.* **68:**275–280.

Ahmed, B., and B. K. Mital. 1990. Effect of magnesium and manganese ions on the growth of *Lactobacillus acidophilus.* *J. Food Sci.* **27:**221–229.

Anal, A. K., and H. Singh. 2007. Recent advances in microencapsulation of probiotics for industrial application and targeted delivery. *Trends Food Sci. Technol.* **18:**240–251.

Anderson, K. I., and A. A. Salyers. 1989. Genetic evidence that outer membrane binding starch is required for starch-utilization by *Bacteroides thetaiotaomicron. J. Bacteriol.* **171:**3199–3204.

Anjani, K., C. Iyer, and K. Kailasapathy. 2004. Survival of co-encapsulated complementary probiotics and prebiotics in yoghurt. *Milchwissenschaft* **59**:396–398.

ANZFA. 2001. *Fermented Milk Products. Standard 2.5.3.* http://www.foodstandards.gov.au.

Arnaud, J. P., C. Lacroix, and L. Choplin. 1992. Effect of agitation on cell release rate and metabolism during continuous fermentation with entrapped growing. *Biotechnol. Tech.* **63**:265–270.

Audet, P., C. Paquin, and C. Lacroix. 1998. Immobilised growing lactic acid bacteria with kappa-carrageenan-locust bean gum gel. *Appl. Microbiol. Biotechnol.* **29**:11–18.

Babu, V., B. K. Mital, and S. K. Garg. 1992. Effects of tomato juice addition on the growth and activity of *Lactobacillus acidophilus.* *Int. J. Food Microbiol.* **17**:67–70.

Backhead, F., R. F. Ley, J. L. Sonnenburg, D. A. Peterson, and J. I. Gordon. 2005. Host bacterial mutualism in the human intestine. *Science* **307**:1915–1920.

Benno, Y., and T. Mitsuoka. 1986. Development of intestinal microflora in human and animals. *Bifidobacteria Microflora* **5**:13–25.

Berg, R. D. 1998. Probiotics, prebiotics or 'conbiotics'? *Trends Microbiol.* **6**:89–92.

Bibiloni, R., A. G. Zavaglin, and G. D. Antoni. 2001. Enzyme-based most probable number method for the enumeration of *Bifidobacterium* in dairy products. *J. Food Prot.* **64**:2001–2006.

Boylston, T. D., C. G. Vinderola, H. B. Ghoddusi, and J. A. Reinheimer. 2004. Incorporation of *Bifidobacterium* into cheese: challenges and rewards. *Int. Dairy J.* **14**:375–387.

Capela, P., T. K. C. Hay, and N. P. Shah. 2006. Effect of cryoprotectants, prebiotics and microencapsulation on survival of probiotic organisms in yoghurt and freeze-dried yoghurt. *Food Res. Int.* **39**:203–211.

Champagne, C. P. 2006. Starter cultures biotechnology: the production of concentrated lactic cultures in alginate beads and their applications in the nutraceuticals and food industries. *Chem. Ind. Eng. Q.* **12**:11–17.

Champagne, C. P., F. Girard, and N. Rodrigue. 1993. Production of concentrated suspensions of thermophilic lactic acid bacteria in calcium-alginate beads. *Int. Dairy J.* **33**:257–275.

Champagne, C. P., C. Lacroix, and I. Sodini-Gallot. 1994. Immobilised cell technologies for the dairy industry. *Crit. Rev. Biochem.* **14**:109–134.

Champagne, C. P., N. Gardiner, and D. Roy. 2005. Challenges in the addition of probiotic cultures to foods. *Crit. Rev. Food Sci. Nutr.* **45**:61–84.

Champagne, C. P., and P. Fustier. 2007. Microencapsulation for the improved delivery of bioactive compounds into foods. *Curr. Opin. Biotechnol.* **18**:184–190.

Chan, E. S., and Z. Zhang. 2002. Encapsulation of probiotic bacteria *Lactobacillus acidophilus* by direct compression. *Food Bio-products Proc.* **80**:78–82.

Chan, E. S., and Z. Zhang. 2005. Bioencapsulation by compression coating of probiotic bacteria for their protection in an acidic medium. *Proc. Biochem.* **40**:3346–3351.

Chandramouli, V., K. Kailasapathy, P. Peiris, and M. Jones. 2004. An improved method of microencapsulation and its

evaluation to protect *Lactobacillus* spp. in simulated gastric conditions. *J. Microbiol. Methods* **56**:27–35.

Charalampopoulos, D., S. S. Pandiella, and C. Webb. 2003. Evaluation of the effect of malt, wheat, and barley extracts on the viability of potentially probiotic lactic acid bacteria under acidic conditions. *Int. Food Microbiol.* **82**:133–141.

Chen, K. N., M. J. Chen, C. W. Liu, and H. Y. Chiu. 2005. Optimisation of incorporated probiotics as coating materials for probiotic microencapsulation. *J. Food Sci.* **70**:M260–M266.

Conrad, P. B., D. P. Miller, P. R. Cielenski, and J. J. Pablo. 2000. Stabilisation and preservation of *Lactobacillus acidophilus* in saccharide matrices. *Cryobiology* **41**:17–24.

Crittenden, R., A. Laitila, P. Forssell, J. Matto, M. Saarela, and T. Mattila-Sandholm. 2001. Adhesion of bifidobacteria to granular starch and its implications in probiotic technologies. *Appl. Environ. Microbiol.* **67**:3469–3475.

Crittenden, R., R. Weerakkody, L. Sanguansri, and M. A. Augustin. 2006. Synbiotic microcapsules that enhance microbial viability during non-refrigerated storage and gastro-intestinal transit. *Appl. Environ. Microbiol.* **72**:2280–2282.

Cui, J. H., J. S. Goh, P. H. Kim, S. H. Choi, and B. J. Lee. 2001. Survival and stability of bifidobacteria loaded in alginate poly-L-lysine microparticles. *Int. J. Pharm.* **210**:51–59.

Cummings, J. H., and G. T. Macfarlane. 1991. The colon and consequences of bacterial fermentation in the human colon. *J. Appl. Bacteriol.* **70**:443–459.

Darukaradhya, J. 2005. Enumeration and survival studies of free and encapsulated *Lactobacillus acidophilus* and *Bifidobacterium lactis* in Cheddar cheese. Master Hons. Thesis, University of Western Sydney, NSW, Australia.

Dave, R. A., and N. P. Shah. 1997. Effect of cysteine on the viability of yoghurt and probiotic bacteria in yoghurts made with commercial starter cultures. *Int. Dairy J.* **7**:537–545.

Dinakar, P., and V. V. Mistry. 1994. Growth and viability of *Bifidobacterium bifidum* in Cheddar cheese. *J. Dairy Sci.* **77**:2854–2864.

FAO/WHO. 2001. Evaluation of health and nutritional properties of powdered milk and live lactic acid bacteria, p. 1–34. *FAO/WHO Expert Consultation Report.* FAO/WHO, Cordoba, Argentina.

FAO/WHO. 2002. Guidelines for the evaluation of probiotics in food, p. 1–11. *FAO/WHO Working Group Report.* FAO/WHO, London, Ontario, Canada.

Fooks, L. J., R. Fuller, and G. R. Gibson. 1999. Prebiotics, probiotics and human gut microbiology. *Int. Dairy J.* **9**:53–61.

Franjione, J., and N. Vasishtha. 1995. The art and science of microencapsulation. *Technol. Today* (Summer). Southwest Research Institute, TX.

Fuller, R. 1989. Probiotics in man and animals. *J. Appl. Bacteriol.* **66**:365–378.

Gardiner, G. E., P. Bouchier, E. O'Sullican, J. Kelly, J. K. Collins, G. F. Fitzgerald, R. P. Ross, and C. Stanton. 2002. A spray-dried culture for probiotic Cheddar cheese manufacture. *Int. Dairy J.* **12**:749–756.

Gibbs, B. F., S. Kermasha, I. Ali, and C. H. Mulligan. 1999. Encapsulation in the food industry: a review. *Int. J. Food Sci. Nutr.* **50**:213–224.

Gibson, G. R., and M. B. Roberfroid. 1995. Dietary modulation of the human colonic microbiota: introducing the concept of prebiotics. *J. Nutr.* **125**:1401–1412.

Gilliland, S. E. 1981. Enumeration and identification of lactobacilli in feed supplements marketed as a source of *Lactobacillus acidophilus. Oklahoma Agricultural Experimental Station Miscellanous Publ.* **108**:61–63.

Gismondo, M. R., J. Drago, and A. Lombardi. 1999. Review of probiotics available to modify gastro-intestinal flora. *Int. J. Antimicrob Agents* **12**:287–292.

Godward, G., K. Sultana, K. Kailasapathy, P. Peiris, R. Arumugaswamy, and N. Reynolds. 2000. The importance of strain selection on the viability and survival of probiotic bacteria in dairy foods. *Milchwissenschaft* **55**:441–445.

Godward, G., and K. Kailasapathy. 2003a. Viability and survival of free, encapsulated and co-encapsulated probiotic bacteria in ice cream. *Milchwissenschaft,* **58**:161–164.

Godward, G., and K. Kailasapathy. 2003b. Viability and survival of free, encapsulated and co-encapsulated probiotic bacteria in yoghurt. *Milchwissenschaft* **58**:396–399.

Godward, G., and K. Kailasapathy. 2003c. Viability and survival of free and encapsulated probiotic bacteria in Cheddar cheese. *Milchwissenschaft* **58**:624–627.

Goldin, B. R. 1996. The metabolic activity of the intestinal microflora and its role in colon cancer. *Nutr. Today Suppl.* **31**:24S–27S.

Goldin, B. R. 1998. Health benefits of probiotics. *Br. J. Nutr.* **80**(Suppl. 2):S203–S207.

Goulet, J., and J. Wozniak. 2002. Probiotic stability: a multifaceted reality. *Innov. Food Technol.* **February**:14–76.

Groboillot, A. F., C. P. Champagne, G. D. Darling, D. Poncelet, and R. J. Neufeld. 1993. Membrane formulation by interfacial cross-linking of chitosan for the microencapsulation of *Lactococcus lactis. Biotechnol. Bioeng.* **42**:1157–1165.

Gronlund, M. M., O. P. Lehtonen, E. Eerola, and P. Kero. 1999. Faecal microflora in healthy infants born by different methods of delivery: permanent changes in intestinal flora after caesarean delivery. *J. Pediatr. Gastroenterol. Nutr.* **28**:19–25.

Guerin, D., J. C. Vuillemand, and M. Subirade. 2003. Protection of bifidobacteria encapsulated in polysaccharide-protein gel beads against gastric juices and bile. *J. Food Prot.* **66**:2076–2084.

He, F., A. Ouwehand, E. Isolauri, M. Hosoda, Y. Benno, and S. Salminen. 2001. Differences in composition and mucosal adhesion of bifidobacteria isolated from healthy adults and healthy seniors. *Curr. Microbiol.* **43**:351–354.

Heasman, M., and J. Mellentin. 2001. *The Functional Foods Revolution—Healthy People, Healthy Profits?* Earthscan Pub., Sterling, VA.

Heenan, C. N. 2001. Application of probiotic micro-organisms in soy-based vegetarian foods. Ph.D. thesis. University of New Castle, NSW, Australia.

Heinzen, C. 2002. Microcapsules solve time dependent problems for food makers. *Eur. Food Drink Rev.* **2002**(3):27–30.

Hilliam, M. A., and J. Young. 2000. *Functional Food Markets, Innovation and Prospects: A Global Analysis.* Leatherhead Pub., Surrey, United Kingdom.

Hoier, E. 1992. Use of probiotic starter cultures in dairy products. *Food Australia* **44**:418–420.

Hsiao, H. C., W. C. Lian, and C. C. Chou. 2004. Efficiency of packaging conditions and temperatures on viability of microencapsulated bifidobacteria during storage. *J. Sci. Food Agric.* **84**:134–139.

Hull, R. R., P. L. Conway, and A. J. Evans. 1992. Probiotic foods—a new opportunity. *Food Australia* **44**:112–113.

Hyndman, C. L., A. F. Groboillot, D. Poncelet, C. P. Champagne, and R. J. Nuefeld. 1993. Microencapsulation of *Lactococcus lactis* with cross-linked gelatin membranes. *J. Chem. Technol. Biotechnol.* **56**:259–263.

International Dairy Federation. 1992. General standard of identity for fermented milks. *Int. Dairy Fed.* **1992**:163–165.

Ishibashi, N., and S. Shimamura. 1993. Bifidobacteria: research and development in Japan. *Food Technol. Eur.* **47**:126–135.

Iwana, H., H. Masuda, H. Fujisama, and T. Mitsuoka. 1993. Isolation and identification of *Bifidobacterium* spp. in commercial yoghurts sold in Europe. *Bifidobacteria Microflora* **12**:39–45.

Iyer, C. 2005. Studies on co-encapsulation of probiotics and prebiotics and its efficacy in survival, delivery, release and immunomodulatory activity in mice intestine. Ph.D. thesis. University of Western Sydney, Sydney, Australia.

Iyer, C., K. Kailasapathy, and P. Peiris. 2004. Evaluation of survival and release of encapsulated bacteria in ex vivo porcine gastrointestinal contents using a green fluorescent protein gene labelled *E. coli. Lebensm. Wiss. Technol.* **37**:639–642.

Iyer, C., and K. Kailasapathy. 2005. Effect of co-encapsulation of probiotics with prebiotics on increasing the viability of encapsulated bacteria under in vitro acidic and bile salt conditions and in yoghurt. *J. Food Sci.* **70**:M18–M23.

Iyer, C., M. Phillips, and K. Kailasapathy. 2005. Release studies of *Lactobacillus casei* strain Shirota from chitosan-coated alginate-starch microcapsules in ex vivo porcine gastro-intestinal contents. *Lett. Appl. Microbiol.* **41**:493–497.

Jankowski, T., M. Zielinska, and A. Wysakowska. 1997. Encapsulation of lactic acid bacteria with alginate/starch capsules. *Biotechnol. Tech.* **11**:31–34.

Kailasapathy, K. 2002. Microencapsulation of probiotic bacteria: technology and potential applications. *Curr. Issues Int. Microbiol.* **3**:39–48.

Kailasapathy, K. 2006. Survival of free and encapsulated probiotic bacteria and their effects on the sensory properties of yoghurt. *Lebensm. Wiss. Technol.* **39**:1221–1227.

Kailasapathy, K., and J. C. Chin. 2000. Survival and therapeutic potential of probiotic organisms with reference to *Lactobacillus acidophilus* and *Bifidobacterium* spp. *Immunol. Cell Biol.* **78**:80–88.

Kailasapathy, K., and S. Rybka. 1997. *Lactobacillus acidophilus* and *Bifidobacterium* spp: their therapeutic potential and survival in yoghurt. *Aust. J. Dairy Technol.* **52**:28–35.

Kailasapathy, K., and K. Sultana. 2003. Survival and beta-D-galactosidase activity of encapsulated and free *Lactobacillus acidophilus* and *Bifidobacterium lactis* in ice cream. *Aust. J. Dairy Technol.* **58**:223–227.

Kailasapathy, K., and D. Supriadi. 1996. Effect of whey protein concentrate on the survival of *L. acidophilus* in lactose hydrolysed yoghurt during refrigerated storage. *Milchwissenschaft* **51**:565–568.

Kailasapathy, K. and B. S. Sureeta. 2004. Effect of storage on shelf life and viability of freeze-dried and microencapsulated *Lactobacillus acidophilus* and *Bifidobacterium infantis* cultures. *Aust. J. Dairy Technol.* **59**:204–208.

Kearney, L., M. Lipton, and A. Loughlin. 1990. Enhancing the viability of *Lactobacillus plantarum* inoculum by immobilizing the cells in calcium-alginate beads. *Appl. Environ. Microbiol.* **56**:3112–3116.

Kebary, K. M. K., S. A. Hussein, and R. M. Badawi. 1998. Improving viability of bifidobacteria and the effect of frozen ice milk. *Egyptian J. Dairy Sci.* **26**:319–337.

Khalil, A. H., and E. H. Mansour. 1998. Alginate-encapsulated bifidobacteria survival in mayonnaise. *J. Food Sci.* **63**:702–705.

Kim, K. I., Y. J. Baek, and Y. H. Yoon. 1996. Effects of rehydration media and immobilisation in calcium alginate on the survival of *Lactobacillus casei* and *Bifidobacerium bifidum*. *Korean J. Dairy Sci.* **18**:193–198.

Klein, G., A. Pack, C. Bonaparte, and G. Reuter. 1998. Taxonomy and physiology of probiotic lactic acid bacteria. *Int. J. Food Microbiol.* **41**:103–125.

Klein, J., J. Stock, and K. D. Vorlop. 1983. Pore size and properties of spherical calcium-alginate biocatalysts. *Eur. J. Appl. Microbiol. Biotechnol.* **18**:86–91.

Kneifel, W., D. Jaros, and F. Erhard. 1993. Microflora and acidification properties of yoghurt and yoghurt-related products fermented with commercially available starter cultures. *Int. J. Food Microbiol.* **18**:179–189.

Krasaekoopt, W., B. Bhandarai, and H. Deeth. 2003. Evaluation of encapsulation techniques of probiotics for yoghurt. *Int. Dairy J.* **13**:3–13.

Krasaekoopt, W., B. Bhandari, and H. Deeth. 2004. The influence of coating material on some properties of alginate beads and survivability of microencapsulated probiotic bacteria. *Int. Dairy J.* **14**:737–743.

Krasaekoopt, W., B. Bhandari, and H. C. Deeth. 2006. Survival of probiotics encapsulated in chitosan-coated alginate beads in yoghurt from UHT-and conventionally treated milk during storage. *Lebensm. Wiss. Technol.* **39**:117–183.

Kushal, R., S. K. Anand, and H. Chandler. 2005. Development of a direct delivery system for a co-culture of *L. acidophilus* and *B. bifidum* based on microentrapment. *Milchwissenschaft* **60**:130–134.

Laine, R., S. Salminen, Y. Benno, and A. C. Ouwenhand. 2003. Performance of bifidobacteria in oat-based media. *Int. J. Food Microbiol.* **83**:105–109.

Lankaputhra, W. E. V., and N. P. Shah. 1995. Survival of *L. acidophilus* and *Bifidobacterium* spp in the presence of acid and bile salts. *Cult. Dairy Products J.* **30**:2–7.

Larisch, B. C., D. Poncelet, C. P. Champagne, and R. J. Neufeld. 1994. Microencapsulation of *Lactococcus lactis* ssp. *Cremoris*. *J. Microencapsul.* **11**:189–193.

Lee, J. S., D. S. Cha, and H. J. Park. 2004. Survival of freeze-dried *Lactobacillus bulgaricus* KFRI 673 in chitosan-coated alginate microparticles. *J. Agric. Food Chem.* **52**:7300–7305.

Lee, K. Y., and T. R. Heo. 2000. Survival of *Bifidobacterium longum* immobilized in calcium alginate beads in simulated gastric juices and bile salt solution. *Appl. Environ. Microbiol.* **66**:869–873.

Lee, Y. K., K. Nomoto, S. Salminen, and S. L. Gorbach. 1999. *Handbook of Probiotics*, p. 25–43. Wiley, New York., NY.

Lilly, D. M., and R. H. Stillwel. 1965. Probiotics: growth-promoting factors produced by micro-organisms. *Science* **147**:747–748.

Lourens-Hattingh, A., and B. C. Viljoen. 2001. Yoghurt as a probiotic carrier in food. *Int. Dairy J.* **11**:1–17.

Mandal, S., A. K. Puniya, and K. Singh. 2006. Effect of alginate concentration on survival of microencapsulated *Lactobacillus casei* NCDC-298. *Int. Dairy J.* **16**:1190–1195.

Marshall, V. M. 1992. Inoculated ecosystems in a milk environment. *J. Appl. Bacteriol.* **73**:127–135.

Marshall, V. M., and A. Y. Tamime. 1997. Starter cultures employed in the manufacture of bio-fermented milk. *Int. J. Dairy Technol.* **50**:35–40.

Marshall, Y. M. 1991. Gut-derived organisms for milk fermentations. Is probiotics fact or fiction? *J. Chem. Technol. Biotechnol.* **51**:548–553.

Mattila-Sandholm, T., P. Myllarinen, R. Crittenden, G. Mogenden, R. Fonden, and M. Saarela. 2002. Technological challenges for future probiotic foods. *Int. Dairy J.* **12**:173–182.

McBrearty, S., R. P. Ross, G. E. Fitzgerald, J. K. Collins, J. M. Wallace, and C. Stanton. 2001. Influence of two commercially available bifidobacteria cultures on Cheddar cheese quality. *Int. Dairy J.* **11**:599–610.

McMaster, L. D., S. A. Kokoh, S. J. Reid, and V. R. Abratt. 2005. Use of traditional African fermented beverages as delivery vehicles for *Bifidobacterium lactis* DSM 10140. *Int. J. Food Microbiol.* **102**:231–237.

Metchnikoff, E. 1907. *The Prolongation of Life: Optimistic Studies*. English translation, P. C. Mitchell. Heinmann, London, United Kingdom.

Micanel, N., I. N. Haynes, and M. J. Playne. 1997. Viability of probiotic cultures in commercial Australian yoghurts. *Aust. J. Dairy Technol.* **52**:24–27.

Miller, C., M. H. Nguyen, M. Rooney, and K. Kailasapathy. 2003. The control of dissolved oxygen content in probiotic yoghurts by alternative packaging materials. *Packaging Technol. Sci.* **16**:61–67.

Mitsuoka. T. 1996. Intestinal flora and human health. *Asia Pacific J. Clin. Nutr.* **5**:2–9.

Modler, H. W., and L. Villa-Garcia. 1993. The growth of *Bifidobacterium longum* in a whey based medium and viability of this organism in frozen yoghurt with low acid and high levels of developed acidity. *Cult. Dairy Prod. J.* **28**:4–8.

Muthukumaraswamy, P., P. Allan-Wojtas, and R. A. Holley. 2006. Stability of *Lactobacillus reuteri* in different types of microcapsules. *J. Food Sci.* **71**:M20–M24.

Myllarinen, P. 2002. *Starches—from Granules to Novel Applications*. VTT Biotechnology, VTT Publications 473. VTT Technical Research Centre of Finland, Vuorimiehentie, Finland. http://www.vtt.fi/inf/pdf/publications/2002/p473.pdf.

Myllarinen, P., P. Forssell, A. von Wright, M. Alander, T. Mattila-Sandholm, and K. Poutnanen. 2000. Starch capsules containing micro-organisms and/or polypeptides or proteins and a process for producing them. Patent WO 9952511. F1104405.

O'Sullivan, M. G., G. Thornton, G. C. O'Sullivan, and J. K. Collins. 1992. Probiotic bacteria: myth or reality? *Trends Food Sci. Technol.* 3:309–314.

Ouwehand, A. C., and S. J. Salminen. 1998. The health effects of cultured milk products with viable and non-viable bacteria. *Int. Dairy J.* 8:749–758.

Parker, R. B. 1974. Probiotics, the other half of the antibiotics story. *Animal Nutr. Health* 29:4–8.

Picot, A., and C. Lacroix. 2004. Encapsulation of bifidobacteria in whey protein based microcapsules and survival in simulated gastrointestinal conditions and in yogurt. *Int. Dairy J.* 14:505–515.

Playne, M. J. 1994. Probiotic foods. *Food Australia* 46:362–366.

Playne, M. J., L. E. Bennet, and G. W. Smithers. 2003. Functional dairy foods and ingredients. *Aust. J. Dairy Technol.* 58:242–264.

Prevost, H., C. Davies, and E. Rousseau. 1985. Continuous yoghurt production with *Lactobacillus bulgaricus* and *Streptococcus thermophilus* entrapped in calcium-alginate. *Biotechnol. Lett.* 7:247–252.

Prevost, H., and C. Davies. 1987. Fresh fermented cheese production with continuous pre-fermented milk by a mixed culture of mesophilic lactic *Streptococci* entrapped in calcium alginate. *Biotechnol. Lett.* 9:789–794.

Prevost, H., and C. Davies. 1988. Continuous pre-fermentation of milk by entrapped yoghurt bacteria. I. Development of the process. *Milchwissenschaft* 43:621–625.

Rao, A. V., N. Shiwnarain, and I. Maharaj. 1989. Survival of microencapsulated *Bifidobacterium pseudolongum* in simulated gastric and intestinal juices. *Can. Inst. Food Sci. Technol.* 22:345–349.

Reid, A. A., C. P. Champagne, N. Gardner, P. Fustier, and J. C. Vuillemard. 2007. Survival in food systems *of Lactobacillus rhamnosus* R011 microentrapped in whey protein gel particles. *J. Food Sci.* 72:M031–M037.

Reid, G., M. E. Sanders, H. R. Gaskins, G. R. Gibson, A. Mercenier, R. Rastall, M. Roberfroid, I. Rowland, C. Cherbut, and T. R. Klaenhammer. 2003. New scientific paradigms for probiotics and prebiotics. *J. Clin. Gastroenterol.* 37:105–118.

Rescigno, M., G. Rotta, B. Valzasina, and P. Riccardi-Castagnoli. 2001. Dendritic cells shuttle microbes across gut epithelial monolayers. *Immunobiology* 204:572–581.

Richardson, D. 1996. Probiotics and product innovation. *Nutr. Food Sci.* 4:27–33.

Roberfroid, M. B. 2000. Prebiotics and probiotics: are they functional food? *Am. J. Clin. Nutr.* 71:1682–1687.

Rybka, S., and G. H. Fleet. 1997. Populations of *Lactobacillus delbrueckii* subsp. *bulgaricus, Streptococcus thermophilus, Lactobacillus acidophilus* and *Bifidobacterium* spp. in Australian yoghurts. *Food Australia* 49:471–475.

Saarela, M., L. Lahteemaki, R. Crittenden, S. Salminen, and T. Mattila-Sandholm. 2002. Gut bacteria and health foods—the European perspective. *Int. J. Food Microbiol.* 78:99–117.

Saarela, M., I. Virkajarvi, H. L. Alakomi, P. Sigvard-Mattila, and J. Matto. 2006. Stability and functionality of freeze-dried probiotic *Bifidobacterium* cells during storage in juice and milk. *Int. Dairy J.* 16:1477–1482.

Sakai, K., C. Mishima, T. Tachiki, H. Kumagi, and T. Tochikura. 1987. Mortality of bifidobacteria in boiled yoghurt. *J. Ferm. Technol.* 65:215–220.

Salminen, S., C. Bouley, M. C. Boutron-Ruault, J. H. Cummings, A. Franck, G. R. Gibson, E. Isolauri, M. C. Moreau, M. Roberfroid, and I. Rowland. 1998. Functional food science and gastro-intestinal physiology and function. *Br. J. Nutr.* 80(Suppl.):141–171.

Sanders, M. E. 1998. Development of consumer probiotics for the US market. *Br. J. Nutr.* 1998(Suppl. 2):S213–218.

Saucier, L., and C. P. Champagne. 2005. Cell immobilisation technology and meat processing, p. 337–350. *In* V. Nedovic and R. Willet (ed.), *Applications of Cell Immobilisation Biotechnology*, Focus on Biotechnology, vol 8B. Spinger Kluwer, Berlin, Germany.

Savard, T., N. Gardner, and C. P. Champagne. 2003. Croissance de cultures de *Lactobacillus* et de *Bifidobacterium* dans jus de légumes et viabilité au cours de l'entreposage dans le jus de légumes fermenté. *Sci. Aliments* 23:273–283.

Saxelin, M., G. Grenov, V. Svensson, R. Fonden, R. Reniero, and T. Mattila-Sandholm. 1999. The technology of probiotics. *Trends Food Sci. Technol.* 10:387–392.

Saxelin, M., R. Korpela, and A. Mayra-Makinen. 2003. Introduction: classifying functional dairy products, p. 1–15. *In* T. Mattila-Sandholm (ed.), *Functional Dairy Products*. CRC Press Woodhead Pub. Ltd., Boca Raton, FL.

Saxena, S. N., B. K. Mital, and S. K. Garg. 1994. Effect of casitone and fructose on the growth of *Lactobacillus acidophilus* and its survival during storage. *Int. J. Food Microbiol.* 21:271–276.

Selmer-Olsen, E., T. Sorhaug, S. E. Birkeland, and R. Pehrson. 1999. Survival of *Lactobacillus helveticus* entrapped in calcium-alginate in relation to water content, storage and rehydration. *J. Ind. Microbiol. Biotechnol.* 23:79–85.

Shah, N. P. 2000. Probiotic bacteria: selective enumeration and survival in dairy foods. *J. Dairy Sci.* 83:894–907.

Shah, N. P., and R. R. Ravula. 2000. Microencapsulation of probiotic bacteria and their survival in frozen fermented desserts. *Aust. J. Dairy Technol.* 55:139–144.

Shah, N. P., J. F. Ali, and R. R. Ravula. 2000. Populations of *Lactobacillus acidophilus, Bifidobacterium* spp and *Lactobacillus casei* in commercial fermented milk products. *BioSci. Microflora* 19:35–39.

Shahidi, F., and X. Q. Han. 1993. Encapsulation of food ingredients. *Crit. Rev. Food Sci. Nutr.* 33:501–547.

Sheu, T. Y., and R. T. Marshall. 1991. Improving culture viability in frozen dairy desserts by micro encapsulation. *J. Dairy Sci.* 74:107–113.

Sheu, T. Y., R. T. Marshall, and A. Heymann. 1993. Improving survival of culture bacteria in frozen desserts by microentrapment. *J. Dairy Sci.* 76:1902–1907.

Shimamura, S. 1982. Milk products containing bifidobacteria. *Jpn. J. Dairy Food Sci.* 31:45–53.

Siuta-Cruce, P., and J. Goulet. 2001. Improving probiotic survival rates: microencapsulation preserves the potency of probiotic micro-organisms in food systems. *Food Technol.* 55:36–42.

Stanton, C., G. Gardiner, P. B. Lynch, J. K. Collins, G. F. Fitzgerald, and R. P. Ross. 1998. Probiotic cheese. *Int. Dairy J.* 8:491–496.

Stanton, C., R. P. Ross, G. F. Fitzgerald, and D. V. Sinderen. 2005. Fermented functional foods based on probiotics and their biogenic metabolites. *Curr. Opin. Biotechnol.* **16:**198–203.

Steenson, L. R., T. R. Klaenhammer, and H. E. Swaisgood. 1987. Calcium-alginate-immobilised cultures of lactic *Streptococci* and protected from bacteriophages. *J. Dairy Sci.* **70:**1121–1127.

Sultana, K., G. Godward, N. Reynolds, R. Arumugaswamy, P. Peiris, and K. Kailasapathy. 2000. Encapsulation of probiotic bacteria with alginate-starch and evaluation of survival in simulated gastro-intestinal conditions and in yoghurt. *Int. Food Microbiol.* **62:**47–55.

Supriadi, D., K. Kailasapathy, and J. A. Hourigan. 1994. Effect of partial replacement of skim milk powder with whey protein concentrate on buffering capacity of yoghurt, p. 112–113. *In* B. Dixon and L. Muller (ed.), *Proceedings of the XXIV Int. Dairy Congress*, Melbourne, 18–22 September. 1994. The Australian National Committee of the International, Dairy Federation, Victoria, Australia.

Svensson, U. 1999. Industrial perspectives, p. 57–66. *In* G. W. Tannock (ed.), *Probiotics: A Critical Review.* Horizon Scientific Press, Norfolk, England.

Tabrizi, C. A., P. Walcher, U. B. Mayr, T. Stiedl, M. Binder, J. McGrath, and W. Lubitz. 2004. Bacterial ghosts—biological particles as delivery systems for antigens, nucleic acids and drugs. *Curr. Opin. Biotechnol.* **15:**530–537.

Talwalkar, A., and K. Kailasapathy. 2003. Effect of microencapsulation and oxygen toxicity in probiotic bacteria. *Aust. J. Dairy Technol.* **58:**36–39.

Talwalkar, A., and K. Kailasapathy. 2004. A review of oxygen toxicity in probiotic yoghurts: influence on the survival of probiotic bacteria and protective techniques. *Comprehensive Rev. Food Sci. Food Safety* **3:**117–124.

Tanaka, T., and K. Hatanake. 1992. Application of hydrostatic pressure to yoghurt to prevent its after acidification. *J. Jpn. Soc. Technol.* **9:**73–77.

Tejada-Simon, M. V., Z. Ustenol, and J. J. Pestka. 1999. Ex vivo effects of lactobacilli, streptococci, and bifidobacteria ingestion on cytokine and nitric oxide production in a murine model. *J. Food Prot.* **62:**162–169.

Tissier, H. 1906. Traitement des infections intestinales par la méthode de transformation de la flore bactérienne de l'intestin. *C. R. Seances Soc. Biol.* **60:**359–361.

Tournut, J. 1993. The digestive flora of the pig and its variations. *Rec. Med. Vet.* **169:**645–652.

Ubbink, J. B., P. Schaer-Zammaretti, and C. Cavandini. 2003. Probiotic delivery system. European patent EP 244 458 A1.

Van den Tempel, T., J. K. Gundersen, and M. S. Nielsen. 2002. The micro-distribution of oxygen in Danablu cheese measured by a microsensor during ripening. *Int. J. Food Microbiol.* **75:**157–161.

Varnam, A. H., and J. P. Sutherland. 1994. *Milk and Milk Products: Technology, Chemistry and Microbiology.* Chapman & Hall, London, United Kingdom.

Vinderola, C. G., N. Bailo, and J. A. Reinheimer. 2000. Survival of probiotic microflora in Argentinian yoghurts during refrigerated storage. *Food Res. Int.* **33:**97–102.

Vinderola, C. G., G. A. Costa, S. Regenhardt, and J. A. Reinheimer. 2002. Influence of compounds associated with fermented dairy products on the growth of lactic acid starter and probiotic bacteria. *Int. Dairy J.* **12:**579–589.

Walter, J., G. W. Tannock, A. Tilsala-Timisjarvi, S. Rodtong, D. M. Loach, K. Munro, and T. Alatossava. 2000. Detection and identification of gastro-intestinal *Lactobacillus* spp. by using denaturing gradient gel electrophoresis and species-specific PCR primers. *Appl. Environ. Microbiol.* **66:**297–303.

Wang, X., I. L. Brown, A. J. Evans, and P. L. Conway. 1999. The protective effects of high amylose maize (amylomaize) starch granules on the survival of *Bifidobacterium* spp in the mouse intestinal tract. *J. Appl. Microbiol.* **87:**631–639.

Wang, Y. C., R. C. Yu, and C. C. Chou. 2002. Growth and survival of bifidobacteria and lactic acid bacteria during the fermentation and storage of cultured soymilk drinks. *Food Microbiol.* **19:**501–508.

Xu, J., and J. I. Gordon. 2003. Honor thy symbionts. *Proc. Natl. Acad. Sci. USA* **100:**10452–10459.

Yuki, N., K. Watanabe, A. Mike, Y. Tagami, R. Tanaka, M. Ohawaki, and M. Morotomi. 1999. Survival of probiotic, *Lactobacillus casei* strain Shirota, in the gastrointestinal tract: selective isolation from faeces and identification using monoclonal antibodies. *Int. J. Food Microbiol.* **48:**51–57.

Zhou, Y., E. Martins, A. Groboillot, C. P. Champagne, and R. J. Neufeld. 1998. Spectrophotometric quantification of lactic acid bacteria in alginate and control of cell release with chitosan coating. *J. Appl. Microbiol.* **84:**342–348.

Therapeutic Microbiology: Probiotics and Related Strategies
Edited by J. Versalovic and M. Wilson
© 2008 ASM Press, Washington, DC

2.3. Prebiotics and Functional Carbohydrates

Helena M. R. T. Parracho, Delphine M. Saulnier,
Anne L. McCartney, Glenn R. Gibson

9

Introduction to Prebiotics

Functional food science evaluates the potential of the diet to promote health and reduce disease risk. Foods touted as being "functional" are thought to exert certain positive properties over and above their normal nutritional value. A functional food is therefore defined as "a food which targets functions in the body, beyond adequate nutrition, in a way that improves health and well-being or reduces the risk of disease." While not universally popular, the concept is certainly commercially successful. As the following list illustrates, some of the terms used to describe functional foods are of variable meaning: "Neutraceutical," "Vitafood," "food for specified health use," "Pharmafood," "Medifood," "designer food," "health foods." Despite this, The Institute of Grocery Distributors (http://www.igd.com) estimates that the value of the functional food market in the United Kingdom alone in 2008 will have annual sales worth around £2,000 million.

It is accepted that the birthplace of functional foods was Japan in the 1980s. Here, foods for specified health use are legislated for, and claims are made regarding particular ingredients. Some examples of these claims are as follows: "Cholesterol busters," "Immunity boosters,"

"Hormone balancers," "Helps menopause," "Women-only: Added calcium," "Helps keep your gums healthy," "Cleans your blood," "Vitalizes the brain," "Keeps your intestines fit," "Makes your tummy work." While many of these claims perhaps suffer from their meaning being lost in translation, it is the case that functional foods have huge commercial, and possible biological, significance. Many of the realistic health properties remain to be determined, and there is a lack of mechanistic data. Examples of functional foods include organic and inorganic micronutrients, vitamins, antioxidants, dietary fiber, some proteins (e.g., lactoferrin), certain bioactive peptides, and polyunsaturated fatty acids.

The concept has now moved markedly towards gastrointestinal (GI) function, in particular the impact of gut bacteria. Possibly this is driven by the ubiquity of GI disorders but also the fact that diet is an important controlling factor with regard to indigenous microbiota activities. The gut microbiota contains pathogenic, benign, and beneficial microbial species/genera. A predominance of the first type of organisms can lead towards gut upset which can be both acute (e.g., gastroenteritis) and chronic (e.g., inflammatory bowel disease).

Helena M. R. T. Parracho, Delphine M. Saulnier, Anne L. McCartney, and Glenn R. Gibson, Department of Food Biosciences, The University of Reading, Whiteknights, Reading, RG6 6AP, United Kingdom.

Functional foods directed towards the gut microbiota would serve to influence the composition of activities towards a more positive metabolism.

THE HUMAN GUT MICROBIOTA

The duodenum receives partly digested food from the stomach, which passes to the small intestine and reaches the colon. Due to gastric acid and the washout effect resulting from rapid passage of digestive substances through the stomach and small intestine, the heaviest colonized area of the human GI tract is the large intestine (Tannock, 1999). This is primarily a result of the slowing down of movement of digestive material in the colon, which allows time for a complex and stable microbial ecosystem to develop. The human GI tract is colonized by a large and complex community of microbes, mostly bacterial species, known collectively as the normal microbiota. The numbers and composition of the resident microbiota vary greatly along the GI tract (Gibson and Collins, 1999). This variability is largely due to the different physicochemical conditions (pH, transit time, and nutrient availability) in these regions (Lambert and Hull, 1996).

The stomach is home to a relatively small number of microorganisms due to acidic conditions (pH 1 to 3), with numbers typically around 10^3 CFU ml^{-1} of contents (Holzapfel et al., 1998). One principal inhabitant of the human stomach is *Helicobacter pylori*, as it is able to attach and invade the mucosal layer and produces ammonia to neutralize the acidic conditions of the stomach (Bury-Moné et al., 2001). In the small intestine, although the pH is higher and more favorable for bacterial growth, bacterial numbers and diversity are limited by a rapid transit time and digestive secretions, such as bile acids and pancreatic juices (ca. 10^4 to 10^6 CFU ml^{-1} of contents). The main inhabitants of the small intestine are streptococci, staphylococci, and lactobacilli, with bacterial numbers showing a progressive increase (Gibson and McCartney, 1998; Salminen et al., 1998). The human large intestine is one of the most diverse and metabolically active organs in the human body. The large intestine is the terminal organ of the GI tract, which also comprises the mouth, pharynx, esophagus, stomach, small intestine (duodenum, jejunum, and ileum), rectum, and anus. The large intestine is approximately 1.5 m long and comprises a number of physiologically distinct regions (Cummings and Macfarlane, 1991).

The richest and most complex part of the human intestinal microbiota resides in the colon, comprising an extremely diverse population that includes several hundred different bacterial species (Eckburg et al., 2005).

Here, microbial populations number approximately 10^{11} to 10^{12} CFU g^{-1} of contents. The colonic environment is favorable for bacterial growth, with a slow transit time, readily available nutrients, and favorable pH (Cummings and Macfarlane, 1991). The majority of microbes in the large intestine are strict anaerobes. The most numerically predominant bacterial group in the colon is bacteroides (Moore and Holdeman, 1974). Other commonly encountered genera include eubacteria, fusobacteria, bifidobacteria, peptostreptococci, clostridia, lactobacilli, and streptococci (Salminen et al., 1998).

The composition and activity of the microbiota have a profound influence on health and disease through its involvement in nutrition, pathogenesis, and immune function of the host (Gibson and Roberfroid, 1995). Most of our understanding of the human colonic microbiota is derived from studying the microbial contents of fecal samples, because it is impractical to access the human large intestine during normal digestion, and as an alternative, bacteria detected in feces are most representative of populations present in distal region of the intestine (Moore et al., 1978; Tannock et al., 2000). At birth, the GI tract is essentially germ free, with initial colonization occurring during birth or shortly afterwards. The GI tract of newborns is inoculated primarily by organisms originating from the maternal microbiota of the genital tract and colon and from the environment (e.g., through direct human contact and hospital surroundings) (Holzapfel et al., 1998; Mountzouris et al., 2002). Bacterial populations develop during the first few days of life (Collins and Gibson, 1999), and the intestinal microbiota develops as a result of the influence of intestinal physiology and diet on acquired bacteria (Drasar and Barrow, 1985). Bacteria such as facultative gram-positive cocci, enterobacteria, and lactobacilli are the first colonizers. These microorganisms rapidly consume any oxygen that is present and subsequently create a more reduced environment that then allows the growth of obligately anaerobic species (Rotimi and Duerden, 1981). Significant differences in the composition of the gut microbiota have also been recognized in response to infant feeding regimens. The microbiota of breast-fed infants is dominated by populations of bifidobacteria, and this may explain the purported healthier outlook of breast-fed infants compared to their formula-fed counterparts (Harmsen et al., 2000). Formula-fed infants have a more complex microbiota, with bifidobacteria, bacteroides, lactobacilli, clostridia, and streptococci all being prevalent (Stark and Lee, 1982; Benno et al., 1984; Harmsen et al., 2000). It is thought that the presence of certain glycoproteins and soluble oligosaccharides in human breast milk is selectively stimulatory for bifidobacteria (Gauhe et al., 1954; Petschow and Talbott, 1991). Moreover, human milk is also known to contain significant amounts of oligosaccharides (human milk oligosaccharides) (i.e., lacto-N-tetraose and lacto-N-neotetraose). Certain human milk oligosaccharides may act as soluble receptors in the mucosa for different pathogens, thus increasing the resistance of breast-fed infants to infections by these organisms (Kunz et al., 2000).

There is a strong indication that diet can influence the ratio between microbial species and strains of the intestinal microbiota (Holzapfel et al., 1998). Following weaning, these differences tend to disappear, the microbiota increases in diversity, and a community resembling the adult microbiota becomes established (Collins and Gibson, 1999). The colonic microbiota of infants is generally viewed as being adult-like after 2 years, although facultative anaerobes are reported to be higher than in adults (Hopkins et al., 2001). Once the climax microbiota has become established, major bacterial groups are relatively stable throughout most of adult life (Mitsuoka, 1992; Kimura et al., 1997; Macfarlane and McBain, 1999).

The numerically predominant species of bacteria in the adult intestinal microbiota are obligately anaerobic. Anaerobes predominate over aerobes 100- to 1,000-fold (Macfarlane and McBain, 1999). On the basis of molecular techniques, over 80% of phylotypes observed in the human fecal microbiota belong to three main groups: the *Bacteroides-Porphyromonas-Prevotella* cluster, phylum *Clostridium* and relatives belonging to the *Eubacterium rectale-Clostridium coccoides* group, and the *Faecalibacterium prausnitzii-Clostridium leptum* subgroup. *Lactobacillus*, *Bifidobacterium*, *Peptostreptococcus*, *Streptococcus*, *Ruminococcus*, *Enterococcus*, and *Enterobacteriaceae* are also frequently encountered, although at lower levels.

The primary role of the colonic microbiota is to salvage energy from dietary material that has escaped digestion in the upper GI tract, through the process of fermentation. Approximately 8 to 10% of the total daily energy requirements of the host are derived from colonic bacterial fermentation (Gibson et al., 2000). Most bacteria in the human colon are saccharolytic and so obtain their energy through the fermentation of carbohydrates. Diet is one of the principal factors that determine the type and amount of bacteria that colonize the bowel, as well as regulatory metabolic processes. Principal substrates for colonic bacterial growth are dietary carbohydrates which have escaped digestion in the upper GI tract. These may be starches, dietary fibers, other nonstarch polysaccharides (e.g., cellulose, hemicellulose, pectins, gums, and nondigestible oligosaccharides), sugars, and nonabsorbable sugar alcohols (Cummings et al., 1987). In addition, proteins and amino acids, such as elastin,

collagen, and albumin, can also be useful substrates for the growth of colonic bacteria (Salminen et al., 1998). Between 10 and 60 g of dietary carbohydrate per day reaches the colon. It is also estimated that around 9 g of available protein per day derives from the diet (Cummings and Macfarlane, 1991).

The principal products of colonic fermentation are short-chain fatty acids (SCFA). It is estimated that over 95% of the SCFA produced is absorbed through the colonic epithelium, indicating that it can potentially be a source of energy to the host (Cummings and Macfarlane, 1991). The most predominant SCFA in the human colon are acetate, butyrate, and propionate. Acetate and propionate are found in portal blood. Acetate is metabolized systemically (brain and muscle tissues), whereas propionate is cleared by the liver (Salminen et al., 1998). Propionate function is still not clear; however, it may lower the hepatic synthesis of cholesterol by interfering with its synthesis in the liver. Butyrate is a major source of fuel for the mucosa (colonic epithelium) and has been shown to be involved in mitosis and mucosal regeneration (Cummings, 1981). Butyrate is almost completely consumed by the colonic epithelium. It plays an important role in the metabolism and normal development of colonic epithelial cells and has been implicated in protection against cancer and ulcerative colitis (UC) (Barcenilla et al., 2000). Lactate, ethanol, and succinate are also important products of carbohydrate fermentation; however, they do not accumulate in the lumen because they are utilized by other bacterial species, i.e., they act as electron sink products in anaerobic metabolism (Cummings et al., 1987).

Another important product of fermentation in the colon is gas, with hydrogen (H_2) and carbon dioxide (CO_2) being predominant. It is estimated that up to 4 liters of gas is produced from fermentation per day, depending on the diet consumed (Levitt and Bond, 1970). This is excreted from the human body mainly via flatus. Undesirable metabolites such as ammonia, phenolic compounds, some amines, and toxins may also be produced during microbial fermentation (Smith and Macfarlane, 1996). Production of such metabolites may impact certain disease states and promote gut disorders (Mykkanen et al., 1998). Vitamins and proteins are also synthesized by certain intestinal bacteria and are partly absorbed and utilized by the host (Conly et al., 1994).

ROLE OF COLONIC MICROBIOTA IN HEALTH AND DISEASE

The human colonic microbiota is a complex and metabolically active ecosystem that exerts a major role on host well-being (Gibson and Roberfroid, 1995). In addition to its role in metabolic activities that results in salvage of energy and absorbable nutrients, the large intestinal microbiota contributes towards health in a number of other ways. The colonic microbiota is suggested to play an important role in protection against pathogens and has important trophic effects on intestinal epithelia and immune structure and function (Guarner, 2006).

The indigenous intestinal bacteria protect the host from infection by exogenous pathogens (Mitsuoka, 1992; Tancrède, 1992) and opportunistic bacteria that are present in the gut (internal harmful bacteria) but have restricted growth (Guarner, 2006). This mechanism of protection is called colonization resistance (Macfarlane and McBain, 1999). The strictly anaerobic components of the microbiota appear to be the most crucial to maintenance of colonization resistance (van der Waaij, 1999). This equilibrium between species of resident bacteria provides a "balanced" gut microbiota, which directly influences GI health and systemically affects host health.

Some indigenous colonic bacteria are thought to be beneficial to health, namely, lactobacilli and bifidobacteria. Among the health-promoting actions of the colonic microbiota, colonization resistance, facilitation of digestion, production of SCFA, anticarcinogenic activity, and stimulation of the immune system of the host are the most important (Guarner and Malagelada, 2003). However, a number of factors influence the composition of the microbiota. These may be related to changes in physiological conditions of the host (age, health status, stress, etc.), composition of the diet, and environmental circumstances, e.g., use of pharmaceutical compounds such as antibiotics. In this way, the conditions underlying digestion (e.g., pH, substrate availability, transit time, immunoglobulin A secretion, etc.) may be modulated. This could result in a decline of beneficial bacteria and an increase in potentially harmful bacteria. Some species are considered benign, such as *Eubacterium* spp., methanogens, bacteroides, and clostridia (Gibson, 1998). Additionally, some species are considered to be detrimental for human health. The most important colonic pathogens are *Clostridium difficile*, *Clostridium perfringens*, and sulfate-reducing bacteria. They have been associated with the production of toxins, carcinogens, precarcinogens, and toxic gases (such as hydrogen sulfide). A predominance of these bacteria may predispose towards a number of clinical disorders such as inflammatory bowel disease, antibiotic-associated diarrhea, gastroenteritis, and colon cancer, while making the host more susceptible to problems from transient enteropathogens such as clostridia (Steer et al., 2001).

DIETARY MODULATION OF THE GUT MICROBIOTA

The concept of a healthy microbiota is not new and probably originates with Metchnikoff (1907), who suggested that the long and healthy life of Bulgarian peasants was due to their consumption of kefir, a fermented milk product. He had previously hypothesized that the complex microbial population in the colon was having an adverse effect on the host through the so-called "autointoxication." During the last century, the role of the intestinal microbiota in health and disease has become increasingly recognized. Much interest exists in modulating the composition of the gut microbiota towards a potentially more beneficial community. This may be achieved through the use of targeted dietary supplementation with functional foods (Collins and Gibson, 1999). Such a functional food would be a dietary ingredient that has a cellular or physiological effect above the basic nutritional value (Gibson, 1998; Playne et al., 2003). Recognition of the health-promoting properties of specific commensal microorganisms has encouraged modulation of the human intestinal microbiota towards a more beneficial composition and metabolism—through probiotics, prebiotics, and synbiotics (Gibson and McCartney, 1998).

METHODS FOR MONITORING THE INTESTINAL MICROBIOTA

The intestinal microbiota of humans is a complex bacterial community in which obligate anaerobic species predominate (Sighir et al., 1999). Therefore, identification and characterization of the microbial composition of the human gut are a complex process. Efficient and highly sophisticated methods are necessary in order to accurately study the gut microbial composition, its functionality, and its activity. Detection and enumeration of bacteria are of primary importance to understand the diversity and role of individual microbes in the intestine, as well as monitoring changes in the microbiota over time, within different disease states, or during different treatments and/or diets.

Traditional Culture Techniques for Analysis of the Intestinal Microbiota

Conventional methods for determining the bacterial composition of fecal samples rely on the cultivation of bacteria on anaerobic selective media. Cultivation methods are mostly based upon phenotypic (morphological and biochemical) rather than genotypic characterization of organisms (O'Sullivan, 2000). Many studies have used culture-based methods for the analysis of the colonic microbiota; however, evidence has accumulated indicating that a significant fraction of the microbiota can escape cultivation (Langendijk et al., 1995; Wilson and Blitchington, 1996; Zoetendal et al., 2001). Since the majority of available media for bacterial culture are not wholly selective and usually account only for the predominant populations present in the sample, it can result in a biased view of the microbial composition. This problem is aggravated by the fact that selective media are not available for most strict anaerobes, which leads to an underestimation of the bacterial diversity and the contribution of specific groups within an ecosystem (Vaughan et al., 2000). Moreover, classical microbiological methodologies of assessing microbiota composition are time-consuming and laborious (Blaut et al., 2002). Therefore, other tools are required to supplement conventional microbiological techniques.

Molecular-Based Techniques for Analysis of the Intestinal Microbiota

Molecular techniques promise a more accurate description of the true diversity, structure, and dynamics of complex microbial communities than cultivation studies. The phylogenetic information encoded by 16S rRNA genes has enabled the development of molecular biological techniques (de Vos et al., 1997). The 16S rRNA gene is approximately 1,500 bases long (nucleotides) and includes several variable regions (some highly variable), as well as conserved regions (Woese, 1987). Analyses of 16S rRNA gene sequences have revealed signature sequences, short stretches of rRNA that are unique to a certain group or groups of organisms, enabling phylogenetic placement and identification of bacteria (Holzapfel et al., 1998; Blaut et al., 2002). Studying the GI microbial composition by using molecular methods has two main advantages over traditional bacteriological techniques. First, specimens do not need to be processed while fresh but can be stored appropriately for future analysis. Second, the methods can detect bacterial species currently noncultivable in microbiological laboratories (Tannock, 1999). A number of molecular-based techniques have been used to study the GI microbial ecology in human health and disease. Different aims have been addressed when studying the microbial ecology of the human gut by using molecular techniques: characterization of bacterial diversity within samples, tracking or monitoring of specific organisms or populations, both quantitatively and qualitatively, and enumeration of phylogenetically related groups of bacteria (McCartney, 2002).

Characterization of Bacterial Diversity within Samples

Variable regions of the 16S rRNA gene can be amplified by using PCR with specific bacterial primers, resulting in a collection of so-called amplicons of similar size that may have a different sequence (de Vos et al., 1997). Profiling techniques, such as denaturing gradient gel electrophoresis (DGGE) or temperature gradient gel electrophoresis, are based on the separation of PCR-amplified fragments or amplicons all having the same length (Muyzer and Waal, 1993). Separation is based on the electrophoretic mobility of PCR amplicons in polyacrylamide gels containing a linear gradient of denaturants or temperature. DGGE analysis of different microbial communities results in DNA banding profiles reflecting the makeup of 16S rRNA gene sequences present in the sample. Each band may reflect a different bacterial species, and the band intensity may be semiquantitative (i.e., demonstrate the relative abundance of that species in the sample) (de Vos et al., 1997). Moreover, cloning and sequencing of excised bands from DGGE gels improve the information obtained concerning identification of the bacterial community. DGGE provides a powerful tool in the initial characterization of the predominant members in a complex ecosystem and also in monitoring bacterial dynamics (i.e., over time) (Duineveld et al., 1998).

Tracking or Monitoring of Specific Organisms or Populations

An alternative approach to PCR and the above techniques is to use DNA fingerprinting to examine specific bacterial strains present in the gut microbiota and to distinguish between strains of ingested organisms and the indigenous microbiota. DNA fingerprinting methods with higher resolution include ribotyping and pulsed-field gel electrophoresis, which have permitted the analysis of the human fecal microbiota at the level of strains (Collins and Gibson, 1999). However, these techniques require isolation of DNA as a first step.

Enumeration of Phylogenetically Related Groups of Bacteria

Fluorescent in situ hybridization (FISH) allows the detection of whole bacterial cells and utilizes fluorescently labeled molecular probes targeting 16S rRNA gene sequences of selected bacteria. Specific probes have proven to be useful for enumeration and identification of fecal bacteria (Langendijk et al., 1995; Franks et al., 1998). Probes that are directed against highly variable regions of the 16S rRNA gene may be species or subspecies specific (Langendijk et al., 1995; Franks et al., 1998; Manz et al., 1996; Harmsen et al., 1999), while probes targeting more conserved regions can target a group that is phylogenetically broader (Zheng et al., 1997; McCartney, 2002).

FISH enables five ecological themes to be addressed simultaneously: (i) to identify subpopulations in natural systems and to locate their niche; (ii) to obtain a structural insight into mixed population communities (using sets of probes); (iii) to bypass cultivation problems; (iv) to determine the in situ cellular rRNA content and "metabolic fitness" of bacteria; and (v) to accurately enumerate defined bacterial populations (Vaughan et al., 2000). Probe design and detection limits are the main disadvantages of FISH. The detection limit of the method is ~10^6 cells per g of feces (Harmsen et al., 1999). Nevertheless, FISH allows accurate quantification of the predominant bacterial species of interest.

Increasing knowledge of the microbial ecology of the human gut will improve our understanding of the important role played by the intestinal microbiota for maintaining health and in the prevention of disease. Investigation of microbial traits in the gut of individuals with autistic spectrum disorders, by using molecular techniques, may elucidate targets for improving gut function in these subjects.

PREBIOTICS

An alternative approach to probiotics for intestinal microbiota modulation is the use of prebiotics. A prebiotic is "a non-digestible food ingredient that beneficially affects the host by selectively stimulating the growth and/or activity of one or a limited number of bacterial species already resident in the colon" (Gibson and Roberfroid, 1995). This definition was updated in 2004, and prebiotics are now defined as "selectively fermented ingredients that allow specific changes, both in the composition and/or activity in the gastrointestinal microflora that confers benefits upon host well-being and health" (Gibson et al., 2004). The latter definition considers the microbiota changes not only in the colonic ecosystem of humans but also in the whole GI tract, and this extrapolates the definition into other areas that may benefit from a selective targeting of particular microorganisms.

Any food that contains carbohydrates, and in particular oligosaccharides, is potentially a prebiotic, but in order to be classified as such it must fulfill the following criteria.

- It must be neither hydrolyzed nor absorbed in the upper part of the GI tract.
- It must be selectively fermented by one or a limited number of potentially beneficial bacteria commensal to the colon, e.g., bifidobacteria and lactobacilli, which are stimulated to grow and/or become metabolically active.

- It must be able to alter the colonic microbiota towards a healthier composition, by increasing, for example, numbers of saccharolytic species while reducing putrefactive microorganisms.

A desirable attribute for prebiotics is the ability to persist towards distal regions of the colon, as this is the site of origin of several chronic disease states including colon cancer and UC (Salminen et al., 1998).

Thus, the prebiotic approach advocates the administration of nonviable entities. Dietary carbohydrates such as fibers are candidate prebiotics, but most promising are nondigestible oligosaccharides because they meet all the current criteria for prebiotic classification (Rycroft et al., 1999).

Although prebiotic and probiotic approaches are likely to share common mechanisms of action since their effect is implemented through the increase of beneficial gut bacteria in both cases, they differ in composition and metabolism. One advantage of the prebiotic over the probiotic approach is that the former does not rely on culture viability. Prebiotics are ingredients in the normal human diet, and as such they do not pose as great a challenge from the aspects of safety and consumer acceptability as do probiotics. The best currently recognized prebiotics in Europe are fructooligosaccharides (FOS), galactooligosaccharides (GOS), and lactulose, which (except for lactulose) are legally classified as food or food ingredients (Coussement, 1999). The European prebiotic market is dominated by FOS and GOS. Table 1 summarizes trials with FOS and GOS. Prebiotics are added to many foods including yogurts, cereals, breads, biscuits, milk desserts, ice creams, spreads, drinks, animal foods, etc.

Types of Prebiotics

The prebiotic approach is currently concentrated towards stimulation/enhancement of the indigenous probiotic microbiota. However, future developments may include more functional aspects especially relative to pathogenic microbiota components. As mentioned above, one of the most extensively studied prebiotics is FOS, and these have proven efficacy (Gibson et al., 1995). The prebiotic activity of FOS has been confirmed in both laboratory and human trials (McCartney and Gibson, 1998; Wang and Gibson, 1993; Williams et al., 1994; Kleessen et al., 1997; Gibson et al., 1995). This is because these carbohydrates have a specific colonic fermentation directed towards bifidobacteria, which are purported to have a number of health-promoting properties (Gibson and Roberfroid, 1995, 1999). Bifidobacteria are able to break down and utilize FOS due to their possession of a β-fructofuranosidase enzyme, providing a

Table 1 Human studies designed to determine the prebiotic effects of FOS and GOS

Prebiotic[a]	Model	Dose (g/day)	Duration	Effect	Reference
Inulin	8 healthy humans, placebo controlled	34	64 days	Significant increase in bifidobacteria established by FISH	Kruse et al., 1999
Short-chain FOS	40 healthy humans	2.5–20	14 days	Significant increase in bifidobacteria levels without excessive gas production	Bouhnik et al., 1999
Inulin and oligofructose	8 healthy humans	15	45 days	Bifidobacteria becoming predominant in feces with both inulin and oligofructose	Gibson et al., 1995
Inulin and lactose	35 elderly constipated humans	20 and 40	19 days	Significant increase in bifidobacteria, decreases in enterococci and fusobacteria. Better laxative effect than lactose	Kleessen et al., 1997
FOS in biscuits	31 healthy humans, double-blind placebo controlled	7	42 days	Significant increase in bifidobacteria established via FISH; no change in total bacterial levels	Tuohy et al., 2003
FOS	12 healthy adult humans	4	42 days	Significant increase in bifidobacteria, no change in total bacteria levels	Buddington et al., 1996
FOS	8 healthy humans, placebo controlled	8	5 wks	Significant increase in fecal bifidobacteria and decrease in fecal pH	Menne et al., 2000
GOS	12 healthy humans	15		Significant increase in fecal lactic acid bacteria	Teuri et al., 1998
GOS plus FOS	90 term infants, placebo controlled	0.4 and 0.8	28 days	Dose-dependent stimulating effect on the growth of bifidobacteria and lactobacilli and softer stool with increasing dosage of supplementation	Moro et al., 2002
Short-chain FOS or GOS or SOS or RS	40 healthy adults, controlled, double-blind, parallel group	10	6 wks	Significant increase in fecal bifidobacteria	Bouhnik et al., 2004

[a]SOS, soybean oligosaccharide; RS, resistant starch.

competitive advantage in a mixed culture environment like the human gut (Imamura et al., 1994).

GOS are another class of prebiotics that are manufactured and marketed in Europe as well as Japan. These consist of a lactose core with one or more galactosyl residues linked via β1→3, β1→4, and β1→6 linkages (Playne and Crittenden, 1996). They have found application in infant formula foods. Recent documents have suggested that FOS and GOS are accepted prebiotics that fulfill current selection criteria (Gibson et al., 2004; Gibson and Rastall, 2006).

A prebiotic dose of 5 g/day should be sufficient to elicit a positive effect on the gut microbiota (in some exceptional cases, this may be nearer to 8 g/day). A possible side effect of prebiotic intake is intestinal discomfort from gas production. However, bifidobacteria and lactobacilli cannot produce gas as part of their metabolic process. Therefore, at a rational dose of up to 20 g/day,

gas distension should not occur. If gas is being generated, then the carbohydrate is not acting as an authentic prebiotic. This is perhaps because dosage is too high and the prebiotic effect is being compromised, i.e., bacteria other than the target organisms are becoming involved in the fermentation (Gibson and Roberfroid, 1995).

Other oligosaccharides are suggested as having a prebiotic effect, although they are not yet widely marketed as such (and evidence of their efficacy is weaker than for FOS or GOS). For example, soybean oligosaccharides, which are composed of galactosyl residues linked α1→6 to a sucrose core (Playne and Crittenden, 1996), are used as prebiotics in Japan. These are isolated from soybean whey. Isomalto-oligosaccharides are comprised of glucosyl residues linked by α1→6 bonds. These oligosaccharides are only partially prebiotic, since they are metabolized by humans. They are, however, very slowly metabolized, and most isomalto-oligosaccharides in the diet would pass through to the colon. Xylo-oligosaccharides are also used as functional foods in Japan. These consist of xylosyl residues linked by $\beta1{\rightarrow}4$ linkages (Playne and Crittenden, 1996) and are much more acid stable than other prebiotics. For this reason, they have found application in soft drinks, which tend to be acidic.

A further possibility in microbiota management is the use of synbiotics, the combination of probiotics and prebiotics. A synbiotic has been defined as "a mixture of probiotics and prebiotics that beneficially affects the host by improving the survival and implantation of live microbial dietary supplements in the GI tract, by selectively stimulating the growth and/or activating the metabolism of one or a limited number of health-promoting bacteria, and thus improving host welfare" (Gibson and Roberfroid, 1995). To date, limited research on the effect of synbiotics is available, although studies (Gmeiner et al., 2000) have shown encouraging evidence of the synbiotic effect.

Beneficial Effects

Historically, documented use of prebiotics is limited to the past decade. Thus, evidence of their efficacy is not as extensive as for probiotics. Prebiotics have been extensively studied as prophylactic food ingredients to maintain or restore a "healthy" gut microbiota, the main targets of this approach being bifidobacteria and lactobacilli. These genera have long been regarded as being among the beneficial members of the human gut microbiota. Because *Bifidobacterium* spp. are susceptible to oxygen and heat, their application in probiotic foods has been limited. Therefore, there has been an increased interest in bifidogenic factors, which endure normal food processing and show effectiveness in the human body when ingested to substitute for the direct application of *Bifidobacterium* spp. in foods.

Increases in bifidobacterial and lactobacillus proportions induced by prebiotics have been extensively studied in vitro (Wang and Gibson, 1993; Gibson and Wang, 1994; Probert and Gibson, 2002). The majority of clinical trials with humans have focused on demonstrating their efficacy in increasing intestinal levels of bifidobacteria and sometimes lactobacilli in fecal samples of healthy subjects (Table 1). Increases in bifidobacteria and lactobacilli have been also reported in gut mucosa of patients waiting for colonoscopy with the ingestion of 15 g/day for 2 weeks of FOS (Langlands et al., 2005). An increase of *Eubacterium* spp. was also reported in this study.

UC and Pouchitis

Preliminary data from animal studies suggest that prebiotic administration can prove as effective as probiotics in UC management (Videla, 1999; Videla et al., 2001; Cherbut et al., 2003). One successful randomized, double-blind, crossover placebo-controlled study of 24 patients with pouchitis has shown that the intake of 24 g of inulin per day for 3 weeks reduced the endoscopic and histological pouchitis disease index score, lowered gut pH, and reduced secondary bile acid and *Bacteroides fragilis* in fecal samples (Welters et al., 2002).

Treatment and Prevention of Diarrhea

AAD

A few clinical studies have been performed to investigate whether prebiotics can prevent antibiotic-associated diarrhea (AAD), and results differ. Daily ingestion of 12 g of FOS made no difference, compared to a placebo, in preventing AAD in a large study involving more than 400 patients aged over 65 years taking broad-spectrum antibiotics (Lewis et al., 2005a), while the same dose of this prebiotic reduced episodes of diarrhea in 142 patients with diarrhea caused by *C. difficile* (Lewis et al., 2005b).

Traveler's diarrhea

Only one clinical study of prebiotic therapy for the treatment and prevention of diarrhea has been published (Cummings et al., 2001). In this study, 244 healthy subjects traveling to high- or medium-risk destinations for traveler's diarrhea received either 10 g of FOS or a placebo for 2 weeks before their departure and then for the 2 weeks they were away. Although it was not significant, the prevalence of diarrhea was less in the prebiotic group (11.2% versus 19.5% in the placebo group). Moreover, less severe attacks of diarrhea were recorded for the group taking the prebiotic than for the one taking the placebo.

Colon Cancer

Research in the field of colon cancer is encouraging (Reddy, 1998; Rowland et al., 1998; Reddy, 1999) but limited to preliminary animal studies or with the identification of earlier biomarkers of risk in humans (Pool-Zobel, 2005). Effects have been reported to be associated with gut microbiota-mediated fermentation and production of protective metabolites such as butyrate.

Calcium Absorption

Although animal studies with rats have uniformly shown enhancement of calcium absorption with certain prebiotics (Delzenne et al., 1995; Roberfroid et al., 2002), results of investigations with humans have been mixed (Coudray and Fairweather-Tait, 1998; van den Heuvel et al., 2000;

Tahiri et al., 2003). However, in one long-term study in which 100 young adolescents received 8 g of short- and long-chain inulin fructans per day for a year, a significant increase in calcium absorption was seen and moreover led to greater bone mineral density (Abrams et al., 2005). In humans, calcium absorption is thought to occur in the proximal gut, but a colonic phase may exist. The mechanism of increase of calcium absorption with ingestion of a prebiotic is not clear, but increased solubility of calcium because of fermentation (which lowers cecal pH and increases SCFA production) or changes in Ca^{2+} concentration (which may enhance paracellular transport) are possible (Scholz-Ahrens et al., 2001). Contradictory results of the effect of prebiotics in the literature may be due to the experimental design because the effect of prebiotics depends on the dose, the time of administration, the content of calcium in the diet, the part of the skeleton investigated, and the age of the subjects studied.

Other Areas of Interest for Prebiotics

There is also a great interest in prebiotics in lipid metabolism, immunomodulation of the gut immune system, glycemic control, and behavioral effects, especially cognitive (Macfarlane et al., 2006). Apart from the increase in beneficial bacteria, prebiotic administration may be beneficial through an entirely different mechanism. Oligosaccharides may act as cellular receptors for intestinal pathogens such as *Escherichia coli* and *Salmonella* spp., which instead of binding to cellular receptors may bind to the "decoy" oligosaccharides (Zopf and Roth, 1996). Although research in this area is still in its infancy, achieving oligosaccharide efficacy at multiple mechanistic levels is indeed intriguing.

The most documented and recognized effect of prebiotics is the promotion of the growth of beneficial bacteria in the colon. However, selectivity of the prebiotics is not always totally established and a stimulation of only beneficial genera may be difficult to achieve. That is why the concept of synbiotics, a mixture of a prebiotic and a probiotic, has been proposed. The main idea is to furnish the specific substrate to the probiotic of interest and to stimulate its growth and/or activity, while at the same time enhancing indigenous beneficial bacteria with the prebiotic component.

References

Abrams, S. A., I. J. Griffin, K. M. Hawthorne, L. Liang, S. K. Gunn, G. Darlington, and K. J. Ellis. 2005. A combination of prebiotic short- and long-chain inulin-type fructans enhances calcium absorption and bone mineralization in young adolescents. *Am. J. Clin. Nutr.* **82**:471–476.

Barcenilla, A., S. E. Pryde, J. C. Martin, S. H. Duncan, C. S. Stewart, C. Henderson, and H. J. Flint. 2000. Phylogenetic relationships of butyrate-producing bacteria from the human gut. *Appl. Environ. Microbiol.* **66**:1654–1661.

Benno, Y., K. Sawada, and T. Mitsuoka. 1984. The intestinal microflora of infants: composition of faecal flora in breast-fed and bottle-fed infants. *Microbiol. Immunol.* **28**:975–986.

Blaut, M., M. D. Collins, G. W. Welling, J. Dore, J. van Loo, and W. M. de Vos. 2002. Molecular biological methods for studying the gut microbiota: the EU human gut flora project. *Br. J. Nutr.* **2**:S203–S211.

Bouhnik, Y., K. Vahedi, L. Achour, A. Attar, J. Salfati, P. Pochart, P. Marteau, B. Flourie, F. Bornet, and J. C. Rambaud. 1999. Short-chain fructo-oligosaccharide administration dose-dependently increases fecal bifidobacteria in healthy humans. *J. Nutr.* **129**:113–116.

Bouhnik, Y., L. Raskine, G. Simoneau, E. Vicaut, C. Neut, B. Flourie, F. Brouns, and F. R. Bornet. 2004. The capacity of nondigestible carbohydrates to stimulate fecal bifidobacteria in healthy humans: a double-blind, randomized, placebo-controlled, parallel-group, dose-response relation study. *Am. J. Clin. Nutr.* **80**:1658–1664.

Buddington, R. K., C. H. Williams, S. C. Chen, and S. A. Witherly. 1996. Dietary supplement of neosugar alters the fecal flora and decreases activities of some reductive enzymes in human subjects. *Am. J. Clin. Nutr.* **63**:709–716.

Bury-Moné, S., S. Skouloubris, A. Labigne, and H. De Reuse. 2001. The *Helicobacter pylori* UreI protein: role in adaptation to acidity and identification of residues essential for its activity and for acid activation. *Mol. Microbiol.* **42**:1021–1034.

Cherbut, C., C. Michel, and G. Lecannu. 2003. The prebiotic characteristics of fructooligosaccharides are necessary for reduction of TNBS-induced colitis in rats. *J. Nutr.* **133**:21–27.

Collins, M. D., and G. R. Gibson. 1999. Probiotics, prebiotics, and synbiotics: approaches for modulating the microbial ecology of the gut. *Am. J. Clin. Nutr.* **69**:1052S–1057S.

Conly, J. M., K. Stein, L. Worobetz, and S. Rutledge-Harding. 1994. The contribution of vitamin K2 (menaquinones) produced by the intestinal microflora to human nutritional requirements for vitamin K. *Am. J. Gastroenterol.* **89**:915–923.

Coudray, C., and S. J. Fairweather-Tait. 1998. Do oligosaccharides affect the intestinal absorption of calcium in humans? *Am. J. Clin. Nutr.* **68**:921–923.

Coussement, P. A. 1999. Inulin and oligofructose: safe intakes and legal status. *J. Nutr.* **129**:S1412–S1417.

Cummings, J. H. 1981. Short chain fatty acids in the human colon. *Gut* **22**:763–779.

Cummings, J. H., E. W. Pomare, W. J. Branch, C. P. E. Naylor, and G. T. Macfarlane. 1987. Short chain fatty acids in human large intestine, portal hepatic and venous blood. *Gut* **28**:1221–1227.

Cummings, J. H., S. Christie, and T. J. Cole. 2001. A study of fructo oligosaccharides in the prevention of travellers' diarrhoea. *Alim. Pharmacol. Ther.* **15**:1139–1145.

Cummings, J. H., and G. T. Macfarlane. 1991. The control and consequences of bacterial fermentation in the human colon. *J. Appl. Bacteriol.* **70**:443–459.

Delzenne, N., J. Aertssens, H. Verplaetse, M. Roccaro, and M. Roberfroid. 1995. Effect of fermentable fructo-oligosaccharides on mineral, nitrogen and energy digestive balance in the rat. *Life Sci.* **57:**1579–1587.

de Vos, W. M., E. Poelwijk, A. Sessitsch, E. G. Zoetendal, L. S. Van-Overbeek, and A. D. L. Akkermeans. 1997. Molecular approaches for analysing the functionality of probiotic lactic acid bacteria in the gastrointestinal tract, p. 51–57. *In Lactic Acid Bacteria. Actes du Colloque LACTIC 1997.* Adria Normandie, Villers-Bocage, France.

Drasar, B. S., and P. A. Barrow. 1985. *Intestinal Microbiology.* Van Nostrand Reinhold Co Limited, London, United Kingdom.

Duineveld, B. M., A. S. Rosado, J. D. van Elsas, and J. A. van Veen. 1998. Analysis of the dynamics of bacterial communities in the rhizosphere of the chrysanthemum via denaturing gradient gel electrophoresis and substrate utilization patterns. *Appl. Environ. Microbiol.* **64:**4950–4957.

Eckburg, P. B., E. M. Bik, C. N. Bernstein, E. Purdom, L. Dethlefsen, M. Sargent, S. R. Gill, K. E. Nelson, and D. A. Relman. 2005. Diversity of the human intestinal microbial flora. *Science* **308:**1635–1638.

Franks, A. H., H. J. M. Harmsen, G. C. Raangs, G. J. Jansen, F. Schut, and G. W. Welling. 1998. Variations of bacterial populations in human feces measured by fluorescent in situ hybridization with group-specific 16S rRNA-targeted oligonucleotide probes. *Appl. Environ. Microbiol.* **64:**3336–3345.

Gauhe, A., P. Gyorgy, J. R. Hoover, R. Kuhn, C. S. Rose, H. W. Ruelis, and F. Zilliken. 1954. Bifidus factor-preparation obtained from human milk. *Arch. Biochem.* **49:**214–224.

Gibson, G. R. 1998. Dietary modulation of the human gut microflora using probiotics. *Br. J. Nutr.* **80:**S209–S212.

Gibson, G. R., and M. D. Collins. 1999. Concept of balanced colonic microbiota, prebiotics, and synbiotics, p. 139–152. *In* L. A. Hanson and R. H. Yolken (ed.), *Probiotics, Other Nutritional Factors, and Intestinal Microflora,* vol. 42. Nestec Ltd, Vevey/Lippincott-Raven Publishers, Philadelphia, PA.

Gibson, G. R., and A. L. McCartney. 1998. Modification of the gut flora by dietary means. *Biochem. Soc. Trans.* **26:**222–228.

Gibson, G. R., and R. A. Rastall (ed.). 2006. *Prebiotics: Development and Application.* John Wiley & Sons Ltd., Chichester, United Kingdom.

Gibson, G. R., and M. B. Roberfroid. 1995. Dietary modulation of the human colonic microflora introducing the concept of probiotics. *J. Nutr.* **125:**1401–1412.

Gibson, G. R., and M. B. Roberfroid (ed.). 1999. *Colonic Microbiota, Nutrition and Health.* Kluwer Academic Publishers, Dordrecht, The Netherlands.

Gibson, G. R., and X. Wang. 1994. Regulatory effects of bifidobacteria on the growth of other colonic bacteria. *J. Appl. Bacteriol.* **77:**412–420.

Gibson, G. R., E. R. Beatty, X. Wang, and J. H. Cummings. 1995. Selective stimulation of bifidobacteria in the human colon by oligofructose and inulin. *Gastroenterology* **108:**975–982.

Gibson, G. R., P. B. Ottaway, and R. A. Rastall. 2000. The gut microflora and its modulation through diet, p. 7–9. *In Probiotics: New Developments in Functional Foods.* Chadwick

House Group, Chandos Publishing Ltd., London, United Kingdom.

Gibson, G. R., H. M. Probert, J. A. E. van Loo, R. A. Rastall, and M. B. Roberfroid. 2004. Dietary modulation of the human colonic microbiota: updating the concept of prebiotics. *Nutr. Res. Rev.* **17:**259–275.

Gmeiner, M., W. Kneifel, K. D. Kulbe, R. Wouters, P. de Boever, L. Nollet, and W. Verstraete. 2000. Influence of a synbiotic mixture consisting of *Lactobacillus acidophilus* 74–2 and a fructooligosaccharide preparation on the microbial ecology sustained in a simulation of the human intestinal microbial ecosystem (SHIME reactor). *Appl. Microbiol. Biotechol.* **53:**219–233.

Guarner, F. 2006. Enteric flora in health and disease. *Digestion* **73:**5–12.

Guarner, F., and J.-R. Malagelada. 2003. Gut flora in health and disease. *Lancet* **361:**512–519.

Harmsen, H. J. M., P. Elfferich, F. Schut, and G. W. Welling. 1999. A 16S rRNA-targeted probe for detection of lactobacilli and enterococci in faecal samples by fluorescent in situ hybridisation. *Microbiol. Ecol. Health Dis.* **11:**3–12.

Harmsen, H. J. M., A. C. M. Wildeboer-Veloo, J. Grijpstra, J. Knol, J. E. Degener, and G. W. Welling. 2000. Development of 16S rRNA-based probes for the *Coriobacterium* group and the *Atopobium* cluster and their application for enumeration of *Coriobacteriaceae* in human feces from volunteers of different age groups. *Appl. Environ. Microbiol.* **66:**4523–4527.

Holzapfel, W. H., P. Haberer, J. Snel, U. Schillinger, and J. H. Huis isn't Veld. 1998. Overview of gut flora and probiotics. *Int. J. Food Microbiol.* **41:**85–101.

Hopkins, M. J., R. Sharp, and G. T. Macfarlane. 2001. Overview of gut flora and probiotics. *Int. J. Food Microbiol.* **41:**85–101.

Imamura, L., K. Hisamitsu, and K. Kobashi. 1994. Purification and characterization of β-fructofuranosidase from *Bifidobacterium infantis.* *Biol. Pharm. Bull.* **17:**596–602.

Kimura, K., A. L. McCartney, M. A. McConnell, and G. W. Tannock. 1997. Analysis of fecal populations of bifidobacteria and lactobacilli and investigation of the immunological responses of their human hosts to the predominant strains. *Appl. Environ. Microbiol.* **63:**3394–3398.

Kleessen, B., B. Sykura, H. J. Zunft, and M. Blaut. 1997. Effects of inulin and lactose on faecal microflora, microbial activity and bowel habit in elderly constipated persons. *Am. J. Clin. Nutr.* **65:**1397–1402.

Kruse, H. P., B. Kleessen, and M. Blaut. 1999. Effects of inulin on faecal bifidobacteria in human subjects. *Br. J. Nutr.* **82:**375–382.

Kunz, C., S. Rudloff, W. Baier, N. Klein, and S. Strobel. 2000. Oligosaccharides in human milk: structural, functional, and metabolic aspects. *Ann. Rev. Nutr.* **20:**699–722.

Lambert, J., and R. Hull. 1996. Upper gastrointestinal disease and probiotics. *Asia Pac. J. Clin. Nutr.* **5:**31–35.

Langendijk, P., F. Schut, G. Jansen, G. C. Raangs, G. R. Kamphuis, M. H. Wilkinson, and G. W. Welling. 1995. Quantitative fluorescent in situ hybridization of *Bifidobacterium* spp. with genus-specific 16S rRNA-targeted probes and its application in fecal samples. *Appl. Environ. Microbiol.* **61:**3069–3075.

Langlands, S. J., M. J. Hopkins, N. Coleman, and J. H. Cummings. 2005. Prebiotic carbohydrates modify the mucosa associated microflora of the human large bowel. *Gut* 53:1610–1616.

Levitt, M. D., and J. H. Bond. 1970. Volume, composition and source of intestinal gas. *Gastroenterology* 59:921–929.

Lewis, S., S. Burmeister, and J. Brazier. 2005a. Effect of the prebiotic oligofructose on relapse of *Clostridium difficile*-associated diarrhea: a randomized, controlled study. *Clin. Gastroenterol. Hepatol.* 3:442–448.

Lewis, S., S. Burmeister, S. Cohen, J. Brazier, and A. Awasthi. 2005b. Failure of dietary oligofructose to prevent antibiotic-associated diarrhoea. *Aliment. Pharmacol. Ther.* 21:469–477.

Macfarlane, G. T., and A. J. McBain. 1999. The human colonic microbiota, p. 1–25. *In* G. R. Gibson and M. B. Roberfroid (ed.), *Colonic Microbiota, Nutrition and Health.* Kluwer Academic Publishers, Dordrecht, The Netherlands.

Macfarlane, S., G. T. Macfarlane, and J. H. Cummings. 2006. Review article: prebiotics in the gastrointestinal tract. *Aliment. Pharmacol. Ther.* 24:701–714.

Manz, W., R. Amann, W. Ludwig, M. Vancanneyt, and K. H. Schleifer. 1996. Application of a suite of 16S rRNA-specific oligonucleotide probes designed to investigate bacteria of the phylum cytophaga-flavobacter-bacteroides in the natural environment. *Microbiology* 142:1097–1106.

McCartney, A. L. 2002. Application of molecular biological methods for studying probiotics and the gut flora. *Br. J. Nutr.* 88:S29–S37.

McCartney, A. L., and G. R. Gibson. 1998. The application of prebiotics in human health and nutrition, p. 59–73. *In Proceedings Lactic 97. Which Strains? For Which Products?* Adria Normandie, Villers-Bocage, France.

Menne, E., N. Guggenbuhl, and M. Roberfroid. 2000. Fn-type chicory inulin hydrolysate has a prebiotic effect in humans. *J. Nutr.* 130:1197–1199.

Metchnikoff, E. 1907. *The Prolongation of Life.* William Heineman, London, United Kingdom.

Mitsuoka, T. 1992. Intestinal flora and aging. *Nutr. Rev.* 50:438–446.

Moore, W. E. C., E. P. Cato, and L. V. Holdeman. 1978. Some current concepts in intestinal bacteriology. *Am. J. Clin. Nutr.* 31:S33–S42.

Moore, W. E. C., and L. V. Holdeman. 1974. Human fecal flora: the normal flora of 20 Japanese-Hawaiians. *Appl. Environ. Microbiol.* 27:961–979.

Moro, G., I. Minoli, M. Mosca, S. Fanaro, J. Jelinek, B. Stahl, and G. Boehm. 2002. Dosage-related bifidogenic effects of galacto- and fructooligosaccharides in formula-fed term infants. *J. Pediatr. Gastroenterol. Nutr.* 34:291–295.

Mountzouris, K. C., A. L. McCartney, and G. R. Gibson. 2002. Intestinal microflora of human infants and current trends for its nutritional modulation. *Br. J. Nutr.* 87:405–420.

Muyzer, G., and E. C. D. Waal. 1993. Profiling of complex microbial populations by denaturing grading gel electrophoresis analysis of polymerase chain reaction-amplified genes coding for 16S rRNA. *Appl. Environ. Microbiol.* 59:695–700.

Mykkanen, H., K. Laiho, and S. Salminen. 1998. Variations in faecal bacterial enzyme activities and associations with bowel function and diet in elderly subjects. *J. Appl. Microbiol.* 85:37–41.

O'Sullivan, D. J. 2000. Methods for analysis of the intestinal microflora. *Curr. Issues. Intest. Microbiol.* 1:39–50.

Petschow, B. W., and R. D. Talbott. 1991. Response of *Bifidobacterium* species to growth promoters in human and cow milk. *Pediatr. Res.* 29:208–213.

Playne, M. J., L. E. Bennett, and G. W. Smithers. 2003. Functional dairy foods and ingredients. *Austr. J. Dairy Technol.* 58:242–264.

Playne, M. J., and R. Crittenden. 1996. Commercially available oligosaccharides. *Bull. Int. Dairy Found.* 313:10–22.

Pool-Zobel, B. L. 2005. Inulin-type fructans and reduction in colon cancer risk: review of experimental and human data. *Br. J. Nutr.* 93:S73–S90.

Probert, H. M., and G. R. Gibson. 2002. Investigating the prebiotic and gas-generating effects of selected carbohydrates on the human colonic microflora. *Lett. Appl. Microbiol.* 35:473–480.

Reddy, B. S. 1998. Prevention of colon cancer by pre- and probiotics: evidence from laboratory studies. *Br. J. Nutr.* 80:S219–S223.

Reddy, B. S. 1999. Possible mechanisms by which pro- and prebiotics influence colon carcinogenesis and tumor growth. *J. Nutr.* 129:1478S–1482S.

Roberfroid, M. B., J. Cumps, and J. P. Devogelaer. 2002. Dietary chicory inulin increases whole-body bone mineral density in growing male rats. *J. Nutr.* 132:3599–3602.

Rotimi, V. O., and B. I. Duerden. 1981. The development of the bacterial flora in normal neonates. *J. Med. Microbiol.* 14:51–62.

Rowland, I. R., C. J. Rumney, J. T. Coutts, and L. C. Lievense. 1998. Effect of *Bifidobacterium longum* and inulin on gut bacterial metabolism and carcinogen-induced aberrant crypt foci in rats. *Carcinogenesis* 19:281–285.

Rycroft, C. E., L. J. Fooks, and G. R. Gibson. 1999. Methods for assessing the potential of prebiotics and probiotics. *Curr. Opin. Clin. Nutr. Metab. Care* 2:1–4.

Salminen, S., C. Bouley, M. C. Boutron-Ruault, J. H. Cummings, A. Franck, G. R. Gibson, E. Isolauri, M. C. Moreau, M. Roberfroid, and I. Rowland. 1998. Functional food science and gastrointestinal physiology and function. *Br. J. Nutr.* 80:S147–S171.

Scholz-Ahrens, K. E., G. Schaafsma, E. van den Heuvel, and J. Schrezenmeir. 2001. Effects of prebiotics on mineral metabolism. *Am. J. Clin. Nutr.* 73:459S–464S.

Sighir, A., J. Doré, and R. I. Mackie. 1999. Molecular diversity and phylogeny of human colonic bacteria. *Molecular Ecology in Gastrointestinal Systems. New Frontiers: Proceedings of the 8th International Symposium on Microbial Ecology, Halifax, Canada.*

Smith, E. A., and G. T. Macfarlane. 1996. Enumeration of human colonic bacteria producing phenolic and indolic compounds: effects of pH, carbohydrate availability and retention on dissimilatory aromatic amino acid metabolism. *J. Appl. Bacteriol.* 81:288–302.

Stark, P. L., and A. Lee. 1982. The microbial ecology of the large bowel of breast-fed and formula-fed infants during the first year of life. *J. Med. Microbiol.* 15:189–203.

Steer, T., H. Carpenter, K. Tuohy, and G. R. Gibson. 2001. Perspectives on the role of the human gut microflora in health and disease and its modulation by pro- and prebiotics. *Nutr. Res. Rev.* **13:**229–254.

Tahiri, M., J. C. Tressol, Y. Arnaud, F. R. J. Bornet, C. Bouteloup-Demange, C. Feillet-Coudray, M. Brandolini, V. Ducros, D. Pepin, F. Brouns, A. M. Roussel, Y. Rayssiguier, and C. Coudray. 2003. Effect of short-chain fructooligosaccharides on intestinal calcium absorption and calcium status in postmenopausal women: a stable-isotope study. *Am. J. Clin. Nutr.* **77:**449–457.

Tancrède, C. 1992. Role of human microflora in health and disease. *Eur. J. Clin. Microbiol. Infect. Dis.* **11:**1012–1015.

Tannock, G. W. 1999. A fresh look at the intestinal microflora, p. 5–12. *In* G. W. Tannock (ed.), *Probiotics: a Critical Review.* Horizon Scientific Press, Wymondham, United Kingdom.

Tannock, G. W., K. Munro, H. J. M Harmsen, G. W. Welling, J. Smart, and P. K. Gopal. 2000. Analysis of the fecal microflora of human subjects consuming a probiotic product containing *Lactobacillus rhamnosus* DR20. *Appl. Environ. Microbiol.* **66:**2578–2588.

Teuri, U., R. Korpela, M. Saxelin, L. Montonen, and S. Salminen. 1998. Increased fecal frequency and gastrointestinal symptoms following ingestion of galacto-oligosaccharide-containing yogurt. *J. Nutr. Sci. Vitaminol.* **44:**465–471.

Tuohy, K. M., H. M. Probert, C. W. Smeijkal, and G. R. Gibson. 2003. Using probiotics and prebiotics to improve gut health. *Ther. Focus* **8:**692–700.

van den Heuvel, E. G., M. H. Schoterman, and T. Muijs. 2000. Transgalactooligosaccharides stimulate calcium absorption in postmenopausal women. *J. Nutr.* **130:**2938–2942.

van der Waaij, D. 1999. Microbial ecology of the intestinal microflora: influence of interactions with the host organism, p. 1–16. *In* L. A. Hanson and R. H. Yolken (ed.), *Probiotics, Other Nutritional Factors, and Intestinal Microflora,* vol. 42. Nestec Ltd, Vevey/Lippincott-Raven Publishers, Philadelphia, PA.

Vaughan, E. E., F. Schut, H. G. J. Heilig, E. G. Zoetendal, W. M. de Vos, and A. D. L. Akkermans. 2000. A molecular view of the intestinal ecosystem. *Curr. Issues Intest. Microbiol.* **1:**1–12.

Videla, S. 1999. Deranged luminal pH homeostasis in experimental colitis can be restored by a prebiotic. *Gastroenterology* **116:**A942.

Videla, S., J. Vilaseca, M. Antolin, A. Garcia-Lafuente, F. Guarner, E. Crespo, J. Casalots, A. Salas, and J. R. Malagelada. 2001. Dietary inulin improves distal colitis induced by dextran sodium sulfate in the rat. *Am. J. Gastroenterol.* **96:**1486–1493.

Wang, X., and G. R. Gibson. 1993. Effects of the *in vitro* fermentation of oligofructose and inulin by bacteria growing in the human large intestine. *J. Appl. Bacteriol.* **75:**373–380.

Welters, C. F., E. Heineman, F. B. Thunnissen, A. E. van den Bogaard, P. B. Soeters, and C. G. Baeten. 2002. Effect of dietary inulin supplementation on inflammation of pouch mucosa in patients with an ileal pouch-anal anastomosis. *Dis. Colon Rectum* **45:**621–627.

Williams, C. H., S. A. Witherly, and R. K. Buddington. 1994. Influence of dietary neosugar on selected bacterial groups of the human fecal microb. *Microb. Ecol. Health Dis.* **7:**91–97.

Wilson, K. H., and R. B. Blitchington. 1996. Human colonic biota studied by ribosomal DNA sequence analysis. *Appl. Environ. Microbiol.* **62:**2273–2278.

Woese, C. R. 1987. Bacterial evolution. *Microbiol. Rev.* **51:**221–271.

Zheng, D., E. W. Alm, D. A. Stahl, and L. Raskin. 1997. Characterization of universal small-subunit rRNA hybridization probes for quantitative molecular microbial ecology studies. *Appl. Environ. Microbiol.* **62:**4505–4513.

Zoetendal, E. G., A. D. L. Akkermans, D. M. Akkermans-van Vilet, J. A. G. M. De Visser, and W. M. De Vos. 2001. The host genotype affects the bacterial community in the human gastrointestinal tract. *Microb. Ecol. Health Dis.* **13:**129–134.

Zopf, D., and S. Roth. 1996. Oligosaccharide anti-infective agents. *Lancet* **347:**1017–1021.

Therapeutic Microbiology: Probiotics and Related Strategies
Edited by J. Versalovic and M. Wilson
© 2008 ASM Press, Washington, DC

Giovanni V. Coppa
Orazio Gabrielli

Human Milk Oligosaccharides as Prebiotics

10

It has been well established that human milk, in addition to its nutritional role, is able to influence the development of the intestinal microbiota and exert beneficial effects on the health of the neonate. It has been known since the beginning of the previous century (Tissier, 1900) that there was a considerable difference between the composition of the fecal microbiota of breast-fed neonates and that of formula-fed neonates—with a prevalence of bifidobacteria and lactobacilli (bifidogenic flora) in the former.

DEVELOPMENT OF THE INTESTINAL MICROBIOTA IN THE NEONATE

Microbial colonization of the human intestine starts at birth, when the neonate moves from a sterile environment to an external environment that is rich in bacterial species. In fact, the composition of the intestinal microbiota during the first days of life is significantly influenced by the type of delivery, environmental contamination, sanitary conditions, and the geographical distribution of bacterial species (Mackie et al., 1999; Mountzouris and Gibson, 2003; Orrhage and Nord, 1999). Naturally

delivered babies experience a period of 2 to 3 days in which, as a consequence of the low selective potential of their stomach and small bowel, bacteria colonize and reproduce in the gut. These bacteria consist mainly of facultatively anaerobic species such as *Enterobacteriaceae*, streptococci, and staphylococci. Their metabolic activities are beneficial to the infant by preparing the gut for colonization by a benign enteric microbiota (Favier et al., 2003). According to data obtained using classical microbiological techniques, it seems that bifidobacteria, lactobacilli, and other anaerobic bacteria reach the gut after 2 to 3 days. Neonates delivered by cesarean section seem to have fewer bacteria than those delivered naturally. Moreover, the appearance of bifidobacteria seems to be delayed in the former (Gronlund et al., 1999).

The sources of bacteria first to arrive in the gut of neonates are the vagina, feces, and skin of the mother, providing an inoculum which is a mixture of intestinal and nonintestinal species. In vaginal delivery, the same serotypes of *Escherichia coli* were found in babies after birth and in their mothers' feces, strongly suggesting that infants are colonized by microbes from their mothers' feces. Vaginal bacteria were also found to be present in

Giovanni V. Coppa and Orazio Gabrielli, Institute of Maternal-Infantile Sciences, Polytechnic University of Marche, 60123 Ancona, Italy.

the gastric content of neonates 5 to 10 min after birth (Brook et al., 1979). Cesarean delivery often results in colonization of infants by bacteria from equipment, air, and nursing staff rather than from maternal bacteria, and this delays the onset of the development of a normal intestinal microbiota. Shortly after birth, environmental microbes and oral and skin microbes from the mother are the major sources of bacteria colonizing the neonate via a range of transfer mechanisms which include suckling, kissing, and caressing. These bacteria are able to create a reduced environment favorable to anaerobic bacteria, which colonize the gut at the end of the first week of life, taking over from the facultative species. After the first week, and regardless of the type of delivery, the development of the intestinal microbiota is significantly influenced by the mode of nutrition. At this time, breast-fed infants have a microbiota characterized by the remarkable prevalence of bifidobacteria and lactobacilli, while bottle-fed babies develop a more heterogeneous microbiota consisting of fewer bifidobacteria together with some species which, in certain situations, may exert pathogenic effects, e.g., clostridia, staphylococci, etc. (Harmsen et al., 2000; Penders et al., 2005). These findings, obtained by traditional cultural techniques, have recently been confirmed, with few exceptions (Fanaro et al., 2003; Kullen and Better, 2005), by more advanced molecular biology techniques.

Many studies have demonstrated the positive influence of a bifidogenic microbiota on the health of neonates, and this has been acknowledged by members of the international community of pediatricians such as the European Society of Pediatric Gastroenteroloy, Hepatology and Nutrition (Agostoni et al., 2004). Briefly, the positive effects of a bifidogenic microbiota include the modulation of mucosal physiology, barrier function, and inflammatory responses. Such a microbiota also plays an important role in developing tolerance of the immune system to self antigens as well as maintaining homeostasis of the intestinal ecosystem by limiting colonization of pathogens and substantially reducing the incidence of intestinal infections and allergies. Moreover, additional data on the enhancement of the intestinal absorption of some minerals and of the synthesis of certain vitamins have recently been published (Macfarlane et al., 2006; Tamine et al., 1995).

SEARCHING FOR THE BIFIDOGENIC FACTORS OF HUMAN MILK

The characteristic composition of the intestinal microbiota of breast-fed neonates is due to the presence of particular substances in human milk. These are resistant to digestive processes and thereby reach the colon, where they exert a prebiotic effect. Cow's milk, which is used in the preparation of infant formula foods, and human milk have significant qualitative and quantitative differences. The bifidogenic effect of human milk is probably not related to a single growth-promoting substance, but rather to a whole complex of interacting factors. Two main lines of investigation of the bifidogenic effect have been undertaken. One aims to identify the components able to promote the prebiotic effect in human milk, and the other is oriented towards modifying the composition of infant formulas in order to obtain an intestinal microbiota similar to that of breast-fed babies. To find the sources of the prebiotic effect, numerous studies of several components of milk have been carried out. In particular, the roles of proteins, phosphorus, lactoferrin, nucleotides, lactose, and oligosaccharides have recently been reviewed (Coppa et al., 2006a).

It has been assumed that the bifidogenic effect of human milk could be ascribed to its optimal buffering properties due to its low phosphate and protein contents with respect to cow's milk. Also, the prevalence of whey proteins has been held as a factor that could play a role in the development of the neonate's intestinal microbiota. The potential influence of an infant formula with reduced phosphate and protein concentrations on the intestinal microbiota has been studied by Radke et al. (1992). Chierici et al. (1997) have carried out a study of full-term neonates, using an experimental milk formula with a reduced protein content and desialylated milk proteins. In both studies the attempts to achieve bifidogenic effects were unsuccessful.

Balmer et al. (1989a) have used a formula in which whey is predominant and obtained a fecal microbiota "generally" closer to that of breast-fed babies, but substantial differences remained. On the other hand, most of the formulas used today in Europe have a protein composition with a predominance of whey proteins. Studies performed with neonates fed such formulas have shown a microbiota that is rather different from that of breast-fed neonates. We also found no bifidogenic effect in a large number of neonates fed on a formula in which whey is predominant. Also, the use of formulas with hydrolyzed proteins has not produced any positive effect on the neonatal intestinal microbiota either. Recently, the prebiotic behavior of a formula enriched with bovine alpha-lactalbulin and casein glycomacropeptide was evaluated (Bruck et al., 2006). An increase in bifidobacteria was observed only in a small number of subjects studied.

In conclusion, the above data do not support a primary role of human milk phosphates and proteins as prebiotics.

Lactoferrin is a major protein in human milk, but there are only traces of it in cow's milk. As a small percentage of lactoferrin (less than 6 to 10%) is estimated not to be digested by breast-fed infants, it could consequently reach the colon and play a role as a prebiotic. Moreover, after the digestion of human milk with pepsin, several bifidogenic peptides have recently been purified by chromatography. Two of these peptides have been found to originate from lactoferrin and have shown bifidogenic activity at very low concentrations in in vitro experiments. The availability of bovine lactoferrin has made it possible to add lactoferrin to infant formulas and to study the effect of feeding such formulas to infants. Balmer et al. (1989b) found that the addition of lactoferrin had little effect on the fecal microbiota and did not shift the pattern of the fecal microbiota in the direction of that observed with breast-fed babies after 2 weeks. In contrast, Roberts et al. (1992) found a predominantly bifidobacterial microbiota in one-half of the infants after 3 months of treatment with a lactoferrin-enriched formula. Lactoferrin, or some peptides derived from its digestion, appear to exert a prebiotic effect. However, data emerging from clinical trials are not yet conclusive.

Another group of substances studied for their possible prebiotic role are nucleotides. Human milk contains relatively high concentrations of preformed nucleotides, whereas cow's milk is usually completely devoid of such substances. First, Gyorgy et al. (1954) showed that nucleotides can exert some stimulating effect on the growth of *Lactobacillus bifidum* in vitro. A role for nucleotides in establishing the fecal microbiota of infants has also been suggested by the work of Gil et al. (1986). In their study, infants fed on a nucleotide-supplemented formula had a fecal microbiota somewhere between that of breast-fed infants and that of standard-formula-fed infants. However, a subsequent study by Balmer et al. (1994) failed to show any positive effects of adding nucleotides to an infant formula in terms of the proportion of bifidobacteria in the fecal microbiota. Neither have we found any bifidogenic effect in neonates fed for 1 month on a nucleotide-enriched formula. The results available to date on the prebiotic effect of nucleotides are inconclusive.

The implication of a prebiotic role for lactose comes from animal studies in which it has been demonstrated that lactose reaching the colon stimulates the growth of bifidobacteria. Furthermore, Szilagyi (2002) has recently drawn attention to the potential prebiotic effect of lactose in humans. In neonates, lactose is not completely digested in the small intestine; therefore, theoretically the unhydrolyzed lactose can reach the colon and can be "salvaged" by bacteria. However, the amount of ingested lactose reaching a neonate's colon is very low.

On the other hand, modern formulas containing the same amount of lactose as human milk do not show any influence on the composition of the intestinal microbiota. However, a certain amount of lactose could remain in the colon after the digestion of human milk oligosaccharides (HMO) by the intestinal microbiota and could be utilized by bifidobacteria because of their peculiar metabolic capacities (Parche et al., 2006).

Other substances proposed as prebiotics are oligosaccharides, which make up one of the most important components of human milk. In contrast, they are present only in small amounts in cow's milk. Over the years, many studies of their prebiotic effect have been carried out. First, Schonfeld (1926) demonstrated that the bifidogenic effect of maternal milk was the result of a "non-protein fraction." Later, Gyorgy et al. (1954) confirmed that the prebiotic effect was related to a mixture of oligosaccharides, and subsequently Kuhn (1958) demonstrated that the addition of N-acetylglucosamine-containing oligosaccharides in cow's milk stimulated the growth of bifidobacteria. Further studies have shown that a considerable percentage of the ingested oligosaccharides resist digestion by the brush border and pancreatic enzymes. Thus, they are able to reach the colon and play a primary role in the development and composition of the microbiota.

Recently, the prebiotic effect of HMO has further been confirmed by in vitro fermentation studies which clearly demonstrated that these substances play a fundamental role in stimulating the selective development of bifidobacteria (Ward et al., 2006).

In conclusion, the prebiotic effect of human milk originates from a combination of several of its components. It is not easy to exactly establish the specific role of each substance. Nevertheless, from an analysis of the literature oligosaccharides clearly emerge as the main substances that promote a predominantly bifidobacterial microbiota in infants.

HMO: HISTORY, SYNTHESIS, AND STRUCTURE

The first studies of the composition of human milk carbohydrates date back to the end of the 19th century (Denigés, 1892). It took more than 40 years before Polonowski and Lespagnol (1933) were able to isolate these carbohydrates from human milk, and it was only in the 1950s that Montreuil (1957) and Kuhn (1958) demonstrated that these substances were a complex mixture of oligosaccharides. Subsequently, the availability of more advanced techniques made it possible to establish the amount of oligosaccharides in human milk.

Montreuil and Mullet (1959), in a single sample of human colostrum, found a concentration of 23 g of oligosaccharides per liter. Subsequently, Viverge et al. (1985) reported the oligosaccharide content of the milk of 15 mothers during their first week of lactation as well as in a group of 11 mothers over a period of 3 months after delivery. Thereafter, in a longitudinal study of a group of 46 lactating mothers, the milk carbohydrate composition during the first 4 months of lactation was analyzed. It was found that the concentration of oligosaccharides was more than 20 g/liter in the colostrum and then decreased during the first month of lactation, stabilizing at around 12 to 14 g/liter (Coppa et al., 1993). Further studies confirmed that oligosaccharides, from a quantitative point of view, are the third most prominent component of human milk, after lactose and lipids (Chaturvedi et al., 1997; Coppa et al., 1999; Kunz et al., 1999, Thurl et al., 1996). In contrast, cow's milk, commonly used for preparing infant formulas, contains only few oligosaccharides, amounting to less than 1.0 g/liter.

HMO are synthesized in the mammary gland by the action of specific glycosyltransferases by the sequential addition of monosaccharide units to the lactose molecule. The monosaccharide building blocks are glucose (Glc), galactose (Gal), N-acetylglucosamine (GlcNAc), fucose (Fuc), and sialic acid (NANA). Oligosaccharides can be classified on the basis of their chemical composition as follows: (i) core-oligosaccharides, made of Glc, Gal, and GlcNAc, representing the starting structures for the synthesis of more complex oligosaccharides; (ii) fucosyl-oligosaccharides, derived from the addition of one or more units of Fuc to the core; (iii) sialyloligosaccharides, ensuing from the addition of one or more units of NANA; (iv) fucosyl-sialyl-oligosaccharides, from the addition of one or more units of both Fuc and NANA. Regardless of their composition, oligosaccharide molecules can have a linear or branched structure (Fig. 1). By using modern analytical methods, over 130 different types of oligosaccharides have been identified. However, it is important to bear in mind that the main quantitative component of HMO is made up of 25 to 30 oligosaccharides, composed of 3 to 10 monosaccharide units—the others are present in only minute amounts.

The presence of the various glycosyltransferases in the mammary gland is genetically determined. Most of them are common to all women (Table 1), the exception being fucosyltransferases, whose presence is linked to the expression of the Secretor (Se) and Lewis (Le) genes.

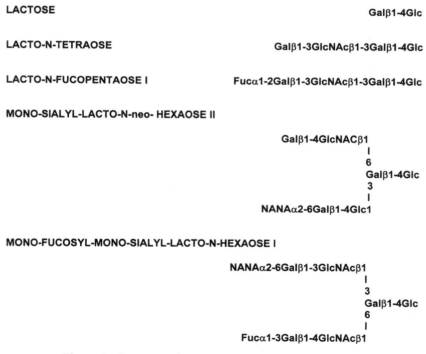

Figure 1 Structure of some human milk oligosaccharides.

Table 1 Glycosyltransferases in the mammary gland

Enzymes	Linkage
Enzymes common to all women	
Galactosyltransferases	β (1-3), β (1-4)
N-acetylglucosaminyltransferases . .	β (1-3), β (1-6)
Sialyltransferases	α (2-3), α (2-6)
Se/Le-dependent enzymes	
Fucosyltransferases	α (1-2), α (1-3), α (1-4)

Depending on the expression of these genes, one or more fucosyltransferases are present in the mammary gland. Depending on their presence, four different groups of human milk have been recognized (Stahl et al., 2001): group 1 (Se+/Le+; 70% of the general population), milk containing all the fucosyl-oligosaccharides as a result of the activity of both the Se gene, which regulates the synthesis of α-1-2 fucosyl-oligosaccharides, and the Le gene, which promotes the synthesis of α-1-3 and 1-4 fucosyl-oligosaccharides; group 2 (Se−/Le+; 20% of the general population), milk without α-1-2 fucosyl-oligosaccharides because of the absence of the Se gene; group 3 (Se+/Le−; 9% of the general population), milk without α-1-4 fucosyl-oligosaccharides because of the inactivity of the Le gene, but containing both α-1-3 fucosyl-oligosaccharides due to the action of an Le gene-independent 1-3 fucosyltransferase and α-1-2 fucosyl-oligosaccharides resulting from the action of the Se gene; group 4 (Se−/Le−; 1% of the general population), milk containing only α-1-3 fucosyl-oligosaccharides because of the presence of the Le gene-independent fucosyltransferase. As a consequence of the presence or absence of specific genes, significant variations in both the qualitative and quantitative contents of HMO occur (Fig. 2).

METABOLISM OF HUMAN MILK OLIGOSACCHARIDES

To date, the presence of specific enzymes for the digestion of HMO in the intestinal wall and pancreas has not been proved. Nevertheless, it is common knowledge that human milk contains several enzymes (Hamosh, 1995). Some of these enzymes have been identified as glycohydrolases (N-acetylglucosaminidase, fucosidase, and galactosidase) potentially capable of degrading oligosaccharides. This is supposed to cause the release of a certain quantity of monosaccharides which are available partially for energy purposes and partially for the synthesis of "noble" molecules (especially Fuc, NANA, and GlcNAc) necessary for the particular needs of the neonate as cerebral glycoproteins and glycolipids. Breast-fed infants ingest several grams of oligosaccharides daily, and these substances have been found in feces in large quantities with a

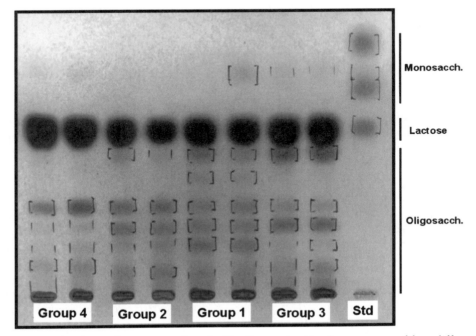

Figure 2 Thin-layer chromatography of milk oligosaccharides from women of four different groups.

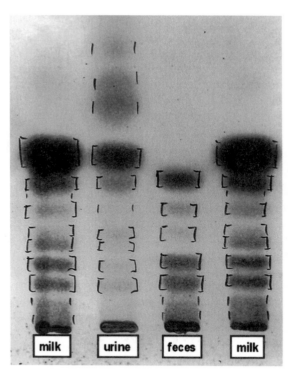

Figure 3 Thin-layer chromatography of carbohydrates from mother's milk and from the urine and feces of a newborn.

pattern that is similar to that of human milk (Chaturvedi et al., 2001; Coppa et al., 2001; Kunz et al., 2000). This is related to the fact that monosaccharide units present in the oligosaccharide molecules are linked with specific bonds resistant to the action of the intestinal enzymes of the neonate (Engfer et al., 2000; Gnoth et al., 2000). As a consequence, large quantities of HMO reach both the small and large intestines of the neonate. In addition to feces, HMO have also been found in the urine of breast-fed infants with the same pattern as in the ingested milk (Coppa et al., 1990). This demonstrates that a quota of oligosaccharides is absorbed as it is in the intestine, reaches the bloodstream, and is excreted in urine (Fig. 3). The explanation of these findings is strictly related to the well-known high permeability to food components of the infant intestine. The mechanism of the uptake and metabolism of oligosaccharides in the various organs once they have passed the intestinal barrier remains to be determined.

PREBIOTIC EFFECT

Throughout human history, a neonate's survival has always been strictly connected with breast-feeding. In fact, its absence in the first months of life is responsible for high mortality due to both severe nutritional deficiencies and infections mainly of the gastrointestinal tract (GIT). It is not to be forgotten that nowadays this is still a sad reality for a large proportion of neonates in several developing countries. Fortunately, the large majority of infants are breast-fed and have a repeated intake of human milk every day for several months. This represents a unique nutritional condition during one's lifetime, and it is easy to understand its fundamental role in the imprinting of the development of the intestinal microbiota. As is well known, the importance of breast-feeding for neonates and infants does not reside solely in its nutritional role but also results from several biological effects linked to the numerous substances present in the milk. These enhance the health status of the neonate as a result of their anti-infective action, their modulation of the antibody response, their control of inflammatory processes, etc. It is in this context that HMO play an important role.

As previously reported, the composition of the intestinal microbiota after the very early days of life is related to the type of feeding. With the intake of human milk, the composition of the intestinal microbiota shifts towards a prevalence of anaerobic bacteria. Among the various other substances, oligosaccharides, due to their peculiar structure, show high resistance to digestion by intestinal enzymes. They reach the colon and stimulate the development of the bifidogenic microbiota, acting as prebiotics (Coppa et al., 2004).

Recent studies of the genomics of the intestinal microbiota have provided important information about the characteristics of the different species of bifidobacteria, differentiating them from other species. However, they also reveal new data for the understanding of the mechanisms involved in the modulation of the intestinal microbiota. Moreover, genomic sequencing gives predictive information about the genetic determinants involved in the adaptive functions specific to the environment in which the bacteria live (Klijn et al., 2005; Ventura et al., 2007). For example, the carbohydrates which reach the GIT may influence the microbiome of the microbiota living in the different regions of the intestine. Moreover, the type of sugar available may influence the composition and abundance of the microbiota along the GIT.

In general, simple sugars are rapidly metabolized in the upper part of the GIT, whereas a large proportion of undigested complex carbohydrates reaches the distal part of the GIT. The ability to degrade complex carbohydrates contributes to the competitiveness of species along the GIT. In the case of breast-fed infants, the first carbohydrates that can play an important role in shaping the microbiome of the intestinal microbiota are represented by lactose and oligosaccharides. Lactobacilli are particularly prevalent in the upper GIT, where they ferment relatively simple sugars. In contrast, bifidobacteria colonize the lower parts of the colon due to their capacity to metabolize complex carbohydrates. In relation to carbohydrate fermentation capabilities, analysis of the genomes of bifidobacteria, and in particular studies performed with *Bifidobacterium longum* NCC2705 (Schell et al., 2002), isolated from the feces of healthy infants, has revealed a number of features that suggest how this bacterium has adapted to its environment and could help us to understand its interactions with the host. In particular, bifidobacteria possess several homologous genes encoding enzymes involved in the metabolism of numerous sugars. It is important to emphasize that, of all the genes contained in the genome of bifidobacteria, nearly 10% encode enzymes which are involved in the metabolism and transport of carbohydrates; in contrast, the genome composition of other intestinal bacteria (*Bacteroides*, *Actinobacteria*, and others) reveals a lower proportion of genes involved in carbohydrate transport and metabolism (3.5 to 5.6%) (Ventura et al., 2007). Moreover, it is important to take into consideration the fact that bifidobacteria are highly endowed with glycohydrolases (β-galactosidase, endo-β-NAc-glucosaminidase, α-fucosidase, and sialidases) able to metabolize monosaccharides that are constituent molecules of HMO (Katayama et al., 2004; Kitaoka et al., 2005; Klijn et al., 2005). In addition, the ability to degrade complex carbohydrates with respect to the level of polymerization and type of glycosidic bonds contributes to the competitiveness of given strains in the different regions of the GIT. Finally, studies have demonstrated that *B. longum* exhibits a preferential metabolic pathway for the use of lactose (Parche et al., 2006). This capability could have an important role as the bacteria can also utilize the lactose contained in oligosaccharide molecules. In conclusion, the significant portion of the genome devoted to sugar metabolism in bifidobacteria could explain their large proportions in the colon, reflecting a specific adaptation to this highly competitive habitat, especially in the breast-fed infant.

Data available on HMO so far have drawn attention mainly to their role as enhancing the growth of bifidobacteria. Only recently, Ward et al. (2006) have demonstrated in vitro, using HMO as a sole carbon source, that growth of *Bifidobacterium infantis* takes place in the presence of a decreased pH and decreased amount of oligosaccharides in the medium as a consequence of their fermentation. In contrast, the same effect was not obtained using *Lactobacillus gasseri*. In particular, *B. infantis* showed more than a 50% reduction in nearly all of the oligosaccharides tested compared with that

observed for *Escherichia coli* (Ninonuevo et al., 2007). These data clearly confirm that bifidobacteria can indeed utilize complex carbohydrates such as HMO, supporting the hypothesis that these substances selectively amplify bacterial population in the infant's GIT. Moreover, fermentation of HMO by bifidobacteria results in the production of short-chain fatty acids (SCFA), lactate, hydrogen, carbon dioxide, and methane. SCFA are absorbed by the colon, salvaging energy which would be lost if excreted with feces. SCFA also favor water and sodium absorption and promote a trophic effect on the intestinal mucosa (Mountzouris et al., 2002; Topping, 1996). Moreover, SCFA, by contributing to a lower colonic pH, prevent the overgrowth of pathogenic bacteria and consequently reduce diarrheal events. Variations in the SCFA pattern reflect changes in the composition of the colonic microbiota. For example, differences in the profile of SCFA in the feces of breast-fed infants compared to formula-fed infants have been found. In fact, the feces of breast-fed infants contain mainly acetic and lactic acid and little or no propionic acid or butyric acid, whereas the feces of formula-fed infants contain mainly acetic and propionic acids with small amounts of butyric acid (Mountzouris et al., 2002; Parrett and Edwards, 1997).

The above-mentioned data clearly show the fundamental role of HMO in modulating the intestinal microbiota. Nevertheless, it is important to emphasize that the quantities of such substances in human milk vary depending on the genetic pattern of fucosyltransferases of the mother. As previously reported, with reference to the presence of fucosyl-oligosaccharides, four different groups of human milk have been recognized. To evaluate the possible role of the different oligosaccharide contents, we investigated the relationship of the four milk groups on the composition of the intestinal microbiota, paying special attention to the bifidobacterial populations. A cohort of breast-fed infants whose feces were sampled on the 30th day of life was recruited. The HMO pattern was established by means of high-performance anion-exchange chromatography, and six species of bifidobacteria (*B. breve*, *B. catenulatum*, *B. longum*, *B. infantis*, *B. bifidum*, and *B. adolescentis*) were characterized by molecular analyses (PCR-denaturing gradient gel electrophoresis and multiple-specific PCR). From a quantitative point of view, in all groups studied, both core- and sialyl-oligosaccharides had a mean concentration of 2 g/liter. In contrast, the total amount of fucosyl-oligosaccharides showed a wide variation, ranging from about 11 g/liter in subjects from group 1 to about 1 g/liter in subjects from group 4. Consequently, the total content of HMO was strictly dependent on the presence or absence of fucosyl-oligosaccharides and showed a large quantitative difference in mature milk, ranging from about 15 g/liter in subjects from group 1 to about 5 g/liter in subjects from group 4. Intermediate values were present in subjects from groups 2 and 3. Preliminary results demonstrate that *B. breve* was the most frequent species among the bifidobacteria (72% of infants), followed by *B. longum* and *B. catenulatum*; *B. infantis* was detected only in one infant. No substantial differences in the presence of bifidobacterial species within the four groups studied were observed. In a control group of bottle-fed infants, the presence of bifidobacteria was significantly lower. In short, the different compositions of oligosaccharides in human milk do not seem to exert any particular influence on the number or type of species belonging to the genus *Bifidobacterium* identified in infants fed with the four types of milk. As the groups differed in their composition of fucosyl-oligosaccharides, it could be speculated that fucosydic residues in the different positions of oligosaccharide molecules are not the only factor involved in the prebiotic effect of human milk. In fact, the core- and sialyl-oligosaccharides are present in almost the same quantities in all four milk groups, and it consequently seems appropriate to believe that they can play an important role in the development of the intestinal microbiota.

In conclusion, within the complex mechanisms that regulate the development of the intestinal microbiota, the ability to utilize complex carbohydrates is believed to exert an important influence on the development of specific bacterial strains over others. It is our opinion that in the GIT of breast-fed neonates, the relationship between HMO and the development of bifidobacteria represents a typical example of this situation.

OTHER FUNCTIONS

As previously mentioned, there is still little knowledge of the digestive-absorptive processes of HMO. Nevertheless, a certain quantity of them is surely absorbed in the GIT, either as monosaccharides resulting from their digestion by glycohydrolases present in human milk, or as unmodified molecules as suggested by their presence in urine. Monosaccharides derived from oligosaccharide degradation can represent a source of calories that is particularly useful for the neonate and as such are considered to be nutrients. It is important to remember that Fuc, GlcNAc, and NANA can be utilized for the synthesis of molecules of biological importance such as cerebral glycolipids and glycoproteins, which play an important role in the maturation process of the central nervous system (Kracun et al., 1992). In particular, in animal studies, the exogenous administration of NANA has resulted in an increase in the concentration of brain gangliosides and glycoproteins, which is linked to an improvement in learning performances (Carlson and House, 1986; Wang et al., 2007). Recently, Wang et al. (2003) demonstrated higher brain ganglioside and glycoprotein sialic acid concentrations in breast-fed infants than in formula-fed ones. These results suggest that exogenous NANA is absorbed and utilized in the process of brain growth and maturation, playing an important role in the neonate as its high requirement corresponds to a limited capacity for its endogenous synthesis in the first months of life.

As shown in Fig. 4 and 5, HMO are present in the sera of breast-fed infants and only traces of oligosaccharides are present in the sera of bottle-fed infants. In this phase of metabolism, the oligosaccharides can play a significant role in the first phase of the inflammatory process. It is well known that the inflammatory reaction in the vasculature starts with the interaction between leukocytes, platelets, and endothelial cells through interactions between specific protein receptors (selectins) and carbohydrate ligands with oligosaccharide structures containing NANA and Fuc. In particular, P-selectin and E-selectin regulate the rolling and adhesion of leukocytes on the vascular wall in the initial phase of the inflammatory process. In vitro studies have shown that some HMO, behaving as soluble analogues of selectin ligands, have the ability to inhibit the adhesion of leukocytes to endothelial cells, contributing to the modulation of the inflammatory process of the neonate (Bode et al., 2004a; Rudloff et al., 2002). In fact, Bode et al. (2004b) have demonstrated that 3'-sialyl-lactose and 3'-sialyl-3-fucosyl-lactose, both present in human milk, may play a role as anti-inflammatory components and might therefore contribute to the lower incidence of inflammatory diseases in breast-fed infants.

As previously reported, a high percentage of undigested HMO reach the neonate's GIT. There is now quite strong evidence that supports the relationship between breast-feeding and a lower incidence of diarrhea. In infants, infections of the GIT are caused by a wide variety of enteropathogens, including bacteria, viruses, and parasites. Breast-feeding offers protection against diarrhea due to the presence in human milk of several anti-infective substances such as secretory antibodies, lactoferrin, lysozyme, etc. (WHO, 2000). In the last few years evidence has also emerged with respect to the significant protective role of oligosaccharides (Newburg, 2000). In fact, at the level of the small intestine, these substances play a role in protection against GIT infections. It is well known that viruses, bacteria, or toxins exert a pathogenic effect as a result of their adhesion to receptors located on the cells of the epithelial surface. Numerous

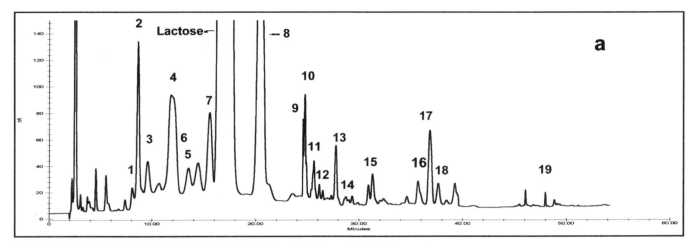

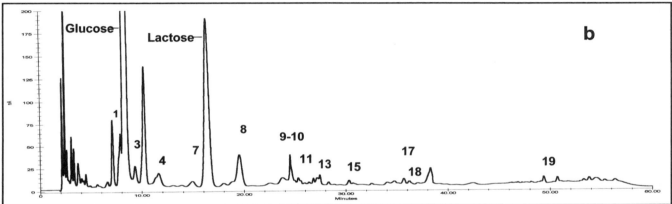

Figure 4 High-performance anion-exchange chromatography of mother's milk (a) and serum of a breast-fed infant (b). Peaks: 1, lacto-*N*-difucohexaose II; 2, trifucosyllacto-*N*-hexaose; 3, difucosyllacto-*N*-hexaose b; 4, difucosyllacto-*N*-hexaose; 5, difucosyllacto-*N*-hexaose I; 6, 3-fucosyllactose; 7, lacto-*N*-fucopentaose II; 8, 2′-fucosyllactose; 9, lacto-*N*-fucopentaose I; 10, monofucosyllacto-*N*-hexaose II; 11, lacto-*N*-neotetraose; 12, lacto-*N*-neohexaose; 13, lacto-*N*-tetraose; 14, lacto-*N*-hexaose; 15, monofucosylmonosialyllacto-*N*-neohexaose; 16, sialyllacto-*N*-tetraose c; 17, 6′-sialyllactose; 18, sialyllacto-*N*-tetraose a; 19, disialyllacto-*N*-tetraose.

receptors are the glycosidic chains of glycoproteins and glycolipids of the intestinal cell membranes, and HMO may compete with these receptors in binding pathogenic agents, hindering their adhesion as well as the subsequent pathological process (Zopf and Roth, 1996). The adhesion of a bacterium to the host cell is an essential prerequisite to exerting a pathogenic effect. The overall process of binding involves the interaction of a solvated polyhydroxylated glycan located on the surface of the cells with a solvated protein-combining site (adhesin) on the pathogenic agent. The forces involved in this bond are represented by hydrogen bonding, van der Waals interactions, and charge and dipole attractions (Varki et al., 1999), suggesting that if the glycan on the surface is complementary to the protein-combining site, water

can be displaced and binding occurs. The antiadhesive effect of HMO in the GIT has been described for a few bacteria such as *Helicobacter pylori* (Simon et al., 1997), *Listeria monocytogenes* (Coppa et al., 2003), *Campylobacter jejuni*, and enteropathogenic *E. coli* (Cravioto et al., 1991). Recently, we demonstrated the ability of HMO to inhibit the adhesion of *Vibrio cholerae* and *Salmonella fyris*, bacteria responsible for severe diarrhea during infancy, to Caco-2 cells (Coppa et al., 2006b). The anti-adhesive role of HMO has also been reported outside the GIT. In the literature, data are available concerning protection against bacteria responsible for infection of the respiratory and urinary systems, such as *Streptococcus pneumoniae* and uropathogenic *E. coli* (Fig. 6) (Andersson et al., 1986; Coppa et al., 1990). Recently,

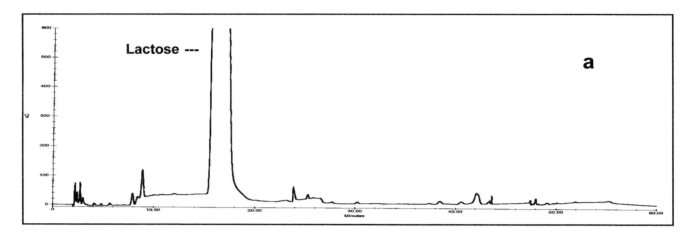

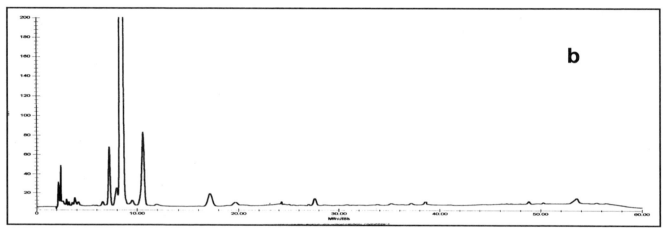

Figure 5 High-performance anion-exchange chromatography of infant formula (a) and serum of a bottle-fed infant (b).

Bode (2006) hypothesized that HMO could also play an important role in other situations where protein-carbohydrate interactions take place, for example, the interaction of galectins with β-galactoside-containing glycans (similar to those in HMO), which regulate cell growth, proliferation, and cell-cell interactions.

Finally, HMO are also important as far as the regulation of intestinal mobility in breast-fed infants is concerned since they behave as soluble dietary fibers. In fact, a consistent quota of undigested HMO is found in the feces of breast-fed infants but not in bottle-fed infants. This fact explains the different number of stool emissions and the different consistency of feces in the two neonate populations. Figure 7 schematically shows the metabolic pathway of HMO and the functions carried out in different regions of the GIT.

FROM HUMAN MILK OLIGOSACCHARIDES TO NONDIGESTIBLE OLIGOSACCHARIDES IN INFANT FORMULAS

The above description clearly shows that oligosaccharides in human milk are the prototypes of natural prebiotics. Their biological effect is closely related to the presence of special bonds in their molecules which offer resistance to digestion in the GIT. No natural substances have the same biochemical composition as that of HMO, nor can they be synthesized in large quantities at acceptable prices. On the other hand, milks from other animals contain very small quantities of oligosaccharides with a structure generally different from that of HMO. To overcome these problems, the industry has focused on the production of several carbohydrates, so-called nondigestible oligosaccharides (NDO), which, although

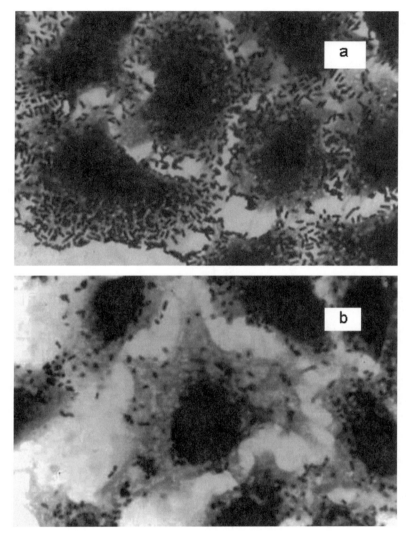

Figure 6 Adherence of uropathogenic *E. coli* to HeLa cells in the absence of (a) and in the presence of (b) HMO.

having compositions different from those of HMO, are able to selectively stimulate the growth of bifidobacteria and lactobacilli in the colon, reproducing the prebiotic effects of HMO.

To date, several NDO preparations are available on the market; they make up a heterogeneous group of substances in terms of composition, type of bonds, and resistance to digestion. Most NDO contain 3 to 10 sugar moieties, although the degree of polymerization, like inulin, could reach up to 60 for some of them. In addition, every commercial product in general contains a mixture of several oligosaccharides with a variable degree of polymerization. The common feature of NDO is represented

by the presence of beta bonds between their monomeric sugar units that are resistant to digestion by gastrointestinal enzymes. For adult use, the market presently offers several types of NDO. In contrast, only fructooligosaccharides (FOS), galactooligosaccharides (GOS), and inulin have been used as NDO to mimic the prebiotic effects of HMO in the preparation of infant formulas.

The first studies on the use of NDO in infant formulas were performed in 2002 and involved both term and preterm neonates. In one study, 90 term neonates (Moro et al., 2002) were divided into three groups: the control group was fed on a normal formula, while the remaining two groups were fed on the same milk supplemented with a

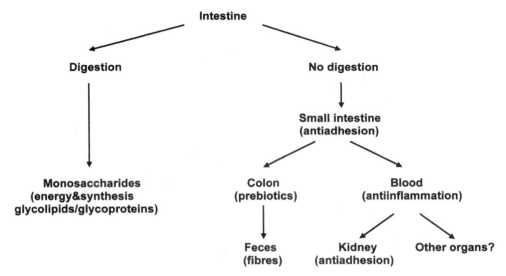

Figure 7   Metabolic fate and biological functions of HMO.

mixture of GOS and inulin in a 9-to-1 ratio at two different concentrations (4 and 8 g/liter, respectively). At the end of the feeding period, the number of bifidobacteria had significantly increased for both groups receiving supplemented formulas. The effect was dose dependent. The number of lactobacilli increased significantly in both groups fed on the supplemented formulas, but there was not a statistical difference related to the doses. A reduced fecal pH, an increase in the number of daily evacuations, and less-consistent feces were reported, as in breast-fed babies. No side effects such as crying, regurgitation, or vomiting were recorded.

In the second study (Boehm et al., 2002), a specific formula, supplemented with the same GOS/inulin mixture, but using a concentration of 10 g/liter, was used in 30 preterm babies divided into two cohorts. The prebiotic effect of the mixture was the same as that in term neonates. Moreover, a tendency towards higher urinary calcium concentrations in the group fed on the supplemented formula was reported, indicating that calcium absorption might be influenced by dietary oligosaccharides.

Other studies have been carried out with neonates and infants fed on supplemented formulas with the same NDO mixture. They have again confirmed a positive effect on the growth of bifidobacteria and lactobacilli, and a variation in the SCFA patterns in the feces was observed. An increase of acetate and lactate with a corresponding pH decrease has actually been observed, similar to what happens in breast-fed infants. A significant decrease of propionate has also been reported, which, on the contrary, is well represented in the feces of bottle-fed infants with traditional formulas. In addition, a reduction in clinically relevant pathogenic bacteria has been described (Knoll

et al., 2005). Very recently, Bakker-Zierikzee et al. (2006) demonstrated that neonates fed on a GOS/inulin-enriched formula showed a trend towards higher fecal secretory immunoglobulin A in feces compared with standard formula-fed infants; this reached statistical significance at the age of 16 weeks. In conclusion, as described above, an NDO mixture is able to match the positive biological effects of HMO. It has also been shown that a portion of the NDO mixture utilized is found in the feces, suggesting it can function as dietary fiber.

Recent studies have shown that the use of a formula containing the same GOS/inulin mixture in the ratio of 9 to 1 has positive clinical effects in the prevention of atopic dermatitis and gastrointestinal infections. Moro et al. (2006), in a prospective double-blind, randomized, placebo-controlled trial, studied infants at risk of atopy during their first 6 months of life: there were 102 infants in the prebiotic group and 104 infants in the placebo group. Atopic dermatitis at the end of the study period was found in 10 infants in the intervention group and 24 infants in the control group. These results have shown, for the first time, a significant beneficial effect of prebiotics in the prevention of atopic dermatitis in a high-risk infant population. Bruzzese et al. (2006) reported the preliminary results of a trial addressed to evaluate the beneficial effects of the 12-month administration to a large population of 1- to 3-month-old infants of a formula that contained the GOS/inulin mixture. The authors observed a significantly lower number of intestinal infections in the infants fed on the supplemented formula than in children receiving a standard formula.

The literature is sparse with regard to studies of the use of formulas containing GOS or FOS exclusively. As far as GOS supplementation is concerned, only two papers have been published. One is a study of a group of 69 neonates with an applied GOS concentration of 2.4 g/liter followed up for 6 months (Ben et al., 2004). The other studied 13 neonates for 3 weeks using a GOS concentration of 7.0 g/liter (Napoli et al., 2003). In both cases, an increased bifidogenic microbiota was observed along with a reduction of fecal pH, proving a GOS prebiotic effect in spite of the limited number of subjects. The ability of GOS to inhibit the in vitro adhesion of enteropathogenic *E. coli* to HEp-2 and Caco-2 cells has recently been demonstrated. The mechanism is analogous to that of HMO (Shoaf et al., 2006). These results offer new possibilities regarding the biological effects of NDO.

With regard to the use of FOS in infant formulas, the first report dates back to 2000. These substances, used in different concentrations for only 2 weeks, did not exhibit any prebiotic effect (Guesry et al., 2000). In 2005, a study carried out by Euler et al. with 58 infants for 5 weeks, using a formula enriched with 1.5 or 3.0 g of FOS per liter, demonstrated minimal effects on the fecal microbiota (Euler et al., 2005). A formula enriched with 2.0 g of FOS per liter used by 44 infants for 13 weeks also had little effect on the host microbiota. Recently, 56 preterm neonates were enrolled to receive either a prebiotic formula containing 4.0 g of FOS per liter or the same formula with maltodextrins as a placebo. In the group fed on the prebiotic formula, the numbers of bifidobacteria and bacteroides were significantly higher than those in the placebo group (Kapiki et al., 2007). The supplemented formula also had a significant influence on the daily stool frequency.

In conclusion, data related to the use of NDO in infant formulas clearly show the efficacy of GOS/inulin mixtures, the capacity of GOS to induce a bifidogenic effect, even if in only a small number of studies, and the positive effects of FOS at a concentration of 4.0 g/liter on the intestinal microbiota. It has been demonstrated that, due to the presence of resistant bonds in their molecules, NDO are able to exert a prebiotic effect. This further confirms that, because of their peculiar structure, HMO have a very significant role in modulating the intestinal microbiota of neonates.

References

Agostoni, C., I. Axelsson, O. Goulet, B. Koletzko, K. F. Michaelsen, J. W. L. Puntis, J. Rigo, R. Shamir, H. Szajewska, and D. Turck. 2004. Prebiotic oligosaccharides in dietetic products for infants: a commentary by the ESPGHAN Committee on Nutrition. *J. Pediatr. Gastroenterol. Nutr.* **39**:465–473.

Andersson, B., O. Porras, L. A. Hanson, T. Lagergard, and C. Svanborg-Eden. 1986. Inhibition of attachment of *Streptococcus pneumoniae* and *Haemophilus influenzae* by human milk and receptor oligosaccharides. *J. Infect. Dis.* **153**:232–237.

Bakker-Zierikzee, A. M., E. A. Tol, H. Kroes, M. S. Alles, F. J. Kok, and J. G. Bindels. 2006. Faecal SIgA secretion in infant fed on pre- or probiotic infant formula. *Pediatr. Allergy Immunol.* **17**:134–140.

Balmer, S. E., P. H. Scott, and B. A. Wharton. 1989a. Diet and the faecal flora in the newborn: casein and whey proteins. *Arch. Dis. Child.* **64**:1678–1684.

Balmer, S. E., P. H. Scott, and B. A. Wharton. 1989b. Diet and faecal flora in the newborn: lactoferrin. *Arch. Dis. Child.* **64**:1685–1690.

Balmer, S. E., L. S. Harvey, and B. A. Wharton. 1994. Diet and faecal flora in the newborn: nucleotides. *Arch. Dis. Child.* **70**:F137–F140.

Ben, X. M., X. Y. Zhou, W. H. Zhao, W. L. Yu, W. Pan, W. L. Zhang, S. M. Wu, C. M. Van Beusekom, and A. Schaafsma. 2004. Supplementation of milk formula with galacto-oligosaccharides improves intestinal micro-flora and fermentation in term infants. *Chin. Med. J.* **117**:927–931.

Bode, L. 2006. Recent advances on structure, metabolism, and function of human milk oligosaccharides. *J. Nutr.* **136:** 2127–2130.

Bode, L., S. Rudloff, C. Kunz, S. Strobel, and N. Klein. 2004a. Human milk oligosaccharides reduce platelet-neutrophil complex formation leading to a decrease in neutrophyl beta 2 integrin expression. *J. Leukoc. Biol.* **76**:820–826.

Bode, L., C. Kunz, M. Muhly-Reinholds, K. Mayer, W. Seeger, and S. Rudloff. 2004b. Inhibition of monocyte, lymphocyte, and neutrophil adhesion to endothelial cells by human milk oligosaccharides. *Thromb. Haemost.* **92**:1402–1410.

Boehm, G., M. Lidestri, P. Casetta, J. Jelinek, F. Negretti, B. Stahl, and A. Marini. 2002. Supplementation of a bovine milk formula with an oligosaccharide mixture increases counts of faecal bifidobacteria in preterm infants. *Arch. Dis. Child. Fetal Neonatal Ed.* **86**:F178–F181.

Brook, I., C. T. Barett, C. R. Brinkman, W. J. Martin, and S. M. Finegold. 1979. Aerobic and anaerobic bacterial flora of the maternal cervix and newborn gastric fluid and conjunctiva: a prospective study. *Pediatrics* **63**:451–455.

Bruck, W. M., M. Redgrave, K. M. Tuohy, B. Lonnerdal, G. Graverholt, O. Hernell, and G. R. Gibson. 2006. Effects of bovine alpha-lactalbumin and casein glycomacropeptide-enriched infant formulae on faecal microbiota in healthy term infants. *J. Pediatr. Gastroenterol. Nutr.* **43**:673–679.

Bruzzese, E., M. Volpicelli, M. Squaglia, A. Tartaglione, and A. Guarino. 2006. Impact of prebiotics on human health. *Dig. Liver Dis.* **38**(Suppl. 2):S283–S287.

Carlson, S. E., and S. G. House. 1986. Oral and intraperitoneal administration of N-acetylneuraminic acid: effect on rat cerebral and cerebellar N-acetylneuraminic acid. *J. Nutr.* **116**:881–886.

Chaturvedi, P., C. D. Warren, G. M. Ruiz-Palacios, L. K. Pickering, and D. S. Newburg. 1997. Milk oligosaccharide profiles by reverse-phase HPLC of their perbenzoylated derivatives. *Anal. Biochem.* **251**:89–97.

Chaturvedi, P., C. D. Warren, C. R. Buescher, L. K. Pickering, and D. S. Newburg. 2001. Survival of human milk oligosaccharides in the intestine of infants. *Adv. Exp. Med. Biol.* 501:315–323.

Chierici, R., G. Sawatzki, S. Thurl, K. Tovar, and V. Vigi. 1997. Experimental milk formula with reduced protein content and desialylated milk proteins: influence on the faecal flora and the growth of term born infants. *Acta Paediatr.* 87:557–563.

Coppa, G. V., O. Gabrielli, P. L. Giorgi, C. Catassi, M. P. Montanari, P. E. Varaldo, and B. L. Nichols. 1990. Preliminary study of breastfeeding and bacterial adhesion to uroepithelial cells. *Lancet* 335:569–571.

Coppa, G. V., O. Gabrielli, P. Pierani, C. Catassi, A. Carlucci, and P. L. Giorgi. 1993. Changes in carbohydrate composition in human milk over 4 months of lactation. *Pediatrics* 91: 637–641.

Coppa, G. V., P. Pierani, L. Zampini, I. Carloni, A. Carlucci, and O. Gabrielli. 1999. Oligosaccharides in human milk during different phases of lactation. *Acta Paediatr.* 430S:89–94.

Coppa, G. V., P. Pierani, L. Zampini, S. Bruni, I. Carloni, and O. Gabrielli. 2001. Characterization of oligosaccharides in milk and feces of breast-fed infants by high-performance anion-exchange chromatography. *Adv. Exp. Med. Biol.* 501: 307–314.

Coppa, G. V., S. Bruni, L. Zampini, T. Galeazzi, R. Facinelli, R. Capretti, A. Carlucci, and O. Gabrielli. 2003. Oligosaccharides of human milk inhibit the adhesion of *Listeria monocytogenes* to Caco 2 cell. *Ital. J. Pediatr.* 29:61–68.

Coppa, G. V., S. Bruni, L. Morelli, S. Soldi, and O. Gabrielli. 2004. The first prebiotics in humans: human milk oligosaccharides. *J. Clin. Gastroenterol.* 38:S80–S83.

Coppa, G. V., L. Zampini, T. Galeazzi, and O. Gabrielli. 2006a. Prebiotics in human milk: a review. *Dig. Liver Dis.* 38(Suppl. 2):S291–S294.

Coppa, G. V., L. Zampini, T. Galeazzi, B. Facinelli, L. Ferrante, R. Capretti, and O. Gabrielli. 2006b. Human milk oligosaccharides inhibit the adhesion to Caco 2 cells of diarrheal pathogens: *Escherichia coli*, *Vibrio cholerae*, and *Salmonella fyris*. *Pediatr. Res.* 59:377–382.

Cravioto, A., A. Tello, H. Villafan, J. Ruiz, S. del Vedovo, and J. R. Neeser. 1991. Inhibition of localized adhesion of enteropathogenic *Escherichia coli* to HEp-2 cells by immunoglobulin and oligosaccharides fractions of human colostrum and breast milk. *J. Infect. Dis.* 163:1247–1255.

Denigés, G. 1892. Contribution à l'étude des lactoses. Thesis. Ecole Supérieure de Pharmacie, Paris, France.

Engfer, M. B., B. Stahl, B. Finke, G. Sawatzki, and H. Daniel. 2000. Human milk oligosaccharides are resistant to enzymatic hydrolysis in the upper gastrointestinal tract. *Am. J. Clin. Nutr.* 71:1589–1596.

Euler, A. R., D. K. Mitchell, R. Kline, and L. K. Pickering. 2005. Prebiotic effect of fructo-oligosaccharide supplemented term infant formula and two concentrations compared with unsupplemented formula and human milk. *J. Pediatr. Gastroenterol. Nutr.* 40:157–164.

Fanaro, S., R. Chierici, P. Guerrini, and V. Vigi. 2003. Intestinal microflora in early infancy: composition and development. *Acta Pediatr.* 91S:48–55.

Favier, C. F., W. M. de Vos, and A. D. L. Akkermans. 2003. Development of bacterial and bifidobacterial communities in feces of newborn babies. *Anaerobe* 9:219–229.

Gil, A., E. Coval, A. Martinez, and J. A. Molina. 1986. Effect of dietary nucleotides on the microbial pattern of faeces of at term newborn infants. *J. Clin. Nutr. Gastroenterol.* 1:38–38.

Gnoth, M. J., C. Kunz, E. Kinne-Saffran, and S. Rudloff. 2000. Human milk oligosaccharides are minimally digested in vitro. *J. Nutr.* 130:3014–3020.

Gronlund, M. M., O. P. Lehtonen, E. Eerola, and P. Kero. 1999. Fecal microflora in healthy infants born by different methods of delivery: permanent changes in intestinal flora after cesarean delivery. *J. Pediatr. Gastroenterol. Nutr.* 28:19–25.

Guesry, P., H. Bodanski, E. Tomsit, and J. Aeschlimann. 2000. Effect of 3 doses of fructo-oligosaccharides in infants. *J. Pediatr. Gastroenterol. Nutr.* 31(Suppl. 2):S252.

Gyorgy, P., R. F. Norris, and C. S. Rose. 1954. Bifidus factor I. A variant of *Lactobacillus bifidus* requiring a special growth factor. *Arch. Biochem. Biophys.* 48:202–208.

Hamosh, M. 1995. Enzymes in human milk, p. 388–427. *In* R. G. Jensen (ed.), *Handbook of Milk Composition.* Academic Press, San Diego, CA.

Harmsen, H. J., A. C. Wildeboer-Veloo, G. C. Raanx, C. Jerwin, A. Wagendorp, N. Klijn, J. G. Bindels, and G. W. Welling. 2000. Analysis of intestinal flora development in breast-fed and formula-fed infants by using molecular identification and detection methods. *J. Pediatr. Gastroenterol. Nutr.* 30:61–70.

Kapiki, A., C. Costalos, C. Oikonomidou, A. Triantafyllidou, E. Loukatou, and V. Pertrohilou. 2007. The effect of a fructo-oligosaccharide supplemented formula on gut flora of preterm infants. *Early Hum. Dev.* 83:335–339.

Katayama, T., A. Sakuma, T. Kimura, Y. Makimura, J. Hiratake, K. Sakata, T. Yamanoi, H. Kumagai, and K. Yamamoto. 2004. Molecular cloning and characterization of *Bifidobacterium bifidum* 1,2-alfa-ʟ-fucosidase (AfcA), a novel inverting glycosidase (glycoside hydrolase family 95). *J. Bacteriol.* 186:4885–4893.

Kitaoka, M., J. Tian, and M. Nishimoto. 2005. Novel putative galactose operon involving lacto-N-biose phosphorylase in *Bifidobacterium longum. Appl. Environ. Microbiol.* 71:3158–3162.

Klijn, A., A. Mercenier, and F. Arigoni. 2005. Lessons from the genomes of bifidobacteria. *FEMS Microbiol. Rev.* 29:491–509.

Knoll, J., P. Scholtens, C. Kafka, J. Steenbakkers, S. Gross, K. Helm, M. Klarczyk, H. Schopfer, H.-M. Bockler, and J. Wells. 2005. Colon microflora in infants fed formula with galacto- and fructo-oligosaccharides: more like breast-fed infants. *J. Pediatr. Gastroenterol. Nutr.* 40:36–42.

Kracun, I., H. Rosner, V. Drnovsek, Z. Vukelic, C. Cosovic, M. Trbojevic-Cepe, and M. Kubat. 1992. Gangliosides in the human brain development and aging. *Neurochem. Int.* 20:421–431.

Kuhn, R. 1958. Les oligosaccharides du lait. *Bull. Soc. Chim. Biol.* 40:297–314.

Kullen, M. J., and J. Bettler. 2005. The delivery of probiotics and prebiotics to infants. *Curr. Pharm. Des.* 11:55–74.

Kunz, C., S. Rudloff, W. Schad, and D. Braun. 1999. Lactose-derived oligosaccharides in the milk of elephants: comparison with human milk. *Br. J. Nutr.* **82**:391–399.

Kunz, C., S. Rudloff, W. Baier, N. Klein, and S. Strobel. 2000. Oligosaccharides in human milk: structural, functional and metabolic aspects. *Annu. Rev. Nutr.* **20**:699–722.

Macfarlane, S., G. T. Macfarlane, and J. H. Cummings. 2006. Review article: prebiotics in the gastrointestinal tract. *Aliment. Pharmacol. Ther.* **24**:701–714.

Mackie, R. I., A. Sghir, and H. R. Gaskins. 1999. Developmental microbial ecology of the neonatal gastrointestinal tract. *Am. J. Clin. Nutr.* **69**:1035S–1045S.

Montreuil, J. 1957. Les glucides du lait de femme. *Bull. Soc. Chim. Biol.* **39**:395–411.

Montreuil, J., and S. Mullet. 1959. Evolution de la constitution glucidique du lait de femme au cours de la lactation. *C. R. Soc. Biol.* **153**:1364–1366.

Moro, G., I. Minoli, F. Mosca, S. Fanaro, J. Jelinek, B. Stahl, and G. Boehm. 2002. Dosage-related bifidogenic effects of galacto- and fructooligosaccharides in formula-fed term infants. *J. Pediatr. Gastroenterol. Nutr.* **34**:291–295.

Moro, G., S. Arslanoglu, B. Stahl, J. Jelinek, U. Wahn, and G. Boehm. 2006. A mixture of prebiotic oligosaccharides reduces the incidence of atopic dermatitis during the first six months of age. *Arch. Dis. Child.* **91**:814–819.

Mountzouris, K. C., A. L. McCartney, and G. R. Gibson. 2002. Intestinal microflora of human infants and current trends for its nutritional modulation. *Br. J. Nutr.* **87**:405–420.

Mountzouris, K. C., and G. R. Gibson. 2003. Colonization of the gastrointestinal tract. *Ann. Nestlé* **61**:43–54.

Napoli, J. E., J. C. Brand-Miller, and P. Conway. 2003. Bifidogenic effects of feeding infant formula containing galacto-oligosaccharides in healthy formula-fed infants. *Asia Pac. J. Clin Nutr.* **12**:S60–S62.

Newburg, D. S. 2000. Oligosaccharides in human milk and bacterial colonization. *J. Pediatr. Gastroenterol. Nutr.* **30**: S8–S17.

Ninonuevo, M. R., R. E. Ward, R. G. LoCascio, J. B. German, S. L. Freeman, M. Barboza, D. A. Mills, and C. B. Lebrilla. 2007. Methods for the quantitation of human milk oligosaccharides in bacterial fermentation by mass spectrometry. *Anal. Biochem.* **361**:15–23.

Orrhage, K., and C. E. Nord. 1999. Factors controlling the bacterial colonization of the intestine in breast-fed infants. *Acta Pediatr.* **430S**:47–57.

Parche, S., M. Beleut, E. Rezzonico, D. Jacobs, F. Arigoni, F. Titgemeyer, and I. Jankovic. 2006. Lactose-over-glucose preference in *Bifidobacterium longum* NCC2705: *glcP*, encoding a glucose transporter, is subject to lactose repression. *J. Bacteriol.* **188**:1260–1265.

Parrett, A. M., and C. A. Edwards. 1997. In vitro fermentation of carbohydrates by breast fed and formula fed infants. *Arch. Dis. Child.* **76**:249–253.

Penders, J., C. Vonk, C. Driessen, N. London, C. Thijs, and E. E. Stobberingh. 2005. Quantification of *Bifidobacterium* spp., *Escherichia coli* and *Clostridium difficile* in faecal samples of breast-fed and formula-fed infants by real-time PCR. *FEMS Microbiol. Lett.* **243**:141–147.

Polonowski, M., and A. Lespagnol. 1933. Nouvelles acquisitions sur les composés glucidiques du lait de femme. *Bull. Soc. Chim. Biol.* **15**:320–349.

Radke, M., C. Mohr, K. D. Wutzke, and W. Heine. 1992. Phosphate concentration. Does reduction in infant formula feeding modify the micro-ecology of the intestine? *Monatsschr. Kinderheilkd.* **140**:S40–S44.

Roberts, A. K., R. Chierici, G. Sawatzki, M. J. Hill, S. Volpato, and V. Vigi. 1992. Supplementation of an adapted formula with bovine lactoferrin. 1. Effect on the faecal flora. *Acta Paediatr.* **81**:119–124.

Rudloff, S., C. Stefan, G. Pohlentz, and C. Kunz. 2002. Detection of ligands for selectins in the oligosaccharide fraction of human milk. *Eur. J. Nutr.* **41**:85–92.

Schell, M. A., M. Karmirantzou, B. Snel, D. Vilanova, B. Berger, G. Pessi, M.-C. Zwahlen, F. Desiere, P. Bork, M. Delley, R. D. Pridmore, and F. Arigoni. 2002. The genome sequence of *Bifidobacterium longum* reflects its adaptation to the human gastrointestinal tract. *Proc. Natl. Acad. Sci. USA* **99**:14422–14427.

Schonfeld, H. 1926. Uber die Beziehungen der einzelnen Bestandteile der Frauenmilch zur bifidus Flora. *Jahrbuch Kinderh.* **113**:19–60.

Shoaf, K., G. L. Mulvey, G. D. Armstrong, and R. W. Hutkins. 2006. Prebiotic galactooligosaccharides reduce adherence of enteropathogenic *Escherichia coli* to tissue culture cells. *Infect. Immun.* **74**:6920–6928.

Simon, P. M., P. L. Goore, A. Mobasseri, and D. Zopf. 1997. Inhibition of *Helicobacter pylori* binding to gastrointestinal epithelial cells by sialic acid-containing oligosaccharides. *Infect. Immun.* **65**:750–757.

Stahl, B., S. Thurl, J. Henker, M. Siegel, B. Finke, and G. Sawatzki. 2001. Detection of four human milk groups with respect to Lewis-blood-group-dependent oligosaccharides by serologic and chromatographic analysis. *Adv. Exp. Med. Biol.* **501**:299–306.

Szilagyi, A. 2002. Lactose—a potential prebiotic. *Aliment. Pharmacol. Ther.* **16**:1591–1602.

Tamine, A. Y., V. M. E. Marshall, and R. K. Robinson. 1995. Microbiological and technological aspects of milks fermented by bifidobacteria. *J. Dairy Res.* **62**:151–187.

Thurl, S., B. Muller-Werner, and G. Sawatzki. 1996. Quantification of individual oligosaccharide compounds from human milk using high-pH anion-exchange chromatography. *Anal. Biochem.* **235**:202–206.

Tissier, H. 1900. Recherches sur la flore intestinale des nourrissons (état normal et pathologique). Thesis. G. Carré and C. Naud, Paris, France.

Topping, D. L. 1996. Short-chain fatty acids produced by intestinal bacteria. *Asia Pacific J. Clin. Nutr.* **5**:15–19.

Varki, A., R. Cummings, J. Esko, H. Freeze, G. Hart, and J. Marth. 1999. Protein-glycan interaction, p. 41–56. *In* A. Varki, R. Cummings, J. Esko, H. Freeze, G. Hart, and J. Marth (ed.), *Essentials of Glycobiology.* Cold Spring Harbor Laboratory Press, Cold Spring Harbor, NY.

Ventura, M., C. Canchaya, G. F. Fitzgerald, R. S. Gupta, and D. van Sinderen. 2007. Genomics as a means to understand bacterial phylogeny and ecological adaptation: the case of bifidobacteria. *Antonie Leeuwenhoek* **91**:351–372.

Viverge, D., L. Grimmonprez, G. Cassanas, L. Bardet, H. Bonnet, and M. Solere. 1985. Variations of lactose and oligosaccharides in milk from women of blood type secretor A or H, secretor Lewis and secretor H/non secretor Lewis during the course of lactation. *Ann. Nutr. Metab.* **29:**1–11.

Wang, B., P. McVeagh, P. Petocz, and J. Brand-Miller. 2003. Brain ganglioside and glycoproteins sialic acid in breast-fed compared with formula-fed infants. *Am. J. Clin. Nutr.* **78:**1024–1029.

Wang, B., B. Yu, M. Karim, H. Hu, Y. Sun, P. McGreevy, P. Petocz, S. Held, and J. Brand-Miller. 2007. Dietary sialic acid supplementation improves learning and memory in piglets. *Am. J. Clin. Nutr.* **85:**561–569.

Ward, R. E., M. Ninonuevo, D. I. Mills, C. B. Lebrilla, and J. B. German. 2006. In vitro fermentation of breast milk oligosaccharides by *Bifidobacterium infantis* and *Lactobacillus gasseri*. *Appl. Environ. Microbiol.* **72:**4497–4499.

WHO Collaborative Study Team on the Role of Breastfeeding on the Prevention of Infant Mortality. 2000. Effect of breastfeeding on infant and child mortality due to infectious diseases in less developed countries: a pooled analysis. *Lancet* **355:**451–455.

Zopf, D., and S. Roth. 1996. Oligosaccharide anti-infective agents. *Lancet* **347:**1017–1021.

Therapeutic Microbiology: Probiotics and Related Strategies
Edited by J. Versalovic and M. Wilson
© 2008 ASM Press, Washington, DC

Jan Van Loo
Douwina Bosscher

Inulin-Type Fructans

11

Inulin-type fructans are the most extensively studied prebiotic compounds with proven efficacy. Inulin is present in many plants, of which a number are edible. On an industrial scale, most of the inulin produced is extracted from chicory roots. Inulin-type fructans are not digested in the upper gastrointestinal tract, are selectively fermented by the endogenous intestinal microbiota, and thereby increase growth and/or activity of certain bacterial populations that are associated with health and well-being (e.g., bifidobacteria and lactobacilli). The prebiotic interaction with the colonic ecosystem of the host results in a wide range of physiological benefits, including improvement of bowel habits; reduced risk of intestinal infections, inflammation, and colonic cancers; immunomodulatory activity; increased mineral absorption and accretion; modulation of lipid metabolism; and regulation of appetite, food intake, and body weight. Inulin-type fructans are nowadays incorporated into a wide range of food products (e.g., bakery, dairy, etc.), where they confer technological benefits, like sugar and fat replacement, emulsion stabilizers, etc. Such technological properties, combined with their science-based nutritional benefits, make them important ingredients for use in foods to improve human health and well-being.

OCCURRENCE

Inulin-type fructans are naturally present as cryoprotectant and energy reserve in a wide variety of plants, a number of which are edible. These cereals (wheat and barley), vegetables (onion and garlic), and fruits (banana and tomato) are still today part of our diet and contribute about 1 g of inulin per day to our daily Western-style diet (Van Loo et al., 1995). Inulin is also present in chicory, which is a biennial plant. During the first season the plants remain in a vegetative phase and make only leaves, taproots, and fibrous roots. The roots look like small oblong sugar beets, which makes them a favorite source of inulin in commercial exploitation. Their inulin content is high and fairly constant from year to year for a given region (between 16.0 to 18.0% or about 60% on dry solids).

CHEMICAL STRUCTURE AND PRODUCTION

Inulin is a polydisperse carbohydrate material consisting mainly, if not exclusively, of $\beta(2\text{-}1)$ fructosyl-fructose links. A starting glucose moiety can be present but

Jan Van Loo and Douwina Bosscher, BENEO-Orafti, Aandorenstraat 1, B3300 Tienen, Belgium.

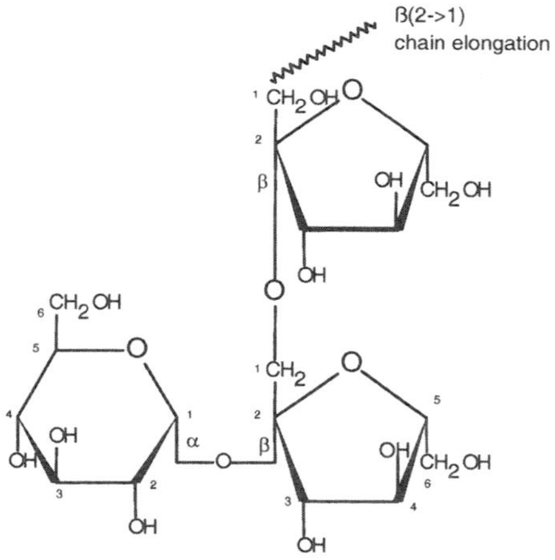

Figure 1   Chemical structure of inulin.

is not necessary. Fructans is a more general name and is used for any compound in which one or more fructosyl-fructose links constitute the majority of linkages (i.e., covering both inulins and levans). Native inulin is a mixture of oligomers and polymers with a degree of polymerization (DP) ranging from 3 to 65 (average DP, 10). "Native" refers to the inulin as it is extracted from the fresh roots, taking precautions to inhibit the plant's own inulinase activity as well as acid hydrolysis. The molecular structure of inulin is shown in Fig. 1.

Industrially, the lengths of the inulin chains can be reduced by means of an endoinulinase to a DP between 2 and 8 (average DP, 4). The resulting product, called oligofructose, is a mixture of GFn (a mnemonic combination of G for glucose, F for fructose, and n for the number of fructose monomers) and Fm fragments, which are, respectively, the sucrose endings and the fragmented polymer tail. Oligofructose can also be chemically synthesized from sucrose by means of invertases (EC 3.1.2.7 from *Aspergillus niger*). The resulting product can have a molecular chain of up to seven fructose moieties (average DP, 3.5). An alternative name for these short-chain inulin-type fructans is fructo-oligosaccharides. By physical separation of the longer chains, a long-chain inulin product can be manufactured which is devoid of any smaller molecules (DP ranges, between 12 and 65; average DP, 25). Oligofructose-enriched inulin (also called Synergy1) is made up of a mixture of oligofructose and long-chain inulin and comprises a preparation with a selected range of chain lengths.

PHYSICAL AND CHEMICAL PROPERTIES

Chicory inulins are available as white and odorless powders with different particle size distribution and density. The use of the different chain length products

differs depending on the target application and desired nutritional effect. The longer chains behave more like polysaccharides and exhibit fat-replacing and stabilizing properties. They have a slower and more sustained fermentation along the large intestine. Oligofructose shows technological properties close to those of sucrose and glucose syrups. It is more rapidly fermented, with a subsequent higher increase in short-chain fatty acids (SCFA) in the proximal part of the large bowel. In oligofructose-enriched inulin (Synergy1) the presence of short and long inulin chains improves the metabolic activity throughout the colon (Van Loo, 2004). The chain length distribution of the different inulin products is given in Fig. 2.

Long-chain inulin has a neutral taste without any off-flavor or aftertaste, whereas native inulin is slightly sweet (10% of the sweetness of sugar). It behaves like a bulk ingredient, contributing to body and mouthfeel, providing a better-sustained flavor with reduced aftertaste (e.g., in combination with high-potency sweeteners) and improving stability. Inulin is moderately soluble in water (maximum solubility, 10% at room temperature), which allows its incorporation into watery systems where the precipitation of other fibers often leads to problems. In very acidic conditions, the $\beta(2-1)$ bonds between the fructose units in inulin can be partially hydrolyzed and fructose is formed. At high concentration (>25% in water for native inulin and >15% for long-chain inulin) it has gelling properties and forms a particle gel network after shearing. When thoroughly mixed with water, or other aqueous liquids, a white creamy structure results which can easily be incorporated into foods to replace fat. Inulin also improves the stability of foams and emulsions, such as aerated dairy desserts, ice creams, table spreads, and sauces. It can, therefore, replace other stabilizers in different food products (Franck, 2002).

Oligofructose is much more soluble than inulin (up to 85% solubility in water at room temperature). It is fairly sweet (35% compared to sucrose) and has a sweetening profile closely approaching that of sugar with a clean taste (no lingering effect). Oligofructose combines with intense sweeteners (such as aspartame and acesulfam K), providing mixtures with rounder mouthfeel and improved flavor with reduced aftertaste (Franck, 2002).

NUTRITIONAL PROPERTIES

Prebiotic Effect

The term "prebiotic" was defined in 1995 as "a nondigestible food ingredient that selectively stimulates growth and/or activity of one or a limited number of bacteria in the colon, thereby improving host health" (Gibson et al., 1995). As research progressed, three criteria that a

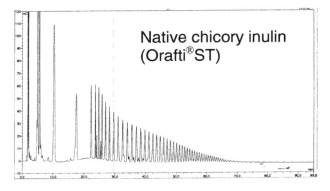

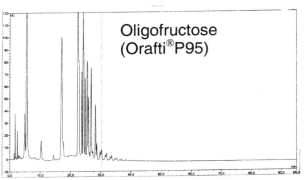

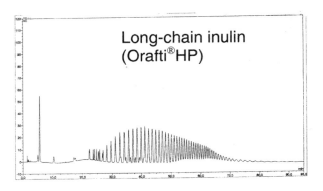

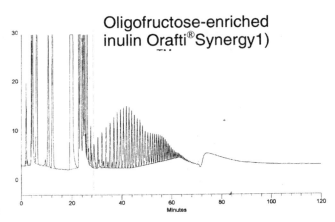

food ingredient should fulfill before it can be classified as a prebiotic were accepted: first, it should be nondigestible and resistant to gastric acidity, hydrolysis by intestinal (brush border/pancreatic) digestive enzymes, and gastrointestinal absorption; second, it should be fermentable; and third, it should, in a selective way, stimulate the growth and/or metabolic activity of intestinal bacteria that are associated with health and well-being. Inulin-type fructans do fulfill all of these criteria and are generally accepted prebiotics (Gibson et al., 2004).

The indigestibility of inulin-type fructans has been demonstrated in ileostomy subjects by their complete recovery (>90%) in the effluent after ingestion (Ellegard et al., 1997). Exploratory in vitro work with fecal slurries, starting in the early 1990s, indicated that inulin and oligofructose are completely fermented by the colonic microbiota and are able to selectively stimulate bifidobacteria and lactobacilli growth and activity at the expense of pathogenic bacteria (e.g., clostridia) (Wang and Gibson, 1993; Gibson and Wang, 1994). This was later confirmed in studies with humans among different age groups (babies, adolescents, adults, and the elderly), after short- and long-term intake, and in health and disease (e.g., inflammatory bowel disease, antibiotic-associated diarrhea, and colonic cancer) (Gibson et al., 1995; Kleessen et al., 1997; Menne et al., 2000; Rao, 2001; Tuohy et al., 2001; Furrie et al., 2005; Lewis et al., 2005; Waligora-Dupriet et al., 2007; Rafter et al., 2007). Interestingly, the magnitude of the prebiotic effect of inulin-type fructans (increase in log CFU of bifidobacteria per gram of colonic content) is dependent on the initial bifidobacteria level of an individual rather than the intake dose (Roberfroid et al., 1998).

Depending on the selection of chain lengths, inulin-type fructans have prebiotic activity at different sites in the colon. Oligofructose is somewhat more rapidly fermented and has a major impact on the composition of the intestinal microbiota in the proximal colon. The longer inulin chains, being fermented more slowly, exert their effect in the more distal parts of the intestines

Figure 2 High-performance anion-exchange chromatographic presentation of different chicory inulin fractions (products). The technique is not quantitative but shows accurately the distribution of various chain lengths. Native inulin (Orafti ST) is the inulin as extracted from the chicory root. The DP varies from 3 to 65; the average DP is 10. Oligofructose (Orafti P95) is partially hydrolyzed chicory inulin (DP, between 2 and 8; average DP, 4). Long-chain inulin (Orafti HP) is devoid of the oligofructose fraction (DP, between 10 and 65; average DP, 25). Oligofructose-enriched inulin (Orafti Synergy1) contains a selected range of chain lengths.

(Langlands et al., 2004). Oligofructose-enriched inulin (Synergy1) combines both properties, maintaining the induced shift in microbial composition in the proximal colon towards the distal colon. This combination has been demonstrated to have distinct physiological properties (Van Loo, 2004). Given the widely studied prebiotic effects of inulin-type fructans, these compounds are nowadays accepted as the "gold standard" of a prebiotic food ingredient.

Effect on Intestinal Metabolism and Function

Inulin-type fructans are completely fermented in the colon by the endogenous microbiota and are converted into bacterial biomass, organic acids, like lactic acid SCFA (acetic, propionic, and butyric acid), and gases (CO_2, H_2, CH_4). Tolerable doses may vary between subjects but are generally above 10 g/day and above the dose necessary to obtain a desirable nutritional effect. Through their fermentation in the large bowel, inulin-type fructans influence metabolism in its lumen (Ohta et al., 1997) and the integrity and functioning of the epithelial cell lining (Osman et al., 2006; Rafter et al., 2007). Increases in stool weight and frequency (also called the "fecal bulking effect") with inulin-type fructans have been observed in humans, having a bulking index (gram of stool weight increase per gram of fiber ingested) of about 1.5 to 2, which can be ascribed to the increase in bacterial biomass (and typically accompanied by a moderate increase in fecal water content). This is comparable with other soluble dietary fiber components, such as pectins and gums (Roberfroid, 1997). This effect has been demonstrated to normalize bowel habits in constipated subjects (Den Hond et al., 1997; Kleessen et al., 1997).

The organic acids that are produced upon inulin and oligofructose fermentation are partly used by the bacteria themselves and partly taken up by the host, and the latter is thought to be the basis of their systemic effects. Also, SCFA and lactic acid are less effective energy substrates than sugars, which explains the reduced caloric value of inulin-type fructans (Roberfroid et al., 1993).

Effect on Intestinal Infection and Inflammation

Intestinal Infection

Several mechanisms have been postulated by which inulin-type fructans and their interaction with the resident microbiota improve resistance of the intestinal tract to (exogenous) pathogen invasion (known as "colonization resistance"). By restricting the availability of substrates within the lumen and adhesion sites on epithelial cells, endogenous bifidobacteria and lactobacilli may inhibit pathogen survival and adherence. Additionally, upon inulin fermentation, lactic acid bacteria produce organic acids (SCFA and lactate), thereby creating an environment unfavorable to pathogen growth. Moreover, butyric acid has been shown to support the barrier function of epithelia (Bosscher et al., 2006).

The protective effects of bifidobacteria have been demonstrated in (gnotobiotic) quails against the development of necrotizing enterocolitis (NEC)-like lesions when inoculated with a pathogenic microbiota (containing *Clostridium butyricum* and *Clostridium perfringens*) from premature newborns. Lesions occurred rapidly after establishment of the NEC microbiota (e.g., thickening of the cecal wall with gas cysts, hemorrhagic ulcerations, and necrotic areas), whereas fewer were formed in the presence of *Bifidobacterium infantis* and *Bifidobacterium longum* (Butel and Roland, 1998). Supplementing the quails' diet with oligofructose induced an increase in the level of bifidobacteria, which prevented overgrowth of bacteria implicated in NEC (e.g., *Escherichia coli*, *Clostridium perfringens*, *Clostridium difficile*, and *Clostridium ramosum*) and reduced NEC-like lesions caused by polymicrobial infection (Catala et al., 1999; Butel et al., 2001). Other experiments showed that supplementation with inulin-type fructans reduced intestinal yeast densities after oral challenge of mice with *Candida albicans*, resulting in an enhanced survival rate (Buddington et al., 2002). A combination of oligofructose and *Lactobacillus paracasei* was also shown to suppress pathogens (*Clostridium*, enterococci, and enterobacteria) in weaning pigs (Bomba et al., 2002). Furthermore, in pigs with cholera toxin-induced secretory diarrhea, oligofructose suppressed the presence of pathogens and increased the numbers of lactobacilli (Oli et al., 1998).

In humans also, inulin-type fructans have been found to protect against pathogen colonization and infection. Critically ill patients have a gut microbial ecology that is in dysbalance and is characterized by high numbers of potential pathogens. Such patients, at risk of developing sepsis (in intensive care units), had lower numbers of pathogens in nasogastric aspirates after they received oligofructose (as a synbiotic) for 10 days (Jain et al., 2004). Treatment with antibiotics, on the other had, also changes the gut microbiota and disrupts the normal ecological balance, which often leads to antibiotic-associated diarrhea. In the study of Orrhage et al. (2000) antibiotic treatment of patients induced a marked decrease in the anaerobic microbiota, mainly with a loss of bifidobacteria and an overgrowth of enterococci. Oligofructose administration (as a synbiotic) for 3 weeks in these patients restored their numbers of lactobacilli and bifidobacteria. Also, in patients with *C. difficile*-associated diarrhea, which frequently occurs after antibiotic therapy, oligofructose suppressed colonization by C. *difficile* and increased bifidobacteria levels. These changes were accompanied by a lower relapse of diarrhea and reduced length of hospital stay (Lewis et al., 2005).

Intestinal Inflammation

Chronic inflammatory intestinal diseases such as inflammatory bowel diseases, ulcerative colitis, Crohn's disease, and pouchitis are thought to have their etiology linked, to some extent, to the composition of the colonic microbial community and its activities. An altered immune response towards normal commensal organisms is estimated to drive the inflammatory process towards a state of chronic inflammation. The effect of inulin-type fructans in modulating the disease process has been repeatedly demonstrated in experimental models, some in which inflammation is induced by chemical agents such as dextran sodium sulfate (Videla et al., 2001) or trinitrobenzene sulfonic acid (Cherbut et al., 2003), as well as in genetically predetermined models (HLA-B27 TG rats) (Hoentjen et al., 2005; Schultz et al., 2004). In each of these, administration of inulin-type fructans (alone or as a synbiotic) in the diets of animals reduced the inflammatory process (e.g., levels of mycloperoxidase, gamma interferon, and prostaglandin E_2), improved clinical and histological markers, and resulted in a reduction in the corresponding lesions. In the study of Hoentjen et al. (2005), using HLA-B27 rats, oligofructose-enriched inulin (Synergy1) decreased gross cecal and inflammatory histological scores in the cecum and colon together with altered mucosal cytokine profiles (decreased interleukin-1β [IL-1β] and increased transforming growth factor β levels).

In humans suffering from ulcerative colitis, it has been described that bifidobacteria populations are about 30-fold lower than those in healthy individuals (Macfarlane et al., 2005). Supplementation of the diet with oligofructose-enriched inulin (Synergy1) together with a probiotic (*B. longum*) for 1 month resulted in a 42-fold increase in bifidobacterial numbers in mucosal biopsy samples (Macfarlane et al., 2005). Administration of the synbiotic improved the full clinical appearance of chronic inflammation, as evidenced by a reduction in sigmoidoscopy scores, a reduction in acute inflammatory activity (cytokines that drive the inflammatory process, e.g., tumor necrosis factor alpha and IL-1 alpha), and a regeneration of the epithelial tissue (Furrie et al., 2005). Also, in patients with Crohn's disease, dietary intervention with a combination of inulin and oligofructose for 3 weeks has been shown to lead towards an improvement in the disease activity (reduction in Harvey Bradshaw Index) and enhanced lamina propria dendritic cell

IL-10 production and Toll-like receptor 2 and 4 expression (Lindsay et al., 2006). A reduction of the inflammation and associated factors was observed also in patients with an ileal pouch-anal anastomosis after therapy with inulin-type fructans (Welters et al., 2002).

Effect on Colon Cancer

Cancer of the colon is one of the most common cancers (together with lung and breast) and among the deadliest ones. Rates of colon cancer are expected to spiral upwards in the future. Diet has a strong influence in its etiology, and appropriate changes in dietary habits are therefore expected to have a major impact on its prevalence. Evidence pinpoints the role of the colonic microbiota in this process. Intestinal bacterial metabolism can generate substances with genotoxic, carcinogenic, and tumor-promoting potential, and human feces have been shown to be genotoxic and cytotoxic to colonic cells. Some bacteria carry specific enzymes that generate carcinogenic substances from food compounds (e.g., clostridia and *Bacteroides*). Therefore, a well-balanced gut microbial ecosystem is important in terms of reducing colorectal cancer risk. Studies in vitro (Klinder et al., 2004a, 2004b) and in animal chemoprevention models have shown that inulin-type fructans (alone or as a synbiotic) are able to inhibit carcinogen (azoxymethane)-induced colonic DNA damage and to suppress the development of colonic preneoplastic lesions (aberrant crypt foci) and tumors in both number and size (Reddy et al., 1997; Femia et al., 2002; Roller et al., 2004, 2007).

In 2001, a collaborative European network (eight partners from seven countries) was initiated on "Synbiotics and Cancer Prevention" (SYNCAN). This project showed for the first time that prebiotics, combined with probiotics (synbiotics), can reduce the risk factors for colon cancer. The core feature of the project involved a 3-month human intervention study with a synbiotic (Synergy1 together with *Bifidobacterium lactis* Bb12 and *Lactobacillus rhamnosus* GG) in patients with a high risk of colon cancer (polypectomized and patients with a history of colon cancer). The synbiotic increased the levels of bifidobacteria in polyp and cancer subjects and of lactobacilli in the polyp group and decreased the numbers of clostridia (*C. perfringens*) in the polyp group. The selectivity of the interaction of the synbiotic with the gut microbiota was further demonstrated by the lack of effect on *Bacteroides* populations. The altered composition of the colonic bacterial ecosystem beneficially affected the metabolic activity in this organ. This was obvious from the decreased DNA damage in the colonic mucosa (measured by the comet assay) and the tendency to a lower level of colorectal proliferation (surrogate biomarker for colon cancer risk) in polyp patients (no measures were taken for cancer patients). The effect of the fecal water on the epithelial barrier function (transepithelial resistance), cell toxicity, and immunology markers was monitored ex vivo in different cell lines. The fecal water is the fecal fraction in most intimate contact with the colonic epithelium and mediates many of the effects of diet on tumorigenesis. A commonly observed effect of tumor promoters is a reduction in the barrier function of the epithelium which results in reduced protection of the mucosa against carcinogenic substances. Interestingly, the synbiotic intervention increased the barrier function of the epithelium which was shown by the higher transepithelial resistance value of the (Caco-2 cell) monolayer when subjected to the fecal water of polyp patients supplemented with the synbiotic. The fecal water of synbiotic-fed polyp patients also showed a lower level of cell necrosis as demonstrated by the lower cytotoxic potential in HCT116 cell types. This indicates that the synbiotic effectively prevented cell death of the colonic epithelium (Rafter et al., 2007).

Impact on Sites beyond the Intestinal Tract

Modulation of Immune Function

To study the effect of a food ingredient on immunity in humans, studies with vaccination (challenge model) or with populations at risk (e.g., individuals at risk of infection or malnourished children) are appropriate and enable the investigation of clinical outcomes after the intervention. Infants are very vulnerable to infections and gastrointestinal tract disturbances. The likelihood of these occurring is increased by attendance at day care centers where infectious diseases are frequent and readily disseminate from one child to another. Saavedra and Tschernia (2002) examined the effect of a daily intake of oligofructose (supplemented to cereal) for 6 months in 123 infants (4 to 24 months of age) attending day care. The consumption of the prebiotic cereal was associated with a decrease in the severity of diarrheal disease. General gut status was improved with decreased bowel movement discomfort, vomiting, and regurgitation. Furthermore, consumption of the prebiotic cereal resulted in adequate growth and led to a reduction in the number of febrile events and cold symptoms, antibiotic prescription (associated with respiratory illness), and day care absenteeism. Such observations were later confirmed in a smaller-scale study of infants of a similar age. Oligofructose intake improved the intestinal bacterial colonization, as characterized by higher levels of bifidobacteria, especially in those infants with lower baseline levels, and a decrease in clostridia. Daily oligofructose administration was well tolerated. Additionally, the number of febrile events and gastrointestinal illness symptoms, such as flatulence, diarrhea, and vomiting, were less often observed (Waligora-Dupriet et al., 2007). Fisberg et al. (2000) evaluated the incidence and duration of sickness in 626 mild to moderately malnourished children (1 to 6 years of age) who received a nutritional supplement with a synbiotic (oligofructose together with *Lactobacillus acidophilus* and *B. infantis*). In a subgroup of children (aged 3 to 5 years), the number of sick days were fewer following synbiotic administration, as were days of constipation. Further investigations have been undertaken by Firmansyah et al. (2000), who examined the immune response in infants after measles vaccination and consumption of a weaning food with oligofructose and inulin. Postvaccination specific immunoglobulin G antibody levels were higher with the synbiotic, indicating a better immune response to vaccination.

Mineral Absorption and Bone Metabolism

Calcium plays an important role in bone development and maintenance, and intakes are well below those recommended across the whole life span (e.g., children and the elderly). Given the increasing prevalence of osteoporosis, increasing calcium absorption from the diet by the addition of inulin-type fructans is an important strategy to improve bone metabolism at all ages (Cashman, 2006). At present there are two approaches to prevent osteoporosis. The first is by optimizing bone mass acquisition in the skeleton during growth, and the second is by minimizing bone loss in later life. Over the past 10 years, studies have repeatedly shown that inulin-type fructans increase calcium absorption from the diet. Initial experiments in growing rats found increased (apparent) calcium absorption, improved bone mineralization (whole-body bone mineral content and density) and accumulation of bone mineral, and improved structure of the trabecular network (Delzenne et al., 1995; Roberfroid et al., 2002). Coudray et al. (2003) showed that oligofructose-enriched inulin (Synergy1) was most effective at increasing calcium absorption and balance when compared to either of the two fractions alone (Coudray et al., 2003).

Following this, a number of intervention studies in adolescents have been carried out using dual stable isotopes to measure true calcium absorption; all showed an increased absorption of calcium from the diet in the presence of oligofructose-enriched inulin (at 8 g of Synergy1 per day) (Griffin et al., 2002, 2003; Abrams et al., 2005). Further study of the subjects' characteristics associated with the beneficial effect found that the most consistent identifiable determinant was the fractional calcium absorption during the placebo period—those individuals with habitual lower calcium absorption showed the greatest increase in response to Synergy1. This finding is important as these adolescents might be most likely to benefit from Synergy1 supplementation in their daily diet (Griffin et al., 2003). In a subsequent long-term (1-year) intervention study in 100 pubertal girls and boys (9 to 12 years of age) Synergy1 was found to enhance bone mineralization, as indicated by the higher change in whole-body bone mineral density and content, the latter corresponding to an additional net accretion of 30 ± 15 mg of calcium per day (Abrams et al., 2005). Given the fact that calcium accretion is at its optimal stage during the pubertal ages and its level determines bone health at later age, higher calcium accretion rates during pubertal growth could maximize peak bone mass, thereby reducing skeletal fragility at an older age.

In women, menopause is a time when estrogen deficiency leads to accelerated bone resorption and negative bone balance. In ovariectomized rats (a model of menopause) the addition of oligofructose-enriched inulin to the diet increased calcium absorption, decreased bone turnover rate, increased accumulation of bone mineral and formation of the trabecular network, and impeded ovariectomy-induced loss of bone structure (Scholz-Ahrens et al., 2002; Zafar et al., 2004). A subsequent intervention study with oligofructose-enriched inulin in postmenopausal women (mean age, 72 years) was carried out. Supplementation with Synergy1 improved calcium (and magnesium) absorption, even when vitamin D status was adequate and calcium intake was good. Markers of bone turnover showed a short-term decrease in bone resorption and a clear increase in bone formation, and this was most pronounced in those women with lower initial spine bone mineral density (Holloway et al., 2007).

Lipid Metabolism

In experimental models, inulin-type fructans have been shown to lower triglyceride levels (Delzenne, 1993) as well as cholesterol levels (Fiordaliso et al., 1995; Trautwein et al., 1998). In rats on high-fat diets, feeding with oligofructose suppressed the observed postprandial increase in triglyceride levels and hepatic triacylglycerol load (both originating from a fat-rich diet) (Kok et al., 1998b). Further studies in genetically obese (fa/fa Zucker) rats showed a similar tendency, with lower body weight, fat mass, and steatosis development when inulin-type fructans were part of the diet. These effects were, however, not seen with other (nonfermentable) dietary fibers (e.g., cellulose). Biochemical studies with isolated hepatocytes have demonstrated that inulin-type fructans reduce the activity of key hepatic enzymes which are related to

lipogenesis (de novo synthesis of fatty acid synthesis) (Kok et al., 1996). Further research revealed that altered gene expression was at the basis of the down-regulation which might have been in response to hormonal changes induced by inulin-type fructans (Kok et al. 1998a). More recently it was demonstrated that the effects of inulin-type fructans on cholesterol and lipid metabolism have beneficial consequences in the process of atherosclerosis given that both are at the basis of disease development. This was demonstrated in mice (ApoE deficient) in which inulin-type fructans inhibited atherosclerotic plaque formation (in the aorta) (Rault-Nania et al., 2006).

In humans, inulin-type fructans have been shown to affect lipid metabolism, although the data are less consistent compared to the results obtained in animal studies. This might be due to a different methodological setup, type of subjects, and duration and dose of inulin-type fructan supplementation. It has been reported that the consumption of inulin-type fructans reduces serum triglycerides and sometimes also cholesterol (mostly the low-density lipoprotein fraction) in healthy volunteers who are (slightly) hyperlipidemic. Lipid parameters in healthy (normolipidemic) young adults, in contrast, appear not to be affected. Also, it appears that the triglyceride-lowering effect might take some time to establish (about 8 weeks) (Davidson and Maki, 1999; Jackson et al., 1999; Brighenti et al., 1999; E. Canzi, F. B. Brighenti, M. C. Casiraghi, E. Del Puppo, and A. Ferrari, presented at the COST '92 Workshop on Dietary Fibre and Fermentation, Helsinki, Finland, 1995).

The mechanisms responsible for the effects of inulin-type fructans on lipid and cholesterol metabolism in the human body are complex and include various interdependent biochemical pathways which take place in the liver, pancreas, intestine, and peripheral tissues (e.g., adipose tissue). Research in this field has evolved, with the primary focus being on endocrine activity in the gut; this is discussed in more detail in the next section.

Appetite, Food Intake, and Body Weight

Obesity is one of the greatest public health challenges of the 21st century. It is characterized by excessive adipose tissue accumulation to an extent that health is impaired. The condition is caused by an imbalance between energy intake and energy expenditure. If energy intake exceeds expenditure for a long period of time, the excess in energy will be stored in the body and will lead to the development of overweight and ultimately obesity. In various animal models (e.g., rats on a normal or high-fat diet, obese and diabetic rats) the addition of inulin-type fructans to the diet has been consistently associated with a significant lower food (and energy) intake and lower body weight and adipose tissue deposition (coming from high-fat diets) and, consequently, a reduction in the development of obesity (and related diseases) (Daubioul et al., 2002; Cani et al., 2004, 2005a, 2005b).

The mechanisms of appetite regulation are complex and involve the interaction of orexigenic (ghrelin) and anorexigenic (e.g., glucagon-like peptide 1 [GLP-1]) hormones that are released by the body (gastrointestinal tract and peripheral tissues) in response to the diet and which send messages to the area of the brain (primarily the hypothalamus) sensing the feeling of hunger and/or being full. Higher colonic expression and blood levels of GLP-1 (appetite-suppressing peptide) and lower levels of ghrelin have been observed in response to the fermentation of inulin-type fructans in the rat colon (Cani et al., 2004, 2005a). The GLP-1 peptide might indeed constitute a link between the outcome of fermentation in the colon and the modulation of food intake (Burcelin, 2005). The role of GLP-1 has been tested in mice by using a GLP-1 receptor antagonist (exendin, Ex 9–39). Administration of the antagonist totally prevented the beneficial systemic effects of oligofructose (e.g., improved glucose tolerance, fasting blood glucose, glucose-stimulated insulin secretion, and insulin-sensitive hepatic glucose production, and lower body weight gain in comparison with the control mice). Also, GLP-1R$^{-/-}$ mice appeared to be totally insensitive to the systemic effects of oligofructose (Cani et al., 2006a).

In healthy men and women (with a normal body mass index), oligofructose intake was found to increase satiety and reduce hunger and prospective food consumption (on a visual analogue scale). This resulted in a lower total energy intake during the day (Cani et al., 2006b). Also, in other human studies, the effects of oligofructose, either alone or in combination with other dietary fibers (pea fiber), on satiety and food intake have been documented (Whelan et al., 2006). Recently it has been shown that long-term (1-year) administration of oligofructose-enriched inulin (Synergy1) to (primarily nonobese) pubertal adolescents (9.0 to 13.0 years of age) benefited the maintenance of an appropriate body mass index during their pubertal growth. The subjects receiving Synergy1 had an increase in their body mass index of about 0.7 kg/m^2 during the supplementation year, which is consistent with the expected increases during puberty, whereas the nonsupplemented group had a higher increase (of 1.2 kg/m^2) (Abrams et al., 2007).

FOOD APPLICATIONS

Inulin-type fructans are used in foods for either their technological properties or their nutritional benefits but are most often applied to offer a double benefit: improved organoleptic quality and a better-balanced nutritional composition. In bakery products and breakfast cereals, the use of inulin-type fructans offers important advantages compared to other fibers. Inulin gives more crispiness and expansion to extruded snacks and cereals, and it increases their bowl life. It also keeps breads and cakes moist and fresh for longer. Its solubility also enables fiber incorporation in watery systems such as drinks, dairy products, and table spreads. Given the specific gelling characteristics of inulin, it can be used in the development of low-fat foods without compromising on taste and texture. In table spreads (both fat and water-continuous), inulin can replace high amounts of fat and can stabilize the emulsion while providing a soft, spreadable texture. In low-fat dairy products, such as fresh cheese, cream cheese, or processed cheese, the addition of a small percentage of inulin increases the body and gives a creamier mouthfeel and a better-balanced round flavor. It can also be used as a fat replacer in frozen desserts, providing easy processing, fatty mouthfeel, excellent melting properties, and freeze-thaw stability, without any off-flavors. Other applications of fat replacement are meal replacers, meat products, sauces, and soups. The synergistic effect of inulin with other gelling agents offers an additional advantage in all of these applications. In some applications, inulin, and more specifically the long-chain inulin, can (partially) replace gelatin, starch, maltodextrin, alginate, caseinate, and other stabilizers. This is particularly interesting for use in dairy desserts, yogurts, cheese products, and table spreads.

Within the yogurt market, low-fat products show the strongest growth and in particular "diet yogurts" with fruit. Incorporation of inulin (1 to 3%) in the fruit preparation improves mouthfeel, reduces syneresis, and offers a synergistic taste effect in combination with high-potency sweeteners such as aspartame, acesulfame K, and sucralose without increasing caloric content. Inulin (1 to 5%) increases the stability of foams and mousses, e.g., dairy-based aerated desserts (chocolate, fruit, yogurt, or fresh cheese-based mousses), improves processability, and upgrades quality. These products retain their typical structure for a longer time and give fat-like feeling even in the case of low-fat or fat-free formulations.

Inulin-type fructans are also used as low-calorie bulk ingredients, e.g., in chocolate without added sugar, to replace sugar and are applied often in combination with polyols. Oligofructose is used as a dietary fiber or sugar replacer in tablets. Also, it is often included in low-calorie dairy products, frozen desserts, and meal replacers. Inulin-type fructans have become key ingredients offering new opportunities to the food industry looking for well-balanced and yet better-tasting products in modern nutrition.

FUTURE PERSPECTIVES

The steadily increasing number of publications relating to inulin-type fructans over the last 2 decades has put the prebiotic concept on the map of well-established functional foods. Knowledge of the mechanisms by which inulin-type fructans exert their physiological effects will shed more light on their effects on health and well-being. The impact of inulin-type fructans on the composition of the colonic microbiota and, more importantly, the implication of such an altered bacterial ecosystem on the host's health status will be better elucidated. Modulation of the immune response and protection against infectious diseases will be thoroughly assessed as potential effects of regular inulin-type fructan consumption. Improving mineral absorption and bone health is another topic which deserves further research. Special efforts will be made to investigate in depth the role of inulin-type fructans in the reduction of (colon) cancer risk and the prevention of obesity. Given the high burden of these diseases in Western societies, functional ingredients such as inulin-type fructans will have a major impact on the health and well-being of populations. Their technological properties, combined with the ease with which inulin-type fructans can be incorporated into foods, mean that they can be readily administered to a large proportion of the population and can, therefore, constitute one of the preventive measures taken by governments to reduce the burden of chronic diseases.

References

Abrams, S. A., I. J. Griffin, K. M. Hawthorne, and K. J. Ellis. 2007. Effect of prebiotic supplementation and calcium intake on body mass index. *J. Pediatr.* **151**:293–298.

Abrams, S. A., I. J. Griffin, K. M. Hawthorne, L. Liang, S. K. Gunn, G. Darlington, and K. J. Ellis. 2005. A combination of prebiotic short- and long-chain inulin-type fructans enhances calcium absorption and bone mineralization in young adolescents. *Am. J. Clin. Nutr.* **82**:471–476.

Bomba, A., R. Nemcova, S. Gancarcikova, R. Herich, P. Guba, and D. Mudronova. 2002. Improvement of the prebiotic effect of micro-organisms by their combination with malto-dextrins, fructo-oligosaccharides and polyunsaturated fatty acids. *Br. J. Nutr.* **88**:(Suppl.):S95–S99.

Bosscher, D., J. Van Loo, and A. Franck. 2006. Inulin and oligofructose as prebiotics in the prevention of intestinal diseases. *Nutr. Res. Rev.* **19**:216–226.

Brighenti, F., M. C. Casiraghi, E. Canzi, and A. Ferrari. 1999. Effect of consumption of a ready-to-eat breakfast cereal containing inulin on the intestinal milieu and blood lipids in healthy male volunteers. *Eur. J. Clin. Nutr.* **53**:726–733.

Buddington, K. K., J. B. Donahoo, and R. K. Buddington. 2002. Dietary oligofructose and inulin protect mice from enteric and systemic pathogens and tumor inducers. *J. Nutr.* **132**:472–477.

Burcelin, R. 2005. The incretins: a link between nutrients and well-being. *Br. J. Nutr.* **93**:S147–S156.

Butel, M., I. Catala, A. Waligora-Dupriet, H. Taper, A. Tessedre, J. Durao, and O. Szylit. 2001. Protective effect of dietary oligofructose against cecitis induced by clostridia in gnotobiotic quails. *Microb. Ecol. Health Dis.* **13**:166–172.

Butel, M., and N. Roland. 1998. Clostridia pathogenicity in experimental necrotising enterocolitis in gnotobiotic quails and protective role of bifidobacteria. *J. Med. Microbiol.* **47**:391–399.

Cani, P., A. Neyrinck, N. Maton, and N. Delzenne. 2005a. Oligofructose promotes satiety in rats fed a high-fat diet: involvement of glucagon-like peptide-1. *Obesity Res.* **13**:1000–1007.

Cani, P., C. Daubioul, B. Reusens, C. Remacle, G. Catillon, and N. Delzenne. 2005b. Involvement of endogenous glucagon-like peptide-1(7–36) amide on glycemia-lowering effect of oligofructose in streptozotocin-treated rats. *J. Endocrinol.* **185**:457–465.

Cani, P. D., C. Dewever, and N. M. Delzenne. 2004. Inulin-type fructans modulate gastrointestinal peptides involved in appetite regulation (glucagon-like peptide-1 and ghrelin) in rats. *Br. J. Nutr.* **92**:521–526.

Cani, P. D., C. Knauf, M. A. Iglesias, D. J. Drucker, N. M. Delzenne, and R. Burcelin. 2006a. Improvement of glucose tolerance and hepatic insulin sensitivity by oligofructose requires a functional glucagon-like peptide 1 receptor. *Diabetes* **55**:1484–1490.

Cani, P. D., E. Joly, Y. Horsmans, and N. M. Delzenne. 2006b. Oligofructose promotes satiety in healthy human: a pilot study. *Eur. J. Clin. Nutr.* **60**:567–572.

Cashman, K. D. 2006. A prebiotic substance persistently enhances intestinal calcium absorption and increases bone mineralization in young adolescents. *Nutr. Rev.* **64**:189–196.

Catala, I., M. J. Butel, M. Bensaada, F. Popot, A. C. Tessedre, A. Rimbault, and O. Szylit. 1999. Oligofructose contributes to the protective role of bifidobacteria in experimental necrotising enterocolitis in quails. *J. Med. Microbiol.* **48**:89–94.

Cherbut, C., C. Michel, and G. Lecannu. 2003. The prebiotic characteristics of fructooligosaccharides are necessary for reduction of TNBS-induced colitis in rats. *J. Nutr.* **133**:21–27.

Coudray, C., J. Bellanger, C. Castiglia-Delavaud, C. Remesy, M. Vermorel, and Y. Rayssignuier. 1997. Effect of soluble or partly soluble dietary fibres supplementation on absorption and balance of calcium, magnesium, iron and zinc in healthy young men. *Eur. J. Clin. Nutr.* **51**:375–380.

Coudray, C., J. C. Tressol, E. Gueux, and Y. Rayssiguier. 2003. Effects of inulin-type fructans of different chain length and type of branching on intestinal absorption and balance of calcium and magnesium in rats. *Eur. J. Nutr.* **42**:91–98.

Daubioul, C., N. Rousseau, R. Demeure, B. Gallez, H. Taper, B. Declerck, and N. Delzenne. 2002. Dietary fructans, but not cellulose, decrease triglyceride accumulation in the liver of obese Zucker fa/fa rats. *J. Nutr.* **132**:967–973.

Davidson, M. H., and K. C. Maki. 1999. Effects of dietary inulin on serum lipids. *J. Nutr.* **129**:1474S–1477S.

Delzenne, N., J. Aertssens, H. Verplaetse, M. Roccaro, and M. Roberfroid. 1995. Effect of fermentable fructo-oligosaccharides on mineral, nitrogen and energy digestive balance in the rat. *Life Sci.* **57**:1579–1587.

Delzenne, N. M. 1993. Dietary fructooligosaccharides modify lipid metabolism in rats. *Am. J. Clin. Nutr.* **57**:820S.

Den Hond, E. M., B. J. Geypens, and Y. F. Ghoos. 1997. Effect of long chain chicory inulin on bowel habit and transit time in constipated persons. *Nutr. Res.* **20**:731–736.

Ellegard, L., H. Andersson, and I. Bosaeus. 1997. Inulin and oligofructose do not influence the absorption of cholesterol, or the excretion of cholesterol, Ca, Mg, Zn, Fe, or bile acids but increases energy excretion in ileostomy subjects. *Eur. J. Clin. Nutr.* **51**:1–5.

Femia, A. P., C. Luceri, P. Dolara, A. Giannini, A. Biggeri, M. Salvadori, Y. Clune, K. J. Collins, M. Paglierani, and G. Caderni. 2002. Antitumorigenic activity of the prebiotic inulin enriched with oligofructose in combination with the probiotics *Lactobacillus rhamnosus* and *Bifidobacterium lactis* on azoxymethane-induced colon carcinogenesis in rats. *Carcinogenesis* **23**:1953–1960.

Fiordaliso, M., N. Kok, J. P. Desager, F. Goethals, D. Deboyser, M. Roberfroid, and N. Delzenne. 1995. Dietary oligofructose lowers triglycerides, phospholipids and cholesterol in serum and very low density lipoproteins of rats. *Lipids* **30**:163–167.

Firmansyah, A., G. Pramita, C. Fassler, F. Haschke, and H. Link-Amster. 2000. Improved humoral immune response to measles vaccine in infants receiving infant cereal with fructooligosaccharides. *J. Pediatr. Gastroenterol. Nutr.* **31**:S134.

Fisberg, M., I. Maulen, E. Vasquez, J. Garcia, G. M. Comer, and P. A. Alarcon. 2000. Effect of oral supplementation with and without synbiotics on catch-up growth in preschool children. *J. Pediatr. Gastroenterol. Nutr.* **31**:A521.

Franck, A. 2002. Technological functionality of inulin and oligofructose. *Br. J. Nutr.* **87**:S287-S291.

Furrie, E., S. Macfarlane, A. Kennedy, J. H. Cummings, S. V. Walsh, D. A. O'Neil, and G. T. Macfarlane. 2005. Synbiotic therapy (*Bifidobacterium longum*/Synergy 1) initiates resolution of inflammation in patients with active ulcerative colitis: a randomised controlled pilot trial. *Gut* **54**:242–249.

Gibson, G. R., E. R. Beatty, X. Wang, and J. H. Cummings. 1995. Selective stimulation of bifidobacteria in the human colon by oligofructose and inulin. *Gastroenterology* **108**:975–982.

Gibson, G. R., H. M. Probert, J. Van Loo, R. A. Rastall, and M. B. Roberfroid. 2004. Dietary modulation of the human colonic microbiota: updating the concept of prebiotics. *Nutr. Res. Rev.* **17**:259–275.

Gibson, G. R., and X. Wang. 1994. Enrichment of bifidobacteria from human gut contents by oligofructose using continuous culture. *FEMS Microbiol. Lett.* **118**:121–127.

Griffin, I. J., P. M. Davila, and S. A. Abrams. 2002. Non-digestible oligosaccharides and calcium absorption in girls with adequate calcium intakes. *Br. J. Nutr.* **87**(Suppl. 2):S187–S191.

Griffin, I. J., P. M. D. Hicks, R. P. Heaney, and S. A. Abrams. 2003. Enriched chicory inulin increases calcium absorption mainly in girls with lower calcium absorption. *Nutr. Res.* **23**:901–909.

Hoentjen, F., G. W. Welling, H. J. Harmsen, X. Zhang, J. Snart, G. W. Tannock, K. Lien, T. A. Churchill, M. Lupicki, and L. A. Dieleman. 2005. Reduction of colitis by prebiotics in HLA-B27 transgenic rats is associated with microflora changes and immunomodulation. *Inflamm. Bowel Dis.* **11**:977–985.

Holloway, L., S. Moynihan, S. A. Abrams, K. Kent, A. R. Hsu, and A. L. Friedlander. 2007. Effects of oligofructose-enriched inulin on intestinal absorption of calcium and magnesium and bone turnover markers in postmenopausal women. *Br. J. Nutr.* **97**:365–372.

Jackson, K. G., G. R. Taylor, A. M. Clohessy, and C. M. Williams. 1999. The effect of the daily intake of inulin on fasting lipid, insulin and glucose concentrations in middle-aged men and women. *Br. J. Nutr.* **82**:23–30.

Jain, P. K., C. E. McNaught, A. D. Anderson, J. MacFie, and C. J. Mitchell. 2004. Influence of synbiotic containing *Lactobacillus acidophilus* La5, *Bifidobacterium lactis* Bb 12, *Streptococcus thermophilus*, *Lactobacillus bulgaricus* and oligofructose on gut barrier function and sepsis in critically ill patients: a randomised controlled trial. *Clin. Nutr.* **23**:467–475.

Kleessen, B., B. Sykura, H. J. Zunft, and M. Blaut. 1997. Effects of inulin and lactose on fecal microflora, microbial activity, and bowel habit in elderly constipated persons. *Am. J. Clin. Nutr.* **65**:1397–1402.

Klinder, A., A. Föster, G. Caderni, A. P. Femia, and B. L. Pool-Zobel. 2004a. Fecal water genotoxicity is predictive of tumor-preventive activities by inulin-type oligofructoses, probiotics (*Lactobacillus rhamnosus* and *Bifidobacterium lactis*), and their synbiotic combination. *Nutr. Cancer* **49**:144–155.

Klinder, A., E. Gietl, R. Hughes, N. Jonkers, P. Karlsson, H. McGlyn, S. Pistoli, K. Tuohy, J. Rafter, I. R. Rowland, J. Van Loo, and B. Pool-Zobel. 2004b. Gut fermentation products of inulin-derived prebiotics beneficially modulate markers of tumour progression in human colon tumour cells. *Int. J. Cancer Prev.* **1**:19–32.

Kok, N., M. Roberfroid, A. Robert, and N. Delzenne. 1996. Involvement of lipogenesis in the lower VLDL secretion induced by oligofructose in rats. *Br. J. Nutr.* **76**:881–890.

Kok, N. N., L. M. Morgan, C. M. Williams, M. B. Roberfroid, J. P. Thissen, and N. M. Delzenne. 1998a. Insulin, glucagon-like peptide 1, glucose-dependent insulinotropic polypeptide and insulin-like growth factor I as putative mediators of the hypolipidemic effect of oligofructose in rats. *J. Nutr.* **128**:1099–1103.

Kok, N. N., H. S. Taper, and N. M. Delzenne. 1998b. Oligofructose modulates lipid metabolism alterations induced by a fat-rich diet in rats. *J. Appl. Toxicol.* **18**:47–53.

Langlands, S. J., M. J. Hopkins, N. Coleman, and J. H. Cummings. 2004. Prebiotic carbohydrates modify the mucosa associated microflora of the human large bowel. *Gut* **53**:1610–1616.

Lewis, S., S. Burmeister, and J. Brazier. 2005. Effect of the prebiotic oligofructose on relapse of *Clostridium difficile*-associated diarrhea: a randomized, controlled study. *Clin. Gastroenterol. Hepatol.* **3**:442–448.

Lindsay, J. O., K. Whelan, A. J. Stagg, P. Gobin, H. O. Al-Hassi, N. Raiment, M. A. Kamm, S. C. Knight, and A. Forbes. 2006. Clinical, microbiological and immunological effects of fructo-oligosaccharides in patients with Crohn's disease. *Gut* **55**:348–355.

Macfarlane, S., E. Furrie, A. Kennedy, J. H. Cummings, and G. T. Macfarlane. 2005. Mucosal bacteria in ulcerative colitis. *Br. J. Nutr.* 93(Suppl. 1):S67–S72.

Menne, E., N. Guggenbuhl, and M. Roberfroid. 2000. Fn-type chicory inulin hydrolysate has a prebiotic effect in humans. *J. Nutr.* 130:1197–1199.

Ohta, A., S. Baba, M. Ohtsuki, T. Takizawa, T. Adachi, and H. Hara. 1997. *In vivo* absorption of calcium carbonate and magnesium oxide from the large intestine in rats. *J. Nutr. Sci. Vitaminol.* 43:35–46.

Oli, M. W., B. W. Petschow, and R. K. Buddington. 1998. Evaluation of fructooligosaccharide supplementation of oral electrolyte solutions for treatment of diarrhea. Recovery of the intestinal bacteria. *Dig. Dis. Sci.* 43:138–147.

Orrhage, K., S. Sjostedt, and C. E. Nord. 2000. Effects of supplements with lactic acid bacteria. *J. Antimicrob. Chemother.* 46:603–611.

Osman, N., D. Adawi, G. Molin, S. Ahrne, A. Berggren, and B. Jeppsson. 2006. *Bifidobacterium infantis* strains with and without a combination of oligofructose and inulin (OFI) attenuate inflammation in DSS-induced colitis in rats. *BMC Gastroenterol.* 6:31.

Rafter, J., M. Bennett, G. Caderni, Y. Clune, R. Hughes, P. C. Karlsson, A. Klinder, M. O'Riordan, G. C. O'Sullivan, B. Pool-Zobel, G. Rechkemmer, M. Roller, I. Rowland, M. Salvadori, H. Thijs, J. Van Loo, B. Watzl, and J. K. Collins. 2007. Dietary synbiotics reduce cancer risk factors in polypectomized and colon cancer patients. *Am. J. Clin. Nutr.* 85:488–496.

Rao, V. A. 2001. The prebiotic properties of oligofructose at low intake levels. *Nutr. Res.* 21:843–848.

Rault-Nania, M. H., E. Gueux, C. Demougeot, C. Demigne, E. Rock, and A. Mazur. 2006. Inulin attenuates atherosclerosis in apolipoprotein E-deficient mice. *Br. J. Nutr.* 96:840–844.

Reddy, B. S., R. Hamid, and C. V. Rao. 1997. Effect of dietary oligofructose and inulin on colonic preneoplastic aberrant crypt foci inhibition. *Carcinogenesis* 18:1371–1374.

Roberfroid, M., G. R. Gibson, and N. M. Delzenne. 1993. The biochemistry of oligofructose, a nondigestible fiber: an approach to calculate its caloric value. *Nutr. Rev.* 51:137–146.

Roberfroid, M. B. 1997. Health benefits of non-digestible oligosaccharides, p. 211. *In* D. Kritchevsky and C. T. Bonfield (ed.), *Dietary Fiber in Health and Disease.* Plenum Press, New York, NY.

Roberfroid, M. B., J. A. Van Loo, and G. R. Gibson. 1998. The bifidogenic nature of chicory inulin and its hydrolysis products. *J. Nutr.* 128:11–19.

Roberfroid, M. B., J. Cumps, and J. P. Devogelaer. 2002. Dietary chicory inulin increases whole-body bone mineral density in growing male rats. *J. Nutr.* 132:3599–3602.

Roller, M., Y. Clune, K. Collins, G. Rechkemmer, and B. Watzl. 2007. Consumption of prebiotic inulin enriched with oligofructose in combination with the probiotics *Lactobacillus rhamnosus* and *Bifidobacterium lactis* has minor effects on selected immune parameters in polypectomised and colon cancer patients. *Br. J. Nutr.* 97:676–684.

Roller, M., G. Rechkemmer, and B. Watzl. 2004. Prebiotic inulin enriched with oligofructose in combination with the probiotics *Lactobacillus rhamnosus* and *Bifidobacterium lactis* modulates intestinal immune functions in rats. *J. Nutr.* 134:153–156.

Saavedra, J., and A. Tschernia. 2002. Human studies with probiotics and prebiotics: clinical implications. *Br. J. Nutr.* 87: S241–S246.

Scholz-Ahrens, K. E., Y. Acil, and J. Schrezenmeir. 2002. Effect of oligofructose or dietary calcium on repeated calcium and phosphorus balances, bone mineralization and trabecular structure in ovariectomized rats. *Br. J. Nutr.* 88:365–377.

Schultz, M., K. Munro, G. W. Tannock, I. Melchner, C. Gottl, H. Schwietz, J. Scholmerich, and H. C. Rath. 2004. Effects of feeding a probiotic preparation (SIM) containing inulin on the severity of colitis and on the composition of the intestinal microflora in HLA-B27 transgenic rats. *Clin. Diagn. Lab. Immunol.* 11:581–587.

Trautwein, E. A., D. Rieckhoff, and H. F. Erbersdobler. 1998. Dietary inulin lowers plasma cholesterol and triacylglycerol and alters biliary bile acid profile in hamsters. *J. Nutr.* 128:1937–1943.

Tuohy, K. M., R. K. Finlay, A. G. Wynne, and G. R. Gibson. 2001. A human volunteer study on the prebiotic effects of HP-Inulin—faecal bacteria enumerated using fluorescent *in situ* hybridisation (FISH). *Anaerobe* 7:113–118.

Van Loo, J. 2004. The specificity of the interaction with intestinal fermentation by prebiotics determines their physiological efficacy. *Nutr. Res. Rev.* 17:89–98.

Van Loo, J., P. Coussement, L. De Leenheer, H. Hoebregs, and G. Smits. 1995. On the presence of inulin and oligofructose as natural ingredients in the western diet. *Crit. Rev. Food Sci. Nutr.* 35:525–552.

Videla, S., J. Vilaseca, M. Antolin, A. Garcia-Lafuente, F. Guarner, E. Crespo, J. Casalots, A. Salas, and J. R. Malagelada. 2001. Dietary inulin improves distal colitis induced by dextran sodium sulfate in the rat. *Am. J. Gastroenterol.* 96:1486–1493.

Waligora-Dupriet, A. J., F. Campeotto, I. Nicolis, A. Bonet, P. Soulaines, C. Dupont, and M. J. Butel. 2007. Effect of oligofructose supplementation on gut microflora and well-being in young children attending a day care centre. *Int. J. Food Microbiol.* 113:108–113.

Wang, X., and G. R. Gibson. 1993. Effects of the in vitro fermentation of oligofructose and inulin by bacteria growing in the human large intestine. *J. Appl. Bacteriol.* 75: 373–380.

Welters, C. F., E. Heineman, F. B. Thunnissen, A. E. van den Bogaard, P. B. Soeters, and C. G. Baeten. 2002. Effect of dietary inulin supplementation on inflammation of pouch mucosa in patients with an ileal pouch-anal anastomosis. *Dis. Colon Rectum* 45:621–627.

Whelan, K., L. Efthymiou, P. A. Judd, V. R. Preedy, and M. A. Taylor. 2006. Appetite during consumption of enteral formula as a sole source of nutrition: the effect of supplementing pea-fibre and fructo-oligosaccharides. *Br. J. Nutr.* 96:350–356.

Zafar, T. A., C. M. Weaver, Y. Zhao, B. R. Martin, and M. E. Wastney. 2004. Nondigestible oligosaccharides increase calcium absorption and suppress bone resorption in ovariectomized rats. *J. Nutr.* 134:399–402.

Therapeutic Microbiology: Probiotics and Related Strategies
Edited by J. Versalovic and M. Wilson
© 2008 ASM Press, Washington, DC

Anthony R. Bird
David L. Topping

Resistant Starch as a Prebiotic

12

The human large bowel harbors an extraordinarily large and taxonomically diverse population of (mostly) anaerobic bacteria comprising more than 500 strains and species in over 50 different genera (Duncan et al., 2007b; Guarner and Malagelada, 2003; Sears, 2005; Vaughan et al., 2002). These microorganisms are present at concentrations of approximately 10^{13} viable cells per g of digesta. Their metabolic activity is considerable and, in terms of total capacity and range of biochemical transformations, may match that of the liver (Hill, 1995; Macfarlane and McBain, 1999). Indeed, this commensal population has been regarded as a functional organ in its own right and is now recognized for its contribution to human health. The constituent organisms of this microbiota generate a wide range of metabolites and end products which influence not only the health of the large bowel and viscera but also the body as a whole. They synthesize certain vitamins and also salvage energy from undigested food and endogenous secretions that would otherwise be voided in the feces. The energy provided to the colonic mucosa by fermentative end products helps to drive the absorption of electrolytes and a considerable volume of water which would otherwise be lost and need replacement.

The commensal microbes of the large bowel also constitute a formidable frontline barrier against colonization of host tissues by potentially harmful exogenous microbes. However, the host-gut microbiota relationship is a dynamic one, and various environmental factors, particularly diet, modulate the composition and metabolic activity of the large-bowel ecosystem in ways that may either benefit or compromise host health. Some of these changes may be manifested directly (e.g., diarrhea), but others may take a long time to become apparent, and bacteria inhabiting the hind gut have been implicated in the pathogenesis of several major large-bowel disorders prevalent in affluent communities. These conditions include inflammatory bowel diseases, irritable bowel syndrome, and colorectal cancer (Bird et al., 2000a). They cause significant morbidity and mortality and are an economic burden through health-related expenditure and loss of productivity. Optimizing the large-bowel microbiota in terms of function

Anthony R. Bird, Commonwealth Scientific and Industrial Research Organization, Food Futures National Research Flagship, and CSIRO Human Nutrition, Adelaide, South Australia. **David L. Topping,** Commonwealth Scientific and Industrial Research Organization, Food Futures National Research Flagship, Adelaide, South Australia.

and products has the potential to improve public and personal health. Prebiotics and probiotics have attracted considerable attention for their potential in this regard.

PROBIOTICS AND THE MICROBIOTA

The use of probiotics is a practice of long standing, but the high level of current interest in probiotic (and prebiotic) foods and supplements by consumers, health professionals, and the food industry is quite novel. Probiosis hinges on the concept that there is an imbalance or deficit in the indigenous bowel microbiota which exogenous live bacteria can correct, giving the host a health benefit. One of the striking features of the phenomenon is that adult consumers seem to have been targeted by manufacturers, but most of the research and development focus has been on bacteria found at their highest level during early human development. These are the lactic acid bacteria (LAB) and bifidobacteria, which are dominant species in milk-fed infants, especially those receiving breast milk. With weaning to solid food, LAB decline in relative numbers as a more "adult" microbiota develops. This raises the question of whether consumption of probiotics by adults can actually deliver some of their anticipated health benefits. In this context, it must be recognized that the majority of health-related claims for probiotics do seem to be largely anecdotal. However, there are now compelling data as to the nutritional merit and clinical efficacy of probiotics for specific limited applications. Not surprisingly, these seem to relate principally to the improvement of problems of lactose digestion and alleviation of the symptoms of lactose intolerance (Santosa et al., 2006; Sullivan and Nord, 2005). However, they also include protection against some types of acute diarrheal diseases, especially in children (Sazawal et al., 2006), and potentiation of humoral and cellular immunity (Saavedra, 2007). There are other areas, for instance, inflammatory bowel disease, where probiotics show some promise, but the evidence is as yet preliminary.

Any consideration of the efficacy of probiotics must take into account the difficulty of maintaining probiotic colonization in adults. Feeding trials have shown consistently that the long-term maintenance of a viable probiotic population requires continual consumption of live organisms (Fujiwara et al., 2001; Brigidi et al., 2003; Mattila-Sandholm et al., 1999; Satokari et al., 2001; Shimakawa et al., 2003; von Wright et al., 2002). This is despite the fact that there is abundant evidence that the composition of the gut microbiota and its metabolic activities are responsive to changes in diet (as measured in

feces). There are also technical difficulties of incorporating probiotic microorganisms into foods and maintaining their shelf stability. Recognition of these two obstacles has prompted interest in the concept of prebiotics, which recognizes that dietary factors, especially macronutrients, are prime determinants of the community structure and fermentation profile of the large bowel ecosystem.

HUMAN LARGE-BOWEL FERMENTATION

It goes almost without saying that the large bowel is the target organ for probiotic foods, and prebiotics are aimed at improving colonization by these bacteria. Most (if not all) current prebiotics are carbohydrates, which is not surprising when one considers that the major metabolic fuels for the colonic microbiota are, in adult humans, undigested dietary carbohydrates (Table 1). Some dietary proteins not digested in the small intestine and endogenous secretions, including small-intestinal enzymes and mucin, which may contribute to the prebiotic action, are also used. The degradation of these substrates is effected in a complex series of reactions which fuel the growth of bacteria and generate short-chain fatty acids (SCFA) as major end products. This fermentation resembles that occurring in obligate herbivores and is found also in other omnivores such as rodents, pigs, and dogs. The main SCFA are acetate, propionate, and butyrate, and their production is accompanied by the evolution of gases (principally H_2, CH_4, and CO_2). SCFA levels are highest in the proximal large bowel, where production predominates due to greatest substrate availability. Levels decline along the colon because of substrate depletion and SCFA uptake with <10% of the total produced appearing in feces (Topping and Clifton, 2001). This distribution is of considerable significance with regard to the risk of

Table 1   Potential substrates for the colonic microbiota of adults on a Western diet[a]

Substrate	Amount (g/day)
RS	1–5
Total NSP	8–18
Insoluble NSP	6–14
Soluble NSP	2–5
Oligosaccharides	2–8
Simple sugars (mainly fructose, sucrose, glucose, and maltose)	2–10
Proteins	3–15

[a]About 5 to 10 g of lipid, 6 to 9 g of endogenous secretions per day, and an unknown quantity of sloughed intestinal cells are substrates for the colonic microbiota. Data from Topping et al. (2003), Cummings and Macfarlane (1991), and Thezee et al., unpublished.

serious diet-related diseases such as colorectal cancer and inflammatory bowel diseases, which predominate in the distal large bowel. It has been suggested that this relationship is causal and that the low SCFA availability in the distal colon is an important factor in disease initiation and progression. There is considerable evidence to support this proposal. While SCFA have nonspecific actions which support a normal colonic environment, one of the major acids (butyrate) seems to have a particular role to play in the promotion of large bowel health. Butyrate is a preferred metabolic substrate for colonocytes, and its metabolism provides energy which helps to drive the salvage of fluid and electrolytes (Topping and Clifton, 2001). However, it also seems to stimulate the production of mucin, which helps to maintain barrier function and to protect against bacterial translocation (Gork et al., 1999; Finnie et al., 1995; Smirnov et al., 2005). Butyrate has a number of other actions including the promotion of DNA repair and the induction of apoptosis, which serve to assist in the maintenance of a normal phenotype in colonocytes (Davie, 2003; Williams et al., 2003). Propionate appears to have many of the beneficial effects of butyrate but at much higher concentrations (Topping and Clifton, 2001).

SCFA are the principal anions in the adult human large-bowel digesta, and the levels of other acids such as lactate and succinate are normally low. This raises interesting questions about the real potential of current probiotics to contribute to improved bowel health and lowered disease risk. As noted, these appear to be mostly preparations containing LAB and bifidobacteria, organisms which predominate in the human gut in early life, when the profile of fermentative products is quite different from that found in adults (Bird et al., 2000a). Propionate and butyrate seem to be virtually absent from the feces of breast-fed infants, and other products (ethanol, formate, and lactate) are the main end products. The point has been made that if current probiotics are effective in promoting bowel health, then it would seem to be via mechanisms other than SCFA (Bird et al., 2000a).

FERMENTATIVE SUBSTRATES FOR THE COLONIC MICROBIOTA

Undigested carbohydrates are the major substrates for the colonic microbiota, supplying up to about 60 g of potentially fermentable material per day for individuals on a "Western" diet (Cummings and Macfarlane, 1991) (Table 1). Nonstarch polysaccharides (NSP), major components of dietary fiber, are quantitatively the most important substrates (10 to 25 g/day for adults)

(Baghurst et al., 1996; Cummings and Englyst, 1987). Much smaller quantities of unabsorbed simple sugars (2 to 10 g/day) and nondigestible oligosaccharides (NDO) (2 to 8 g/day) also contribute to total carbohydrate flow from the terminal ileum. NDO are generally minor dietary contributors. However, they have a major influence on the composition of the colonic microbiota due to their capacity to selectively stimulate bifidobacteria, giving them their preeminent status as prebiotics (Gibson et al., 2004). Undigested dietary protein (about 5 to 15 g/day) is also another important influence on the composition and metabolic activity of the colonic microbiota. Lipids and plant secondary metabolites (e.g., polyphenols) as well as endogenous secretions and sloughed epithelial cells, as mentioned previously, are also substrates but are quantitatively minor entities compared to carbohydrates and proteins (Cummings and Englyst, 1987). Recently, evidence has been gathered that mucins may contribute SCFA (as acetate) as well as substrate to the large bowel (Clarke et al., 2007).

There is widespread recognition that carbohydrate fermentation creates a luminal environment favorable to mucosal health. Conversely, large-bowel bacterial protein degradation is considered to be deleterious. Indeed, it has been described as a "putrefactive" process through the production of potentially toxic compounds such as phenols, cresols, and amines. Although the precise effects of these end products are yet to be determined, the perception remains that they are undesirable. There is some support for this view from animal studies where high-protein diets have been shown to increase genetic damage in colonocytes (Toden et al., 2006, 2007).

CURRENT PREBIOTICS

The widespread use of dietary supplements to promote the growth and activity of "beneficial" bacteria specifically is a relatively recent phenomenon (Gibson and Roberfroid, 1995). It is considered to be more attractive than using probiotics alone because it is simpler, cheaper, and more versatile as to the range of possible food applications. It also offers technological advantages through improved flavor and texture and other food-related functional attributes.

One of the key issues in the development of prebiotics is consideration of the means of effecting benefit. Prebiotics are defined in terms of selective stimulation of the activities and/or numbers of bacteria (Gibson et al., 2004). This definition has been crafted to differentiate a prebiotic from a colonic food (which promotes the activities of the colonic microbiota in general). However, if the end products of colonic fermentation are of major health benefit, this makes the distinction somewhat questionable. In terms of documented prebiotic action, the only substances claimed to qualify fully as prebiotics are a relatively limited number of oligomeric and polymeric fructans (Gibson et al., 2004). There are several other candidate prebiotics which are also short-chain carbohydrate polymers. Larger polysaccharides, such as NSP and resistant starch (RS), have been discounted because they are viewed as colonic foods. This is not entirely unexpected given that both are collective terms encompassing a broad range of structural and/or chemical variants. However, a recent study with pigs has shown that one type of RS (high-amylose maize starch [HAMS]) can function as a prebiotic by promoting selective proliferation of bifidobacteria and also lactobacilli (Bird et al., 2007). The same study showed that this RS stimulated SCFA production considerably, consistent with other human and animal studies.

An understanding of the biology of dietary starches, their digestion in the upper gut, and their interaction with the microbiota of the large bowel is essential in ascertaining the full prebiotic potential of RS. It is easy to think that all forms of RS are the same. This is not so, and it is critical to realize that RS is a physiological concept and not a simple chemical one. Some RS-rich ingredients can function as prebiotics and enhance the delivery of ingested probiotics to the large bowel. These effects may be obtained at dietary intakes which are reasonable in terms of daily food consumption. However, it is our conclusion that RS occurs for diverse reasons and not all forms can act as prebiotics. Nevertheless, the evidence available suggests also that different forms of RS modify the activity of the large-bowel microbiota and (through SCFA) promote host health. Some data suggest that fructan prebiotics, when combined with RS, have greatly enhanced physiological functionality compared to when used alone and may prove particularly effective in delivering beneficial health outcomes for the consumer (Topping et al., 1997; Bird et al., submitted).

DIETARY STARCH AND RESISTANT STARCH

The historic importance of starchy staple foods to human diets is well recognized. However, increasing affluence and the ready availability of convenience foods have led to starch becoming progressively less significant. Per capita starch consumption has declined steadily over the last century in westernized affluent countries, where adults now consume between 120 and 150 g of starch daily compared with the much larger relative and absolute quantities consumed in traditional agrarian societies

(Baghurst et al., 1996). Refined cereal starches, principally from wheat, rice, and maize, and starches from roots, tubers, pulses, legumes, and a few fruits are the major sources of starch for humans. Starchy foods are commonly highly processed before consumption, especially in economically developed countries, and uncooked starches are eaten only rarely by humans.

Starch digestion starts in the mouth through the actions of salivary α-amylase and continues in the stomach until the enzyme is inactivated by gastric acid (pH, <4). Amylolysis continues in the small intestine through the actions of pancreatic α-amylase, and this digestive phase accounts for the bulk of starch that is assimilated by the gut. Salivary and pancreatic α-amylases (endoamylases) attack internal 1,4-α-glucosidic bonds randomly, i.e., those not located at the ends of starch molecules or adjacent to branch points. The process produces a mixture of di- and trisaccharides (maltose and maltotriose) and dextrins (branched-chain oligosaccharides). These relatively small molecules are hydrolyzed to completion at the apical or brush border enterocyte membrane by α-glucosidase (maltase), which splits off one glucose at a time, and isomaltase, a debranching enzyme which targets α-1,6 linkages. High-affinity, energy-dependent (active) transporters (SGLT1) in the brush border of the small intestine ensure the rapid removal of glucose from the lumen. The almost immediate and substantial postprandial rise in blood glucose levels commonly caused by many modern (highly refined) starchy foods (Cordain et al., 2005) suggests that starch is extensively digested and absorbed in the proximal small bowel.

Until recently, the prevailing view was that starch was digested completely in the small intestine. This belief was based largely on the fact that only starch, unlike all other polysaccharides of plant origin, can be digested to completion by human small-intestinal enzymes. Coupled to the fact that human fecal starch excretion is normally extremely low, the natural conclusion was that ileal starch digestibility was very close to 100%. There is evidence of long standing showing that this is not the case. Early in vitro analytical studies demonstrated that certain starches were resistant to robust in vitro digestion procedures (Englyst et al., 1996). An even earlier study with healthy humans (where breath H_2 evolution was increased following consumption of a starchy convenience food) provided indirect evidence that some dietary starch could resist small intestinal digestion and was fermented in the large bowel (Anderson et al., 1981). More recently, studies with intubated healthy humans and subjects with ileostomy and animal models have all confirmed that a metabolically significant fraction of starch can enter the large bowel from the small intestine.

RS

RS is defined as that fraction of ingested starch which, along with its digestion products (glucose and maltooligosaccharides), enters the colon of healthy individuals (Asp, 1992). It occurs to some degree in all starchy foods but is normally low in processed consumer foods. The amount of RS actually present is determined by the quantity of starch consumed and its residence time in the upper gastrointestinal tract. It is a key point that RS is intrinsically digestible, unlike NSP or oligosaccharides such as fructans. For example, the rapid transit of a highly digestible starch through the small intestine may mean that its time of exposure to luminal hydrolases is too short to allow complete digestion. Conversely, a slower rate of passage for the same starch would allow sufficient time for digestion and absorption to proceed to completion. Thus, the functional capacity of the gut and various physiological factors have a major influence on the amount of starch reaching the colon. Chewing facilitates starch digestion by disrupting food structure, which has the effect of increasing exposure of the starch to luminal hydrolases. This is through a reduction in particle size and slowing of the rate of transit (smaller particles pass along the gut more slowly than larger ones). Food-related factors, mainly particle size, starch physicochemical composition, and interaction with other food constituents, especially plant cell wall structures, also determine the amount of starch escaping the small intestine (Champ et al., 2003; Champ, 2004). The proportion of the starch that escapes digestion also depends on the methods used to manufacture, cook, and store foods. As a corollary, food-processing methods may be used to manipulate the content and fermentative properties of resistant starches.

Types of RS

RS has been classified into five major types (Table 2) (Brown et al., 2006). RS_1 is physically inaccessible starch where the food matrix itself may simply shield dietary starch from intestinal hydrolases. NSP and other structural elements of plant cell walls (dietary fiber) cannot be digested by mammalian enzymes and so contribute to RS_1 formation. Some grains contain soluble NSP that increase the viscosity of digesta, thereby hindering the activity of α-amylase and also luminal diffusion of starch oligosaccharides to the absorptive surface of the epithelium lining the intestinal tract. Soluble NSP are used in food processing for their technological attributes (e.g., to prevent syneresis), but they can also contribute to RS generation. Whole grains can provide RS, and it has been proposed that this is one of the mechanisms for some of their health benefits (Topping et al., 2007). In economically

Table 2 Nutritional classification of RS

Type of RS	Mode of resistance	Common dietary sources
RS_1	Physically inaccessible	Whole or partly milled grains
RS_2	Raw (granular) starches	High-amylose and certain leguminous starches
RS_3	Retrograded starches	Starchy foods that have been cooked and cooled, e.g., potato salad
RS_4	Chemically modified	Etherized, esterified, or cross-bonded starches
RS_5	V-form	Inclusion complexes formed by amylose and polar lipids

developed countries, cereals are eaten mainly as refined (white) flours or polished grains and so contribute little to RS intake. Obviously, chewing has an impact on the RS content of a food which is difficult to quantify, but any RS resulting from inadequate mastication would be classified as RS_1.

RS_2 comprises granular (i.e., raw) starches (Bird et al., 2000a). In this group (as in RS_3, retrograded starches) starch molecular architecture is an important contributor to its level in a food. Starches are homopolysaccharides composed of α-1,4 or α-1,6 linked glucose monomers, found in two major structural forms—amylose and amylopectin (Annison and Topping, 1994). Amylose, which is the lesser contributor to most food starches, consists of long, essentially linear, glucose chains that are arranged in a helical conformation. Various compounds, for instance monoglycerides, can be sequestered in this cavity to form inclusion complexes (V-form starch; see below). Amylopectin is a much larger, highly branched molecule (>1,000 kDa compared to 60 kDa for amylose) with a more complex structure (Topping and Clifton, 2001). Starches are laid down as granules in seeds, tubers, and other reserve tissues of plants. X-ray diffraction analysis indicates that granular starch has a semicrystalline character resulting from the regular branching of the constituent molecules of amylopectin. Amylose has a more densely packed structure, whereas the more open and lattice-like structure of amylopectin renders it more susceptible to amylolysis (Annison and Topping, 1994). Accordingly, the relative proportions of amylose and amylopectin have a major bearing on the

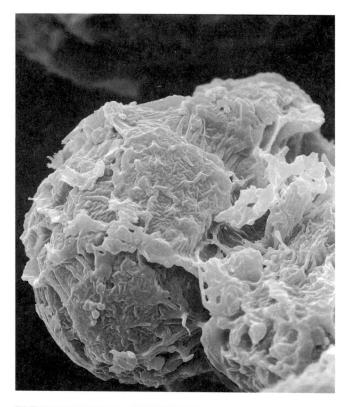

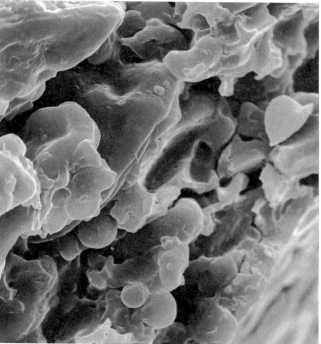

Figure 1 Scanning electron micrographs of starch particles in commercially processed foods. (a) Commercial muesli containing multiple whole-grain cereals and other starch sources; (b) starch from commercial four-bean mix (canned). Bar, 10 μm.

susceptibility of a starch to amylolysis. Amylose is much slower to gelatinize when heated with water, meaning that it is more likely to raise the content of RS_2 in a food. Generally, amylose contributes <30% to standard starches but >50% to high-amylose starches. These high-amylose starches are relatively new and have been generated by selective breeding (Brown et al., 1995, 2006). The first to find general food use was a HAMS, but a range of related starches (e.g., tapioca) are available commercially (Brown et al., 1995; Brown, 2004). CSIRO is developing novel high-amylose cereals to exploit the physiological properties and health benefits of RS (Ahmed et al., 2007; Rahman et al., 2007). These include a high-amylose barley generated as part of a conventional barley breeding program and a high-amylose wheat produced using RNA interference to modify key enzymes of starch synthesis to increase the amylose content of grains. In the case of the barley (cultivar Himalaya 292) the activity of starch synthase IIa was inhibited, giving less total starch but a higher content of amylose (Morell et al., 2003; Topping et al., 2003b). The activities of two branching enzymes (SBE IIa and SBE IIb), which play a pivotal role in starch biosynthesis, were suppressed in wheat, yielding a grain with a high proportion of amylose. Animal studies have confirmed favorable changes in indices of bowel health for both grains, i.e., more RS. Collectively, these data add weight to the point that RS is a complex phenomenon and that there are multiple routes to increasing its content in grains and the foods made from them.

Food processing is an important factor in determining the RS level of finished products. Hydrothermal processing and recrystallization produces RS_3 (retrograded starch). Application of moist heat disrupts the structure of starch granules (gelatinization), rendering the constituent glucan chains more susceptible to hydrolysis. Complete gelatinization depends on the amount of heat and moisture used and the duration of cooking (Gidley, 1992). As consumed, most processed foods contain starch granules in various stages of disintegration (Fig. 1) and any RS would most likely be RS_2. High-amylose starches, such as HAMS, not only gelatinize at much higher temperatures than standard starches but also retrograde more readily (Brown, 2004). This property is responsible in part for the greater RS content of consumer foods containing these ingredients. Retrogradation occurs in foods that have been cooled and stored after cooking, a process characterized by the molecular reassociation of linear amylose chains or the side chains of amylopectin (Tang and Copeland, 2007). RS_3 is retrograded starch, mainly retrograded amylose. Reheating retrograded starches usually results in a loss of RS content, and repeated cycles involving heating and cooling starchy foods can increase their RS content (Ahmed et al., 2000; Bird et al., 2000a; Brown, 2004).

One of the interesting recent developments in the field is the growing awareness that chemically modified starches can contribute to the RS content of foods. These starches are used widely by the food industry to impart desired texture and other properties to processed foods (Brown, 2004). They are classified as RS_4 and include etherized, esterified, and cross-bonded starches, and the radicals involved include acyl (e.g., acetyl), hydroxypropyl, and methoxyl groups. These modifications result in a reduced small-intestinal digestibility with the fraction of the modified starch that is resistant to digestion varying depending on the substituent and degree of chemical modification. The actual physiological effects of the particular RS_4 depend on the same factors. For example, dietary hydroxypropylated distarch phosphates increase large-bowel digesta mass with increasing degrees of cross bonding and substitution (Kishida et al., 2001). However, SCFA were not increased as much, indicating greater resistance to bacterial degradation. This is not surprising given that some modifications (e.g., etherization) are likely to be very resistant to bacterial breakdown and, by analogy with lignin, would require O_2 to be degraded. Conversely, knowledge of starch chemistry has been exploited to develop starches acylated with specific SCFA to a high degree of substitution for the express purpose of delivering those acids to targeted sites in the large bowel (Annison and Topping, 1994). These particular acylated starches have markedly reduced ileal digestibility in humans (Clarke et al., 2007) and animals (Bird et al., 2006) but also are fermented extensively in the large bowel and improve several indices of large-bowel health in rats (Bird et al., 2006; Bajka et al., 2006).

V-form starch has been suggested as a possible new category of RS (RS_5) (Brown et al., 2006). Amylose is known to interact with polar lipids to form molecular structures which are considered more resistant to hydrolysis. However, there is as yet little information on the structural, digestion, or physiological properties of this candidate RS.

RS INTAKE AND PREBIOTIC ACTION

The classification of RS into groups RS_1 through RS_5 and the widely diverse types that are consumed in foods show that it is very difficult to link consumption directly to prebiotic action. One of the obstacles to progress is the lack of an internationally accepted and validated analytical method for RS in human foods. Consequently there is very little reliable information on the amount of RS that humans consume on a daily basis. RS is a physiological

concept, and the best methodologies use in vivo techniques such as humans with ileostomy or after intestinal intubation (Champ, 2004). These approaches are slow and laborious and require a considerable investment in specialized resources. They also raise ethical issues and hence are impractical for routine analyses (see Champ, 2004).

In vitro laboratory techniques are based on conventional enzymatic and spectrophotometric methods of analysis and essentially simulate digestion in the human gastrointestinal tract. The more recent in vitro methods are comparatively less complicated and yield consistent results, but their accuracy has not been confirmed (Champ et al., 2003; Madrid and Arcot, 2000). Indeed, some of these methods do not measure resistant starch as defined (Birkett et al., 1997; Danjo et al., 2003). We are developing a reliable in vitro method that predicts the resistant starch content of a range of everyday foods with acceptable accuracy ($r^2 = 0.80$ for values obtained with the in vitro test versus in vivo values derived using humans with ileostomy; see Topping et al., 2007). For Western diets, about 5% of starch intake is considered resistant to digestion, which is comparable to about 5 g/day (Baghurst et al., 1996; Roberts et al., 2004). However, accurate data on RS intake are not available for the reasons just mentioned. Given that foods which are rich sources of RS, such as intact cereal grains and beans, are uncommon in industrialized societies, and modern starchy foods are mostly highly processed (refined) products incorporating pregelatinized starches and low-amylose starches or polished grains, the above is likely to be an overestimate. We (and others) have reported that the RS content of some common everyday starchy foods consumed in Australia is low (Muir et al., 1995, Topping et al., 2007). By extrapolating this information, the RS intake of Australians and, presumably, other Western populations is unlikely to exceed 2 g/day. It certainly appears that modern commercial food processing and dietary habits have almost eliminated RS from the Western diet.

Clearly, RS is a relatively minor carbon and energy source for the large bowel microbiota in individuals consuming a typical Western diet. There is epidemiological evidence that in certain populations RS is of considerable significance and may rival NSP as a fermentable substrate for the large bowel microbiota (Bird et al., 2000a; Bird and Topping, 2001; Cassidy et al., 1994; Topping and Bird, 1999). Estimated dietary fiber intake (predominantly NSP) provides insufficient carbohydrate to account for metabolic activities of the large bowel microbiota or fecal biomass excretion. It has been estimated that 60 g of fermentable carbohydrate is required to sustain the colonic microbiota, yet fiber intakes in many countries account for about ~20 g of this requirement per day. This leaves a deficit of about 40 g/day, which is referred to as the "carbohydrate gap" (Cummings and Macfarlane, 1991). RS is considered a potential candidate to fill this gap (Cummings and Englyst, 1991; Stephen, 1991; Topping et al., 2003a). Indeed, there have been numerous controlled trials relating intakes of specific high-RS foods or starches to biomarkers, e.g., fecal SCFA or colonocyte genetic damage or proliferation. However, it is worth noting that the human studies to date have been driven by the low habitual intakes of RS in human populations at high risk of large-bowel disease and not any investigation of prebiotic action.

There is growing supportive evidence of the health potential of RS from the study of low-risk groups and a reappraisal of its importance relative to NSP. Interest in the health benefits of dietary fiber is of long standing. However, systematic investigations of its potential benefits can be said to have started with the pioneering observational studies of British colonial medical officers in East Africa over 50 years ago (Burkitt, 1970). They noted the high consumption of unrefined cereal grains (principally maize corn) by the native Africans who were at low risk of diseases such as coronary heart disease, diabetes, and colorectal cancer. The rarity of these conditions was such that any reported cases were deemed noteworthy. In contrast, Europeans living in the same environment ate refined foods and were at much greater risk. With time, the focus shifted from the whole-grain aspect of the native Africans' diet to its fiber content. Since then, the health benefits of dietary fiber through its bulking action have been well established. Like RS, NSP are also fermented (to a variable degree) by the microbiota of the human colon, and the resultant changes in the intracolonic environment, notably production of SCFA, have a positive influence on bowel physiology and mucosal health as well as systemic effects (Topping and Clifton, 2001). It might have been expected that fiber would have proved to be of clear benefit in serious large-bowel disease. However, fiber has proved to be rather disappointing in the prevention of colorectal cancer and inflammatory bowel disease. Population studies have given conflicting findings on the protective value of fiber, with some prospective studies showing no effect (Schatzkin et al., 2007). This apparent conflict can be resolved if one considers that the current analytical methods include a variable fraction of RS (depending on the food) plus NSP and other indigestible material. Further, reexamination of the traditional African diets using modern methodologies reveals that their (assumed) high-fiber intakes

are actually less than those of Europeans (Segal, 2002). The native foods are whole grain, which would be expected to generate RS_1, while their culinary practices (cooking and cooling of corn) would be likely to raise RS_3. Indeed, it has been confirmed that traditional African maize porridge is high in RS as measured by large-bowel SCFA (Ahmed et al., 2000). Differences in cooking practice may also explain the failure of Chinese foods to improve indices of bowel health in a study conducted in Australia (Birkett et al., 1997).

RS and Colonic Fermentation

It is well established that the microbiota of the colon, especially in the proximal segment, consists of predominantly saccharolytic bacteria and that reducing carbohydrate intake alters markedly the population structure of the fecal microbiota of humans (Duncan et al., 2007a). That very little starch normally appears in feces of healthy individuals consuming diets rich in RS is clear evidence that the microbiota is well capable of utilizing resistant starch (Cummings and Englyst, 1991). Indeed, the capacity of the microbiota to salvage energy from starch is apparently acquired at an early age and may actually be more efficient in children than in adults (Christian et al., 2003). Various in vitro studies have shown that several constituents of the human large bowel microbiota, including *Eubacterium* spp., *Bacteroides* spp., *Escherichia coli*, several species of *Bifidobacterium*, and *Clostridium butyricum*, are equipped with the necessary hydrolases to efficiently utilize starch (Brown et al., 1998; Wang and Gibson, 1993). In vitro studies have shown that although bifidobacteria may use starch, their ability to do so is apparently limited (Brown et al., 1998; Wang et al., 1999b).

That starch is fermented by the colonic microbiota is also evidenced by postprandial increases in breath hydrogen evolution and changes in bowel habit and fecal properties not too dissimilar to those produced by other carbohydrate substrates, notably, soluble NSP. These include increased concentrations and fecal excretion of SCFA, a reduction in pH, and greater stool bulk in response to the consumption of foods containing RS (Topping and Bird, 1999; Bird et al., 2000a; Topping et al., 2003a).

RS and the Demonstration of Its Prebiotic Effects

The prebiotic concept has been updated recently since its derivation more than 10 years ago by Gibson and Roberfroid (1995) and a prebiotic is defined now as "a selectively fermented ingredient that allows specific changes, both in the composition and/or activity in the gastrointestinal microflora that confers benefits upon host well-being and health" (Gibson et al., 2004). Accordingly, to qualify as a prebiotic a food ingredient must be shown to (i) escape digestion and absorption in the small intestine, whereupon reaching the large bowel it (ii) changes the composition or activity of the microbiota selectively, which results in (iii) demonstrable health benefits for the consumer.

By definition, RS satisfies the first criterion and there is ample evidence from in vivo studies that starch reaching the colon stimulates fermentation and is readily and extensively utilized by the colonic microbiota, as presented earlier. The second requirement, i.e., that RS must have a selective effect on the growth or activity of the colonic microbiota, is really the defining characteristic of a prebiotic. Indeed, one might say that if this criterion is met, the first is redundant. Although appearing quite straightforward, the task of confirming unequivocally that a particular RS encourages the proliferation or activity of a select subset of the microbial population of the large bowel microbiota is a difficult one. Demonstration of an association between the compositional and metabolic changes in the large bowel ecosystem and any associated health benefits that may result is also difficult.

There are several methodological and conceptual considerations when evaluating the prebiotic potential of candidate resistant starches.

In Vivo Testing Is Essential

A prebiotic effect can be substantiated only by performing sound, controlled studies in the target species. In vitro testing provides useful insights but is of limited physiological significance and may not necessarily reflect the situation in vivo. Animal models are instructive in defining and characterizing activities of candidate prebiotics. The pig is a well-established model for investigating human large-bowel metabolism of polysaccharides (Topping and Clifton, 2001) and is an especially useful research tool for gathering a comprehensive picture of regional differences in microbial composition and activity in the gut. Pigs have the advantage of willingly eating human foods, a behavioral attribute of immediate relevance to the study of RS, as its level and physiological functionality in food are sensitive to preparation and processing methods. Another advantage of the pig model is its excellent predictive power owing to similarities in the anatomical form and physiological functioning of the porcine and human gastrointestinal tracts (Topping and Clifton, 2001). However, demonstration of a prebiotic effect in one species does not necessarily translate to another. Hence, studies with humans are essential, but

they are inconvenient and expensive to perform and there are various technical matters to deal with. The inaccessibility of the human gastrointestinal tract often means that demonstration of a prebiotic effect is based on an analysis of feces, unless, of course, invasive techniques are deployed. Feces are considered to provide a true indication of luminal conditions in the distal colon but not higher up the bowel. It is known from studies of subjects with colostomies that the SCFA profile of digesta varies markedly according to sampling sites along the large bowel (Mitchell et al., 1985). The collection (and analysis) of fresh stool specimens is also critical, but this is difficult to arrange especially in large dietary interventions studies involving free-living subjects.

Intracolonic Microcosms

Analysis of feces (and digesta) may provide a reasonable representation of the overall composition and metabolic activity of the luminal microbiota, but such samples are not necessarily indicative of the microbial community in closer proximity to host tissues, i.e., those adhering to the epithelial lining of the bowel or resident in the mucus layer. Although invasive sampling, i.e., biopsy specimens, can be performed, studies of this nature are much more difficult to conduct and there are ethical issues in obtaining endoscopic biopsy samples from healthy volunteers as opposed to those undergoing medical intervention.

The composition of bacterial populations associated with the colonic epithelium differs from that in the fecal stream (Zoetendal et al., 2002) and also appears less responsive to alterations in the luminal environment (Macfarlane and Dillon, 2007). Evidence that the mucosal microbiota is nonetheless responsive to diet is accumulating. Kleessen et al. (2003) showed that fructans could be used to raise the numbers of colonic mucosa-associated bifidobacteria in gnotobiotic rats. This response was accompanied by favorable changes in mucosal architecture as well as an increase in mucin secretion. Consumption of a comparable prebiotic mixture (7.5 g/day each of inulin and oligofructose) by volunteers produced selective increases in surface cell counts of bifidobacteria and lactobacilli in biopsy specimens from the proximal and distal colon (Langlands et al., 2004). That the population structure of the microbiota on the surface of the bowel is responsive to dietary constituents is pertinent in that it is this microbial community, through its intimate association with the mucosa, which is likely to play a crucial role in health and disease of the host. There are, as yet, no published results of studies on the effects of RS on the mucosa-associated microbiota.

An increase in mucin secretion has been reported in humans (Ten Bruggencate et al., 2006) and rats consuming rapidly fermentable carbohydrates (e.g., fructo-oligosaccharides [FOS]), and this has been associated with mucosal irritation and weakened intestinal barrier function (Ten Bruggencate et al., 2005; Bovee-Oudenhoven et al., 2003). However, various fibers increase mucin section in the colon (and small intestine), most likely in response to the need for mucus to lubricate the greater digesta mass (mechanical effect of fiber) and a direct stimulatory action of SCFA (Barcelo et al., 2000). Toden et al. (2007) have shown in rats that feeding RS increases large-bowel SCFA and reverses colonic DNA damage and a thinning of the colonic mucus layer induced by feeding high-protein diets.

Enumeration Methodology and Experimental Procedures

The prebiotic concept was established at a time when classical culturing techniques using semiselective growth media were state of the art. The methodological limitations of culture techniques for enumerating bacteria are well documented. The imprecision and inaccuracy of these techniques necessitated that a major increase in cell counts of probiotic bacteria, i.e., bifidobacteria and lactobacilli, of the order of at least 1 log unit was usually required to achieve a statistically significant treatment effect. Changes of this magnitude certainly reflect a major (selective) shift in colonic microbial populations. Quantitative molecular techniques (such as fluorescence in situ hybridization), being more specific, sensitive, and precise, allow more subtle changes in the microbiota to be detected (Mai and Morris, 2004).

Dose response

Intakes of established prebiotics such as FOS to obtain effects are of the order of 5 to 10 g/day, depending on the specific product (Gibson, 2004). Although the dose-response association is not well defined, it is clear that the quantity of prebiotic consumed is important and that, for an effect, the threshold is quite low. These prebiotics are reasonably stable food ingredients, and as most of the ingested dose (>80%) is recovered in ileal effluent, the amount delivered to the colon for fermentation can be tightly controlled. This is not the case for RS. For a given starchy food, the amount of RS it contains (and hence its fermentative properties) is not intrinsic but dependent on how the food is processed, stored, and prepared prior to consumption. In addition, the digestive capacity of the upper GI tract, especially the rate at which food passes through the small intestine, varies greatly between individuals (Faulks et al., 2004; Bratten and Jones, 2007). Aside from these physiological factors, between-individual and day-to-day variation

in colonic starch fermentation is considerable. Although the number of relevant studies is small, the amount of RS required to elicit a demonstrable effect on the composition of the large bowel microbiota appears to be of the order of 10 g, which is comparable to that of short-chain carbohydrate prebiotics.

Minimum response

What is not yet defined is the extent of the shift in the microbiota sufficient to exert a discernible (and meaningful) health benefit. The traditional view of a prebiotic effect is an increase in the proportion of LAB and/or bifidobacteria (considered synonymous with a positive health outcome). Conversely, the balance of the microbiota could also presumably be altered favorably simply by selectively repressing species or genera of bacteria that are undesirable because they are, or have the potential to be, pathogenic or their activity elaborates metabolites which may be harmful to mucosal health. This aspect of the prebiotic effect has received comparatively little attention. However, it may be quite relevant in the case of RS.

Preprandial microbiota

The prebiotic concept is largely predicated first on the target (desirable) bacterial species being present already in the colonic ecosystem and, second, that there is an existing imbalance in the microbiota in favor of undesirable bacteria. The magnitude of the response depends on the size of the bifidobacteria population prior to prebiotic treatment (Bouhnik et al., 2004; Tuohy et al., 2001). Demonstration of a prebiotic effect becomes increasingly difficult if the large bowel microbiota is already in a healthy state, i.e., replete with bifidobacteria (or lactic bacteria). Diets rich in fermentable carbohydrates increase intestinal motility and reduce retention time, and these changes are associated with a reduction in colonic protein fermentation and consequent lowering of luminal concentrations of putrefactive products such as phenols and cresols (Birkett et al., 1996).

RS as a Prebiotic

Most research on RS, especially its fermentative properties, has focused on HAMS, quite possibly because it can be obtained commercially as a purified ingredient. There is much less published information on the effects of other types of RS, and studies with humans are scant. The first in vivo evidence that RS was a potential prebiotic was provided in a study by Brown et al. (1997), which showed that a specific HAMS fed to pigs with a live culture of bifidobacteria resulted in a substantial increase in fecal bifidobacterial excretion. There are now a number of animal studies demonstrating similar findings for various HAMS products as well as other sources of RS. Studies with pigs (Bird et al., 2007) and mice (Brown et al., 1998) have shown that this particular RS increases colonic populations of bifidobacteria severalfold. Brown et al. (1997) also demonstrated the synbiotic (a combination of a probiotic and a prebiotic) potential of HAMS in pigs orally administered *Bifidobacterium longum*. An RS and FOS mixture was more effective in raising fecal bifidobacterial numbers in pigs than when these products were fed separately (A. R. Bird, M. Vuaran, R. Crittenden, T. Hayakawa, M. J. Playne, I. L. Brown, and D. L. Topping, unpublished observations). That the prebiotic responses were additive suggests different mechanisms were operating (Topping et al., 2003a). It appears that HAMS functions through physical adherence of exogenous bacteria to the granule which protects them on passage through the gastrointestinal tract. Chemical modification of HAMS (which converts it from RS_2/RS_3 to RS_4) has been shown to alter its prebiotic properties (Brown et al., 1998), suggesting that starch molecular structure and, in this case, chemical composition are important factors determining its utilization by the gut microbiota. Carboxymethylated and acetylated amylomaize starches (both RS_4) fed to mice raised colonic bifidobacterial numbers, but the modified starches were not as bifidogenic as the corresponding (unmodified) amylomaize (Wang et al., 2002). The bifidogenic potency of HAMS appears comparable to that of FOS and several other oligosaccharides.

Although HAMS appears to yield consistent changes in the composition of the microbiota, it is clear that not all other RS are prebiotics. We found that in young pigs, rice-based diets that resulted in greater quantities of starch (RS_1 and RS_3) entering the cecum had no effect on proximal-colonic populations of bifidobacteria or lactobacilli (Bird et al., 2000b), although these diets greatly (and selectively) suppressed coliform counts, especially those of *E. coli* (Topping et al., 2003a). Kleessen and colleagues (1997) showed that hydrothermal treatment of potato starch altered its large-bowel bifidogenicity. Another important finding from this study was that retrograded potato starch (RS_3), but not native potato starch (RS_2), raised lactobacilli numbers in cecal digesta and feces. The type of RS also altered the species profile of the *Lactobacillus* population.

These animal studies provide an insight into the interactions of RS and the colonic microbiota. It is apparent that not all RS function as prebiotics and that molecular structure and morphology are an important determinant of prebiosis. Accordingly, the type of RS, as per the current classification system, bears little relevance to

the impact of RS on the composition of the microbiota. Also, RS vary in their effects, and certain types of RS support the growth of lactobacilli as well as bifidobacteria and therefore may be especially potent prebiotics. Most prebiotics are effective bifidogenic agents but have little or no effect on the growth of other desirable groups of bacteria. Furthermore, some types of RS may not fit the bill as a prebiotic in the classical (bifidogenic) sense, but their ability to drastically reduce numbers of undesirable bacteria suggests that they may nevertheless have considerable potential for improving host health.

There is evidence that RS creates an environment in the colon that is conducive to the growth and metabolic activity of desirable bacteria but perhaps unfavorable to less desirable species, thereby lessening their competitiveness. In addition to functioning as a synbiotic as mentioned earlier, the inclusion of HAMS in the diet has been shown to attenuate the customary decline in colonic populations of probiotic bacteria that accompanies probiotic withdrawal from the diet (Brown et al., 1997). HAMS may act by affording protection to probiotic bacteria as they move through the upper gut, thereby facilitating delivery of greater numbers of probiotic cells to the colon. Bifidobacteria are known to attach strongly to granular starches (Wang et al., 1999a, 1999b; Crittenden et al., 2001; O'Riordan et al., 2001), and this may be relevant to observations that probiotic viability in yogurts can be maintained longer by including small amounts of HAMS in the product (Brown et al., 1998). The study of Le Leu et al. (2005) underscores the utility of RS in creating conditions in the large-bowel ecosystem that enable probiotic bacteria (*Bifidobacterium lactis*) to modulate epithelial biology through the promotion of apoptosis.

A small molecular size is considered a prerequisite property for prebiosis (as with short-chain carbohydrates). For maltooligosaccharides, a degree of polymerization (DP) of 3 to 6 effectively promoted growth of bifodobacteria while larger malto-oligosaccharides (DP, >7) did not (Sanz et al., 2006). Yet it is clear from animal studies to date that RS is capable of functioning as a prebiotic whereas nonstarch polysaccharides apparently are not. However, RS is a collective term for glucans whose sizes range from several thousand daltons to several million. Significant quantities of starch and products of partial starch digestion reach the terminal small intestine of ileostomates eating certain common starchy foods (J. Thezee, K. Konietzska, M. Kutschera, Z. Zhou, D. L. Topping, and A. R. Bird, unpublished observations). Hence, this RS fraction, although differing in chemical composition, could well have molecular and physical properties comparable to those of short-chain carbohydrate prebiotics, such as FOS and inulin. Furthermore, hydrolysis of starch polymers is such that short-chain glucans would be released when starch granules are fermented in the colon. The staggered release of prebiotic starch fractions may have important implications for mucosal health, as many degenerative diseases of the gut occur in the distal colon (Topping and Clifton, 2001). From this perspective, RS may be more efficacious than NDO prebiotics throughout the length of the colon, owing to the sequential release of bioactive fractions from starch polysaccharides as they are fermented. Conversely, NDO are most likely fermented to completion in the proximal reaches of the large bowel and so may be capable of modulating the microbiota only in this region of the gut.

Despite the data being limited to relatively few animal feeding trials and even fewer studies with humans, there is still reasonable evidence that certain RS, notably HAMS, are capable of modulating the composition of the colonic microbiota in ways considered conducive to host health. The results also suggest that these effects are dependent not only on the amount, but in particular on the molecular and morphological properties, of starch reaching the colon. It is also apparent that the classification system for RS bears little relevance to prebiotic capacity or physiological functionality.

One of the most important questions remaining open relates to the nature of prebiotics. If the products of LAB and bifidobacterial fermentation are important in milk-fed children, then it remains to be established whether the stimulation of the production of these is equally as important in adults.

We thank Zhong Kai Zhou for kindly providing the electron micrographs and Ross Crittenden for reviewing the manuscript critically.

References

Ahmed, R., A. R. Bird, Z. Li, S. Rahman, G. Mann, W. Chanliaud, P. Berbezy, D. Topping, and M. K. Morell. 2007. Bioengineering cereal carbohydrates to improve human health. *Cereal Foods World* 52:182–187.

Ahmed, R., I. Segal, and H. Hassan. 2000. Fermentation of dietary starch in humans. *Am. J. Gastroenterol.* 95:1017–1020.

Anderson, L. H., A. S. Levine, and M. D. Levitt. 1981. Incomplete absorption of the carbohydrate in all purpose wheat flour. *New Engl. J. Med.* 304:891–892.

Annison, G., and D. L. Topping. 1994. Nutritional role of resistant starch: chemical structure vs physiological function. *Annu. Rev. Nutr.* 14:297–320.

Asp, N.-G. 1992. Resistant starch. *Eur. J. Clin. Nutr.* 46(Suppl. 2): S1.

Baghurst, P. A., K. I. Baghurst, and S. J. Record. 1996. Dietary fibre, non-starch polysaccharides and resistant starch—a review. *Food Aust.* 48(Suppl.):S3–S35.

Bajka, B. H., D. L. Topping, L. Cobiac, and J. M. Clarke. 2006. Butyrylated starch is less susceptible to enzymic hydrolysis and increases large-bowel butyrate more than high-amylose maize starch in the rat. *Br. J. Nutr.* 96:276–282.

Barcelo, A., J. Claustre, F. Moro, J. A. Chayvialle, J. C. Cuber, and P. Plaisancie. 2000. Mucin secretion is modulated by luminal factors in the isolated vascularly perfused rat colon. *Gut* 46:218–224.

Bird, A. R., I. L. Brown, and D. L. Topping. 2000a. Starches, resistant starches, the gut microflora and human health. *Curr. Issues Intest. Microbiol.* 1:25–37.

Bird, A. R., I. L. Brown, and D. L. Topping. 2006. Low and high amylose maize starches acetylated by a commercial or a laboratory process both deliver acetate to the large bowel in rats. *Food Hydrocolloids* 20:1135–1150.

Bird, A. R., T. Hayakawa, Y. Marsono, J. M. Gooden, I. R. Record, R. L. Correll, and D. L. Topping. 2000b. Coarse brown rice increases fecal and large bowel short-chain fatty acids and starch but lowers calcium in the large bowel of pigs. *J. Nutr.* 130:1780–1787.

Bird, A. R., and D. L. Topping. 2001. Resistant starch, fermentation, and large bowel health, p. 147–158. *In* S. S. Cho and M. L. Dreher (ed.), *Handbook of Dietary Fiber*. Marcel Dekker, New York, NY.

Bird, A. R., M. Vuaran, I. Brown, and D. L. Topping. 2007. Two high-amylose maize starches with different amounts of resistant starch vary in their effects on fermentation, tissue and digesta mass accretion, and bacterial populations in the large bowel of pigs. *Br. J. Nutr.* 97:134–144.

Bird, A. R., M. Vuaran, R. Crittenden, T. Hayakawa, M. J. Playne, I. L. Brown, and D. L. Topping. A high amylose starch and a fructooligosaccharide promote fecal and colonic bifidobacteria numbers in pigs fed *Bifidobacterium longum* but only high amylose starch raises short chain fatty acids. Submitted for publication.

Birkett, A. M, G. P. Jones, A. M. de Silva, G. P. Young, and J. G. Muir. 1997. Dietary intake and faecal excretion of carbohydrate by Australians: importance of achieving stool weights greater than 150 g to improve faecal markers relevant to colon cancer risk. *Eur. J. Clin. Nutr.* 51:625–632.

Birkett, A., J. Muir, J. Phillips, G. Jones, and K. O'Dea. 1996. Resistant starch lowers fecal concentrations of ammonia and phenols in humans. *Am. J. Clin. Nutr.* 63:766–772.

Bouhnik, Y., L. Raskine, G. Simoneau, E. Vicaut, C. Neut, B. Flourie, F. Brouns, and F. R. Bornet. 2004. The capacity of nondigestible carbohydrates to stimulate fecal bifidobacteria in healthy humans: a double-blind, randomized, placebo-controlled, parallel-group, dose-response relation study. *Am. J. Clin. Nutr.* 80:1658–1664.

Bovee-Oudenhoven, I. M., S. J. Ten Bruggencate, M. L. Lettink-Wissink, and R. van der Meer. 2003. Dietary fructo-oligosaccharides and lactulose inhibit intestinal colonisation but stimulate translocation of salmonella in rats. *Gut* 52:1572–1578.

Bratten, J. R., and M. P Jones. 2007. Small intestinal motility. *Curr. Opin. Gastroenterol.* 23:127–133.

Brigidi, P., E. Swennen, B. Vitali, M. Rossi, and D. Matteuzzi. 2003. PCR detection of *Bifidobacterium* strains and

Streptococcus thermophilus in feces of human subjects after oral bacteriotherapy and yogurt consumption. *Int. J. Food Microbiol.* **81**:203–209.

Brown, I. L. 2004. Applications and uses of resistant starch. *J. AOAC Int.* **87**:727–732.

Brown, I. L., K. J. McNaught, and E. Moloney. 1995. Hi-maize™: new directions in starch technology and nutrition. *Food Aust.* **47**:272–275.

Brown, I. L., X. Wang, D. L. Topping, M. J. Playne, and P. L. Conway. 1998. High amylose maize starch as a versatile prebiotic for use with probiotic bacteria. *Food Aust.* **50**:602–609.

Brown, I., M. Warhurst, J. Arcot, M. Playne, R. J. Illman, and D. L. Topping. 1997. Faecal numbers of bifidobacteria are higher in pigs fed *Bifidobacterium longum* with a high amylose cornstarch than with a low amylose cornstarch. *J. Nutr.* **127**:1822–1827.

Brown, I. L., M. Yotsuzuka, A. Birkett, and A. Henriksson. 2006. Prebiotics, synbiotics and resistant starch. *J. Jpn. Assoc. Dietary Fiber Res.* **10**:1–9.

Burkitt, D. P. 1970. Relationship as a clue to causation. *Lancet* **2**:1237–1240.

Cassidy, A., S. A. Bingham, and J. H. Cummings. 1994. Starch intake and colorectal-cancer risk—an international comparison. *Br. J. Cancer* **69**:937–942.

Champ, M., A.-M. Langkilde, F. Brouns, B. Kettlitz, and Y. L. Bail-Collet. 2003. Advances in dietary fibre characterisation. 2. Consumption, chemistry, physiology and measurement of resistant starch; implications for health and food labelling. *Nutr. Res. Rev.* **16**:143–161.

Champ, M. M. 2004. Physiological aspects of resistant starch and in vivo measurements. *J. AOAC Int.* **87**:749–755.

Christian, M. T., C. A. Edwards, T. Preston, L. Johnston, R. Varley, and L. T. Weaver. 2003. Starch fermentation by faecal bacteria of infants, toddlers and adults: importance for energy salvage. *Eur. J. Clin. Nutr.* **57**:1486–1491.

Clarke, J. M., A. R. Bird, D. L. Topping, and L. Cobiac. 2007. Excretion of starch and esterified short chain fatty acids by ileostomists after the ingestion of acylated starches. *Am. J. Clin. Nutr.* **86**:1146–1151.

Cordain, L., S. B. Eaton, A. Sebastian, N. Mann, S. Lindeberg, B. A. Watkins, J. H. O'Keefe, and J. Brand-Miller. 2005. Origins and evolution of the Western diet: health implications for the 21st century. *Am. J. Clin. Nutr.* **81**:341–354.

Crittenden, R., A. Laitila, P. Forssell, J. Mättö, M. Saarela, T. Mattila-Sandholm, and P. Myllärinen. 2001. Adhesion of bifidobacteria to granular starch and its implications in probiotic technologies. *Appl. Environ. Microbiol.* **67**:3469–3475.

Cummings, J. H., and H. N. Englyst. 1987. Fermentation in the human large intestine and the available substrates. *Am. J. Clin. Nutr.* **45**(5 Suppl.):1243–1255.

Cummings, J. H., and H. N. Englyst. 1991. Measurement of starch fermentation in the human large intestine. *Can. J. Physiol. Pharmacol.* **69**:121–129.

Cummings, J. H., and G. T. Macfarlane. 1991. The control and consequences of bacterial fermentation in the human colon. *J. Appl. Bacteriol.* **70**:443–459.

Danjo, K., S. Nakaji, S. Fukuda, T. Shimoyama, J. Sakamoto, and K. Sugawara. 2003. The resistant starch level of heat moisture-treated high amylose cornstarch is much lower when measured in the human terminal ileum than when estimated in vitro. *J. Nutr.* **133**:2218–2221.

Davie, J. R. 2003. Inhibition of histone deacetylase activity by butyrate. *J. Nutr.* **133**:2485S–2493S.

Duncan, S. H., A. Belenguer, G. Holtrop, A. M. Johnstone, H. J. Flint, and G. E. Lobley. 2007a. Reduced dietary intake of carbohydrates by obese subjects results in decreased concentrations of butyrate and butyrate-producing bacteria in feces. *Appl. Environ. Microbiol.* **73**:1073–1078.

Duncan, S. H., P. Louis, and H. J. Flint. 2007b. Cultivable bacterial diversity from the human colon. *Lett. Appl. Microbiol.* **44**:343–350.

Englyst, H. N., S. M. Kingman, G. J. Hudson, and J. H. Cummings. 1996. Measurement of resistant starch in vitro and in vivo. *Br. J. Nutr.* **75**:749–755.

Faulks, R. M., D. J. Hart, G. M. Brett, J. R. Dainty, and S. Southon. 2004. Kinetics of gastro-intestinal transit and carotenoid absorption and disposal in ileostomy volunteers fed spinach meals. *Eur. J. Nutr.* **43**:15–22.

Finnie, I. A., A. D. Dwarakanath, B. A. Taylor, and J. M. Rhodes. 1995. Colonic mucin synthesis is increased by sodium-butyrate. *Gut* **36**:93–99.

Fujiwara, S., Y. Seto, A. Kimura, and H. Hashiba. 2001. Intestinal transit of an orally administered streptomycin-rifampicin-resistant variant of *Bifidobacterium longum* SBT2928: its long-term survival and effect on the intestinal microflora and metabolism. *J. Appl. Microbiol.* **90**:43–52.

Gibson, G. R. 2004. Fibre and effects on probiotics (the prebiotic concept). *Clin. Nutr. Suppl.* **1**:25–31.

Gibson, G. R., and M. B. Roberfroid. 1995. Dietary modulation of the human colonic microbiota: introducing the concept of prebiotics. *J. Nutr.* **125**:1401–1412.

Gibson, G. R., H. M. Probert, J. Van Loo, R. A. Rastall, and M. B. Roberfroid. 2004. Dietary modulation of the human colonic microbiota: updating the concept of prebiotics. *Nutr. Res. Rev.* **17**:259–275.

Gidley, M. J. 1992. Structural order in starch granules and its loss during gelatinisation, p. 87–92. In G. O. Phillips, P. A. Williams, and G. J. Wedlock (ed.), *Gums and Stabilisers for the Food Industry.* IRL Press, Oxford, United Kingdom.

Gork, A. S., N. Usui, E. Ceriati, R. A. Drongowski, M. D. Epstein, A. G. Coran, and C. M. Harmon. 1999. The effect of mucin on bacterial translocation in I-407 fetal and Caco-2 adult enterocyte cultured cell lines. *Pediatr. Surg. Int.* **15**:155–159.

Guarner, F., and J. R. Malagelada. 2003. Gut flora in health and disease. *Lancet* **361**:512–519.

Hill, M. J. 1995. Bacterial fermentation of complex carbohydrate in the human colon. *Eur. J. Cancer Prev.* **4**:353–358.

Kishida, T., Y. Nakai, and K. Ebihara. 2001. Hydroxypropyl-distarch phosphate from tapioca starch reduces zinc and iron absorption, but not calcium and magnesium absorption, in rats. *J. Nutr.* **131**:294–300.

Kleessen, B., L. Hartmann, and M. Blaut. 2003. Fructans in the diet cause alterations of intestinal mucosal architecture, released mucins and mucosa-associated bifidobacteria in gnotobiotic rats. *Br. J. Nutr.* **89**:597–606.

Kleessen, B., G. Stoof, J. Proll, D. Schmiedl, J. Noack, and M. Blaut. 1997. Feeding resistant starch affects faecal and cecal microflora and short-chain fatty acids in rats. *J. Anim. Sci.* 75:2453–2462.

Langlands, S. J., M. J. Hopkins, N. Coleman, and J. H. Cummings. 2004. Prebiotic carbohydrates modify the mucosa associated microflora of the human large bowel. *Gut* 53:1610–1616.

Le Leu, R. K., I. L. Brown, Y. Hu, A. R. Bird, M. Jackson, A. Esterman, and G. P. Young. 2005. A synbiotic combination of resistant starch and *Bifidobacterium lactis* facilitates apoptotic deletion of carcinogen-damaged cells in rat colon. *J. Nutr.* 135:996–1001.

Macfarlane, S., and J. F. Dillon. 2007. Microbial biofilms in the human gastrointestinal tract. *J. Appl. Microbiol.* 102:1187–1196.

Macfarlane, G. T., and A. J. McBain. 1999. The human colonic microbiota, p. 1–25. *In* G. R. Gibson and M. B. Roberfroid (ed.), *Colonic Microbiota, Nutrition and Health*. Kluwer Academic Publishers, Dordrecht, The Netherlands.

Madrid, J., and J. Arcot. 2000. Comparison of two in vitro analyses of resistant starch of some carbohydrate containing foods. *Proc. Nutr. Soc. Aust.* 24:208.

Mai, V., and J. G. Morris. 2004. Colonic bacterial flora: changing understandings in the molecular age. *J. Nutr.* 134:459–464.

Mattila-Sandholm, T., S. Blum, J. K. Collins, R. Crittenden, W. de Vos, C. Dunne, R. Fondén, B. Grenov, E. Isolauri, B. Kiely, P. Marteau, L. Morelli, A. Ouwehand, R. Reniero, M. Saarela, S. Salminen, M. Saxelin, E. Schiffrin, F. Shanahan, E. Vaughan, and A. von Wright. 1999. Probiotics: towards demonstrating efficacy. *Trends Food Sci. Technol.* 10:393–399.

Mitchell, B. L., M. J. Lawson, M. Davies, A. Kerr-Grant, W. E. W. Roediger, R. J. Illman, and D. L. Topping. 1985. Volatile fatty acids in the human intestine: studies in surgical patients. *Nutr. Res.* 5:1089–1092.

Morell, M. K., B. Kosar-Hashemi, M. Cmiel, M. S. Samuel, P. Chandler, S. Rahman, A. Buleon, I. L. Batey, and Z. Li. 2003. Barley sex6 mutants lack starch synthase IIa activity and contain a starch with novel properties. *Plant J.* 34:173–185.

Muir, J. G., A. Birkett, I. Brown, G. Jones, and K. O'Dea. 1995. Food processing and maize variety affects amounts of starch escaping digestion in the small intestine. *Am. J. Clin. Nutr.* 61:82–89.

O'Riordan, K., N. Muljadi, and P. Conway. 2001. Characterization of factors affecting attachment of *Bifidobacterium* species to amylomaize starch granules. *J. Appl. Microbiol.* 90:749–754.

Rahman, S., M. Morell, D. Topping, A. Bird, Z. Li, E. Dennis, and J. Peacock. 2007. Low glycaemic response cereals for enhanced human health. *Int. Diabetes Monit.* 19:21–25.

Roberts, J., G. P. Jones, I. H. E. Rutihauser, A. Birkett, and C. Gibbons. 2004. Resistant starch in the Australian diet. *Nutr. Diet* 61:98–104.

Saavedra, J. M. 2007. Use of probiotics in pediatrics: rationale, mechanisms of action, and practical aspects. *Nutr. Clin. Pract.* 22:351–365.

Santosa, S., E. Farnworth, and P. J. Jones. 2006. Probiotics and their potential health claims. *Nutr. Rev.* 64:265–274.

Sanz, M. L., G. L. Cote, G. R. Gibson, and R. A. Rastall. 2006. Influence of glycosidic linkages and molecular weight on the fermentation of maltose-based oligosaccharides by human gut bacteria. *J. Agric. Food Chem.* 27:9779–9784.

Satokari, R. M., E. E. Vaughan, A. D. L. Akkermans, M. Saarela, and W. M. de Vos. 2001. Polymerase chain reaction and denaturing gradient gel electrophoresis monitoring of fecal *Bifidobacterium* populations in a prebiotic and probiotic feeding trial. *Syst. Appl. Microbiol.* 24:227–231.

Sazawal, S., G. Hiremath, U. Dhingra, P. Malik, S. Deb, and R. E. Black. 2006. Efficacy of probiotics in prevention of acute diarrhoea: a meta-analysis of masked, randomised, placebo-controlled trials. *Lancet Infect. Dis.* 6:374–382.

Schatzkin, A., T. Mouw, Y. Park, A. F. Subar, V. Kipnis, A. Hollenbeck, M. F. Leitzmann, and F. E. Thompson. 2007. Dietary fiber and whole-grain consumption in relation to colorectal cancer in the NIH-AARP Diet and Health Study. *Am. J. Clin. Nutr.* 85:1353–1360.

Sears, C. L. 2005. A dynamic partnership: celebrating our gut flora. *Anaerobe* 11:247–251.

Segal, I. 2002. Physiological small bowel malabsorption of carbohydrates protects against large bowel diseases in Africans. *J. Gastroenterol. Hepatol.* 17:249–252.

Shimakawa, Y., S. Matsubara, N. Yuki, M. Ikeda, and F. Ishikawa. 2003. Evaluation of *Bifidobacterium breve* strain Yakult-fermented soymilk as a probiotic food. *Int. J. Food Microbiol.* 81:131–136.

Smirnov, A., R. Perez, E. Amit-Romach, D. Sklan, and Z. Uni. 2005. Mucin dynamics and microbial populations in chicken small intestine are changed by dietary probiotic and antibiotic growth promoter supplementation. *J. Nutr.* 135:187–192.

Stephen, A. M. 1991. Starch and dietary fibre: their physiological and epidemiological interrelationship. *Can. J. Physiol. Pharmacol.* 69:116–120.

Sullivan, A., and C. E. Nord. 2005. Probiotics and gastrointestinal diseases. *J. Intern. Med.* 257:78–92.

Tang, M. C., and L. Copeland. 2007. Investigation of starch retrogradation using atomic force microscopy. *Carbohydr. Polym.* 70:1–7.

Ten Bruggencate, S. J., I. M. Bovee-Oudenhoven, M. L. Lettink-Wissink, M. B. Katan, and R. van der Meer. 2006. Dietary fructooligosaccharides affect intestinal barrier function in healthy men. *J. Nutr.* 136:70–74.

Ten Bruggencate, S. J., I. M. Bovee-Oudenhoven, M. L. Lettink-Wissink, and R. van der Meer. 2005. Dietary fructooligosaccharides increase intestinal permeability in rats. *J. Nutr.* 135:837–842.

Toden, S., A. R. Bird, D. L. Topping, and M. A. Conlon. 2007. Differential effects of dietary whey, casein and soy on colonic DNA damage in rats. *Br. J. Nutr.* 97:535–543.

Toden, S., A. R. Bird, D. L. Topping, and M. A. Conlon. 2006. Resistant starch abolishes increased colonic DNA damage induced by high dietary cooked red meat or casein in rats. *Cancer Biol. Ther.* 5:267–272.

Topping, D. L., and P. Clifton. 2001. Short chain fatty acids and human colonic function—roles of resistant starch and non starch polysaccharides. *Physiol. Rev.* 81:1031–1064.

Topping, D. L., M. Fukushima, and A. R. Bird. 2003a. Resistant starch as a prebiotic and synbiotic: state of the art. *Proc. Nutr. Soc.* 62:171–176.

Topping, D. L., M. Warhurst, R. J. Illman, I. L. Brown, M. J. Playne, and A. R. Bird. 1997. A high amylose (amylomaize) starch and fructooligosaccharide increase faecal excretion of bifidobacteria in pigs fed live *Bifidobacterium longum*. *Proc. Nutr. Soc. Aust.* **21:**134.

Topping, D., A. Bird, S. Toden, M. Conlon, M. Noakes, R. King, G. Mann, Z. Li, and M. Morell. 2007. Resistant starch as a contributor to the health benefits of whole grains, p. 219–227. *In* L. Marquart, D. Jacobs, G. McIntosh, K. Poutanen, and M. Reicks (ed.), *Whole Grains and Health*. Blackwell Publishers, Ames, IA.

Topping, D. L., M. K. Morell, R. A. King, L. Zhongyi, A. R. Bird, and M. Noakes. 2003b. Resistant starch and health—Himalaya 292, a novel barley cultivar to deliver benefits to consumers. *Starch/Stärke* **55:**539–545.

Topping, D. L., and A. R. Bird. 1999. Food, nutrients and digestive health. *Aust. J. Nutr. Diet.* **56**(Suppl.)**:**S22–S34.

Tuohy, K. M., R. K. Finlay, A. G. Wynne, and G. R. Gibson. 2001. A human volunteer study on the prebiotic effects of HP-inulin—faecal bacteria enumerated using fluorescent in situ hybridisation (FISH). *Anaerobe* **7:**113–118.

Vaughan, E. E., M. C. de Vries, E. G. Zoetendal, K. Ben-Amor, A. D. Akkermans, and W. M. de Vos. 2002. The intestinal LABs. *Antonie Leeuwenhoek* **82:**341–352.

von Wright, A., T. Vilpponen-Salmela, M. P. Llopis, K. Collins, B. Kiely, F. Shanahan, and C. Dunne. 2002. The survival and colonic adhesion of *Bifidobacterium infantis* in patients with ulcerative colitis. *Int. Dairy J.* **12:**197–200.

Wang, X., I. L. Brown, A. J. Evans, and P. L. Conway. 1999a. The protective effects of high amylose maize (amylomaize) starch granules on the survival of *Bifidobacterium* spp. in the mouse intestinal tract. *J. Appl. Microbiol.* **87:**631–639.

Wang, X., I. L. Brown, D. Khaled, M. C. Mahoney, A. J. Evans, and P. L Conway. 2002. Manipulation of colonic bacteria and volatile fatty acid production by dietary high amylose maize (amylomaize) starch granules. *J. Appl. Microbiol.* **93:**390–397.

Wang, X., P. L. Conway, I. L. Brown, and A. J. Evans. 1999b. In vitro utilization of amylopectin and high-amylose maize (Amylomaize) starch granules by human colonic bacteria. *Appl. Environ. Microbiol.* **65:**4848–4854.

Wang, X., and G. R. Gibson. 1993. Effects of the in vitro fermentation of oligofructose and inulin by bacteria growing in the human large intestine. *J. Appl. Bacteriol.* **75:**373–380.

Williams, E. A., J. M. Coxhead, and J. C. Mathers. 2003. Anti-cancer effects of butyrate: use of micro-array technology to investigate mechanisms. *Proc. Nutr. Soc.* **62:**107–115.

Zoetendal, E. G., A. von Wright, T. Vilpponen-Salmela, K. Ben-Amor, A. D. Akkermans, and W. M. de Vos. 2002. Mucosa-associated bacteria in the human gastrointestinal tract are uniformly distributed along the colon and differ from the community recovered from feces. *Appl. Environ. Microbiol.* **68:**3401–3407.

Therapeutic Microbiology: Probiotics and Related Strategies
Edited by J. Versalovic and M. Wilson
© 2008 ASM Press, Washington, DC

Steven A. Abrams

Effects of Prebiotic Supplementation on Bone Mineral Metabolism and Weight in Humans

13

The ability of prebiotics to enhance calcium absorption and bone mineralization has become an important rationale for their use. This chapter reviews the key human studies related to this potential effect and considers the role prebiotics may play in bone health. In addition, recent evidence that prebiotics may be beneficial in weight management is discussed. Finally, potential applications of prebiotics in nutritional planning, especially for children and adolescents, are considered.

WHY SHOULD WE CONSIDER PREBIOTICS AND BONE HEALTH?

The first question to be considered is "Why does this matter?" The health benefits of prebiotics are diverse and would be of considerable importance even if there were no benefits to mineral metabolism or bone health. Furthermore, the likely benefits of prebiotics on increasing the amount of absorbed calcium, although important, could potentially be accomplished by other interventions including higher calcium or vitamin D intakes. Evaluation of these considerations requires a critical under-

standing both of the data related to prebiotics and the relative benefits and risks and of the costs of bone health-related interventions.

Ultimately, however, as with all forms of health promotion, it is crucial to have multiple approaches that can be effective. In this case, using prebiotics can be one important tool to enhance the amount of calcium available for skeletal growth and maintenance. Furthermore, the multiple health benefits of prebiotics, when combined with the bone and potential weight benefits, may allow for the development of "value added" products which are important both for consumers and in the marketplace.

NUTRITION AND BONE HEALTH

Public policy in the United States and elsewhere has largely been based on the concept that optimizing bone mineralization in all age groups can best be achieved by increasing dietary intake of calcium and enhancing its absorption with supplemental vitamin D (Standing Committee on the Scientific Evaluation of Dietary

Steven A. Abrams, USDA/ARS Children's Nutrition Research Center, and Department of Pediatrics, Texas Children's Hospital, Baylor College of Medicine, 1100 Bates St., Houston, TX 77030.

Reference Intakes, 1997; Greer and Krebs, 2006). Despite these policies, the efforts to enhance calcium intake within the population, especially among adolescents, have met with relatively little success in recent years. Strategies and public policy focusing only on intake of a single nutrient (or two, if one includes vitamin D) do not lead to clear health benefits perceived by the consumer and have been difficult to maintain. Furthermore, secular trends away from drinking fluid milk have made it especially challenging to increase population intakes of calcium (Abrams, 2005). On the whole, it is impossible to perceive the public health campaign related to increasing calcium intake as having been successful in any age group, but most especially in children and adolescents. As such, new approaches are clearly necessary.

Guidelines for optimal calcium intake, especially for children and adolescents, are vague. There is no "Estimated Adequate Requirement" or "Recommended Dietary Allowance" for calcium. These standard nutritional terms provide information needed to assess the population and individual intakes of nutrients such as calcium. The current recommended dietary intake of calcium is referred to as an "adequate intake" (AI) (Standing Committee on the Scientific Evaluation of Dietary Reference Intakes, 1997). For example, this value is 1,300 mg/day for adolescents based on data suggesting that this intake would maximize calcium absorption and retention. This intake, however, is not achieved by the vast majority of young adolescents in the United States, including over 80% of adolescent females (Greer and Krebs, 2006). Therefore, it is important to consider other factors, such as calcium absorptive efficiency, that may affect total calcium absorption and improve bone mineral mass accumulation at a calcium intake less than the current AI.

Additionally, the value of 1,300 mg/day is not well defined, nor is it clear that there truly is an asymptotic value above which additional calcium cannot be absorbed. Ultimately, it is likely that the net amount of calcium that can be retained by the skeleton is determined by a variety of influences and is different based on genetic, dietary, and hormonal factors even within a defined population group such as adolescents.

Specifically, guidelines for calcium intake do not specifically take into account genetic or dietary factors that impact calcium absorption. These factors, which affect solubility as well as the vitamin D-dependent transport mechanism, may have a large effect on the rate at which dietary calcium is absorbed (Abrams et al., 2005a). As the current "gold standard" for bone mineral evaluation is whole-body and regional measurement of bone mineral content and density, it is necessary to consider all factors in determining bone mineral status.

For example, in studies of both adults and adolescents it has been shown that height is an important cofactor in determining calcium absorption and utilization of calcium supplements (Abrams et al., 2005b; Barger-Lux and Heaney, 2005). This may be related to gut length or other factors not clearly understood. However, prebiotics may interact with these genetic factors by changing the rate and location at which calcium is absorbed in the intestine (Cashman, 2006). As such, there may be an interactive effect of genetic factors such as height and prebiotic supplementation. Understanding these factors, which were not principal aspects in the formation of the current dietary recommendations for calcium intake, may further enhance individualization of mineral and dietary recommendations.

CLINICAL STUDIES OF PREBIOTICS AND BONE HEALTH: OVERVIEW

There have been approximately 15 studies published evaluating the effects of prebiotics on bone health in humans. These early studies have been reviewed by Griffin and Abrams (2005). Of note is that many of these studies evaluated oligofructose as the prebiotic source designed to enhance calcium absorption or bone mineral outcome (Lopez-Huertas et al., 2006). However, in a direct comparison of the calcium-absorption benefits of oligofructose compared to oligofructose-enriched inulin, we did not find any effect on calcium absorption (Griffin et al., 2002). Rather, we reported that an enriched product, which had a mixture of long- and short-chain fructans, had a greater benefit than those consisting of only short-chain oligofructose (Griffin et al., 2002, 2003). This differential was further supported by data showing that only inulin, but not fructo-oligosaccharides, increased the density of bone in growing rats (Nzeusseu et al., 2006).

Several of the human studies performed are difficult to interpret due to their use of inadequate techniques (only a single tracer) or their use of inadequate sample collection time (van den Heuvel et al., 1999). As such, there are only a small number of human studies that have used the prebiotic products most likely to be beneficial and have utilized adequate methodology to evaluate bone health-related outcomes. Furthermore, all except one of these studies was very short term and there are no long-term (>1-yr) follow-up data. Additionally, dose-response studies of prebiotics and calcium absorption in humans are not available. The minimal effective dose and the "maximum tolerable dose" have not been systematically evaluated, nor have the differences in these among population groups been considered. Thus, although the data provide solid evidence for a benefit to calcium absorption and mineral metabolism from some prebiotics, they are far from a complete dataset that ultimately will be important in furthering the clinical use of these products in nutritional planning.

METHODOLOGICAL ISSUES

The most important studies and how they relate to our understanding of the effects of prebiotics on calcium metabolism are considered next. In order to understand these data, it is necessary to appreciate some methodological issues involved in determining calcium absorption and how these may be affected by prebiotics.

The classic method to determine calcium absorption is by mass balance. In this method the total daily intake of calcium and the urinary and fecal excretion are determined for a fixed period of time, usually at least 7 days. This method is inexpensive but is very difficult to conduct, especially with adolescents, due to the challenges of both controlling intake and obtaining fecal collections. It requires in-patient care throughout the time to ensure complete collection and strict adherence to dietary regulation. It does not permit the easy identification of the effects of individual dietary components. It is therefore not useful for conducting large-sized studies of prebiotic effects on calcium absorption.

A second method is the use of short-term markers such as changes in blood calcium, or parathyroid hormone levels, or increases in urinary calcium before and after therapy. This approach is of limited value for several reasons. First, especially in children, it is impossible to correlate absorption changes with these biochemical or urinary changes. Second, other difficult-to-control factors such as salt intake can have a profound effect on the results. Finally, although some comparisons can be made, this method does not provide an actual measure of calcium absorption. It is poorly suited therefore to understanding the effects of prebiotics on calcium absorption.

The gold standard method for determining calcium absorption is the dual-tracer isotope technique. Originally performed in the 1950s using radioactive calcium, the technique has evolved, and methods for the safe use of nonradioactive (stable) isotopes have been in use since about 1970 and well developed since about 1990. For children and adolescents, all research is performed with stable isotopes, which have absolutely no risks associated with their use as long as the usual medical sterility and infusion protocols are maintained. We have performed over 5,000 such studies in the past 20 years with individuals of all ages without any complications.

In this method, a stable calcium isotope is given with a meal (Abrams, 1999) and a second isotope is given intravenously. A urine sample is collected 24 h after the dosing, the relative recovery of the oral and the intravenous isotopes is determined, and absorption is calculated. This is a robust method, well demonstrated to be as accurate as mass balances with much greater tolerance by subjects, as there is no need for prolonged fecal collections. A version of this may be done using only an oral isotope, but, especially in children, this has no real advantages and is unlikely to be accurate.

A particular issue in the case of prebiotics is that the 24-h urine method assumes that virtually all of the calcium is absorbed in the upper small intestine (van den Heuvel et al., 2000; Griffin and Abrams, 2005). However, it is hypothesized that calcium absorption is enhanced by prebiotics primarily via an effect in the colon (Cashman, 2006). As such, it is likely that the usual 24-h urine collection period is inadequate to fully evaluate this effect. Therefore, studies using this method or methods in which isotope enrichment is determined from blood samples taken shortly after dosing will almost certainly lead to a failure to identify a prebiotic effect on calcium absorption. A 36-h urine collection was used in our studies in order to identify a prebiotic effect on calcium absorption.

It is important to consider the impact of such data on our understanding of dietary requirements for calcium. One useful way of evaluating this is to ask the question, "Based on the baseline usual calcium absorption of the subject population, how much additional calcium would have needed to be consumed to achieve the effect of the prebiotic?" To determine this, one can take the total benefit from the prebiotic (in milligrams per day) and divide it by the expected fractional absorption.

For example, if calcium absorption increased in a study of a prebiotic from 25 to 30% and the usual study intake of calcium was 1,000 mg/day, then the net benefit to the subjects was 5% × 1,000 mg/day = 50 mg/day. To achieve the same benefit by increasing calcium intake without using a prebiotic, one would need to ingest an additional 50/25% = 200 mg/day.

SPECIFIC CLINICAL STUDY: GALACTO-OLIGOSACCHARIDES

The first study to be considered is that of van den Heuvel et al. (2000). In this investigation, a stable-isotope method was used to evaluate the effects of a transgalacto-oligsaccharide on calcium absorption in a group of 12 postmenopausal women. Calcium absorption increased from 20.6% ± 7.0% to 23.9% ± 6.9% during treatment

$(P = 0.04)$. One of the key aspects of this study was the use of a prolonged urinary collection period of 36 h to assess calcium absorption.

A substantial limitation of this study, as well as many of the studies in this area, is the very small sample size. It remains challenging to interpret studies involving groups of fewer than approximately 20 to 30 subjects. Population variation in calcium absorption is substantial as are variations in tolerance, natural inulin intake, and similar factors. Such very small subject numbers pose a risk, especially of false-negative results.

The population of elderly adults reported in this investigation was also characterized by a very low rate of calcium absorption such as might be expected in postmenopausal women. It can be most useful to consider the absorption benefit as a fraction of the baseline absorption. In this case, the benefit (increase in calcium absorption in the prebiotic-treated group) was 3.3% compared to the baseline absorption of 20.6%. Therefore, the absorption benefit was $(100 \times 3.3)/20.6 = 16.0\%$.

Another useful way of looking at these data is to consider the total increase in calcium absorption and whether there was any change in urinary calcium excretion. In this case, the increase in total absorption is not calculable, as the dietary calcium intakes were not provided in the published manuscript. However, making the reasonable assumption of calcium intakes of 900 mg/day, the net benefit would be about 30 mg/day (=3.3% × 900 mg/day). Urinary excretion of calcium was essentially identical at about 205 mg/day in the two groups, demonstrating that the increased absorbed calcium led to an increase in calcium available for bone.

Although useful as a starting place to consider benefits in calcium absorption, this calculation is imprecise for several reasons. First, there is an inverse relationship between calcium intake and absorption fraction. Thus, the calculation underestimates the actual amount of calcium intake benefit from the prebiotic. Second, calcium

intake is often increased by individuals by ingesting calcium in the form of vitamin/mineral supplements taken at a single time each day. The bioavailability of the calcium both from those supplements and from the use of a single dose is likely to be lower than the usual daily absorption. Even further, the solubility of the supplement would need to be considered. Finally, whether the subject was a child or an adult, their genetic makeup, their vitamin D status, and their urinary and sweat calcium excretion would all affect these relationships.

Recognizing these limitations, however, the magnitude of the effect shown in the study of galacto-oligosaccharides (i.e., total absorbed calcium of 30 mg/day) would require an additional calcium intake of at least 145 mg (assuming 20.6% absorption) (Table 1). On a population basis, this is a very substantial amount. Although individuals might adjust their intake accordingly, on a population basis, having the equivalent effect of that magnitude of increase would be substantial.

In summary, this study demonstrated the potential use of a galacto-oligosaccharide to increase calcium absorption. This is a short-chain product and has not been subjected to extensive animal investigations. Nonetheless, galacto-oligosaccharides may be important biologically and may also be combined with fructo-oligosaccharides in products. Further investigations, especially with infants and children, might be useful. Further cost-benefit considerations regarding different prebiotics would also be important in this regard.

CLINICAL STUDIES: FRUCTO-OLIGOSACCHARIDES

In adolescents, calcium absorption after supplementation with oligofructose was compared with supplementation with a mixed short- and long-chain inulin-type fructan (enriched chicory). The enriched chicory was a mixture of a long- and short-chain inulin, Beneo Synergy1 (Orafti,

Table 1 Determination of the equivalent daily intake of calcium needed to achieve the same benefit as inclusion of a prebiotic on calcium absorption[a]

Study	Population	Calcium intake (mg)	Calcium absorption: baseline (%)	Prebiotic increase in calcium absorption % (mg)	Increased calcium intake needed for same effect as prebiotic (mg)
van den Heuvel et al., 2000	Adult	900[b]	20.6	3.3 (30)	145
Griffin et al., 2003	Pediatric	1,340	33.1	2.9 (40)	115
Holloway et al., 2007	Adult	1,086	22.2	5.1 (55)	250
Abrams, 2005c	Pediatric	933	29.9	8.5 (80)	265

[a]Prebiotic increase in calcium absorption and increased calcium intake needed values are rounded to the nearest 5 mg. Benefit to prebiotic is calculated as the product of calcium intake and prebiotic increase in calcium absorption. Increased calcium intake needed for same effect as prebiotic is calculated as prebiotic increase in calcium absorption divided by the calcium absorption: baseline.
[b]Estimated intake.

Tienen, Belgium), henceforth referred to as Synergy1. Synergy1 is an oligofructose-enriched inulin produced through selection of the chain length distribution. This distribution is achieved by coprocessing a long-chain inulin with a pure oligofructose, at approximately a 1:1 ratio.

Groups of 30 girls were studied before and after daily supplementation for 6 to 8 weeks with 8 g of either oligofructose or Synergy1 per day. The results of this study demonstrated a significant benefit to calcium absorption only in the subjects who received Synergy1, not the group receiving oligofructose. This unique effect of Synergy1 was consistent with animal investigations demonstrating a greater effect of prebiotics on calcium absorption when mixtures of long- and short-chain fructans are used.

The magnitude of the effect is best considered using the pooled data in which the data from the 29 subjects who received the Synergy1 were combined with the data of a cohort of 25 similar subjects from a second site (Griffin et al., 2003). Overall the mean calcium intake was 1,340 mg/day in the group, and calcium absorption increased from $33.1\% \pm 9.2\%$ to $36.1\% \pm 9.8\%$ ($P = 0.027$), or a change of 2.9%. The total increase in calcium absorption therefore was $100 \times 2.9/33.1 = 8.8\%$. The total increase in absorption was $2.9 \times 1,340 =$ approximately 40 mg/day, slightly higher than the approximately 30-mg benefit described above based on the study of van den Heuvel et al. (2000).

Compared to earlier studies, this study had the benefit of a much larger sample size, comparison with an alternative prebiotic source, and provision of detailed dietary data. However, its limitations are its short-term nature and the use of the single outcome variable of calcium absorption.

EFFECTS OF SYNERGY1 ON MULTIPLE OUTCOMES IN ADULTS

Two recent studies have taken advantage of multiple outcome measures to evaluate the effects of prebiotics on calcium and bone mineral metabolism. The first to be considered is that of Holloway et al. (2007). In this study involving a group of 15 postmenopausal women (mean age, 72 years), stable isotopes were used to look at both calcium and magnesium absorption. A benefit was shown for both of these in a short-term intervention study. Furthermore, bone resorption markers were assessed, and supplementation with Synergy1 had a significant effect on bone resorption (urinary deoxypridinoline cross-links).

In considering the magnitude of effect that was demonstrated, calcium absorption efficiency increased in the Synergy1 group by 5.1% (22.2% versus 27.3%) after supplementation in subjects with a mean calcium intake of 1,086 mg/day. This net benefit was therefore about

55 mg/day, a magnitude somewhat greater than in the earlier studies. One can estimate, using a calcium absorption of 22%, that achieving the same net increase in absorbed calcium would require a 250-mg/day calcium supplement (Table 1). As noted, this is undoubtedly a low estimate as absorption efficiency of the supplement would likely be less than the dietary absorption efficiency of 22%.

The principal limitations of this study were its small sample size and the short-term duration of intervention. In addition, usual calcium intake was somewhat higher than is typical for women in this age group. Nonetheless, these data are some of the few that demonstrate an effect of prebiotics on calcium absorption in adults.

EFFECTS OF SYNERGY1 ON MULTIPLE OUTCOMES IN ADOLESCENTS

By far the largest study with humans of the effects of prebiotics on calcium absorption and bone mineral metabolism was reported by Abrams et al. in 2005 with further data analysis reported in 2007 (Abrams et al., 2005c, 2007a). In this study, calcium absorption and total body bone mineral content (TBBMC) and density (TBBMD) were measured in 49 boys and 49 girls before and after a 1-year intervention study. All subjects were between 9.0 and 13.0 years of age when enrolled. To be enrolled, subjects had to be healthy and at Tanner Stage 2 or 3, and girls had to be premenarcheal. After a baseline study of calcium absorption and measurement of TBBMC and TBBMD, subjects were randomized, in a double-blinded fashion, and stratified by gender to either 8 g/day of Synergy1 or maltodextrin (placebo control).

After 8 weeks of receiving the carbohydrate supplement to which they had been randomized, subjects returned for a calcium absorption study. Twelve months after the initial baseline study, they returned for a follow-up visit in which measurements of calcium absorption and TBBMC and TBBMD were performed.

In comparing the groups who had received the Synergy1 versus the maltodextrin, there was a significant difference in calcium absorption shown after both 8 weeks and 1 year of supplementation. The difference at 8 weeks was $8.5\% \pm 1.6\%$ ($P < 0.001$), and the difference at 1 year was $5.9\% \pm 2.8\%$ ($P = 0.03$). Similarly, Synergy1 subjects had a greater increment in both TBBMC (35 ± 16 g/year ($P = 0.03$) and TBBMD (0.015 ± 0.004 g/cm^2/year [$P = 0.01$]) than those who had received the placebo. Overall these represented an approximately 20% increase in calcium absorption efficiency for the study population.

In calculating overall benefit to total calcium absorption, based on average calcium intakes of approximately

930 mg/day, these differences corresponded to a net increase in calcium absorption of about 80 mg/day. For the calcium absorptive effects, the 80 mg/day would require a supplement of about 265 mg/day to have the same net increase in absorbed calcium (Table 1).

In a further analysis of these data, the effects on calcium absorption specific to the approximately two-thirds of the study subjects who responded to the Synergy1 were evaluated. We found a net increase in calcium absorption of 12.4% during the first 8 weeks of supplementation. This would, based on an intake of approximately 900 mg/day, amount to about 110 mg/day. To achieve this benefit would, at 30% absorption, require an increased intake of about 300 mg/day.

MECHANISMS BY WHICH PREBIOTICS INCREASE CALCIUM ABSORPTION

The exact mechanisms by which prebiotics affect calcium absorption are unknown. It is furthermore unknown why about two-thirds of subjects appear to respond with an increase in absorption and others do not respond.

As outlined by Cashman (2006) and Scholz-Ahrens et al. (2007), possible mechanisms include, but are not limited to, the following: (i) increased passive absorption in the colon due to increased solubility of calcium associated with pH and microbial changes in the colon, (ii) direct effect of short-chain fatty acids in increasing transcellular calcium absorption, and (iii) increased cell growth and adaptive surface area in the small and large intestines. These findings are supported by a series of animal studies (Ohta et al., 1995; Mineo et al., 2002). Furthermore, Raschka and Daniel (2005) demonstrated the possibility that an inulin-type fructan (ITF) could affect calbindin or other transcellular absorption-related proteins. In Caco-2 cells, a 300 to 400% increase in paracellular calcium absorption was associated with ITF in human intestinal cells (Suzuki and Hara, 2004). Taken together, it appears that the increase in absorption is most likely principally in the large intestine and primarily related to non-vitamin-D-related mechanisms. However, some effect in the small intestine or effect on vitamin-D-related active calcium absorption is possible.

Reasons for a differential response in which some individuals increase their calcium absorption after prebiotics and others do not are likely to fall into two primary categories. First are genetic differences. A differential effect of Synergy1 based on polymorphisms of the vitamin D receptor gene, Fok1, has been demonstrated (Abrams et al., 2005a). The reasons for this are unknown. Specific ethnic and gender differences in effect have not been identified in our studies.

The second reason is likely to be the differences in usual diet and colonic flora between individuals. Although the usual intake of prebiotics is small in the United States, some are part of the diet and these are not well identified in dietary questionnaires. As such, it is not clear from the published studies what the usual level of intake was in the subjects. Furthermore, the available studies have not included fecal analysis to determine what changes in fecal flora occurred with prebiotic supplementation. Both the natural flora and the prebiotic changes may vary between responders and nonresponders.

EFFECTS OF PREBIOTICS ON WEIGHT

In the 1-year study described above (Abrams et al., 2005c), Synergy1 supplementation was found to have significant benefits in the maintenance of an appropriate body mass index (BMI) during pubertal growth. This effect was significantly modified in a nonlinear fashion by the dietary intake of calcium such that the maximum benefit to the prebiotic occurred when low calcium intakes were avoided. Calcium intakes of <800 mg/day were associated with a greater increase in BMI than intakes of ≥800 mg/day, and the benefit to ITF supplementation was greater when low calcium intakes were avoided. A highly significant effect of Synergy1 occurred on BMI Z-score (difference versus control, 0.13 ± 0.06, $P = 0.048$), BMI (difference versus control, 0.52 ± 0.21 kg/m^2, $P = 0.016$), weight (difference versus control, 1.3 ± 0.6 kg, $P = 0.048$), and total fat mass (difference versus control, 0.84 ± 0.36 kg, $P = 0.022$). BMI normally increases during puberty at a yearly rate of about 0.6 to 0.8 kg/m^2 (Maynard et al., 2001). The ITF group was found to have an increase in BMI of about 0.7 kg/m^2 during the supplementation year, consistent with expected increases during puberty, while the control group had an increase of 1.2 kg/m^2. The effect on the age- and gender-normalized BMI, the BMI Z-score, was also considered. The changes in BMI Z-score demonstrated no significant change in the ITF group compared to a significant increase in the control group during the study year. Thus, the overall greater increase in BMI during the supplementation year in the control group was likely not desirable.

The mechanism of the prebiotic effect on BMI and body fat has only minimally been evaluated to date. In a rat model, ITF regulates appetite via increases in gastrointestinal peptides that modulate food intake such as glucagon-like peptide-1 (Cani et al., 2004). A recent pilot study involving 10 young adults suggested that prebiotics reduce hunger and food consumption (Cani et al., 2006). The lack of a significant increase in BMI Z-score in the prebiotic group despite the supplementation both with the prebiotic and with juice implies an overall regulatory effect on energy intake associated with the diet or with the prebiotic. In the study of Abrams et al. (2005c), although energy intake was assessed at the beginning and end of the study, the tools used and the assessment methods would not have been able to identify small changes in intake over a long period of time.

In the study of Abrams et al. (2005c) there was a relative benefit over 1 year for healthy pubertal children of approximately 2.0 kg or 0.8 kg/m² in BMI from maintaining an appropriate calcium intake and receiving a daily prebiotic supplement. Interpreting the clinical importance of this magnitude of an effect is not easily done. This is because relatively few intervention studies have considered the consequences of interventions in diet or behavior on a nonobese young adolescent population. A recent study of extensive counseling of families of middle school children found a net benefit in BMI to 2 years of intervention that was smaller than that found in this study and statistically significant in girls but not boys (Haerens et al., 2006). Therefore, these outcome data likely represent a biologically important benefit and should be further tested in a controlled trial in which BMI Z-score and fat mass changes are a primary study outcome and in a population (prepubertal children) at high risk for undesired increases in BMI Z-score.

PLACING THESE DATA IN CONTEXT

It is important to place the findings related both to mineral metabolism and to weight management in context and to consider future areas of investigation. First, there is little doubt that prebiotics can enhance the absorption of minerals in both animals and humans. This alone is important as it provides a clear rationale for their use in products beyond immunological benefits. For many, the clear rationale of increased mineral absorption itself is evidence for the use of these products and their incorporation into "value-added" foods, such as yogurts.

The concept that the same benefit can be obtained through less expensive means such as increasing mineral intake is oversimplified for a number of reasons. First, several decades of evidence has shown a secular trend towards a decrease in calcium intake. This has occurred despite a large effort to enhance milk and dairy product intake, especially among children and adolescents. Second, it is likely that the benefit of a prebiotic on absorption occurs regardless of intake. That is, it can serve to help balance the nutrient needs for calcium over time. No approach to increasing intake consistently is followed, and thus, a fundamental change in absorptive capacity is beneficial. Third, it is far from clear that there actually is a readily achieved asymptote for maximal calcium absorbed. That is, even among those who do maintain a relatively high calcium intake, there is likely a benefit to the net amount of calcium absorbed using prebiotics.

Fourth, the effects of prebiotics on calcium absorption almost certainly extend to other minerals of importance as well. Magnesium is critical for bone and overall health and is deficient in the diets of many, especially children. A possible benefit to iron and zinc bioavailability is a further benefit of prebiotics.

Finally, increasing calcium absorption is one of a multitude of health benefits described for prebiotics. Using nutritional approaches to enhance health in multiple simultaneous ways is important both from a public health perspective and from the perspective of the individual making a dietary choice. Certainly, if further data support a benefit to weight maintenance, this would be of crucial public health importance.

IMPLEMENTATION

From a calcium and bone health perspective, especially in children and adolescents, it is necessary to consider how prebiotics may be integrated into the diet. The research studies described in this chapter have generally focused on prebiotics given in packets (sachets). This approach is used due to the clear simplicity of conducting research, especially that involving a placebo control such as maltodextrin. However, dietary strategies are much more likely to utilize food-based prebiotics. In the United States, it is likely that this will be through their addition to dairy products, such as yogurts. Other potential products could be considered as well. For use in children and adolescents, it is likely that yogurts would be a primary source as these are increasingly consumed in place of fluid milk by these age groups.

A special case to be considered is that of infants and very young children. Human milk contains a large quantity of oligosaccharides, and it is possible that these have important health benefits not obtained by infants receiving routine commercial formulas. The possibility that benefits to calcium or other mineral absorption would occur in infants needs to be evaluated.

FURTHER RESEARCH

Research into the mineral benefits of prebiotics has only begun. Findings that different products may have greater benefits than others, especially that long-chain inulin or mixtures of short- and long-chain inulin increase calcium absorption, whereas oligosaccharides may not, need replication. It is crucial to evaluate infants, to use a variety of products, and to test multiple minerals.

Regarding weight management, the available data have just begun to provide evidence for the use of prebiotics. Studies are needed that are long-term, are conducted across a range of body weights and body mass indices, and are multiethnic. Consideration of the effects of prebiotics on satiety and of the interaction of prebiotics and behavioral modifications and exercise is also needed.

References

Abrams, S. A. 1999. Using stable isotopes to assess mineral absorption and utilization by children. *Am. J. Clin. Nutr.* 70:955–964.

Abrams, S. A. 2005. Long-term benefits of calcium supplementation during childhood on bone mineralization. *Nutr. Rev.* 63:251–255.

Abrams, S. A., I. J. Griffin, K. M. Hawthorne, Z. Chen, S. K. Gunn, M. Wilde, G. Darlington, R. Shypailo, and K. Ellis. 2005a. Vitamin D receptor *Fok1* polymorphisms affect calcium absorption, kinetics and bone mineralization rates during puberty. *J. Bone Miner. Res.* 20:945–953.

Abrams, S .A., I. J. Griffin, K. M. Hawthorne, S. K. Gunn, C. M. Gundberg, and T. O. Carpenter. 2005b. Relationships among vitamin D levels, PTH, and calcium absorption in young adolescents. *J. Clin. Endocrinol. Metab.* 90:5576–5581.

Abrams, S. A., I. J. Griffin, K. M. Hawthorne, L. Liang, S. K. Gunn, G. Darlington, and K. J. Ellis. 2005c. A combination of prebiotic short-and long-chain inulin-type fructans enhances calcium absorption and bone mineralization in young adolescents. *Am. J. Clin. Nutr.* 82:471–476.

Abrams, S. A., I. J. Griffin, and K. M. Hawthorne. 2007a. Young adolescents who respond to an inulin-type fructan (ITF) substantially increase total absorbed calcium and daily calcium accretion to the skeleton. *J. Nutr.* 137(11 Suppl.): 2524S–2526S.

Abrams, S. A., I. J. Griffin, K. M. Hawthorne, and K. J. Ellis. 2007b. Effect of prebiotic supplementation and calcium intake on body mass index. *J. Pediatr.* 151:293–298.

Barger-Lux, M. J., and R. P. Heaney. 2005. Calcium absorptive efficiency is positively related to body size. *J. Clin. Endocrinol. Metab.* 90:5118–5120.

Cani, P. D., C. Dewever, and N. M. Delzenne. 2004. Inulin-type fructans modulate gastrointestinal peptides involved in appetite regulation (glucagon-like peptide-1 and ghrelin) in rats. *Br. J. Nutr.* 92:521–526.

Cani, P. D., E. Joly, Y. Horsmans, and N. M. Delzenne. 2006. Oligofructose promotes satiety in healthy human: a pilot study. *Eur. J. Clin. Nutr.* 60:567–572.

Cashman, K. D. 2006. A prebiotic substance persistently enhances intestinal calcium absorption and increases bone mineralization in young adolescents. *Nutr. Rev.* 64:189–196.

Greer, F. R., and N. F. Krebs. 2006. Optimizing bone health and calcium intakes of infants, children and adolescents. *Pediatrics* 117:578–585.

Griffin, I. J., P. M. Davila, and S. A. Abrams. 2002. Non-digestible oligosaccharides and calcium absorption in girls with adequate calcium intakes. *Br. J. Nutr.* 87(Suppl. 2):S187–S191.

Griffin, I. J., P. M. D. Hicks, R. P. Heaney, and S. A. Abrams. 2003. Enriched chicory inulin increases calcium absorption in girls with lower calcium absorption. *Nutr. Res.* 23:901–909.

Griffin, I. J., and S. A. Abrams. 2005. Methodological issues in assessing calcium absorption in humans: relevance to study the effects of inulin-type fructans. *Br. J. Nutr.* 93(Suppl. 1): S105–S110.

Haerens, L., B. Deforche, L. Maes, V. Stevens, G. Cardon, and I. De Bourdeaudhuij. 2006. Body mass effects of a physical activity and healthy food intervention in middle schools. *Obesity* 14:847–854.

Holloway, L., S. Moynihan, S. A. Abrams, K. Kent, A. R. Hsu, and A. L. Friedlander. 2007. Effects of oligofructose enriched inulin on calcium and magnesium intestinal absorption and bone turnover markers in postmenopausal women. *Br. J. Nutr.* 97:365–372.

Lopez-Huertas, E., B. Teucher, J. J. Boza, A. Martinez-Ferz, G. Majsak-Newman, L. Baro, J. J. Carrero, M. Gonzalez-Santiago, J. Fonolla, and S. Fairweather-Tait. 2006. Absorption of calcium from milks enriched with fructo-oligosaccharides, caseinophosphopeptides, tricalcium phosphate, and milk solids. *Am. J. Clin. Nutr.* 83:310–316.

Maynard, L. M., W. Wisemandle, A. F. Roche, W. C. Chumlea, S. S. Guo, and R. M. Siervogel. 2001. Childhood body composition in relation to body mass index. *Pediatrics* 107:344–350.

Mineo, H., H. Hara, N. Shigematsu, Y. Okuhara, and F. Tomita. 2002. Melibiose, difructose anhydride III and difructose anhydride IV enhance net calcium absorption in rat small and large intestinal epithelium by increasing the passage of tight junctions in vitro. *J. Nutr.* 132:3394–3399.

Nzeusseu, A., D. Dienst, V. Haufroid, G. Depresseux, J. P. Devogelaer, and D. H. Manicourt. 2006. Inulin and fructo-oligosaccharides differ in their ability to enhance the density of cancellous and cortical bone in the axial and peripheral skeleton of growing rats. *Bone* 38:394–399.

Ohta, A., M. Ohtsuki, S. Baba, T. Adachi, T. Sakata, and E. Sakaguchi. 1995. Calcium and magnesium absorption from the colon and rectum are increased in rats fed fructo-oligosaccharides. *J. Nutr.* 125:2417–2424.

Raschka, L., and H. Daniel. 2005. Mechanisms underlying the effects of inulin-type fructans on calcium absorption in the large intestine of rats. *Bone* 37:728–735.

Scholz-Ahrens, K. E., P. Ade, B. Marten, P. Weber, W. Timm, Y. Acil, C. C. Gluer, and J. Schrezenmeir. 2007. Prebiotics, probiotics, and synbiotics affect mineral absorption, bone mineral content, and bone structure. *J Nutr.* 137(3 Suppl. 2): 838S–846S.

Standing Committee on the Scientific Evaluation of Dietary Reference Intakes, Food and Nutrition Board, Institute of Medicine. 1997. *Dietary Reference Intakes for Calcium, Magnesium, Phosphorus, Vitamin D, and Fluoride.* National Academy Press, Washington, DC.

Suzuki, T., and H. Hara. 2004. Various nondigestible saccharides open a paracellular calcium transport pathway with the induction of intracellular calcium signaling in human intestinal Caco-2 cells. *J. Nutr.* 134:1935–1941.

van den Heuvel, E. G., G. Schaafsma, T. Muys, and W. van Dokkum. 1999. Nondigestible oligosaccharides do not interfere with calcium and nonheme-iron absorption in young, healthy men. *Am. J. Clin. Nutr.* 67:445–451.

van den Heuvel, E. G., M. H. Schoterman, and T. Muijs. 2000. Transgalactooligosaccharides stimulate calcium absorption in postmenopausal women. *J. Nutr.* 130:2938–2942.

Therapeutic Microbiology: Probiotics and Related Strategies
Edited by J. Versalovic and M. Wilson
© 2008 ASM Press, Washington, DC

Nathalie M. Delzenne
Patrice D. Cani
Audrey M. Neyrinck

Prebiotics and Lipid Metabolism

14

EFFECT OF PREBIOTICS ON FATTY ACID METABOLISM

Triacylglycerols (TAG) have important physiological roles, and abnormalities in their metabolism are implicated in major pathologies such as obesity, insulin resistance, type 2 diabetes, dyslipidemia, and atherosclerosis. The main sites of endogenous TAG synthesis from glycerol-3-phosphate and fatty acids are the liver and adipose tissue. Most of the fatty acids used for this synthesis are provided by breaking down other TAG, whereas de novo lipogenesis, the synthesis of new molecules of fatty acids from nonlipid substrates, is a minor pathway. In rats fed a lipid-rich diet containing 10% fructans, a decrease in triglyceridemia occurs without any protective effect on hepatic TAG accumulation and lipogenesis, suggesting a possible peripheral mode of action (Roberfroid and Delzenne, 1998). In contrast, in obese Zucker rats, dietary supplementation with fructans reduces hepatic steatosis, with no effect on postprandial triglyceridemia. This effect is likely to result mainly from a lower availability of nonesterified fatty acids coming from adipose tissue, since fat mass and body weight are decreased by the treatment (Daubioul et al., 2000).

A decrease in hepatic and serum TAG is observed when inulin-type fructans (Delzenne and Kok, 2001), fermented resistant rice starch (Cheng and Lai, 2000), or raw potato or high-amylose corn starch (Lopez et al., 2001) is added for several weeks to the standard diet of rats or hamsters—which is rich in carbohydrates. The doses required to obtain such an effect are relatively high (3 to 20% [wt/wt] in the diet), and depending on the model, the effect appears to be dose dependent (Tokunaga et al., 1986; Hokfelt et al., 1999). The TAG-lowering effect is also found in beagle dogs receiving 5% of a short-chain inulin-type fructan associated with 10% sugar beet fiber (Diez et al., 1997). The TAG-lowering effect of inulin type fructans has also been shown in apolipoprotein E (apo-E)-deficient mice. In this model, the inhibition of plaque formation was more pronounced with long-chain inulin than with shorter ones (Rault-Nania et al., 2006). A decrease in serum TAG is even more pronounced in animal models in which the diet is enriched with dietary fructose (Kok et al., 1996; Busserolles et al., 2003).

Short-chain fructo-oligosaccharides also decrease hepatic TAG accumulation (steatosis) in models in which

Nathalie M. Delzenne, Patrice D. Cani, and **Audrey M. Neyrinck,** Université Catholique de Louvain, School of Pharmacy, MD/FARM/PMNT 7369 UCL, 73 Avenue Mounier, B-1200 Brussels, Belgium.

TAG synthesis in the liver is promoted, either induced by a fructose-rich diet in rats or due to leptin receptor defect (Delzenne and Kok, 1998; Daubioul et al., 2000, 2002; Busserolles et al., 2003). They also protect rats fed a high-sucrose/high-fat diet against hepatic steatosis, and in this model, they decrease susceptibility to the hepatotoxic effect of phenobarbital treatment (Sugatani et al., 2006).

In most studies involving animals (rats and mice), the decrease in triglyceridemia and/or in hepatic TAG level due to feeding of fructans is accompanied by a decrease in fat mass development, observed after 2 to 4 weeks of treatment in mice or rats (depending on the model), and a lower body weight after a prolonged treatment (more than 4 weeks in rats). Subcutaneous and visceral fat mass are both decreased by prebiotics.

It has been reported that chronic resistant starch (RS) feeding in rats causes a decrease in adipocyte cell size, a decrease in fatty acid synthase expression, and reduced whole-body weight gain relative to digestible starch feeding (Lerer-Metzger et al., 1996). On a whole-body level, this attenuation of fat deposition in white adipose tissue in response to an RS diet could be significant for the prevention of weight gain in the long term (Higgins et al., 2006). The decrease in fat mass development is clearly linked to a decrease in energy intake. Besides this effect on fat mass development, no effect on serum non-esterified fatty acids is observed in the animals receiving prebiotics.

The decrease in serum TAG due to prebiotics such as fructans results mainly from a decrease in very low density lipoproteins as shown in rats or hamsters (Fiordaliso et al., 1995; Trautwein et al., 1998). In animals, the reduced triglyceridemia observed after fructans feeding is often linked to a decrease in de novo lipogenesis in the liver, but not in adipose tissue (Delzenne and Kok, 2001). The activities and mRNA levels of key enzymes involved in fatty acid synthesis (acetyl coenzyme A carboxylase [ACC], glucose-6-phosphate dehydrogenase, ATP citrate lyase, and fatty acid synthase [FAS]) are lower in animals fed fructans, suggesting that a lower lipogenic gene expression is involved in the decreased lipogenic capacity after supplementation with fructans (Kok et al., 1996). This effect on hepatic de novo lipogenesis was also shown in rats fed RS (Takase et al., 1994). Moreover, following an overnight fast, male Wistar rats ingesting a meal with an RS content of 2 or 30% of total carbohydrate exhibited a lower rate of lipogenesis in white adipose tissue (Higgins et al., 2006).

The decrease in glycemia and/or insulinemia observed in animals fed synthetic (from saccharose) or chicory root-derived inulin has been proposed as a mechanism explaining the lower de novo lipogenesis (Delzenne and Williams, 2002; Sugatani et al., 2006). In fact, glucose and insulin promote lipogenesis through the activation of several key peptides or nuclear factor (activation of sterol response element binding protein [SREBP-1C] and phosphorylation of AMP kinase) (Ferre and Foufelle, 2007). No data have been published to date to support a relationship between a lower SREBP-1C or AMP kinase in the antilipogenic effect of inulin-type fructans and other nondigestible carbohydrates.

Levan from *Zymomonas mobilis*, which is largely fermented in the cecocolon by bifidobacteria, also reduces the expression of genes coding FAS and ACC in the liver (but not in the adipose tissue) of rats fed a high-fat/high-sucrose diet; this phenomenon correlates with a decrease in the insulin level (Kang et al., 2006). The authors, in view of their experimental results, suggested that, in addition to the lower glucose-induced lipogenesis, prebiotics could also promote fatty acid oxidation via an activation of hepatic peroxisome proliferator-activated receptor alpha (PPARα). Some recent data obtained in our laboratory support a role for PPARα in oligofructose effects, since PPARα KO (−/−) mice treated with oligofructose had the same hepatic and serum TAG level as the one measured in the controls (P. D. Cani, E. Dewulf, A. Neyrinck, and N. Delzenne, personal communication, 2007).

EFFECT ON CHOLESTEROL HOMEOSTASIS

Cholesterol is an important constituent of cell membranes, where it is implicated in the control of important cellular functions. There are two sources of the compound at the whole-body level: dietary intake and endogenous synthesis, the latter being quantitatively the most important in humans. Type 2 (high-amylose) RS (200 g/kg of food) lowers the cholesterol content in total serum and triglyceride-rich lipoprotein in rats (Lopez et al., 2001). This fact is in accordance with the lower cholesterol absorption observed in rats fed with soluble corn bran arabinoxylans or fermentable starch (Lopez et al., 1999, 2001). Increased low-density lipoprotein (LDL) receptor mRNA content could also contribute to the decrease in serum total cholesterol occurring in rats receiving bean RS in their diet for 4 weeks (Fukushima et al., 2001). Other fermentable soluble dietary fibers, such as pectin, low-viscosity guar gum, and beta-glucan from oat bran, have been shown to lower serum cholesterol in rats (Delzenne and Williams, 1999; Slavin, 2005; Queenan et al., 2007).

Several studies have also reported a decrease in total serum cholesterol after dietary supplementation with inulin (10%) in mice or rats (Levrat et al., 1991; Fiordaliso et al., 1995; Delzenne et al., 2002; Mortensen et al., 2002; Fava et al., 2006; Rault-Nania et al., 2006). Experiments with apo-E-deficient mice support the fact that dietary inulin (mainly long-chain inulin) significantly lowers the total cholesterol level by about one-third. This is accompanied by a significant decrease in the hepatic cholesterol content. The authors suggest that the decrease in serum cholesterol could reflect a decrease in TAG-rich lipoproteins, which are also rich in cholesterol in apo-E-deficient animals (Rault-Nania et al., 2006).

With regard to the hypocholesterolemic effect of prebiotics, several mechanisms have been proposed which are often related to a modulation of the intestinal metabolism of bile acids, but other properties (e.g., steroid-binding properties) may be involved, which are independent of the fermentation of the prebiotic in the lower intestinal tract (Trautwein et al., 1999; Delzenne and Williams, 1999; Adam et al., 2001; Lopez et al., 2001).

ROLE OF SHORT-CHAIN FATTY ACIDS IN THE MODULATION OF LIPID METABOLISM BY PREBIOTICS

Gut fermentation of prebiotics leads to the production of short-chain fatty acids, mostly acetate, propionate, and butyrate, which are almost completely absorbed along the digestive tract. Whereas butyrate is widely metabolized by enterocytes, propionate and acetate reach the liver through the portal vein (Demigne et al., 1999). When acetate enters the hepatocyte, it is activated mainly by the cytosolic acetyl coenzyme A synthetase 2 and then enters the cholesterogenesis and lipogenesis pathways. This effect has been proposed as a rationale for the hypercholesterolemic effect of those nondigestible carbohydrates such as lactulose whose fermentation in the colon results in enhanced acetate, but not propionate, production. Conversely, propionate is a competitive inhibitor of the protein controlling the entrance of acetate into liver cells (N. M. Delzenne, N. Kok, A. Neyrinck, and C. Daubioul, unpublished results), a phenomenon which contributes to a decrease in lipogenesis and cholesterogenesis, at least in vitro in rat hepatocytes. The production of a high concentration of propionate, through fermentation, has been proposed as a mechanism to explain the reduction in serum and hepatic cholesterol in rats fed RS or fructans (Levrat et al., 1994; Demigne et al., 1995; Jenkins et al., 1998; Cheng and Lai, 2000; Lopez et al., 2001; Delzenne and Kok, 2001). It thus appears that the pattern of fermentation of prebiotics, and mostly the ratio of acetate to propionate reaching the liver through the portal vein, is a putative intermediate marker that could be used

to predict the potential lipid-lowering properties of prebiotics and other nondigestible fermentable carbohydrates. Oligofructose fermentation by human fecal bacteria can increase butyrate production in vitro (Morrison et al., 2006). However, oligofructose appears to be fermented by mainly acetate- and lactate-producing bacteria rather than butyrate-producing bacteria (Morrison et al., 2006). As bacterial acetate conversion to butyrate and lactate conversion to acetate, propionate, and butyrate were observed, carbohydrates with similar properties represent a refinement of the prebiotic definition, termed butyrogenic prebiotics, because of their additional functionality.

Interestingly, acetate, when supplied in the diet of diabetic mice at a dose of 0.5% for 8 weeks, activates AMP kinase in the liver, a phenomenon that is related to the inhibition of de novo lipogenesis (Sakakibara et al., 2006). The incubation of rat hepatocytes with acetate (0.2 mM) activates AMP kinase and decreases SREBP-1c expression, two factors clearly implicated in the regulation of lipogenesis. Therefore, the classical deleterious role attributed to acetate as a precursor of lipogenesis might be modulated, taking into account its regulatory effect on key molecular factors involved in fatty acid synthesis in the liver.

In humans, key experimental data are lacking, with regard to the quantitative contribution of acetate and propionate, produced in the colon through prebiotic fermentation, in the regulation of lipid synthesis in vivo.

IMPLICATION OF ENERGY INTAKE AND ENERGY EXPENDITURE IN THE FAT-REDUCING EFFECT OF PREBIOTICS

The analysis of food intake behavior reveals that feeding of fructans decreases the total energy intake by about 5 to 10% throughout the period of treatment (Delzenne et al., 2007). This effect explains the relevance of these prebiotics to the control of fat mass development in different animal models. The "satietogenic" effect of nondigestible carbohydrates results from the overproduction of anorexigenic gut peptides (GLP-1 and PYY) and a decrease in orexigenic peptides (ghrelin) (Cani et al., 2004). We have shown, in high-fat-fed mice, that the antiobesity effect of fructans is clearly dependent on the higher production of GLP-1 by L cells in the colon and requires a functional GLP-1 receptor (Cani et al., 2006; Delmée et al., 2006; Cani et al., 2007b). In mice exhibiting a functional GLP-1 receptor, the following beneficial effects of oligofructose were observed: (i) a decrease in food intake, fat mass, and body weight gain; (ii) an improved glucose tolerance during oral glucose tolerance testing; and (iii) an improved hepatic insulin resistance.

The disruption of GLP-1R function, by chronic infusion of exendin 9-39, prevented the majority of those beneficial effects observed following oligofructose treatment. The importance of GLP-1R-dependent pathways was confirmed using GLP-1R$^{-/-}$ mice fed a high-fat diet: no beneficial effects of oligofructose treatment were observed in GLP-1R$^{-/-}$ mice. Moreover, in some specific experimental models, oligofructose did not have any effect on body weight and glucose homeostasis: those models were also characterized by a lack of effect of oligofructose on GLP-1 production in the colon (Delmée et al., 2006) or were characterized by a lack of GLP-1.

Leptin is another peptide known to control food intake. The acute administration of propionate has been shown to increase circulating leptin in mice, through the interaction with the orphan G protein-coupled receptor GRP41 (Xiong et al., 2004). However, the administration of oligofructose in rats receiving a diet rich in fructose led to a decrease in serum leptin (Busserolles et al., 2003). The administration of levan, which is largely fermented by bifidobacteria in the colon, also decreases, in a dose-dependent manner, the level of serum leptin in rats fed a high-fat diet for 4 weeks (Kang et al., 2006). This decrease in leptin correlated with a decrease in serum insulin. Although few data are available, it would appear that feeding of prebiotics lowers serum leptin, probably as a consequence of the decrease in fat mass observed in prebiotic-fed animals. Leptin is thus not involved in the control of food intake by prebiotics; in accordance with this hypothesis, several studies with mice or rats lacking leptin (receptor) expression or functionality showed that these animals' intake of energy was less throughout the treatment with nondigestible prebiotic carbohydrates, such as fructans, than that of control animals receiving the corresponding control diet (Daubioul et al., 2002).

THE ROLE OF THE INTESTINAL MICROBIOTA IN THE CONTROL OF LIPID HOMEOSTASIS BY PREBIOTICS

The gut microbiota may affect hepatic lipid metabolism involved in energy homeostasis. Germfree mice colonized with the gut microbiota derived from conventionally reared mice have a higher expression of factors/enzymes promoting de novo lipogenesis in the liver (increase in SREBP-1c and carbohydrate response element binding protein, ACC, and FAS) (Backhed et al., 2004). These data suggest that the gut microbiota may affect the pathophysiology of obesity. In fact, recent data have been published showing that the composition of the gut microbiota is different in obese and nonobese individuals (Ley et al., 2006). In humans, the relative proportion of *Bacteroidetes* versus *Firmicutes* is decreased in obese people in comparison with lean people, and this proportion increases with weight loss on two types of low-calorie diet (low-carbohydrate or low-fat diet). In obese mice (leptin-deficient ob/ob mice), the proportion of *Bacteroidetes* is also decreased compared to their lean siblings (Ley et al., 2005). These changes in bacterial composition—observed both in obese humans and animals—were division-wide, whereas bacterial diversity remained constant over time; no blooms or extinctions of specific bacterial species were observed in obese versus lean individuals, or after dietary (low-calorie) intervention (Ley et al., 2006). The composition of the microbiota has an impact on calorie sparing from food and on fat mass development. The ingestion of the same quantity of food allows ob/ob mice to harvest more calories than the corresponding lean animals: the "energy sparing" phenomenon is transmissible to germfree recipients when they are colonized with an "obese microbiota," suggesting that the microbiota composition seems relevant to explain this difference. It is important to note that this colonization results also in a greater increase in total body fat than the colonization with a "lean microbiota" (Turnbaugh et al., 2006). In contrast to mice with a gut microbiota, germfree animals are protected against the obesity that develops after consuming a high-fat/high-sugar diet (Backhed et al., 2007). Therefore, the presence of the gut microbiota itself controls the metabolic response to energy-dense food. This protection against fat mass development in germfree mice is attributable to a higher level of fasting-induced adipocyte factor (FIAF), which both inhibits lipoprotein lipase (and therefore limits fat storage of dietary fatty acids) and promotes fatty acid oxidation in muscles by inducing peroxisomal proliferator-activated receptor coactivator (PGC-1α). FIAF expression may be modulated by specific microbial determinants: when germfree mice are colonized by saccharolytic and methanogenic species (*Bacteroides thetaiotaomicron* and *Methanobrevibacter smithii*), intestinal FIAF expression is suppressed and de novo lipogenesis and host adiposity increase (Backhed et al., 2004; Rawls et al., 2006). Moreover, germfree animals exhibit a higher AMP kinase activity in the liver and in muscles, which promotes fatty acid β-oxidation (carnitine palmitoyltransferase I activity) and favors the inhibition of anabolism via inhibition of key enzymes controlling fatty acid and glycogen synthesis; those events are independent of FIAF expression (Backhed et al., 2007).

We have recently shown that specific modulation of the gut microbiota by prebiotics influences fat mass development and lipid metabolic disorders associated with obesity (Cani et al., 2007c). We reported that high-fat feeding was associated with a higher endotoxemia and a lower *Bifidobacterium* spp. cecal content in mice (Cani et al., 2007a). Therefore, we tested whether restoration of the number of cecal *Bifidobacterium* spp. could modulate metabolic endotoxemia, the inflammatory tone, and the development of diabetes. Since bifidobacteria have been reported to reduce intestinal endotoxin levels and improve mucosal-barrier function (Griffiths et al., 2004; Wang et al., 2004, 2006), we specifically increased the gut bifidobacterial content of high-fat-diet-fed mice through the use of a prebiotic (oligofructose). We demonstrated that high-fat feeding significantly reduced intestinal gram-negative and gram-positive bacteria including levels of bifidobacteria, a dominant member of the intestinal microbiota which is regarded as physiologically positive, compared to normal-chow-fed mice. As expected, in prebiotics-fed mice the numbers of bifidobacteria were completely restored. High-fat feeding significantly increased endotoxemia, which was normalized to normal-chow-fed mice in prebiotics-treated mice. Multiple-correlation analyses showed that endotoxemia significantly and negatively correlated with the number of *Bifidobacterium* spp. in prebiotics-treated mice; *Bifidobacterium* spp. significantly and positively correlated with improved glucose tolerance, glucose-induced insulin secretion, and normalized inflammatory tone (decreased endotoxemia and plasma and adipose-tissue proinflammatory cytokines). Together, these findings suggest that the gut microbiota contributes towards the pathophysiological regulation of endotoxemia and sets the tone of inflammation for the occurrence of diabetes/obesity. Thus, it would be useful to develop specific strategies for modifying the gut microbiota in favor of bifidobacteria to prevent the deleterious effect of high-fat-diet-induced metabolic diseases.

COULD AN EFFECT BE MEDIATED BY PROBIOTICS THEMSELVES THROUGH THE MODIFICATION OF THE INTESTINAL MICROBIOTA?

Most prebiotics promote lactic acid-producing bacteria. The possibility that modification of the intestinal microbiota may have beneficial effects on lipid metabolism is equivocally supported by studies using lactic acid-producing probiotics (live microbial feed supplements, e.g., fermented dairy products) (Taylor and Williams, 1998; St Onge et al., 2000; Whelan et al., 2001; Andersson et al., 2001; McNaught and MacFie, 2001). The influence of probiotics on TAG homeostasis is only poorly documented. An interesting review suggests a moderate

cholesterol-lowering effect associated with the consumption of dairy products fermented with specific strains of *Lactobacillus* and/or *Bifidobacterium* (Fava et al., 2006). The regular consumption of both probiotic and conventional yogurt for 4 weeks exerted a positive effect on the lipid profile (increase in high-density lipoproteins [HDL]/LDL ratio) in the plasma of healthy women (Fabian and Elmadfa, 2006).

In animals, a cholesterol-lowering action of certain fermented dairy products indicates that the bacterial content, and more precisely the combination of different types of bacteria such as *Lactobacillus acidophilus*, *Lactobacillus casei*, and *Bifidobacterium bifidum*, is responsible for the cholesterol-lowering action of dairy products (Andersson et al., 2001). Bifidobacterial proliferation does not seem to play an exclusive role in the hypocholesterolemic effect of prebiotics, since levan β-2-6, which is not bifidogenic, decreases serum cholesterol in rats (Yamamoto et al., 1999). An enhanced bile acid deconjugation and the subsequent enhanced fecal bile acid excretion have been implicated in the cholesterol reduction associated with certain probiotics and prebiotics (St Onge et al., 2000). Another hypothesis is that cholesterol from the growth medium of the fermented product is incorporated into the bacterial cell membrane and thus escapes digestion (Fava et al., 2006). The intestinal colonization potency of the probiotics, which is strongly dependent on the strain, seems a crucial factor in determining a hypocholesterolemic effect (Usman and Hosono, 2000). This may explain why a combination of probiotics (lactobacillus) and prebiotics (fructans) promotes a decrease in cholesterolemia (−0.23 mol/liter) in healthy people (Schaafsma et al., 1998). The positive effects of an altered intestinal microbiota have also been reported in studies in which no probiotic addition is given: in a four-phase randomized crossover study in healthy people, a higher HDL cholesterol level and a lower LDL cholesterol level were correlated with lower fecal output of fusobacteria and bacteroides, due to RS treatment (Jenkins et al., 1999).

EFFECT OF PREBIOTICS ON LIPID METABOLISM IN HUMANS

A small number of well-designed human studies have reported some positive outcomes with regard to the effects of prebiotics on blood lipids (Delzenne and Williams, 1999; Daubioul et al., 2000; Williams and Jackson, 2002; Daubioul et al., 2005; Beylot, 2005; Fava et al., 2006). Relevant studies reported in the literature with inulin-type fructans are presented in Table 1; the authors have investigated the response of blood lipids

Table 1 Effects of inulin-type fructans on lipid metabolism in humans[a]

Reference	Prebiotic	Dose (g/day)	Duration (weeks)	Effect on blood lipids
Yamashita et al., 1984	OFS	8	2	↓ T-Chol, ↓ LDL-Chol
Hidaka et al., 1991	OFS	8	5	↓ T-Chol
Luo et al., 1996	OFS	20	4	NS
Pedersen et al., 1997	Inulin	14	4	NS
Davidson et al., 1998	Inulin	18	6	↓ LDL-Chol, ↓ T-Chol
Jackson et al., 1999	Inulin	10	8	↓ TAG
Brighenti et al., 1999	Inulin	9	4	↓ TAG, ↓ LDL-Chol
Alles et al., 1999	OFS	15	3	NS
Havenaar et al., 1999	Inulin, OFS	15	3	NS
Luo et al., 2000	OFS	20	4	NS
Causey et al., 2000	Inulin	20	3	↓ TAG
Balcazar-Munoz et al., 2003	Inulin	7	4	↓ TAG, ↓ T-Chol
Letexier et al., 2003	Inulin	10	3	↓ TAG
Giacco et al., 2004	OFS	10.6	8	NS
Daubioul et al., 2005	OFS	16	8	NS
Forcheron and Beylot, 2007	Inulin, OFS	10	24	NS

[a]OFS, oligofructose; T-Chol, total cholesterol; LDL-Chol, LDL cholesterol; NS, no significant effect; ↓, decrease.

(usually total and LDL cholesterol and TAG) to prebiotic supplementation in human volunteers.

Studies have been conducted with both normal and moderately hyperlipidemic subjects. Inulin-type fructans tended to decrease TAG and cholesterol levels. No clear conclusion can be drawn concerning the influence of the duration of the treatment and the efficacy of prebiotics to lower blood lipids (Delzenne and Williams, 1999, 2002). However, in human studies performed with inulin-type fructans, lower doses (from 7 to 10 g/day) seem more efficacious than higher doses (15 to 20 g) in decreasing blood lipids (Beylot, 2005).

Some studies have shown that dietary supplementation with 15 or 20 g of fructo-oligosaccharides per day for 4 weeks had no effect on serum cholesterol or triglycerides in type 2 diabetic patients (Alles et al., 1999; Luo et al., 2000), whereas positive outcomes have tended to be observed more frequently in those studies conducted with subjects with moderate hyperlipidemia. In men with hypercholesterolemia, daily intake of 20 g of inulin significantly reduces serum triglycerides by 40 mg/dl (Causey et al., 2000), as previously shown in moderate hyperlipidemic patients receiving 9 g of inulin per day (Jackson et al., 1999). Subjects with a serum cholesterol above 250 mg/dl tended to have the greatest reduction of cholesterol after inulin supplementation. The effect of fructan (long-chain inulin) supplementation on hepatic lipogenesis and cholesterogenesis has been analyzed (deuterated water incorporation into lipids) in healthy subjects in a double-blind, placebo-controlled crossover study (Letexier et al., 2003; Forcheron and Beylot, 2007). It confirms the experimental data obtained with animals, namely that hepatic de novo lipogenesis is reduced by feeding fructans at a moderate dose (10 g of inulin per day for 3 weeks). However, there is no significant modification of cholesterol synthesis (Letexier et al., 2003). The analysis of mRNA concentrations from genes coding key enzymes or proteins involved in the regulation of lipid synthesis (FAS, ACC, and SREBP1c) in the adipose tissue revealed no differences between the placebo and inulin groups. This supports the fact that, at least for inulin-type prebiotics, the hypolipidemic effect is linked to modulation of liver rather than adipose-tissue metabolism. Contrary to what was observed in short-term studies, no significant beneficial effect of a long-term (6-month) administration of inulin-type fructans on plasma lipids was observed in healthy human subjects (Forcheron and Beylot, 2007).

In a pilot study performed with patients presenting nonalcoholic steatohepatitis, 16 g of oligofructose per day for 8 weeks led to a decrease in serum aminotransferases, thus suggesting a hepatoprotective effect of prebiotic treatment in that context; a slight decrease in serum TAG was observed, but it was not significant (Daubioul et al., 2005).

Other nondigestible fermentable carbohydrates with prebiotic properties have been studied. Glucomannans are prone to decrease TAG and cholesterol (LDL cholesterol) levels; these effects could be linked to their influence on fecal steroid excretion (Gallaher et al., 2002).

The effect of RS on lipid homeostasis in humans is controversial. Certain classes of RS (called type 1 RS) have been associated in humans with reduced postprandial insulin and higher HDL cholesterol levels, but these effects are more related to the sustained release of carbohydrate within the small intestine, rather than to an effect linked to fermentation (Jenkins and Kendall, 2000). A lack of effect of low doses of β-glucan (3 g/day for 8 weeks) on total and LDL cholesterol and triglyceridemia in volunteers with mild-to-moderate hyperlipidemia was also recently reported—a negative result—which is in contrast to some other previous positive studies that have employed higher daily doses of β-glucan (Lovegrove et al., 2000). The fact that higher doses of β-glucan are required to induce an effect on lipidemia is supported by a recent single-blind crossover study showing a significant lowering of serum LDL cholesterol (reduced by 9%) in hyperlipidemic subjects consuming 7 g of oat β-glucans incorporated in various foods for 3 weeks (Pomeroy et al., 2001).

In humans, data show that a decrease in plasma glucose after a meal containing β-glucan is not related to a decrease in de novo lipogenesis (Battilana et al., 2001). Lactulose is also able to decrease serum TAG (Vogt et al., 2006). In overweight subjects, a short-term decrease in free fatty acids level and glycerol turnover after lactulose ingestion corresponded to a decrease of lipolysis which was closely related to an increase in acetate production (Ferchaud-Roucher et al., 2005).

CONCLUSION

Several oligosaccharides which strictly correspond to the definition of prebiotics exhibit interesting effects on lipid metabolism. The resulting changes in the intestinal microbiota composition or fermentation activity could be implicated in the modulation of fatty acid and cholesterol metabolism. There is not a single biochemical locus through which prebiotics modulate serum, hepatic, and whole-body lipid content in animals. The effects observed depend on the pathophysiological and nutritional conditions. This may help to explain why in humans, where such conditions cannot be so rigorously controlled (namely, in terms of nutrient intake), the reported effects of prebiotics on circulating blood lipids are much more variable.

Most of the data described to date have been obtained in animal studies; the relevance of such observations on obesity and cardiovascular disease risk in humans remains a key question also addressed in this chapter. Fundamental research devoted to understanding the biochemical and physiological events (on glucose and lipid

homeostasis, on gut hormone secretion, on satiety, etc.), as well as clinical research focusing on the target population, is required to achieve progress in the new area of the nutritional management of metabolic syndromes, based on modulation of the gut microbiota and intestinal function by specific food components.

References

Adam, A., M. A. Levrat-Verny, H. W. Lopez, M. Leuillet, C. Demigne, and C. Remesy. 2001. Whole wheat and triticale flours with differing viscosities stimulate cecal fermentations and lower plasma and hepatic lipids in rats. *J. Nutr.* 131:1770–1776.

Alles, M. S., N. M. De Roos, J. C. Bakx, E. van de Lisdenk, P. L. Zock, and G. A. Hautvast. 1999. Consumption of fructooligosaccharides does not favorably affect blood glucose and serum lipid concentrations in patients with type 2 diabetes. *Am. J. Clin. Nutr.* 69:64–69.

Andersson, H., N. G. Asp, and A. Bruce. 2001. Health effects of probiotics and prebiotics. A literature review on human studies. *Scand. J. Nutr.* 45:48–75.

Backhed, F., H. Ding, T. Wang, L. V. Hooper, G. Y. Koh, A. Nagy, C. F. Semenkovich, and J. I. Gordon. 2004. The gut microbiota as an environmental factor that regulates fat storage. *Proc. Natl. Acad. Sci. USA* 101:15718–15723.

Backhed, F., J. F. Manchester, C. F. Semenkovich, and J. I. Gordon. 2007. Mechanisms underlying the resistance to diet-induced obesity in germ-free mice. *Proc. Natl. Acad. Sci. USA* 104:979–984.

Balcazar-Munoz, B. R., E. Martinez-Abundis, and M. Gonzalez-Ortiz. 2003. Effect of oral inulin administration on lipid profile and insulin sensitivity in dyslipidemic obese subjects. *Rev. Med. Chil.* 131:597–604.

Battilana, P., K. Ornstein, K. Minehira, J. M. Schwarz, K. Acheson, P. Schneiter, J. Burri, E. Jequier, and L. Tappy. 2001. Mechanisms of action of beta-glucan in postprandial glucose metabolism in healthy men. *Eur. J. Clin. Nutr.* 55:327–333.

Beylot, M. 2005. Effects of inulin-type fructans on lipid metabolism in man and in animal models. *Br. J. Nutr.* 93(Suppl. 1): S163–S168.

Brighenti, F., M. C. Casiraghi, E. Canzi, and A. Ferrari. 1999. Effect of consumption of a ready-to-eat breakfast cereal containing inulin on the intestinal milieu and blood lipids in healthy male volunteers. *Eur. J. Clin. Nutr.* 53:726–733.

Busserolles, J., E. Gueux, E. Rock, C. Demigne, A. Mazur, and Y. Rayssiguier. 2003. Oligofructose protects against the hypertriglyceridemic and pro-oxidative effects of a high fructose diet in rats. *J. Nutr.* 133:1903–1908.

Cani, P. D., C. Dewever, and N. M. Delzenne. 2004. Inulin-type fructans modulate gastrointestinal peptides involved in appetite regulation (glucagon-like peptide-1 and ghrelin) in rats. *Br. J. Nutr.* 92:521–526.

Cani, P. D., C. Knauf, M. A. Iglesias, D. J. Drucker, N. M. Delzenne, and R. Burcelin. 2006. Improvement of glucose tolerance and hepatic insulin sensitivity by oligofructose requires a functional glucagon-like peptide 1 receptor. *Diabetes* 55:1484–1490.

Cani, P. D., J. Amar, M. A. Iglesias, M. Poggi, C. Knauf, D. Bastelica, A. M. Neyrinck, F. Fava, K. M. Tuohy, C. Chabo, A. Waget, E. Delmee, B. Cousin, T. Sulpice, B. Chamontin, J. Ferrieres, J. F. Tanti, G. R. Gibson, L. Casteilla, N. M. Delzenne, M. C. Alessi, and R. Burcelin. 2007a. Metabolic endotoxemia initiates obesity and insulin resistance. *Diabetes* **56**:1761–1772.

Cani, P. D., S. Hoste, Y. Guiot, and N. M. Delzenne. 2007b. Dietary non-digestible carbohydrates promote L-cell differentiation in the proximal colon of rats. *Br. J. Nutr.* **98**: 32–37.

Cani, P. D., A. M. Neyrinck, F. Fava, C. Knauf, R. G. Burcelin, K. M. Tuohy, F. K. Gibbons, and N. M. Delzenne. 2007c. Selective increases of bifidobacteria in gut microflora improve high-fat diet-induced diabetes in mice through a mechanism associated with endotoxaemia. *Diabetologia* **50**:2374–2380.

Causey, J. L., J. M. Feirtag, D. D. Gallaher, B. C. Tungland, and J. L. Slavin. 2000. Effects of dietary inulin on serum lipids, blood glucose, and the gastrointestinal environment in hypercholesterolemic men. *Nutr. Res.* **20**:191–201.

Cheng, H. H., and M. H. Lai. 2000. Fermentation of resistant rice starch produces propionate reducing serum and hepatic cholesterol in rats. *J. Nutr.* **130**:1991–1995.

Daubioul, C., N. Rousseau, R. Demeure, B. Gallez, H. Taper, B. Declerck, and N. Delzenne. 2002. Dietary fructans, but not cellulose, decrease triglyceride accumulation in the liver of obese Zucker fa/fa rats. *J. Nutr.* **132**:967–973.

Daubioul, C. A., Y. Horsmans, P. Lambert, E. Danse, and N. M. Delzenne. 2005. Effects of oligofructose on glucose and lipid metabolism in patients with nonalcoholic steatohepatitis: results of a pilot study. *Eur. J. Clin. Nutr.* **59**:723–726.

Daubioul, C. A., H. S. Taper, L. D. De Wispelaere, and N. M. Delzenne. 2000. Dietary oligofructose lessens hepatic steatosis, but does not prevent hypertriglyceridemia in obese zucker rats. *J. Nutr.* **130**:1314–1319.

Davidson, M. H., K. C. Maki, C. Synecki, S. A. Torri, and K. B. Drennan. 1998. Effects of dietary inulin on serum lipids in men and women with hypercholesterolemia. *Nutr. Res.* **18**:503–517.

Delmée, E., P. D. Cani, G. Gual, C. Knauf, R. Burcelin, N. Maton, and N. M. Delzenne. 2006. Relation between colonic proglucagon expression and metabolic response to oligofructose in high fat diet-fed mice. *Life Sci.* **79**:1007–1013.

Delzenne, N. M., and N. Kok. 1998. Effect of non-digestible fermentable carbohydrates on hepatic fatty acid metabolism. *Biochem. Soc. Trans.* **26**:228–230.

Delzenne, N. M., and C. Williams. 1999. Actions of non-digestible carbohydrates on blood lipids in humans and animals, p. 213–232. *In* G. Gibson, and M. Roberfroid (ed.), *Colonic Microbiota, Nutrition and Health.* Kluwer Academic Publisher, Dordrecht, The Netherlands.

Delzenne, N. M., and N. Kok. 2001. Effects of fructans-type prebiotics on lipid metabolism. *Am. J. Clin. Nutr.* **73**:456S–458S.

Delzenne, N. M., and C. M. Williams. 2002. Prebiotics and lipid metabolism. *Curr. Opin. Lipidol.* **13**:61–67.

Delzenne, N. M., C. Daubioul, A. Neyrinck, M. Lasa, and H. S. Taper. 2002. Inulin and oligofructose modulate lipid metabolism in animals: review of biochemical events and future prospects. *Br. J. Nutr.* **87**(Suppl. 2):S255–S259.

Delzenne, N., and P. D. Cani. 2005. A place for dietary fibres in the management of metabolic syndrome. *Curr. Opin. Clin. Nutr. Metab. Care* **8**:638–640.

Delzenne, N. M., P. D. Cani, and A. Neyrinck. 2007. Modulation of glucagon-like peptide 1 and energy metabolism by inulin and oligofructose: experimental data. *J. Nutr.* **137**(11 Suppl.):2547S–2551S.

Demigne, C., C. Morand, M. A. Levrat, C. Besson, C. Moundras, and C. Remesy. 1995. Effect of propionate on fatty acid and cholesterol synthesis and on acetate metabolism in isolated rat hepatocytes. *Br. J. Nutr.* **74**:209–219.

Demigne, C., C. Remesy, and C. Morand. 1999. Short chain fatty acids, p. 55–63. *In* G. Gibson and M. Roberfroid (ed.), *Colonic Microbiota, Nutrition and Health.* Kluwer Academic Publisher, Dordrecht, The Netherlands.

Diez, M., J. L. Hornick, P. Baldwin, and L. Istasse. 1997. Influence of a blend of fructo-oligosaccharides and sugar beet fiber on nutrient digestibility and plasma metabolite concentrations in healthy beagles. *Am. J. Vet. Res.* **58**:1238–1242.

Fabian, E., and I. Elmadfa. 2006. Influence of daily consumption of probiotic and conventional yoghurt on the plasma lipid profile in young healthy women. *Ann. Nutr. Metab.* **50**:387–393.

Fava, F., J. A. Lovegrove, R. Gitau, K. G. Jackson, and K. M. Tuohy. 2006. The gut microbiota and lipid metabolism: implications for human health and coronary heart disease. *Curr. Med. Chem.* **13**:3005–3021.

Ferchaud-Roucher, V., E. Pouteau, H. Piloquet, Y. Zair, and M. Krempf. 2005. Colonic fermentation from lactulose inhibits lipolysis in overweight subjects. *Am. J. Physiol. Endocrinol. Metab.* **289**:E716–E720.

Ferre, P., and F. Foufelle. 2007. SREBP-1c transcription factor and lipid homeostasis: clinical perspective. *Horm. Res.* **68**:72–82.

Fiordaliso, M., N. Kok, J. P. Desager, F. Goethals, D. Deboyser, M. Roberfroid, and N. Delzenne. 1995. Dietary oligofructose lowers triglycerides, phospholipids and cholesterol in serum and very low density lipoproteins of rats. *Lipids* **30**:163–167.

Forcheron, F., and M. Beylot. 2007. Long-term administration of inulin-type fructans has no significant lipid-lowering effect in normolipidemic humans. *Metabolism* **56**:1093–1098.

Fukushima, M., T. Ohashi, M. Kojima, K. Ohba, H. Shimizu, K. Sonoyama, and M. Nakano. 2001. Low density lipoprotein receptor mRNA in rat liver is affected by resistant starch of beans. *Lipids* **36**:129–134.

Gallaher, D. D., C. M. Gallaher, G. J. Mahrt, T. P. Carr, C. H. Hollingshead, R. Hesslink, Jr., and J. Wise. 2002. A glucomannan and chitosan fiber supplement decreases plasma cholesterol and increases cholesterol excretion in overweight normocholesterolemic humans. *J. Am. Coll. Nutr.* **21**:428–433.

Giacco, R., G. Clemente, D. Luongo, G. Lasorella, I. Fiume, F. Brouns, F. Bornet, L. Patti, P. Cipriano, A. A. Rivellese, and G. Riccardi. 2004. Effects of short-chain fructo-oligosaccharides on glucose and lipid metabolism in mild hypercholesterolaemic individuals. *Clin. Nutr.* **23**:331–340.

Griffiths, E. A., L. C. Duffy, F. L. Schanbacher, H. Qiao, D. Dryja, A. Leavens, J. Rossman, G. Rich, D. Dirienzo, and P. L. Ogra. 2004. In vivo effects of bifidobacteria and lactoferrin on gut endotoxin concentration and mucosal immunity in Balb/c mice. *Dig. Dis. Sci.* **49:**579–589.

Havenaar, R., S. Bonnin-Marol, W. Van Dokkum, S. Petitet, and G. Schaafsma. 1999. Inulin: fermentation and microbial ecology in the intestinal tract. *Food Rev. Int.* **15:**109–120.

Hidaka, H., Y. Tashiro, and T. Eida. 1991. Proliferation of bifidobacteria by oligosaccharides and their useful effect on human health. *Bifidobacteria Microflora* **10:**65–79.

Higgins, J. A., M. A. Brown, and L. H. Storlien. 2006. Consumption of resistant starch decreases postprandial lipogenesis in white adipose tissue of the rat. *Nutr. J.* **5:**25.

Hokfelt, T., C. Broberger, M. Diez, Z. Q. Xu, T. Shi, J. Kopp, X. Zhang, K. Holmberg, M. Landry, and J. Koistinaho. 1999. Galanin and NPY, two peptides with multiple putative roles in the nervous system. *Horm. Metab. Res.* **31:**330–334.

Jackson, K. G., G. R. J. Taylor, A. M. Clohessy, and C. M. Williams. 1999. The effect of the daily intake of inulin on fasting lipid, insulin and glucose concentrations in middle-aged men and women. *Br. J. Nutr.* **82:**23–30.

Jenkins, D. J., and C. W. Kendall. 2000. Resistant starches. *Curr. Opin. Gastroenterol.* **16:**178–183.

Jenkins, D. J., V. Vuksan, C. W. Kendall, P. Wursch, R. Jeffcoat, S. Waring, C. C. Mehling, E. Vidgen, L. S. Augustin, and E. Wong. 1998. Physiological effects of resistant starches on fecal bulk, short chain fatty acids, blood lipids and glycemic index. *J. Am. Coll. Nutr.* **17:**609–616.

Jenkins, D. J., V. Vuksan, A. V. Rao, E. Vidgen, C. W. Kendall, N. Tariq, P. Wursch, B. Koellreutter, N. Shiwnarain, and R. Jeffcoat. 1999. Colonic bacterial activity and serum lipid risk factors for cardiovascular disease. *Metabolism* **48:**264–268.

Kang, S. A., K. Hong, K. H. Jang, Y. Y. Kim, R. Choue, and Y. Lim. 2006. Altered mRNA expression of hepatic lipogenic enzyme and PPARalpha in rats fed dietary levan from *Zymomonas mobilis. J. Nutr. Biochem.* **17:**419–426.

Kok, N., M. Roberfroid, and N. Delzenne. 1996. Dietary oligofructose modifies the impact of fructose on hepatic triacylglycerol metabolism. *Metabolism* **45:**1547–1550.

Lerer-Metzger, M., S. W. Rizkalla, J. Luo, M. Champ, M. Kabir, F. Bruzzo, F. Bornet, and G. Slama. 1996. Effects of long-term low-glycaemic index starchy food on plasma glucose and lipid concentrations and adipose tissue cellularity in normal and diabetic rats. *Br. J. Nutr.* **75:**723–732.

Letexier, D., F. Diraison, and M. Beylot. 2003. Addition of inulin to a moderately high-carbohydrate diet reduces hepatic lipogenesis and plasma triacylglycerol concentrations in humans. *Am. J. Clin. Nutr.* **77:**559–564.

Levrat, M. A., M. L. Favier, C. Moundras, C. Remesy, C. Demigne, and C. Morand. 1994. Role of dietary propionic acid and bile acid excretion in the hypocholesterolemic effects of oligosaccharides in rats. *J. Nutr.* **124:**531–538.

Levrat, M. A., C. Remesy, and C. Demigne. 1991. High propionic acid fermentations and mineral accumulation in the cecum of rats adapted to different levels of inulin. *J. Nutr.* **121:**1730–1737.

Ley, R. E., F. Backhed, P. Turnbaugh, C. A. Lozupone, R. D. Knight, and J. I. Gordon. 2005. Obesity alters gut microbial ecology. *Proc. Natl. Acad. Sci. USA* **102:**11070–11075.

Ley, R. E., P. J. Turnbaugh, S. Klein, and J. I. Gordon. 2006. Microbial ecology: human gut microbes associated with obesity. *Nature* **444:**1022–1023.

Lopez, H. W., M. A. Levrat, C. Guy, A. Messager, C. Demigne, and C. Remesy. 1999. Effects of soluble corn bran arabinoxylans on cecal digestion, lipid metabolism, and mineral balance (Ca, Mg) in rats. *J. Nutr. Biochem.* **10:**500–509.

Lopez, H. W., M. A. Levrat-Verny, C. Coudray, C. Besson, V. Krespine, A. Messager, C. Demigne, and C. Remesy. 2001. Class 2 resistant starches lower plasma and liver lipids and improve mineral retention in rats. *J. Nutr.* **131:**1283–1289.

Lovegrove, J. A., A. Clohessy, H. Milon, and C. M. Williams. 2000. Modest doses of beta-glucan do not reduce concentrations of potentially atherogenic lipoproteins. *Am. J. Clin. Nutr.* **72:**49–55.

Luo, J., S. W. Rizkalla, C. Alamowitch, A. Boussairi, A. Blayo, J. L. Barry, A. Laffitte, F. Guyon, F. R. Bornet, and G. Slama. 1996. Chronic consumption of short-chain fructooligosaccharides by healthy subjects decreased basal hepatic glucose production but had no effect on insulin-stimulated glucose metabolism. *Am. J. Clin. Nutr.* **63:**939–945.

Luo, J., M. Van Yperselle, S. W. Rizkalla, F. Rossi, F. R. Bornet, and G. Slama. 2000. Chronic consumption of short-chain fructooligosaccharides does not affect basal hepatic glucose production or insulin resistance in type 2 diabetics. *J. Nutr.* **130:**1572–1577.

McNaught, C. E., and J. MacFie. 2001. Probiotics in clinical practice: a critical review of the evidence. *Nurs. Res.* **21:**343–353.

Morrison, D. J., W. G. Mackay, C. A. Edwards, T. Preston, B. Dodson, and L. T. Weaver. 2006. Butyrate production from oligofructose fermentation by the human faecal flora: what is the contribution of extracellular acetate and lactate? *Br. J. Nutr.* **96:**570–577.

Mortensen, A., M. Poulsen, and H. Frandsen. 2002. Effect of a long-chained fructan Raftiline HP on blood lipids and spontaneous atherosclerosis in low density receptor knockout mice. *Nutr. Res.* **22:**473–480.

Pedersen, A., B. Sandstrom, and J. M. M. VanAmelsvoort. 1997. The effect of ingestion of inulin on blood lipids and gastrointestinal symptoms in healthy females. *Br. J. Nutr.* **78:**215–222.

Pomeroy, S., R. Tupper, M. Cehun-Aders, and P. Nestel. 2001. Oat beta-glucan lowers total and LDL-cholesterol. *Aust. J. Nutr. Diet.* **58:**51–55.

Queenan, K. M., M. L. Stewart, K. N. Smith, W. Thomas, R. G. Fulcher, and J. L. Slavin. 2007. Concentrated oat beta-glucan, a fermentable fiber, lowers serum cholesterol in hypercholesterolemic adults in a randomized controlled trial. *Nutr. J.* **6:**6.

Rault-Nania, M. H., E. Gueux, C. Demougeot, C. Demigne, E. Rock, and A. Mazur. 2006. Inulin attenuates atherosclerosis in apolipoprotein E-deficient mice. *Br. J. Nutr.* **96:**840–844.

Rawls, J. F., M. A. Mahowald, R. E. Ley, and J. I. Gordon. 2006. Reciprocal gut microbiota transplants from zebrafish and mice to germ-free recipients reveal host habitat selection. *Cell* **127:**423–433.

Roberfroid, M. B., and N. M. Delzenne. 1998. Dietary fructans. *Annu. Rev. Nutr.* **18**:117–143.

Sakakibara, S., T. Yamauchi, Y. Oshima, Y. Tsukamoto, and T. Kadowaki. 2006. Acetic acid activates hepatic AMPK and reduces hyperglycemia in diabetic KK-A(y) mice. *Biochem. Biophys. Res. Commun.* **344**:597–604.

Schaafsma, G., W. J. Meuling, W. Van Dokkum, and C. Bouley. 1998. Effects of a milk product, fermented by *Lactobacillus acidophilus* and with fructo-oligosaccharides added, on blood lipids in male volunteers. *Eur. J. Clin. Nutr.* **52**:436–440.

Scheppach, W., H. Luehrs, and T. Menzel. 2001. Beneficial health effects of low-digestible carbohydrate consumption. *Br. J. Nutr.* **85**(Suppl. 1):S23–S30.

Slavin, J. L. 2005. Dietary fiber and body weight. *Nutrition* **21**:411–418.

St Onge, M. P., E. R. Farnworth, and P. J. Jones. 2000. Consumption of fermented and nonfermented dairy products: effects on cholesterol concentrations and metabolism. *Am. J. Clin. Nutr.* **71**:674–681.

Sugatani, J., T. Wada, M. Osabe, K. Yamakawa, K. Yoshinari, and M. Miwa. 2006. Dietary inulin alleviates hepatic steatosis and xenobiotics-induced liver injury in rats fed a high-fat and high-sucrose diet: association with the suppression of hepatic cytochrome P450 and hepatocyte nuclear factor 4alpha expression. *Drug. Metab. Dispos.* **34**:1677–1687.

Takase, S., T. Goda, and M. Watanabe. 1994. Monostearoylglycerol-starch complex: its digestibility and effects on glycemic and lipogenic responses. *J. Nutr. Sci. Vitaminol.* (Tokyo) **40**:23–36.

Taylor, G. R. J., and C. M. Williams. 1998. Effects of probiotics and prebiotics on blood lipids. *Br. J. Nutr.* **80**:S225–S230.

Tokunaga, T., T. Oku, and N. Hosoya. 1986. Influence of chronic intake of new sweetener fructooligosaccharide (Neosugar) on growth and gastrointestinal function of the rat. *J. Nutr. Sci. Vitaminol.* (Tokyo) **32**:111–121.

Trautwein, E. A., K. Forgbert, D. Rieckhoff, and H. F. Erbersdobler. 1999. Impact of beta-cyclodextrin and resistant starch on bile acid metabolism and fecal steroid excretion in regard to their hypolipidemic action in hamsters. *Biochim. Biophys. Acta* **1437**:1–12.

Trautwein, E. A., D. Rieckhoff, and H. F. Erbersdobler. 1998. Dietary inulin lowers plasma cholesterol and triacylglycerol and alters biliary bile acid profile in hamsters. *J. Nutr.* **128**:1937–1943.

Turnbaugh, P. J., R. E. Ley, M. A. Mahowald, V. Magrini, E. R. Mardis, and J. I. Gordon. 2006. An obesity-associated gut microbiome with increased capacity for energy harvest. *Nature* **444**:1027–1031.

Usman, K. E., and A. Hosono. 2000. Effect of administration of *Lactobacillus gasseri* on serum lipids and fecal steroids in hypercholesterolemic rats. *J. Dairy Sci.* **83**:1705–1711.

Vogt, J. A., K. B. Ishii-Schrade, P. B. Pencharz, P. J. Jones, and T. M. Wolever. 2006. L-rhamnose and lactulose decrease serum triacylglycerols and their rates of synthesis, but do not affect serum cholesterol concentrations in men. *J. Nutr.* **136**:2160–2166.

Wang, Z., G. Xiao, Y. Yao, S. Guo, K. Lu, and Z. Sheng. 2006. The role of bifidobacteria in gut barrier function after thermal injury in rats. *J. Trauma* **61**:650–657.

Wang, Z. T., Y. M. Yao, G. X. Xiao, and Z. Y. Sheng. 2004. Risk factors of development of gut-derived bacterial translocation in thermally injured rats. *World J. Gastroenterol.* **10**:1619–1624.

Whelan, K., G. R. Gibson, P. A. Judd, and M. A. Taylor. 2001. The role of probiotics and prebiotics in the management of diarrhoea associated with enteral tube feeding. *J. Hum. Nutr. Diet.* **14**:423–433.

Williams, C. M., and K. G. Jackson. 2002. Inulin and oligofructose: effects on lipid metabolism from human studies. *Br. J. Nutr.* **87**:S261–S264.

Xiong, Y., N. Miyamoto, K. Shibata, M. A. Valasek, T. Motoike, R. M. Kedzierski, and M. Yanagisawa. 2004. Short-chain fatty acids stimulate leptin production in adipocytes through the G protein-coupled receptor GPR41. *Proc. Natl. Acad. Sci. USA* **101**:1045–1050.

Yamamoto, Y., Y. Takahashi, M. Kawano, M. Iizuka, T. Matsumoto, S. Saeki, and H. Yamaguchi. 1999. In vitro digestibility and fermentability of levan and its hypocholesterolemic effects in rats. *J. Nutr. Biochem.* **10**:13–18.

Yamashita, K., M. Itakura, and K. Kawai. 1984. Effects of fructo-oligosaccharides on blood glucose and serum lipids in diabetic subjects. *Nutr. Res.* **4**:961–966.

Therapeutic Microbiology: Probiotics and Related Strategies
Edited by J. Versalovic and M. Wilson
© 2008 ASM Press, Washington, DC

2.4. GENOMICS OF LACTIC ACID BACTERIA

Tri Duong
Todd R. Klaenhammer

15

Functional Genomics of Lactic Acid Bacteria

The lactic acid bacteria (LAB) are a diverse group of microorganisms related by their common metabolic and physiological characteristics and named for the major end product of their primary metabolism. While not a taxonomical classification, the LAB are composed of various genera primarily of the order *Lactobacillales* (Fig. 1). The LAB are gram-positive, acid-tolerant, anaerobic, nonsporulating bacteria found naturally in a wide range of environments including dairy products, meats, and vegetable and plant matter and associated with animal/human mucosal surfaces. Metabolically, LAB can be classified according to the hexose fermentation pathway used as part of their primary metabolism. Homofermentative LAB use the Embden-Meyerhof-Parnas pathway, producing primarily lactic acid, while heterofermentative LAB utilize the pentose phosphoketolase pathway to produce lactic acid (~50%), acetic acid, ethanol, carbon dioxide, and formic acid.

The LAB are important in the production and preservation of foods because of their abilities to produce lactic acid and impart important flavor, texture, and nutritional properties (Stiles, 1996). These microbes are used as starter cultures for the fermentation of dairy products, meats, and vegetables and are also important for the production of coffee, chocolate, and wine. In addition to their role in food production, the LAB are involved in the production of bulk ingredients and fine chemicals as well. L-Lactic acid is an important building block for the synthesis of biodegradable polymers and is the substrate for the production of other compounds such as propionic acid, acrylic acid, acetic acid, propylene glycol, ethanol, and acetaldehyde.

The long history of use and consumption of LAB by humans has resulted in their formal status as "generally recognized as safe" (GRAS) organisms. LAB have long been considered beneficial to human health. The lactobacilli, in particular, occupy important niches in the gastrointestinal (GI) tracts of humans and animals and are increasingly recognized as modulators of human and animal health. Currently, LAB are used as functional food ingredients in numerous probiotic products. This segment of the food and pharmaceutical industry has

Tri Duong, Genomic Sciences Graduate Program, Department of Food, Bioprocessing and Nutrition Sciences, North Carolina State University, Raleigh, NC 27695. **Todd R. Klaenhammer**, Dept. of Food, Bioprocessing and Nutrition Sciences, and Southeast Dairy Foods Research Center, North Carolina State University, Raleigh, NC 27695.

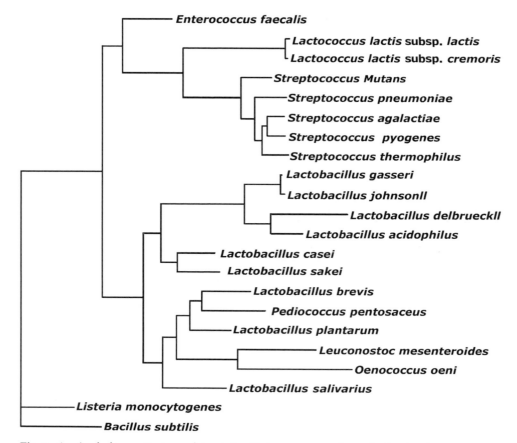

Figure 1 A phylogenetic tree of *Lactobacillales* constructed on the basis of concatenated alignments of genes encoding four subunits of the DNA-dependent RNA polymerase. Reprinted from *Journal of Bacteriology* (Makarova and Koonin, 2007) with permission of the publisher.

been rapidly expanding due to increased public awareness of the role of nutrition and microbiota in maintaining health. Recently, engineered strains of LAB have been employed as oral delivery vectors for vaccines and other biotherapeutics (Braat et al., 2006; Wells et al., 1996).

Recently, major advances have been made in the genomic characterization of the LAB. A number of LAB genomes have been sequenced and are publicly available, while more genomes are being sequenced. Genome features of sequenced LAB appear in Table 1. The LAB are low-GC organisms, between 33 and 50%, with relatively small genomes, ranging in size from 1.78 Mb for *Oenococcus oeni* to 3.31 Mb for *Lactobacillus plantarum* (Table 1). The availability of genome sequences has enabled researchers to study and compare the genomic content of these organisms, providing insights into the

evolution, physiology, and metabolism underlying their beneficial functionalities.

COMPARATIVE AND EVOLUTIONARY GENOMIC ANALYSIS

The loss and decay of ancestral genes have played a major role in the evolution of these organisms. Phyletic reconstruction suggests that the common ancestor of the *Lactobacillales* had 2,100 to 2,200 genes and incurred a loss of 600 to 1,200 genes after the divergence from the *Bacilli*. Many of the genes lost in lactobacilli, particularly those relating to cofactor biosynthesis and sporulation, are indicative of a shift in lifestyle to a nutrient-rich environment (Makarova and Koonin, 2007). Comparisons with pathogenic streptococci

Table 1 Features of sequenced LAB genomes

Species and strain	Size (Mb)	%GC	No. of proteins	No. of plasmids	No. of prophages	Relevance/use	Reference
Lactobacillus acidophilus NCFM	1.99	34.7	1,864	0	0	GI/probiotic tract	Altermann et al., 2005
Lactobacillus brevis ATCC 367	2.34	46.1	2,221	2	1	Plant/meat fermentation	Makarova et al., 2006a
Lactobacillus casei ATCC 334	2.92	46.6	2,776	1	2	Dairy fermentation (cheese)	Makarova et al., 2006a
L. delbrueckii subsp. *bulgaricus* ATCC 11842	1.86	49.7	1,562	1	0	Dairy fermentation (yogurt)	van de Guchte et al., 2006
L. delbrueckii subsp. *bulgaricus* ATCC BAA-365	1.86	49.7	1,721	0	0	Dairy fermentation (yogurt)	Makarova et al., 2006a
Lactobacillus gasseri ATCC 33323	1.89	35.3	1,755	0	1	GI tract/probiotic	Makarova et al., 2006a
L. johnsonii NCC 533	1.99	34.6	1,821	0	2	GI tract/probiotic	Pridmore et al., 2004
L. plantarum WCFS1	3.31	44.5	3,009	3	2	Plant/meat fermentation	Kleerebezem et al., 2003
Lactobacillus sakei 23K	1.88	41.3	1,879	0	0	Meat fermentation	Chaillou et al., 2005
L. salivarius subsp. *salivarius* UCC 118	1.83	33.0	1,717	3	2	GI tract/probiotic	Claesson et al., 2006
L. lactis subsp. *cremoris* MG1363	2.50	35.7	2,434	0	2	Dairy fermentation (cheese)	Wegmann et al., 2007
L. lactis subsp. *cremoris* SK11	2.40	35.9	2,384	5	4	Dairy fermentation (cheese)	Makarova et al., 2006a
L. lactis subsp. *lactis* IL1403	2.37	35.4	2,310	0	6	Dairy fermentation (cheese)	Bolotin et al., 2001
Leuconostoc mesenteroides subsp. *mesenteroides* ATCC 8293	2.08	37.7	2,009	1	1	Plant fermentation	Makarova et al., 2006a
O. oeni PSU-1	1.78	37.9	1,701	0	0	Wine fermentation	Makarova et al., 2006a
Pediococcus pentosaceus ATCC 25745	1.83	37.4	1,757	0	2	Plant/meat fermentation	Makarova et al., 2006a
S. thermophilus CNRZ1066	1.80	39.1	1,915	0	1	Dairy fermentation (yogurt)	Bolotin et al., 2004
S. thermophilus LMD-9	1.86	39.1	1,710	2	1	Dairy fermentation (yogurt)	Makarova et al., 2006a
S. thermophilus LMG183111	1.80	39.0	1,889	0	0	Dairy fermentation (yogurt)	Bolotin et al., 2004

suggest that *Streptococcus thermophilus* adapted to a dairy environment through gene decay (10% pseudogenes) and gene loss, particularly the loss of virulence determinants relating to adhesion and antibiotic resistance. The presence of a specific lactose symporter absent from pathogenic streptococci further corroborates the adaptation of *S. thermophilus* to life in a dairy environ-

ment and supports its GRAS status for use in foods (Bolotin et al., 2004). The genome sequence of *Lactobacillus delbrueckii* subsp. *bulgaricus* (*L. bulgaricus*) revealed the presence of an unusually high number of pseudogenes (17%), suggesting an ongoing process of evolution through gene degradation (van de Guchte et al., 2006). *L. bulgaricus* was also found to share significant synteny

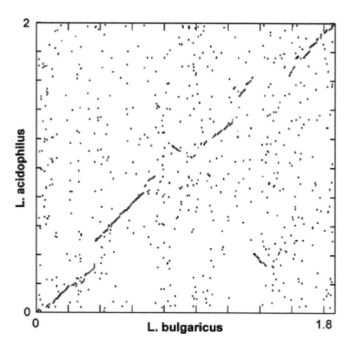

Figure 2 Synteny between *L. bulgaricus* and *L. acidophilus* genomes. *x* axis, position on *L. bulgaricus* genome (unit, megabase pairs); *y* axis, position on *L. acidophilus* genome (unit, megabase pairs). 0, replication origin. Dots indicate windows of significant protein similarity by BLAST scores. Adapted from *Proceedings of the National Academy of Sciences of the United States of America* (van de Guchte et al., 2006) with permission of the publisher.

with *Lactobacillus acidophilus* (Fig. 2) and *Lactobacillus johnsonii*. BLAST analyses indicate that ~55 to 60% of *L. bulgaricus* proteins have homologs in *L. acidophilus* and *L. johnsonii*. Genes encoding homologous proteins constitute the common backbone of these related genomes. Differences in gene content reflect their respective ecological niches and involve genes related to the biosynthesis of cofactors and fatty acids, carbohydrate transport and metabolism, and predicted intestinal functions (e.g., bile salt hydrolase and mucin binding proteins) which are absent in *L. bulgaricus* (van de Guchte et al., 2006).

Gene gain through horizontal gene transfer or gene duplication appears to have contributed to the evolution of LAB. *L. plantarum's* ability to utilize a wide range of carbohydrates and reside in diverse environments is reflected in the relatively large size of its genome. Many genes for carbohydrate transport and metabolism are clustered in a region of lower GC content, suggesting that many of these genes were acquired by horizontal gene transfer (Kleerebezem et al., 2003). Horizontal gene

transfer appears to have been important in the adaptation of LAB to environmental niches. Plasmid conjugation was clearly responsible for the transfer of genes related to growth of *Lactococcus lactis* in milk (McKay, 1983; Siezen et al., 2005). Particularly, genes related to lactose metabolism and proteolysis have been shown to be carried on plasmids (McKay, 1983).

The 2.13-Mb genome of *Lactobacillus salivarius* UCC 118 is composed of a 1.83-Mb chromosome, a 242-kb megaplasmid, and two smaller plasmids. While no essential genes appear to be carried on the megaplasmid, it is predicted to confer a number of metabolic capabilities and traits related to GI tract survival and competitiveness including bacteriocin production and heterofermentative traits. Additionally, the variation in megaplasmid size found in other *L. salivarius* strains suggests that this multireplicon architecture provides the species with a flexible genetic complement and a possible mechanism for adaptation to different environments via genome expansion or contraction (Claesson et al., 2006).

PHAGE GENOMICS

The era of genomics began with the sequencing of the genome of bacteriophage φX174 in 1977 (Sanger et al., 1977). Bacteriophages (phages) are viruses that infect prokaryotes and can enter either a lytic or lysogenic life cycle. A lytic phage infection results in phage replication followed by cell lysis. During a lysogenic infection the viral genome integrates into host DNA and replicates harmlessly until host conditions deteriorate. At that time, the integrated phage (prophage) may be induced, initiating an active lytic infection (Sturino and Klaenhammer, 2006).

A lytic phage infection during a fermentation process can result in loss of efficiency and product quality. Because of their economic impact on industrial dairy fermentations, many virulent and temperate phages that infect LAB have been isolated and sequenced (Brussow and Desiere, 2001). Comparative genomic analyses of *S. thermophilus* phages revealed four independently evolving modules encoding specific phage-related functions (Brussow and Desiere, 2001; Lucchini et al., 1999). The analysis of phage genomes has streamlined the selection of targets for the development of phage defense systems (Sturino and Klaenhammer, 2006). Specifically, genes in the DNA replication module of *S. thermophilus* phages were highly conserved. Expression of antisense RNA complementary to the helicase (Sturino and Klaenhammer, 2002) and primase (Sturino and Klaenhammer, 2004) genes provided effective phage protection for one of the two major *S. thermophilus* phage groups. Comparative genomic analyses of closely related *S. thermophilus* strains revealed genetic polymorphisms concentrated in loci called Clustered Regularly Interspaced Short Palindromic Repeats (CRISPR) (Bolotin et al., 2004), consisting of several noncontiguous direct repeats separated by variable spacer regions (Jansen et al., 2002). In silico analyses of these regions revealed sequence homologies with foreign DNA elements including plasmids and phages, suggesting their extrachromosomal origins (Bolotin et al., 2005). Functional analyses of these regions along with CRISPR-associated (*cas*) genes suggest a possible mechanism of phage resistance in which specificity is mediated by the CRISPR spacer content and resistance is provided by the *cas* genes (Barrangou et al., 2007) possibly through a mechanism based on RNA interference (Makarova et al., 2006a, 2006b). While further study is required to determine the exact mechanism of action, CRISPR-*cas* systems might be exploited to enhance phage resistance in LAB involved in industrial fermentations.

In addition to their economic importance, phages have had an important impact on bacterial genomes and their evolution. Sequencing has revealed the presence of both intact prophage and phage remnants in the genomes of many LAB, which can comprise a significant portion (3 to 10%) of the gene content of host genomes (Brussow and Hendrix, 2002). As mobile DNA elements, phage DNA can be an efficient vector for horizontal gene transfer between bacteria, having been involved in the transfer of virulence factors among pathogens (Ohnishi et al., 2001). With the increase in metabolic load placed upon the host to replicate prophage DNA, it has been proposed that prophages may contribute to the evolutionary fitness of LAB (Brussow and Hendrix, 2002).

FUNCTIONAL GENOMICS

Whole-genome sequencing and comparative genomic analyses have provided much insight into the genetic content of LAB and offered many clues into possible gene functions. While genomic analyses of LAB have identified features important for the functionality of these organisms in bioprocessing and health (Klaenhammer et al., 2005), further characterization of genes and gene products remains important for understanding cell physiology, metabolic and signaling networks, and molecular interactions of LAB with their environments. This information is rapidly providing a mechanistic understanding of these microorganisms and identifying important gene sets critical to their functionality. Examples include the

discovery of many plasmid elements encoding key fermentative functions in lactococci (McKay, 1983; et al., Siezen et al., 2005) and identification of genes encoding adhesive traits in probiotic lactobacilli (Altermann et al., 2005; Buck et al., 2005; Pridmore et al., 2004). Such traits are absent from *L. bulgaricus* (van de Guchte et al., 2006), which has evolved with milk as its natural habitat.

Gene expression analyses using microarrays have enabled the profiling of gene expression patterns of tens of thousands of genes in a single experiment (Duggan et al., 1999). Global gene expression analysis has been used to study the transcriptional response of LAB to acid stress (Azcarate-Peril et al., 2005; Pieterse et al., 2005), hydrostatic pressure (Pavlovic et al., 2005), and cell-cell signaling (Sturme et al., 2005). Transcriptional analysis of global gene expression in *L. acidophilus* during growth on eight different carbohydrates revealed that genes of the glycolytic pathway, responsible for the conversion of carbohydrates to lactic acid, were among the most highly expressed coding sequences in the genome. Additionally, this analysis identified genes involved in the transport and catabolism of the prebiotics fructo-oligosaccharide (FOS) and raffinose and the metabolism of lactose via the Leloir pathway (Barrangou et al., 2006). The ability of LAB to use substrates not digested by the host, including FOS and raffinose, may contribute to their ability to compete in the GI tract. Functional analysis of FOS utilization in *Lactobacillus paracasei* suggests that FOS may be hydrolyzed extracellularly into fructose and sucrose by a cell wall-bound β-fructosidase with uptake occurring via fructose and sucrose phosphotransferase system transporters (Goh et al., 2006). In contrast, *L. acidophilus* FOS utilization was shown to occur via an ATP-binding cassette (ABC) transporter and an intracellular β-fructosidase, allowing the organism to transport FOS into the cell, where it is hydrolyzed internally (Barrangou et al., 2003). It was suggested that strains able to hydrolyze FOS intracellularly may have a selective advantage relative to organisms that hydrolyze FOS extracellularly. Microarray analyses can also be used to study host responses to LAB. Tao et al. (2006) showed that soluble factors from *Lactobacillus rhamnosus* GG induced heat shock proteins in intestinal epithelial cells.

In addition to gene expression analysis, comparative genomic hybridization using DNA microarrays (Array-CGH) can be used to obtain a detailed comparison of the gene content of closely related microorganisms, particularly in strains of closely related species or of the same species (Murray et al., 2001). Array-CGH was used to compare the genomic content of 20 *L. plantarum* strains, using the genome of the sequenced *L. plantarum* WCFS1

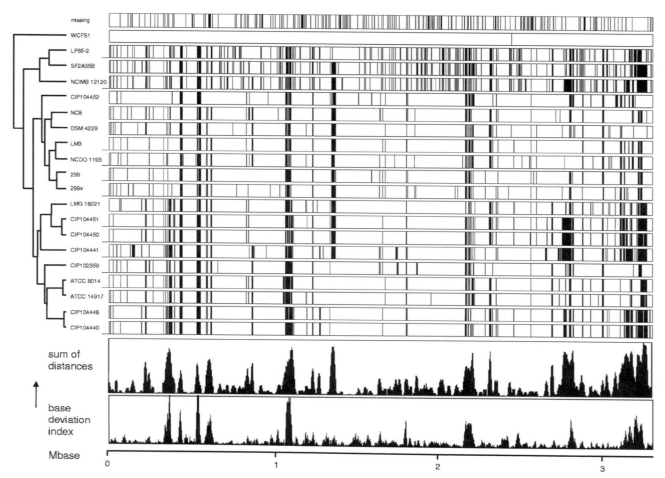

Figure 3 A comparison of the gene contents of 20 *L. plantarum* strains. Strains are indicated on the left. Gene content is indicated in a rectangle mapping onto the *L. plantarum* WCFS1 genome sequence: the presence (no line) and absence (black line) of fragments are indicated. The upper rectangle, labeled "missing," shows in black the fragments of the genome that were not spotted on the microarray. Sum of distances indicates genotypic variation mapping onto the loci of the WCFS1 genome. The lower panel shows the base deviation index along the chromosome of *L. plantarum* WCFS1. A phylogenetic tree of the strains compared is shown on the left. Reprinted from the *Journal of Bacteriology* (Molenaar et al., 2005) with permission of the publisher.

as a reference (Molenaar et al., 2005) (Fig. 3). This study found genes related to biosynthesis or degradation of proteins, nucleotides, and lipids to be very highly conserved among *L. plantarum* strains. While genes related to glycolysis were almost completely conserved, genes involved in the transport and catabolism of specific carbohydrates demonstrated significant variation. Additionally, genes of the pentose phosphate pathway were not conserved. Genes unique to *L. plantarum* WCFS1 were mainly concentrated in two clusters involved in

nonribosomal peptide synthesis and exopolysaccharide biosynthesis. The unusual base composition at these loci suggests that these genes were acquired via horizontal gene transfer. Additionally, the high degree of genomic variation and unusual base composition in two regions of the WCFS1 genome further corroborates their identification as lifestyle adaptation islands (Kleerebezem et al., 2003).

While genome and gene expression analyses have contributed much to the understanding of LAB physiology, gene expression studies in vivo are important in identification of genes important for probiotic functionality. In vivo expression technology has been used in both *Lactobacillus reuteri* (Walter et al., 2003) and *L. plantarum* (Bron, 2004a) in order to identify a total of 75 genes specifically induced during passage through the murine GI tract. In vivo-inducible (*ivi*) genes include coding sequences involved in nutrient metabolism, cofactor and intermediate biosynthesis, and stress responses. Quantitative PCR analyses of 15 *ivi* genes in *L. plantarum* during passage through the mouse GI tract found *copA* and *adhE* to be the most highly induced genes in vivo (Marco et al., 2007). While these genes were upregulated up to 350-fold in the murine GI tract, several genes including four extracellular proteins potentially involved in host-microbe interactions were preferentially induced in the small intestine. Two of these genes encoding an integral membrane protein and argininosuccinate synthase were induced in response to bile salts, suggesting that these genes may be responding to host-derived compounds in the small intestine (Bron, 2004b).

Adherence to the human intestinal epithelium may be required for probiotic effects including immunomodulation (Valeur et al., 2004) and pathogen exclusion (Bernet et al., 1994). Buck et al. (2005) identified five genes in *L. acidophilus* encoding proteins putatively involved in adhesion including two R28 homologs, a fibronectin-binding protein (FbpA), a mucin binding protein (Mub), and a surface layer protein (SlpA). Insertional mutagenesis in these loci identified FbpA, Mub, and SlpA as contributing significantly to adherence of *L. acidophilus* to intestinal epithelial cells (Caco-2) in vitro (Buck et al., 2005).

Lactobacilli altered cytokine profiles and induced maturation of human immune cells (Christensen et al., 2002; Mohamadzadeh et al., 2005). The composition of teichoic acids on the cell surface of *L. plantarum* was shown to affect cytokine expression profiles of peripheral blood mononuclear cells and monocytes (Grangette et al., 2005). Disruption of the *dlt* operon, involved in the D-alanylation of teichoic acids, resulted in reduction of D-alanine incorporation into teichoic acids of the bacterial cell wall. This change in cell wall composition resulted in reduced secretion of proinflammatory cytokines and increased secretion of the anti-inflammatory cytokine interleukin-10 (IL-10) by peripheral blood mononuclear cells when exposed to the mutant lacking *dlt*. Additionally, this mutant was significantly more protective in a murine colitis model than wild-type *L. plantarum*.

METABOLIC ENGINEERING

While the primary contribution to fermentation by LAB is acidification, the production of additional metabolites by LAB contributes to the flavor (diacetyl) and nutrition (B complex vitamins) of fermented food products. An understanding of genes directing important metabolic pathways combined with the tools available for the inactivation of undesirable genes and overexpression of existing or novel genes (de Ruyter et al., 1996) will certainly aid in the production of important food ingredients or food products with improved flavor and nutritional properties.

Folic acid (vitamin B_{11}) is an essential component in the human diet, serving as a cofactor in a number of metabolic reactions including the biosynthesis of nucleotides. The genome sequence of *L. lactis* revealed a gene cluster encoding all of the enzymes of the folic acid biosynthesis pathway (Fig. 4). Using metabolic engineering approaches, Sybesma et al. were able to overexpress *folKE* to increase folic acid production threefold (Sybesma et al., 2003).

VACCINE AND BIOTHERAPEUTIC DELIVERY

Because of their acid tolerance, record of safety, and ability to modulate the immune system, considerable interest has developed for using LAB as live vectors for the delivery of vaccines and other biotherapeutics to the intestinal mucosa (Wells et al., 1996). Oral ingestion of bioactive molecules can result in denaturation, degradation, and loss of biological activity during passage through the stomach. Biotherapeutic molecules can be protected by viable or nonviable cells for their eventual release in the small intestine. Orally administered recombinant *L. lactis* expressing tetanus toxin fragment C was able to elicit a potent immune response in mice (Robinson et al., 1997). Using tetanus toxin fragment C as a model antigen, Grangette et al. (2004) were able to show that alanine racemase mutants (lacking *alr*) of *L. plantarum* and *L. lactis* were dramatically more immunogenic than their wild-type counterparts when administered orally or vaginally to mice. *L. lactis* secreting IL-10 was shown to decrease GI inflammatory responses of mice with colitis, demonstrating the potential of LAB for the delivery of biotherapeutic compounds. More recently, researchers have developed recombinant *Lactobacillus jensenii* expressing cyanovirin-N, a potent antiviral compound, to interfere with the infectivity of human immunodeficiency virus in vitro (Liu et al., 2006).

A

Purine Metabolism

GTP

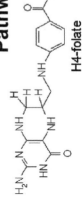
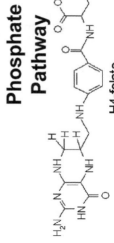

folE GTP Cyclohydrolase

HCOO⁻

H2-neopterintriphosphate

Pase

PPi
Pi

H2-neopterin

folB H2-neopterinaldolase

HOCH2CHO

6-Hydroxymethyl-H2-pterin

folK

AMP ATP
6-Hydroxymethyl-H2-pterinpyrophosphokinase

6-Hydroxymethyl-H2-pterinpyrophosphate

Glycolysis

Pentose Phosphate Pathway

Shikimate Pathway

chorismate

p-Aminobenzoate

H2-pteroate synthase *folP*

PPi

H2-pteroate

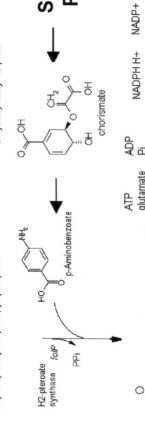
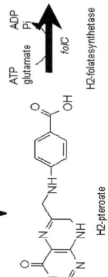

ATP
glutamate
folC

ADP
Pi

H2-folate

H2-folatesynthetase

NADPH H+
folA

NADP+

H2-folatereductase

H4-folate

B

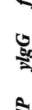
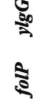
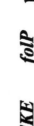

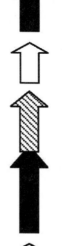

folA   *clpX*   *ysxc*   *folB*   *folKE*   *folP*   *ylgG*   *folC*   *dukB*   *hom*

~10 kb

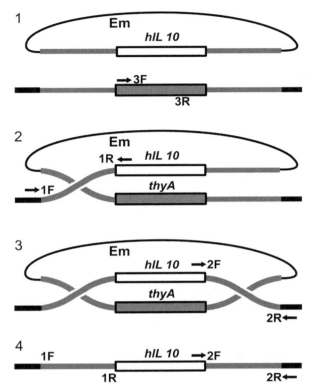

Figure 5 Schematic diagram of a *thyA* replacement strategy. Gray lines represent target areas for recombination, thick black lines represent nontarget chromosome fragments, and thin black lines represent the exchange vector. 1, 2, and 3 represent PCR primer pairs. Stages include the following: (1) introduction of the nonreplicative vector; (2) 5′ crossover event, facilitated by erythromycin (Em) selection; (3) second crossover event in the absence of Em; (4) acquisition of desired transgenic chromosome organization. *hIL10*, human IL-10 gene; *thyA*, thymidylate synthase gene. Reprinted from *Nature Biotechnology* (Steidler et al., 2003) with permission from Macmillan Publishers Ltd.

The use of genetically modified organisms raises concerns about their release and propagation in the environment and the potential transfer of genes to other microorganisms. Relying on genomic information of nucleotide biosynthesis pathways in lactococci, Steidler et al. (2003) described a strategy for biological containment of genetically modified microorganisms. A recombinant *L. lactis* strain auxotrophic for thymidine was made by replacing the thymidylate synthase gene (*thyA*) with a construct driving the expression of IL-10 (Fig. 5). The resulting strain was able to produce potentially therapeutic IL-10 but dies rapidly in the environment when deprived of thymine or thymidine. A phase I clinical trial using this strain showed evidence of reduced disease activity in patients, with only minor adverse effects. Additionally, fecally recovered bacteria were dependent upon thymidine for growth, indicating that the containment strategy was effective (Braat et al., 2006).

CONCLUDING REMARKS

Genome sequencing has yielded an abundance of DNA, evolutionary, and metabolic information about LAB. This information has provided considerable insight into the physiology of these organisms and has made it possible to understand their genetic content, predict important capabilities, and manipulate them for expanded and improved beneficial activities. Microarray analyses of LAB have generated significant contributions to the understanding of global gene expression in response to diverse environmental conditions, and functional genomic analyses have facilitated the identification and characterization of genes and gene products critical to cell growth, metabolism, survival, cell–cell communication, and probiotic functionality. The continued application and ongoing advancement of genomics and other "omics" technologies will contribute to a comprehensive mechanistic understanding of the physiology of LAB and can only positively impact the ability to utilize these organisms for practical benefit.

Tri Duong was supported by a National Science Foundation Integrated Graduate Education and Research Traineeship in Functional Genomics and a North Carolina State University Genomics Fellowship. Research activities at North Carolina State University on LAB are supported by the North Carolina Dairy Foundation, Danisco USA, Inc., Dairy Management, Inc., The Southeast Dairy Foods Research Center, and CREES-USDA-NRI project number 2005-35503-16167. We thank Erika Pfeiler for insightful discussion.

Figure 4 (A) Chemical structures of intermediates and end products in the tetrahydrofolate and folate biosynthesis pathways. Thick arrows indicate enzymatic reactions that are controlled in metabolic engineering experiments. (B) Schematic representation of folate biosynthesis genes in *L. lactis*. *folKE* encodes a bifunctional protein. Hatched arrows represent genes involved in folate biosynthesis, black arrows represent genes involved in folate biosynthesis that are overexpressed by metabolic engineering, and white arrows represent genes that are not expected to be involved in folate biosynthesis. Reprinted from *Applied and Environmental Microbiology* (Sybesma et al., 2003) with permission of the publisher.

References

Altermann, E., W. M. Russell, M. A. Azcarate-Peril, R. Barrangou, B. L. Buck, O. McAuliffe, N. Souther, A. Dobson, T. Duong, M. Callanan, S. Lick, A. Hamrick, R. Cano, and T. R. Klaenhammer. 2005. Complete genome sequence of the probiotic lactic acid bacterium *Lactobacillus acidophilus* NCFM. *Proc. Natl. Acad. Sci. USA* 102:3906–3912.

Azcarate-Peril, M. A., O. McAuliffe, E. Altermann, S. Lick, W. M. Russell, and T. R. Klaenhammer. 2005. Microarray analysis of a two-component regulatory system involved in acid resistance and proteolytic activity in *Lactobacillus acidophilus*. *Appl. Environ. Microbiol.* 71:5794–5804.

Barrangou, R., E. Altermann, R. Hutkins, R. Cano, and T. R. Klaenhammer. 2003. Functional and comparative genomic analyses of an operon involved in fructooligosaccharide utilization by *Lactobacillus acidophilus*. *Proc. Natl. Acad. Sci. USA* 100:8957–8962.

Barrangou, R., M. A. Azcarate-Peril, T. Duong, S. B. Conners, R. M. Kelly, and T. R. Klaenhammer. 2006. Global analysis of carbohydrate utilization by *Lactobacillus acidophilus* using cDNA microarrays. *Proc. Natl. Acad. Sci. USA* 103:3816–3821.

Barrangou, R., C. Fremaux, H. Deveau, M. Richards, P. Boyaval, S. Moineau, D. A. Romero, and P. Horvath. 2007. CRISPR provides acquired resistance against viruses in prokaryotes. *Science* 315:1709–1712.

Bernet, M. F., D. Brassart, J. R. Neeser, and A. L. Servin. 1994. *Lactobacillus acidophilus* LA 1 binds to cultured human intestinal cell lines and inhibits cell attachment and cell invasion by enterovirulent bacteria. *Gut* 35:483–489.

Bolotin, A., B. Quinquis, P. Renault, A. Sorokin, S. D. Ehrlich, S. Kulakauskas, A. Lapidus, E. Goltsman, M. Mazur, G. D. Pusch, M. Fonstein, R. Overbeek, N. Kyprides, B. Purnelle, D. Prozzi, K. Ngui, D. Masuy, F. Hancy, S. Burteau, M. Boutry, J. Delcour, A. Goffeau, and P. Hols. 2004. Complete sequence and comparative genome analysis of the dairy bacterium *Streptococcus thermophilus*. *Nat. Biotechnol.* 22:1554–1558.

Bolotin, A., B. Quinquis, A. Sorokin, and S. D. Ehrlich. 2005. Clustered regularly interspaced short palindrome repeats (CRISPRs) have spacers of extrachromosomal origin. *Microbiology* 151:2551–2561.

Bolotin, A., P. Wincker, S. Mauger, O. Jaillon, K. Malarme, J. Weissenbach, S. D. Ehrlich, and A. Sorokin. 2001. The complete genome sequence of the lactic acid bacterium *Lactococcus lactis* ssp. *lactis* IL1403. *Genome Res.* 11:731–753.

Braat, H., P. Rottiers, D. W. Hommes, N. Huyghebaert, E. Remaut, J. P. Remon, S. J. van Deventer, S. Neirynck, M. P. Peppelenbosch, and L. Steidler. 2006. A phase I trial with transgenic bacteria expressing interleukin-10 in Crohn's disease. *Clin. Gastroenterol. Hepatol.* 4:754–759.

Bron, P. A., C. Grangette, A. Mercenier, W. M. de Vos, and M. Kleerebezem. 2004a. Identification of *Lactobacillus plantarum* genes that are induced in the gastrointestinal tract of mice. *J. Bacteriol.* 186:5721–5729.

Bron, P. A., M. Marco, S. M. Hoffer, E. Van Mullekom, W. M. de Vos, and M. Kleerebezem. 2004b. Genetic characterization of the bile salt response in *Lactobacillus plantarum*

and analysis of responsive promoters in vitro and in situ in the gastrointestinal tract. *J. Bacteriol.* 186:7829–7835.

Brussow, H. 2001. Phages of dairy bacteria. *Annu. Rev. Microbiol.* 55:283–303.

Brussow, H., and F. Desiere. 2001. Comparative phage genomics and the evolution of Siphoviridae: insights from dairy phages. *Mol. Microbiol.* 39:213–222.

Brussow, H., and R. W. Hendrix. 2002. Phage genomics: small is beautiful. *Cell* 108:13–16.

Buck, B. L., E. Altermann, T. Svingerud, and T. R. Klaenhammer. 2005. Functional analysis of putative adhesion factors in *Lactobacillus acidophilus* NCFM. *Appl. Environ. Microbiol.* 71:8344–8351.

Chaillou, S., M. C. Champomier-Verges, M. Cornet, A. M. Crutz-Le Coq, A. M. Dudez, V. Martin, S. Beaufils, E. Darbon-Rongere, R. Bossy, V. Loux, and M. Zagorec. 2005. The complete genome sequence of the meat-borne lactic acid bacterium *Lactobacillus sakei* 23K. *Nat. Biotechnol.* 23:1527–1533.

Christensen, H. R., H. Frokiaer, and J. J. Pestka. 2002. Lactobacilli differentially modulate expression of cytokines and maturation surface markers in murine dendritic cells. *J. Immunol.* 168:171–178.

Claesson, M. J., Y. Li, S. Leahy, C. Canchaya, J. P. van Pijkeren, A. M. Cerdeno-Tarraga, J. Parkhill, S. Flynn, G. C. O'Sullivan, J. K. Collins, D. Higgins, F. Shanahan, G. F. Fitzgerald, D. van Sinderen, and P. W. O'Toole. 2006. Multireplicon genome architecture of *Lactobacillus salivarius*. *Proc. Natl. Acad. Sci. USA* 103:6718–6723.

de Ruyter, P. G., O. P. Kuipers, and W. M. de Vos. 1996. Controlled gene expression systems for *Lactococcus lactis* with the food-grade inducer nisin. *Appl. Environ. Microbiol.* 62:3662–3667.

Duggan, D. J., M. Bittner, Y. Chen, P. Meltzer, and J. M. Trent. 1999. Expression profiling using cDNA microarrays. *Nat. Genet.* 21:10–14.

Goh, Y. J., C. Zhang, A. K. Benson, V. Schlegel, J. H. Lee, and R. W. Hutkins. 2006. Identification of a putative operon involved in fructooligosaccharide utilization by *Lactobacillus paracasei*. *Appl. Environ. Microbiol.* 72:7518–7530.

Grangette, C., H. Muller-Alouf, P. Hols, D. Goudercourt, J. Delcour, M. Turneer, and A. Mercenier. 2004. Enhanced mucosal delivery of antigen with cell wall mutants of lactic acid bacteria. *Infect. Immun.* 72:2731–2737.

Grangette, C., S. Nutten, E. Palumbo, S. Morath, C. Hermann, J. Dewulf, B. Pot, T. Hartung, P. Hols, and A. Mercenier. 2005. Enhanced antiinflammatory capacity of a *Lactobacillus plantarum* mutant synthesizing modified teichoic acids. *Proc. Natl. Acad. Sci. USA* 102:10321–10326.

Jansen, R., J. D. Embden, W. Gaastra, and L. M. Schouls. 2002. Identification of genes that are associated with DNA repeats in prokaryotes. *Mol. Microbiol.* 43:1565–1575.

Klaenhammer, T. R., R. Barrangou, B. L. Buck, M. A. Azcarate-Peril, and E. Altermann. 2005. Genomic features of lactic acid bacteria effecting bioprocessing and health. *FEMS Microbiol. Rev.* 29:393–409.

Kleerebezem, M., J. Boekhorst, R. van Kranenburg, D. Molenaar, O. P. Kuipers, R. Leer, R. Tarchini, S. A. Peters, H. M. Sandbrink, M. W. Fiers, W. Stiekema, R. M. Lankhorst,

P. A. Bron, S. M. Hoffer, M. N. Groot, R. Kerkhoven, M. de Vries, B. Ursing, W. M. de Vos, and R. J. Siezen. 2003. Complete genome sequence of *Lactobacillus plantarum* WCFS1. *Proc. Natl. Acad. Sci. USA* 100:1990–1995.

Liu, X., L. A. Lagenaur, D. A. Simpson, K. P. Essenmacher, C. L. Frazier-Parker, Y. Liu, D. Tsai, S. S. Rao, D. H. Hamer, T. P. Parks, P. P. Lee, and Q. Xu. 2006. Engineered vaginal *Lactobacillus* strain for mucosal delivery of the human immunodeficiency virus inhibitor cyanovirin-N. *Antimicrob. Agents Chemother.* 50:3250–3259.

Lucchini, S., F. Desiere, and H. Brussow. 1999. Comparative genomics of *Streptococcus thermophilus* phage species supports a modular evolution theory. *J. Virol.* 73:8647–8656.

Makarova, K., A. Slesarev, Y. Wolf, A. Sorokin, B. Mirkin, E. Koonin, A. Pavlov, N. Pavlova, V. Karamychev, N. Polouchine, V. Shakhova, I. Grigoriev, Y. Lou, D. Rohksar, S. Lucas, K. Huang, D. M. Goodstein, T. Hawkins, V. Plengvidhya, D. Welker, J. Hughes, Y. Goh, A. Benson, K. Baldwin, J. H. Lee, I. Diaz-Muniz, B. Dosti, V. Smeianov, W. Wechter, R. Barabote, G. Lorca, E. Altermann, R. Barrangou, B. Ganesan, Y. Xie, H. Rawsthorne, D. Tamir, C. Parker, F. Breidt, J. Broadbent, R. Hutkins, D. O'Sullivan, J. Steele, G. Unlu, M. Saier, T. Klaenhammer, P. Richardson, S. Kozyavkin, B. Weimer, and D. Mills. 2006a. Comparative genomics of the lactic acid bacteria. *Proc. Natl. Acad. Sci USA* 103:15611–15616.

Makarova, K. S., N. V. Grishin, S. A. Shabalina, Y. I. Wolf, and E. V. Koonin. 2006b. A putative RNA-interference-based immune system in prokaryotes: computational analysis of the predicted enzymatic machinery, functional analogies with eukaryotic RNAi, and hypothetical mechanisms of action. *Biol. Direct.* 1:7.

Makarova, K. S., and E. V. Koonin. 2007. Evolutionary genomics of lactic acid bacteria. *J. Bacteriol.* 189:1199–1208.

Marco, M. L., R. S. Bongers, W. M. de Vos, and M. Kleerebezem. 2007. Spatial and temporal expression of *Lactobacillus plantarum* genes in the gastrointestinal tracts of mice. *Appl. Environ. Microbiol.* 73:124–132.

McKay, L. L. 1983. Functional properties of plasmids in lactic streptococci. *Antonie Leeuwenhoek* 49:259–274.

Mohamadzadeh, M., S. Olson, W. V. Kalina, G. Ruthel, G. L. Demmin, K. L. Warfield, S. Bavari, and T. R. Klaenhammer. 2005. Lactobacilli activate human dendritic cells that skew T cells toward T helper 1 polarization. *Proc. Natl. Acad. Sci. USA* 102:2880–2885.

Molenaar, D., F. Bringel, F. H. Schuren, W. M. de Vos, R. J. Siezen, and M. Kleerebezem. 2005. Exploring *Lactobacillus plantarum* genome diversity by using microarrays. *J. Bacteriol.* 187:6119-6127.

Murray, A. E., D. Lies, G. Li, K. Nealson, J. Zhou, and J. M. Tiedje. 2001. DNA/DNA hybridization to microarrays reveals gene-specific differences between closely related microbial genomes. *Proc. Natl. Acad. Sci. USA* 98:9853–9858.

Ohnishi, M., K. Kurokawa, and T. Hayashi. 2001. Diversification of *Escherichia coli* genomes: are bacteriophages the major contributors? *Trends Microbiol* 9:481–485.

Pavlovic, M., S. Hormann, R. F. Vogel, and M. A. Ehrmann. 2005. Transcriptional response reveals translation machin-

ery as target for high pressure in *Lactobacillus sanfranciscensis*. *Arch. Microbiol.* 184:11–17.

Pieterse, B., R. J. Leer, F. H. Schuren, and M. J. van der Werf. 2005. Unravelling the multiple effects of lactic acid stress on *Lactobacillus plantarum* by transcription profiling. *Microbiology* 151:3881–3894.

Pridmore, R. D., B. Berger, F. Desiere, D. Vilanova, C. Barretto, A. C. Pittet, M. C. Zwahlen, M. Rouvet, E. Altermann, R. Barrangou, B. Mollet, A. Mercenier, T. Klaenhammer, F. Arigoni, and M. A. Schell. 2004. The genome sequence of the probiotic intestinal bacterium *Lactobacillus johnsonii* NCC 533. *Proc. Natl. Acad. Sci. USA* 101:2512–2517.

Robinson, K., L. M. Chamberlain, K. M. Schofield, J. M. Wells, and R. W. Le Page. 1997. Oral vaccination of mice against tetanus with recombinant *Lactococcus lactis*. *Nat. Biotechnol.* 15:653–657.

Sanger, F., G. M. Air, B. G. Barrell, N. L. Brown, A. R. Coulson, C. A. Fiddes, C. A. Hutchison, P. M. Slocombe, and M. Smith. 1977. Nucleotide sequence of bacteriophage phi X174 DNA. *Nature* 265:687–695.

Siezen, R. J., B. Renckens, I. van Swam, S. Peters, R. van Kranenburg, M. Kleerebezem, and W. M. de Vos. 2005. Complete sequences of four plasmids of *Lactococcus lactis* subsp. *cremoris* SK11 reveal extensive adaptation to the dairy environment. *Appl. Environ. Microbiol.* 71:8371–8382.

Steidler, L., S. Neirynck, N. Huyghebaert, V. Snoeck, A. Vermeire, B. Goddeeris, E. Cox, J. P. Remon, and E. Remaut. 2003. Biological containment of genetically modified *Lactococcus lactis* for intestinal delivery of human interleukin 10. *Nat. Biotechnol.* 21:785–789.

Stiles, M. E. 1996. Biopreservation by lactic acid bacteria. *Antonie Leeuwenhoek* 70:331–345.

Sturino, J. M., and T. R. Klaenhammer. 2002. Expression of antisense RNA targeted against *Streptococcus thermophilus* bacteriophages. *Appl. Environ. Microbiol.* 68:588–596.

Sturino, J. M., and T. R. Klaenhammer. 2004. Antisense RNA targeting of primase interferes with bacteriophage replication in *Streptococcus thermophilus*. *Appl. Environ. Microbiol.* 70:1735–1743.

Sturino, J. M., and T. R. Klaenhammer. 2006. Engineered bacteriophage-defense systems in bioprocessing. *Nat. Rev. Microbiol.* 4:395–404.

Sturme, M. H., J. Nakayama, D. Molenaar, Y. Murakami, R. Kunugi, T. Fujii, E. E. Vaughan, M. Kleerebezem, and W. M. de Vos. 2005. An *agr*-like two-component regulatory system in *Lactobacillus plantarum* is involved in production of a novel cyclic peptide and regulation of adherence. *J. Bacteriol.* 187:5224–5235.

Sybesma, W., M. Starrenburg, M. Kleerebezem, I. Mierau, W. M. de Vos, and J. Hugenholtz. 2003. Increased production of folate by metabolic engineering of *Lactococcus lactis*. *Appl. Environ. Microbiol.* 69:3069–3076.

Tao, Y., K. A. Drabik, T. S. Waypa, M. W. Musch, J. C. Alverdy, O. Schneewind, E. B. Chang, and E. O. Petrof. 2006. Soluble factors from *Lactobacillus* GG activate MAPKs and induce cytoprotective heat shock proteins in intestinal epithelial cells. *Am. J. Physiol. Cell Physiol.* 290:C1018–C1030.

Valeur, N., P. Engel, N. Carbajal, E. Connolly, and K. Lade-foged. 2004. Colonization and immunomodulation by *Lactobacillus reuteri* ATCC 55730 in the human gastrointestinal tract. *Appl. Environ. Microbiol.* 70:1176–1181.

van de Guchte, M., S. Penaud, C. Grimaldi, V. Barbe, K. Bryson, P. Nicolas, C. Robert, S. Oztas, S. Mangenot, A. Couloux, V. Loux, R. Dervyn, R. Bossy, A. Bolotin, J. M. Batto, T. Walunas, J. F. Gibrat, P. Bessieres, J. Weissenbach, S. D. Ehrlich, and E. Maguin. 2006. The complete genome sequence of *Lactobacillus bulgaricus* reveals extensive and ongoing reductive evolution. *Proc. Natl. Acad. Sci. USA* 103:9274–9279.

Walter, J., N. C. Heng, W. P. Hammes, D. M. Loach, G. W. Tannock, and C. Hertel. 2003. Identification of *Lactobacillus reuteri* genes specifically induced in the mouse gastrointestinal tract. *Appl. Environ. Microbiol.* 69:2044–2051.

Wegmann, U., M. O'Connell-Motherway, A. Zomer, G. Buist, C. Shearman, C. Canchaya, M. Ventura, A. Goesmann, M. J. Gasson, O. P. Kuipers, D. van Sinderen, and J. Kok. 2007. Complete genome sequence of the prototype lactic acid bacterium *Lactococcus lactis* subsp. *cremoris* MG1363. *J. Bacteriol.* 189:3256–3270.

Wells, J. M., K. Robinson, L. M. Chamberlain, K. M. Schofield, and R. W. Le Page. 1996. Lactic acid bacteria as vaccine delivery vehicles. *Antonie Leeuwenhoek* 70:317–330.

Therapeutic Microbiology: Probiotics and Related Strategies
Edited by J. Versalovic and M. Wilson
© 2008 ASM Press, Washington, DC

2.5. PROTEOMICS OF LACTIC ACID BACTERIA

David P. A. Cohen, Elaine E. Vaughan,
Willem M. de Vos, Erwin G. Zoetendal

Proteomic Approaches To Study Lactic Acid Bacteria

16

Biology aims to describe, understand, and predict the functionality of living cells, tissues, organisms, and ecosystems. While biological studies for a long time have been based on a reductionistic approach, in recent years more global approaches have been developed. In a reductionistic approach, a complex biological system is analyzed by reducing it into smaller subunits, making it easier to study its properties (Romero et al., 2006). However, analyzing a single trait (gene, protein, or metabolic process) will not automatically lead to a complete understanding of a living organism (Strange, 2005). High-throughput approaches that allow simultaneous investigation of more than one parameter will ultimately lead to better understanding of the organism's behavior. Examples of such high-throughput approaches are genomics, transcriptomics, proteomics, and metabolomics. The suffix "-omics" refers to the study of aggregates of an entity, group, or mass, like genome, proteome, transcriptome, or metabolome (Romero et al., 2006). Genomics is the (systematic) study of the (entire) genome of an organism, which provides information on its genetic potential. On the other hand, transcriptomics, proteomics, and metabolomics focus on total gene expression, protein synthesis, and metabolite production, respectively, of the organism of interest under certain conditions and, therefore, reflect its aggregate functional properties.

In this chapter, we focus on the application of proteomics in microbiological research in which special attention is given to the lactic acid bacteria (LAB). LAB are ubiquitous bacteria that inhabit the human gastrointestinal tract, are marketed as probiotics, and are important in the food industry because of their long history of safe use as starter cultures for industrial food fermentations.

LAB are ubiquitous bacteria that inhabit a wide variety of habitats, which include the gastrointestinal tract of animals and decomposing plants, and they are traditionally used in the manufacture of fermented and functional foods (Enan et al., 1996; Ercolini et al., 2003; Yoon et al., 2006). Among the various LAB, notably *Lactobacillus* strains are also marketed as probiotics, being often claimed to have a beneficial effect on gut functionality (Molin, 2001).

LAB consist of a heterogeneous group of bacteria, including the genera *Lactobacillus*, *Lactococcus*, *Leuconostoc*, *Oenococcus*, *Pediococcus*, *Streptococcus*, and *Weissella*, which all share the common property that

David P. A. Cohen, Elaine E. Vaughan, Willem M. de Vos, and Erwin G. Zoetendal, Laboratory of Microbiology, Wageningen University, Dreijenplein 10, 6703 HB, Wageningen, The Netherlands.

they are able to produce lactic acid by fermenting a wide variety of carbon sources (Bonestroo et al., 1992). Furthermore, they are gram-positive, nonmotile, nonspore-forming bacteria and have either a rod or coccus morphology. Among the LAB, the genus *Lactobacillus* includes 32 species that are members of the commensal microbiota of humans (Rajilić-Stojanović, 2007), being attached to or closely associated with body surfaces covered by epithelial cells (Tlaskalova-Hogenova et al., 2004). Like other commensal bacteria, these LAB can contribute to and regulate host processes such as nutrition and development, immunomodulation, overall health status, and disease susceptibility (Hooper and Gordon, 2001). In general, lactobacilli may be present in quantities of 10^7 to 10^8 cells per g of feces, and therefore, they do not constitute dominant populations in the colon (Vaughan et al., 2002). On the other hand, lactobacilli have been proposed as dominant members of the small intestine. However, this suggestion should be viewed cautiously, since the relative dominance of lactobacilli has been demonstrated only in a few studies based on cultivation and has not been confirmed by culture-independent approaches (Finegold et al., 1970).

As LAB have a robust adaptation capacity in order to survive a variety of stress conditions in the host, the secrets of these survival strategies may be reflected in their proteomes. Proteomics has been used to investigate the functionality of LAB during preparation or fermentation of foods or their responses towards certain stress conditions (e.g., bile salts and acid) that these organisms encounter during passage through the human gastrointestinal tract. Proteomic approaches make it possible to gain insights into the relative abundance of proteins under certain conditions, and this knowledge may help predict which proteins of LAB are involved in survival under harsh conditions. This information can be important for some members of the LAB group, which have potential health claims and medical applications. By knowing the relative abundance of proteins during acid shock, a similar proteome can be expected when the same organism is exposed to gastric acid during passage through the human gastrointestinal tract. Following an introduction regarding recent developments in proteomics, we describe major findings obtained by studying the proteomes of LAB, especially under physiological stress conditions.

GENOMICS, TRANSCRIPTOMICS, AND PROTEOMICS

During the past decade, the determination of genome sequences of a wide variety of organisms has increased explosively. Because of their relatively small size, most sequenced genomes derive from microbial species. As of October 2007, 593 bacterial genomes (http://www.ncbi.nlm.nih.gov/genomes/static/eub_g) and 48 genomes of archaeal species (http://www.ncbi.nlm.nih.gov/genomes/static/a_g.html) have been fully sequenced. This genomic explosion has resulted in a new research area, termed genomics, which is the study of the entire genome of an organism. So far, complete genome sequences of a wide variety of LAB species used in the food industry or marketed as probiotic cultures have been reported (see chapter 15). Since more genomic sequences are being unraveled, comparative genomics can yield insights into phylogenetic and functional diversity of these bacteria and facilitate reconstruction of ancestral gene sets and molecular evolution including gene losses and gains. Comparative genomics may contribute to insights regarding the genetic organization, dynamics and control of gene expression, and advancements in predicted functions of LAB in the gastrointestinal tract (Altermann et al., 2005; Makarova et al., 2006).

Genomics forms the basis of functional or postgenomic studies, such as transcriptomics and proteomics. Subsets of genes transcribed in an organism are called transcriptomes, which represent dynamic links between genomes, proteins, and cellular phenotypes (Singh and Nagaraj, 2006). Transcriptomic approaches facilitate studies of gene expression profiles and have been successful in enabling the determination of changes in gene expression using specifically designed microarrays (Pieterse et al., 2005; Bron et al., 2006). Although transcriptomics has been used for functional analyses that are rapid, easy to apply, and data rich, several drawbacks of this approach are noted. Transcriptomics data represent snapshots in time as these methods monitor relative mRNA concentrations, and because of fast turnover rates of mRNA in prokaryotes, sampling methods can be limiting for isolation of mRNA needed for microarray hybridization. Furthermore, environmental contamination of samples can affect the quality of microarray hybridization studies (Zhou and Thompson, 2002). On the other hand, because the concentration ranges of most mRNA are not as wide as that of proteins, the detection and quantification of many mRNAs are easier to perform. Consequently, the detection of many mRNA molecules can be achieved more easily, and transcriptomics may provide a more comprehensive view of gene expression of the whole genome in comparison to other -omics technologies (Singh and Nagaraj, 2006).

Proteomics is a very powerful tool to study cellular functionality because of the direct link between the phenotype of an organism and its proteins. Fitness and adaptation to the environment are more immediately reflected by relative protein abundance and aggregate activities than the quantities of mRNA molecules (Feder and Walser, 2005). Transcriptomics may not accurately predict the relative abundance of proteins because protein concentrations depend partly on relative rates of protein synthesis and degradation. Important phenomena that cannot be extrapolated from transcriptomics data are posttranslational modifications of proteins such as phosphorylation, glycosylation, and acetylation. Posttranslational modifications affect the physicochemical properties of proteins, protein conformations, cellular location, and macromolecular interactions. These properties depend on parameters of protein context such as the cell type, the tissue, and the environmental conditions. Although investigating posttranslational modifications remains challenging, several effective proteomic strategies addressing posttranslational modifications have been developed (Jensen, 2006).

The relative concentrations and posttranslational modifications of proteins have major impacts on many cellular processes. Simple deductions from mRNA transcript analyses to quantitative analyses of proteins may be insufficient (Gygi et al., 1999). The proteome is a fundamental basis to study functionality in relation to phenotype, adaptation, and fitness. Proteins are major contributors to functionality and represent the predominant end products of gene expression.

From Proteins to Proteomics

The biochemical analyses of proteins and their functions started to evolve around 1940 (Fraenkel-Conrat, 1994). These studies resulted in the development of protein biochemistry, which is an example of a reductionistic approach as it provides the link between the activity of a pure protein and its corresponding gene (Patterson and Aebersold, 2003). The subsequent development of analytical protein chemistry resulted in technical improvements of protein separation and improved sensitivity of methods for identifying proteins. A major technical breakthrough was the Edman degradation for the identification of N-terminal sequences of proteins, and this method could be used for identification of proteins isolated by one-dimensional and two-dimensional electrophoresis (1-DE and 2-DE, respectively) (Aebersold et al., 1987; Graves and Haystead, 2002). Initially this method had poor sensitivity and was slow, but further optimization allowed the identification of micrograms of proteins separated by isoelectric focusing in immobilized pH gradients (Aebersold et al., 1988). Simultaneously, the number of databases containing protein or gene sequences expanded, and therefore, the identification of proteins by Edman degradation and subsequent

database comparison have become more accurate and reliable (Patterson and Aebersold, 2003). Meanwhile other methods were investigated to facilitate rapid protein identification, as the Edman degradation was relatively slow. Mass spectrometry was already used intensively for identification of small molecules, and by the late 1980s, two methods were developed, making it possible to analyze peptides and proteins by mass spectrometry (MS) with high sensitivity and without excessive molecular fragmentation. These methods included matrix-assisted laser desorption ionization (MALDI) and electron spray ionization (ESI). Because of successful approaches that enabled ionization of large molecules, a process essential for MS, robust ESI and MALDI mass spectrometers became commercially available and enhanced the toolkit available to the protein chemistry community. MS is much more sensitive than the Edman degradation method and currently allows identification of proteins in the femtomolar range (Graves and Haystead, 2002).

Since 1993, several groups were able to correlate the data obtained by MS with protein sequence databases (Andersen and Mann, 2000), and in 1994, it was possible to use fragmentation spectra for peptide identification (Eng et al., 1994). This methodology is still used and is known as peptide mass fingerprinting. In addition, during the First Siena Meeting: From Genome to Proteome in Siena (Italy) in 1994, the term proteome was coined, and the process of studying the proteome became known as "proteomics" (Patterson and Aebersold, 2003). Nowadays, the term proteomics can be defined as "the large-scale characterization of the entire protein complement of a cell line, tissue, or organism" (Graves and Haystead, 2002).

Proteomics

Several techniques can be used to characterize the proteome of any cell type or unicellular organism. All methods consist of two main steps including separation of individual proteins within a mixture and identification of target proteins. In principle, two mainstream separation methods used in proteomics include gel-based and non-gel approaches. For gel-based methods, sodium dodecyl sulfate-polyacrylamide gel electrophoresis is used as the primary strategy for separation of protein mixtures. For non-gel approaches, chromatography-based methods are applied to separate proteins from mixtures.

Gel-Based Methods

In many cases, 1-DE by sodium dodecyl sulfate-polyacrylamide gel electrophoresis is used for resolving relatively simple protein mixtures obtained after purification of desired protein fractions. With this method, proteins will be separated only based on molecular weight. The protein bands can be easily excised from the gel and identified by MS. The major advantages of this method are its speed, simplicity, and reproducibility, but in cases of more complex protein mixtures, this method is not desirable because of limited resolution.

To enhance the abilities to resolve proteins in complex biological mixtures, protein separation in two dimensions (2-DE) was developed. The 2-DE method is an established and robust technique that was first developed by O'Farrell (O'Farrell, 1975) and continues to be refined. For highly complex protein mixtures, such as crude cell lysates, 2-DE has the advantage that it separates proteins in two dimensions. The first dimension is based on isoelectric points or isoelectric focusing of individual proteins, and the second dimension is based on molecular size or weight. Consequently, the resolving power is increased dramatically with 2-DE. Hundreds of different proteins can be separated individually and

visualized by 2-DE. With thorough analyses, up- and down-regulation of proteins including those that have undergone posttranslational modifications can be detected. A widely applied work flow for gel-based proteomics is depicted in Fig. 1.

By applying different pH ranges in the first dimension, one can zoom into areas of interest. Using a pH range between 4 and 7, only proteins that have an isoelectric point between 4 and 7 will be separated and visualized on the gel. The use of a smaller pH range when performing isoelectric focusing results in increased resolving power of the gel. By simply choosing the desired pH range, enhanced separation of a portion of the complex protein mixture can be performed in this way. The resolution of 2-DE is enhanced by increasing the gel size in the second dimension, resulting in greater numbers of protein spots per gel, as demonstrated by Inagaki and colleagues (Inagaki and Katsuta, 2004). For example, a gel (93 by 103 cm) composed of several long gels (24 cm

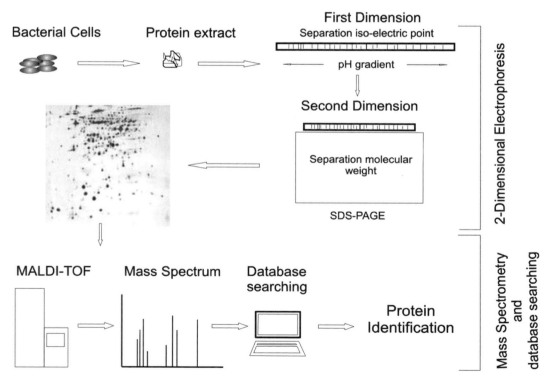

Figure 1 The gel-based proteomic method can be divided into two main parts, separation of protein complexes and identification of individual proteins. The separation of proteins in mixtures is based on the protein's isoelectric point and its molecular weight. Identification of the proteins is commonly achieved using MALDI-TOF MS and mass fingerprinting prior to database searching.

by 70 cm by 1 mm) displayed more than 11,000 protein spots with a dynamic range from 10^0 to 10^5 in cells versus a standard (18 by 20 cm) gel display of approximately 800 spots with silver staining. By increasing the resolution (gel size), a larger part of the proteome can be visualized and analyzed.

The next step following protein separation for gel-based approaches is the visualization of protein spots in the gels. Many methods are available, but one approach should be chosen on the basis of intended use of the visualized samples. For quantification of protein spots, the detection method should have a wide dynamic range and linear correlation between the amount of protein and the intensity of the staining (Westermeier and Marouga, 2005). Detection methods should be compatible with MS so that target spots can be identified. Staining methods that are commonly used include Coomassie brilliant blue-based staining, silver staining, staining by fluorescent dyes, and autoradiography. These staining methods have advantages and disadvantages (Table 1), and their choice, therefore, depends on the study design.

MALDI-TOF MS
After visualization of protein spots in gels, identification of the protein (of interest) spots is generally desired. By 1989, fast atom bombardment to ionize peptides had been developed, and the new method of peptide mass fingerprinting for faster identification of proteins was described (Henzel et al., 2003). When a peptide/protein is digested with a known enzyme, the sizes of the resulting fragments can be predicted, forming a fingerprint for that protein. With the development of MALDI time of flight (TOF) and ESI-MS (Table 2) techniques, it was possible to ionize fragments larger than 20 kDa. In the case of MALDI, a laser beam is adsorbed by samples embedded in a matrix, yielding sufficient energy to form ions. The generated ions have a reduced charge state

(m/z) resulting in less complex spectra when mixtures of proteins and peptides are used (Lahm and Langen, 2000). Furthermore, MALDI-TOF can be automated, resulting in high-throughput proteomics.

Non-Gel Methods
The main advantage of non-gel techniques is that hydrophobic and basic proteins may be separated with enhanced resolution. Moreover, non-gel techniques can be automated, leading to high-throughput analyses. Using non-gel methods, protein mixtures are digested in solution with several specific proteases, including trypsin, generating an assortment of different peptides. These peptides are analyzed by liquid chromatography (LC), using a reverse-phase capillary column, coupled with nano-ESI-MS. The dynamic range of this analytic technique is similar to that of gel-based 2-DE. Currently, this non-gel method is being refined in order to increase the separation efficiency by including more columns. However, protein quantification and detection of posttranslational modifications are poorly detected with this method (Roe and Griffin, 2006).

Another non-gel chromatography technique is the use of a surface enhanced laser desorption ionization (SELDI)-TOF MS (Tang et al., 2004). The chromatography is performed on a solid-phase affinity surface. The surface is designed to have affinity for proteins based on chemical (anionic, cationic, hydrophilic, etc.) or biochemical (antibody, receptor, enzyme, etc.) properties. In the case of surfaces coated with antibodies, receptors, or other biochemical agents, specific proteins bind to the solid-phase extractors. Captured proteins are detected by laser desorption ionization-TOF MS, and these proteins are displayed as a series of peaks. The generated output shows the relative abundance versus the molecular weight of detected proteins, and the data can be visualized in a simulated 1-DE gel using multivariate analyses

Table 1 Methods used to visualize proteins by two-dimensional gel electrophoresis[a]

Detection method	Detection limit	Advantage	Disadvantage	Reference
Coomassie brilliant blue	0.1 µg	Very easy to apply	Not sensitive	Wayne, 2000
Fluorescent labeling	1 ng	Sensitive	Requires laser scanner	Ünlü et al., 1997
Fluorescent stains	2–8 ng	Easy to apply	Expensive	Wayne, 2000
Negative stains	15 ng	Fast and easy	Not suitable for quantification	Matsui et al., 1997
Radioactive labeling	<1 pg	Sensitive	More difficult to handle	Westermeier and Marouga, 2005
Silver staining	0.05–0.2 ng	Sensitive	Small dynamic range	Jin et al., 2006
Stable-isotope labeling	6–8 ng	Sensitive	Need living cells	Roe and Griffin, 2006

[a]All these methods are compatible with MS for identification of proteins.

Table 2 Ionization methods and available mass spectrometers commonly used in proteomics studies[a]

Method	Short description	Reference(s)
Ionization method		
MALDI	The energy of the laser will ionize the sample	Tanaka et al., 1988
ESI	Analyte exists as an ion in solution and leaves the charged capillary as an aerosol	Fenn et al., 1989
Desorption ESI	Collision of charged particles on surface of compound produces gaseous ions	Takats et al., 2004
Fast atom bombardment	Sample is ionized by bombardment of atoms from inert gas	Barber et al., 1981
Mass spectrometer		
TOF	Measures the time of ions to travel from the sample to the detector	Wollnik, 1993
Quadrupole	Filters ions based on mass-to-charge ratio by selectively stabilizing or destabilizing ions	Mann et al., 2001
Quadrupole ion trap	Same principle as "normal" quadrupole but ions are trapped and sequentially ejected	Krutchinsky et al., 2001
Linear quadrupole ion trap	Similar to quadrupole ion trap but traps ions in a two-dimensional quadrupole field	Cha et al., 2000
Fourier transform ion cyclotron resonance	Detects the current produced by ions traveling cyclotronic in magnetic field	Marshall et al., 1998; Martin et al., 2000
Orbitrap	Ions are trapped electrostatically and orbit around a central electrode	Hu et al., 2005

[a]These instruments can be used as a single apparatus for MS or as combinations of mass spectrometers for tandem MS/MS analyses.

and artificial neural networks (Grus et al., 2005). The end result of SELDI-TOF MS is a list of molecular weights of proteins whose relative abundance differs significantly between the analyzed samples. The next step is to actually identify the proteins that are differentially produced. Protein identification is achieved by molecular-weight-based selection and purification of proteins that are differentially produced by SELDI-TOF MS analyses. After purification of desired proteins, standard MS-based techniques like peptide mass fingerprinting or tandem MS can be applied to identify proteins. SELDI-TOF MS is a powerful method, which is used regularly for diagnostic purposes, such as identifying biomarkers produced by specific tissues/organisms.

Tandem MS

In certain cases, peptide mass fingerprinting is not sufficient to identify the peptide digest. This limitation can be due to the low amounts of peptides of interest in mixtures, the unknown origins of proteins, or the presence of unknown or undiscovered proteins. Tandem MS can select, isolate, and sequence a single peptide ion in the presence of other detected peptides (Peng and Gygi, 2001). By de novo peptide sequencing, the amino acid sequences of peptides allow in silico analyses of newly

identified proteins. Furthermore, tandem MS allows the identification of posttranslational modifications (Anderson et al., 2002).

In principle, tandem MS is sequential mass analyses by different mass spectrometers. For peptide ionization, ESI is commonly used because it generates multiple charged ions of peptide fragments. Furthermore, multicharging of larger macromolecules by ESI facilitates ion dissociation and produces more peptide fragmentation than singly charged ions generated by MALDI. In the first mass spectrometer, different ions are selected based on their *m/z* value. Selected ions are brought into a collision chamber where the target ions are fragmented by collisions. In the second mass spectrometer, fragments are further analyzed.

Many combinations of tandem MS instruments (Table 2) are possible, and the most recent commercially available instrument is the Orbitrap mass spectrometer (Thermo Fisher Scientific, Waltham, MA). In the Orbitrap mass analyzer, ions travel in a rapidly changing electric field where the ions move in rings around an inner electrode. Furthermore, the ions oscillate along the central electrode and by measuring the oscillations, as in a transform ion cyclotron resonance mass spectrometer, the Orbitrap can be used as a mass spectrometer with a high degree of sensitivity and mass accuracy and a robust dynamic range (Hu et al., 2005; Makarov et al., 2006).

STATE OF THE ART OF PROTEOMICS OF LAB

In this section, we highlight the major results that were obtained by studying the proteomes of LAB under various conditions. Two separate proteomic research strategies have been applied frequently to LAB. These approaches include the construction of protein reference maps, systematic indexing of proteins, and analyses of bacterial stress responses culminating in induced changes in different proteomes.

Proteome Reference Maps

Systematic identification of proteins during studies of microorganisms or cells under specific conditions will result in the construction of proteome reference maps containing subsets of the total proteome. These maps provide insights into protein production under specific conditions such as adaptation, stress, and growth, and such maps will provide fundamental knowledge of metabolic states of different bacteria. Furthermore, these maps are powerful tools for rapid indexing of known proteins in gels for future experiments. Predicted proteins

without assigned functions or hypothetical proteins can be traced back to proteome reference maps, confirming the presence of these specific proteins. In addition, proteins not predicted by genomics analyses may be discovered by proteomics approaches, as was the case for four proteins in *Mycoplasma pneumoniae* (Regula et al., 2000).

The first proteome reference map of LAB was documented for *Lactobacillus bulgaricus* (Chervaux et al., 2000). More than 700 proteins of the proteome of *L. bulgaricus*, cultured in exponential growth phase in a defined medium known as milieu proche du lait (Chervaux et al., 2000), were visualized in gels. No protein identification was performed (Lim et al., 2000). Recently, the proteomes of *Lactobacillus* sp. 30a (ATCC 33222) and *Lactobacillus* sp. W53, two strains isolated from amine-contaminated wine, yielded 22 spots (Table 3) that were identified (pH range, 4 to 7) after culturing in MRS medium until exponential- or early-stationary-growth phase (Pessione et al., 2005). A more extensive proteome reference map of *Lactobacillus plantarum* strain WCFS1 cytosolic fractions isolated from mid- and late-log and early- and late-stationary-phase cells grown on MRS medium was constructed. Approximately 200 spots (Table 3) were identified within a pH range between 3 and 10 (Cohen et al., 2006). More recently, the proteomes of two other

Table 3 Proteome reference map of lactic acid bacteria

Functional class of identified proteins	No. of protein spots identified				
	L. plantarum (Cohen et al., 2006)	*L. lactis* NCDO763 (Anglade et al., 2000; Gitton et al., 2005)	*L. lactis* (Drews et al., 2004)	*Lactobacillus* species strain 30a and w53 (Pessione et al., 2005)	*L. delbrueckii* (Lim et al., 2000)
Amino acid metabolism	20	71			
Carbohydrate metabolism	36	64		12	
Cell envelope			5		
Cell growth and death	7	5	10		
Cofactors metabolism	1	4			
Energy metabolism	9	5		3	
Fatty acid metabolism	5	9	4		
Folate metabolism		2			
Folding	5	6			
Membrane transport	7	23	6	4	
Miscellaneous	30	44	6	4	
Nucleotide metabolism	14	29	2		
Replication and repair	4	10	4		
Signal transduction	3				
Stress proteins	10	11			3
Transcription	6	9	3		
Translation	14	14	47		
Unknown function	20	43	20		

L. plantarum strains (REB1 and MLBPL1) were investigated using the pH range of 4 to 7, and 231 proteins were identified and indexed (Koistinen et al., 2007). Furthermore, 39 and 64 protein spots were found to be differentially regulated during growth of the REB1 and MLBPL1 strains, respectively. The combination of these two studies will give extensive information about the proteomes of *L. plantarum* in terms of a comprehensive pH range.

The proteome reference map of the *Lactococcus lactis* (*Lc. lactis*) NCDO763 proteome was isolated after growing the cells in a defined medium (Jensen and Hammer, 1993) until mid-exponential phase (Anglade et al., 2000). By using a pH range between 4 and 7, approximately 400 spots were visualized and 18 spots were identified by MALDI-TOF or N-terminal (protein) sequencing. By focusing on more-specific pH ranges (e.g., pH ranges of 4 to 7 and 4.5 to 5) of the *Lc. lactis* proteome, approximately 800 spots were visualized, and 335 spots (Table 3) were identified (Gitton et al., 2005). The proteome reference map was applied to identify differentially produced proteins when *Lc. lactis* was grown in different media including synthetic medium M17lac (Difco, Sparks, MD) with lactose, skim milk microfiltrates, and milk. The acidic part of the *Lc. lactis* proteome has been effectively visualized. Numerous proteins were identified including enzymes involved in glycolysis and glutamine synthetase, an essential enzyme needed for survival of *Lc. lactis* in dairy products.

A proteome reference map of the alkaline part of the *Lc. lactis* proteome (pH range, 6 to 12) has also been constructed. More than 200 protein spots were visualized, and 152 protein spots were identified (Drews et al., 2004). Because the alkaline part of the proteome contains mainly hydrophobic proteins, no proteins associated with glycolysis were identified. Instead, most of the identified proteins were involved in translation or their function could not yet be predicted (Table 3).

The proteins identified in proteome reference maps of various *Lactobacillus* and *Lactococcus* species can be indexed systematically into functional groups according to the KEGG database (http://www.genome.jp/kegg) (Kanehisa and Goto, 2000). By comparative analyses of these reference maps, metabolic and functional processes were demonstrated despite the use of different bacteriologic media and variable physiological growth phases of bacteria, indicating that a "core proteome" may address key essential functions. However, the major advantage of proteome reference maps is that such knowledge bases can be applied to a series of experiments, facilitating rapid protein identification. This advantage was demonstrated with proteomic analyses during different growth phases of *L. plantarum* WCFS1 in MRS medium (Cohen et al., 2006). Proteins that were differentially regulated during

early log, mid-log, and early and late stationary phases of growth were initially identified via proteome reference maps, and the majority of the growth phase-regulated proteins were identified by MS. Each growth phase yielded different sets of proteins. During mid-log phase, the highest priority was energy generation, and during late log phase, biosynthesis of many macromolecules and cell division proteins became predominant. During early stationary phase alternative pathways to generate pyruvate became more important, and during the late stationary phase cell wall biosynthesis and production of stress proteins were key activities. Proteomic analyses of *L. plantarum* strains REB1 and MLBPL1 revealed differences in protein regulation which might be explained by specific environmental growth conditions (Koistinen et al., 2007). However, key similarities between the two strains included metabolic activities during the lag phase, abilities to produce energy, increased metabolism of nucleotides for cell division, and induction of stress responses.

In conclusion, systematic analyses of the proteomes of *Lc. lactis* and various *Lactobacillus* spp. have unraveled aspects of the basic metabolism of these organisms. Construction of proteome reference maps and subsequent monitoring of proteome dynamics constitute a fundamental approach of proteomics to study basic concepts such as focusing on metabolic activities during growth in a standardized medium. Differential regulation of organismal proteomes under different conditions may be studied by analyses of protein regulation during exposure or adaptation to certain stimuli.

Microbial Adaptation and Responses to Stress

Much research regarding stress responses of LAB has been performed in order to investigate the changes in proteomes during harsh environmental exposure of bacteria, their passage through the gastrointestinal tract, and food processing. Gastric and other organic acids in addition to bile salts and enzymatic secretions in the duodenum represent physiological stressors in the gastrointestinal tract. Acidic environments may also be encountered by microbes during food preparation or preservation, and LAB metabolize carbon sources to lactic acid during growth. In order to survive reductions in pH, these bacteria alter their gene expression programs and generate inducible acid tolerance responses, first reported and described in *Lc. lactis* (Frees et al., 2003; Budin-Verneuil et al., 2005). The acid tolerance response was induced by challenging *Lc. lactis* initially in a mildly acidic environment prior to exposure to extremely acidic conditions. Analyses of 2-DE gels revealed that several functional protein classes were induced by acid stress in *Lc. lactis*, including proteins involved in carbohydrate metabolism, regulation of translation or amino acid metabolism, and pH homeostasis and stress responses (Table 4). Stress response proteins may be associated with heat shock, oxidative stress, osmotic challenge, cold shock and DNA repair, and quorum-sensing pathways (Frees et al., 2003). The *ahpC* and *sodA* genes coding for alkyl hydroperoxide reductase and superoxide dismutase, respectively, were found to be involved in oxidative stress. Low pH also induced LuxS, a component of the autoinducers mediating bacterial intercellular communication (Schauder et al., 2001). DnaK and GroEL, induced during acid stress, are typical heat shock proteins involved in refolding of proteins during heat stress and have been induced in

lactobacilli (Table 4) during heat stress (De Angelis et al., 2004; Di Cagno et al., 2006). The up-regulation of these proteins during acid stress has been confirmed in *L. lactis* MG1363 by proteomics (Table 4) (Budin-Verneuil et al., 2005). In *Lc. lactis* CNRZ 157, proteomics and transcriptomics approaches showed that DnaK was induced in the stationary phase due to increased lactic acid concentrations (Larsen et al., 2006). In addition to stress proteins, proteins involved in basic metabolic pathways were differentially regulated by adaptation to acid stress. Remarkably, low pH induced a switch to alternative carbon sources other than glucose, and the formation of acids to neutral compounds was up-regulated. The genes coding for the proteins involved in the acid

Table 4 Proteins produced by LAB as responses to different stress challenges

Stress	Organism	Proteins	Reference(s)
Acid stress	*Lc. lactis*	AhpC; ArcA, B; AtpA, F; BusAA; Cfa; ClpB, C, E, P; CspE; Dnak; EraL; GadB; GroEL; GrpE; Hpr; LuxS; RecA; SodA; Tig; Tpx; YxbE	Frees et al., 2003; Budin-Verneuil et al., 2005
	P. freudenreichii	BCCP, EF-Tu, enolase, GroEL, GroES, malate dehydrogenase, RecR, RepB	Jan et al., 2001; Leverrier et al., 2003
	L. delbrueckii	DnaK, GroEL, GroES	Lim et al., 2000
Heat stress	*L. helveticus*	DnaK, thioredoxin reductase, TuaH, acetyltransferase, DbpII, Dps, enolase, GapDH, GroEL, Hsp20, pyruvate kinase, ribosomal proteins	Di Cagno et al., 2006
	L. plantarum	CspC, DbpII, DnaK, GroEL, ribosomal proteins, trigger factor	De Angelis et al., 2004
	P. freudenreichii	ClpA, B; Dnak; GroEL; SSB	Leverrier et al., 2003; Anastasiou et al., 2006
	Lc. lactis	GroEL, GroES	Hartke et al., 1996
Oxidative stress	*Lc. lactis*	Alkylhydroperoxide reductase, malonyl-CoA acyl carrier protein, NADH oxidase, β-phosphoglucomutase, pyrroline-5-carboxylate reductase, acetylcoenzyme A acetyltransferase, pyruate dehydrogenase, transcription elongation factor, GapDH, SodA	Vido et al., 2005
High hydrostatic pressure	*L. sanfranciscensis*	ClpL, CspE, DnaK, EF-Tu, GMP synthase, GroEL, maltose hydrolase, RbsK, thioredoxin reductase, YudG	Drews et al., 2002; Hörmann et al., 2006
Bile salt	*P. freudenreichii*	ClpB, cysteine synthase, DnaK, Hsp20, OppD, oxidoreductase, signal transducer, SodA	Leverrier et al., 2003, 2004
Cold/NaCl shock	*L. sakei*	Asp-23, GAPDH, MsrA, Ohr, PFK, Usp	Marceau et al., 2004

tolerance response have been shown to be up-regulated by transcriptomics (Budin-Verneuil et al., 2005). The production of stress proteins and alterations of metabolism towards production of neutral end products at low pH occur during the acid tolerance response.

The acid tolerance response has also been reported in organisms such as *Propionibacterium freudenreichii* and *Lactobacillus delbrueckii* subsp. *bulgaricus* (Table 4). For these microorganisms it was demonstrated using 2-DE that GroES/EL and DnaK proteins were up-regulated during exposure to acidic conditions (Lim et al., 2000; Jan et al., 2001). Furthermore, transcriptomic analyses of acid responses of *L. plantarum* WCFS1 yielded a reduced transcription ratio of the gene coding for GroEL suppressor protein SugE (Pieterse et al., 2005), confirming that relative concentration of the stress protein GroES during acid stress increased. During acid adaptation, it was confirmed that heat shock proteins DnaK and GroEL were induced in *P. freudenreichii* (Table 4) together with increased RecR and RepB proteins (Jan et al., 2001). In *Bacillus subtilis*, RecR is involved in DNA recombination and can be induced by bile salts (Alonso et al., 1990). In *Escherichia coli*, these genes are involved in DNA repair and replication, respectively, and were induced by stationary-phase entry, nutrient starvation, mutagenic agent exposure, and bile salt challenge (Nyström and Neidhardt, 1994; Bernstein et al., 1999).

After passage through the stomach, another physiological stress is bile in the small intestine, which the LAB must survive in order to transit or colonize the intestine. The heat shock protein DnaK and another typical heat shock protein, Hsp20, were induced when *P. freudenreichii* was exposed to bile salts. Only the proteome of *P. freudenreichii* has been investigated during bile salt stress (Table 4) (Leverrier et al., 2003). Analysis of gels revealed 24 distinct protein spots that were associated with protein protection and degradation, heat shock, oxidative stress, signal sensing and transduction, and an alternative sigma factor. These results suggest that, during bile salt adaptation, general stress and signal-sensing responses are induced. When *P. freudenreichii* was subjected to acid, heat, and bile salt stress, six proteins were induced including DnaK, ClpB, and SodA. It was suggested that *P. freudenreichii* has the ability to produce homologous tolerance-associated proteins to different forms of stresses (Leverrier et al., 2004).

For *L. plantarum*, proteomics studies to investigate effects of bile salts have not been performed. However, comparative transcriptomics data show discordances between *L. plantarum* and *P. freudenreichii*. The homolog RecF in *L. plantarum* was down-regulated upon bile

exposure (Bron et al., 2006), while it has been shown by proteomics that this protein was up-regulated in *P. freudenreichii*. Other stress responses have been observed, including induced amino acid metabolism and pH homeostasis (Bron et al., 2006). After passage through the small intestine, genes encoding proteins involved in amino acid metabolism and genes encoding stress proteins were up-regulated by exposure to acidic conditions in the small intestine (de Vries, 2006).

Key proteins involved in stress adaptation were investigated by proteomics and included DnaK, GroEL/ES, SodA, and members of the Clp protein family. The proteins GroEL/ES and DnaK have been found to be produced in increased amounts following exposure to acid, heat, and elevated hydrostatic pressure (Table 4). The evidence of potential crossover protection towards different kinds of stresses has been shown in *Lc. lactis* (Hartke et al., 1997; O'Sullivan and Condon, 1997) and *P. freudenreichii* (Leverrier et al., 2004). Exposure to heat, acid, and UV irradiation resulted in the up-regulation of the GroEL and GroES, although quantitative analyses of the 2-DE gels indicated that the magnitude of induction is dependent on the nature of the stress. GroES was up-regulated 12-fold during heat stress, but this protein was up-regulated only 3.8-fold after exposure to acidic pH (Hartke et al., 1997). However, in *P. freudenreichii* cross-protection from acid pretreatment to heat stress did not occur, and acidic pretreatment sensitized the cells to bile salt stress (Leverrier et al., 2004). These results suggest that cross-protection is not necessarily reciprocal. Bile salt adaptation resulted in protection against acid and heat, but adaptation to acid stress did not culminate in protection against bile salt or heat stress. Furthermore, these results indicate that cross-protection to stress differs in various bacteria.

Regulation of Stress Proteins

The regulation of stress responses in LAB in response to several stressors can be divided into three main groups (Fig. 2). One group includes proteins regulated by specific stress factors. The second group includes proteins regulated by nonspecific responses to certain stimuli and may not be considered to be stress proteins (e.g., glycolytic proteins), and the third group includes general stress proteins (Fig. 2). Indeed, proteins known to be regulated by the general stress response regulator, σ^B, have been visualized by proteomics during several different stress inducers. The σ^B-dependent genes are induced by heat, ethanol, acid, bile salts, and carbon starvation and in the presence of phosphate or oxygen (Drews et al., 2002; Spano et al., 2005). Proteomics has shown that the heat shock proteins DnaK and GroEL/ES are examples

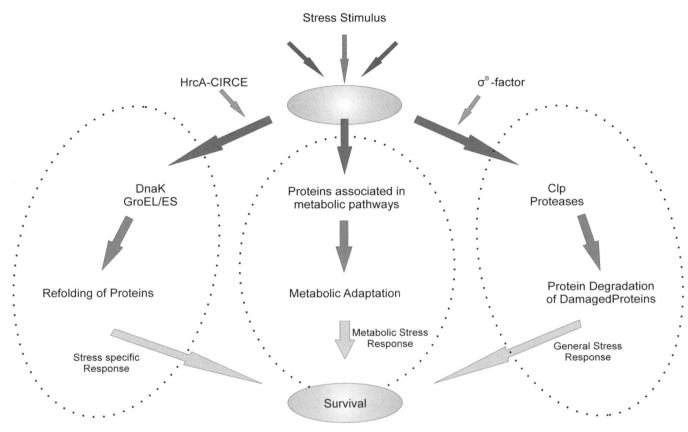

Figure 2 A schematic overview of stress responses in LAB (based on Drews et al., 2002, and van de Guchte et al., 2002). Proteins within the dashed circles are associated with several stress responses visualized by two-dimensional gel electrophoresis. DnaK and GroES/EL are induced during specific stress challenges, while Clp is a general stress protein. The third group consists of proteins found to be differentially regulated during stress, changing the metabolism of the bacterium towards adaptation to the stress inducer.

of stress-specific responses that are normally induced during heat shock. The genes *dnaK* and *groE*, coding for DnaK and GroES/EL, respectively, are controlled by the HrcA-CIRCE repression system which, in turn, can be controlled by GroEL/ES (van de Guchte et al., 2002). The Clp protein family was shown by proteomics to be induced by different stress-associated stimuli.

Clp proteins are ATP-dependent proteases involved in the repair or protein degradation under normal and stress conditions and are under the control of the stress response regulator σ^B (Drews et al., 2002). Although the stress proteins are highly conserved and the responses are similar in different microorganisms, the regulation of specific stress proteins is complex in nature. Proteins involved in metabolic pathways and not obviously associated with stress responses may be up-regulated by specific stress inducers. The production of known stress proteins may not be sufficient to respond to physiological stresses for prolonged periods. As an example, the glycolytic proteins glyceraldehyde-3-phosphate dehydrogenase (GAPDH), 6-phosphate-fructokinase (PFK), and enolase are produced in greater abundance during heat and cold shock, oxidative stress, and acid stress, respectively (Table 4).

Upon cold shock in *Lc. lactis*, the production of CcpA and HPr was up-regulated two- to threefold (Wouters et al., 2000). The *pfk* gene is under control of the *las* operon, and this operon is subjected to catabolite activation by CcpA-HPr(Ser-P). However, increased quantities of CcpA and HPr did not lead to greater abundance of PFK or GAPDH in *Lc. lactis* (Wouters et al., 2000). It was proposed that factors other than CcpA-HPr alone are needed to regulate cold shock and glycolysis. These results indicate that investigation of a few proteins (reductionism) alone is not sufficient to predict the metabolic behavior of LAB during stress, and it is expected that proteomics approaches will provide a more holistic view of microbial and cellular phenotypes under a variety of environmental conditions.

METAPROTEOMICS

Proteomics is a high-throughput methodology and provides a more complete understanding of the changes that are occurring in an organism's proteome under specific environmental conditions. Up to now, single organisms and monocellular tissues have been investigated using proteomics, and these studies have provided novel insights into relatively simple ecosystems. Analyses of proteomes of bacteria cultivated under controlled laboratory conditions will not result in the understanding of their collective functions in any host ecosystem. In fact, studying the details of a single bacterium from an ecosystem is comparable to studying a single protein from a proteome, and therefore, studying a single bacterium can be seen again as a form of reductionism when the complete ecosystem is considered. Studying samples of a complex ecosystem will provide a more complete overview of metabolic networks and interactions between different organisms and their environments. The new term "metaproteomics" has been proposed by Wilmes and Bond and can be defined as large-scale characterization of the entire protein complement of an environmental microbiota at a given point in time (Wilmes and Bond, 2004).

Applications of metaproteomics have been described for analyzing mixed microbial communities in samples including sludge, saltwater such as the Chesapeake Bay, natural microbial biofilms grown on surfaces of sulfuric acid-rich solutions, and the human infant gastrointestinal tract (Wilmes and Bond, 2004; Kan et al., 2005; Ram et al., 2005; Klaassens et al., 2007). Applications of 2-DE studies to the metaproteome of the complex human infant gastrointestinal tract ecosystem yielded more than 200 protein spots including 21 proteins that were differentially regulated in time (Klaassens et al., 2007). However, only one protein spot was identified as a transaldolase, which is used in the pentose phosphate pathway to obtain D-fructose-6-phosphate and NADPH (KEGG database, http://www.genome.jp/keg) (Kanehisa and Goto, 2000). NADPH provides the proton motive force for the synthesis of ATP (Friedrich and Scheide, 2000). The low number of protein spots identified from the metaproteome of the human infant gastrointestinal tract is in accordance with metaproteomics study samples obtained from the Chesapeake Bay in North America. This study yielded significant identifications of seven proteins visualized in 2-DE gels (Kan et al., 2005). However, proteomics of a natural microbial biofilm present in acid mine drainage yielded identifications of 5,994 proteins corresponding to 2,003 unique proteins (Ram et al., 2005). The success of this study is based on a slightly different approach that is described below.

Although 2-DE gels and the use of two-dimensional nano-LC have been established to resolve complex protein mixtures, facile identification of proteins by mass fingerprinting is unlikely. Greater than 97% amino acid sequence identity is required to provide a positive, statistically relevant match when searching protein databases with MALDI-TOF MS data (Kan et al., 2005). In order to overcome this problem, tandem MS can be used to identify protein spots by performing de novo peptide sequencing. Amino acid sequences will provide a highly statistically relevant identification of the protein. Complementary analyses of the pI and molecular weight of the identified protein with de novo sequencing can generate confidence in identification of the protein of interest. The differentially produced transaldolase, which has a high probability to be derived from *Bifidobacterium infantis* in the human infant gastrointestinal tract when analyzed by metaproteomics, has been identified using this combination methodology (Klaassens et al., 2007).

A basis for studying the metaproteome of the human gastrointestinal tract is to obtain a metagenomic data set of proteins likely to be produced in the intestine (Fig. 3). The predicted proteins can be used for the construction of new protein databases which can serve protein identification strategies in additional metaproteomics studies. A metagenomic database of a biofilm has been analyzed, and from this database, a new protein database has been constructed containing 12,148 proteins. This protein database has been used to identify new proteins by two-dimensional nano-LC tandem MS (Ram et al., 2005).

FUTURE PERSPECTIVES

In order to investigate the functionality of LAB that can have beneficial health effects on the human host, analyses of proteomes using 2-DE may provide insights into the metabolic activities and regulation, microbial survival, and possible interactions between microbes and host. Proteins are a key dynamic link between genotype and phenotype. To generate a global view of the interplay between microbes and their ecosystems, metaproteomics may be able to elucidate key insights. A possible work flow of metaproteomics studies is depicted

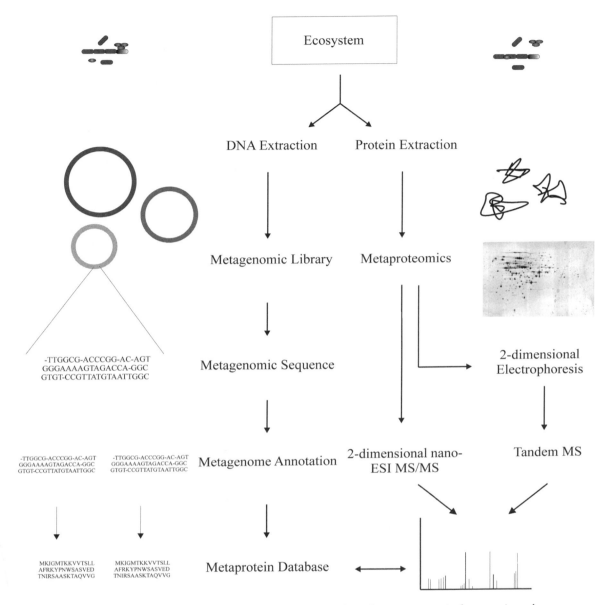

Figure 3 A schematic diagram combines metagenomic and metaproteomic data sets in order to address gut functionality of LAB. With metagenomics, identification of bacterial genes is feasible. Protein predictions of active genes by metagenomics will facilitate protein identification by metaproteomics.

in Fig. 3. By establishing databases of proteins predicted to be generated by microbes in particular ecosystems such as the intestine based on metagenomic data, more proteins will be identified by analyses of different spots. The first metagenomic libraries from the human gastrointestinal tract have been described (Gill et al., 2006; Manichanh et al., 2006; Jones and Marchesi, 2007; Kurokawa et al., 2007) and have provided a wealth of information about the genetic diversity within the human gastrointestinal microbiota. Moreover, transcriptomics analyses of the human gastrointestinal microbiota are being performed and indicate that genes involved in carbohydrate transport and metabolism are dominantly expressed, especially in the small intestine (C. Booijnk, personal communication).

Combinations of metagenomics and metaproteomics data sets should be used for future experiments to address the functionality of LAB in gut health. Moreover, to have detailed insights regarding interactions between LAB and epithelial cells in the intestine, genomic data sets of eukaryotic cells and bacterial communities should be combined into comprehensive databases of proteins engaged in microbial-host interactions. The ultimate metaproteomics studies of eukaryotic and prokaryotic cells can be applied simultaneously to obtain insights into the interactions between microbes and humans for an enhanced understanding of beneficial health effects delivered by microbes in the host.

Ultimately, complete integration of -omics technologies is needed to fully understand the complex behaviors of microorganisms in complex ecosystems. These investigations of systems biology will result from applications of high-throughput methodologies and the integration of experimental techniques. The successful capture and integration of experimental data generated by genomics, transcriptomics, proteomics, and metabolomics may be combined with theoretical models to predict the behavior of cells or microorganisms (Romero et al., 2006). Indeed, integration of transcriptomics and proteomics data is an ongoing process, and a holistic understanding of organisms in the context of ecosystems may require large-scale biological studies applying metagenomics, metatranscriptomics, and metaproteomics. Such approaches should be combined in the future to develop more complete portraits of microbial-host interactions for the benefit of animal and human health.

References

Aebersold, R. H., J. Leavitt, R. A. Saavedra, L. E. Hood, and S. B. H. Kent. 1987. Internal amino acid sequence analysis of proteins separated by one- or two-dimensional gel electrophoresis after in situ protease digestion on nitrocellulose. *Proc. Natl. Acad. Sci. USA* 84:6970–6974.

Aebersold, R. H., G. Pipes, L. E. Hood, and S. B. H. Kent. 1988. N-terminal and internal sequence determination of microgram amounts of proteins separated by isoelectric focusing in immobilized pH gradients. *Electrophoresis* 9:520–530.

Alonso, J. C., K. Shirahige, and N. Ogasawara. 1990. Molecular cloning, genetic characterization and DNA sequence analysis of the *recM* region of *Bacillus subtilis*. *Nucleic Acids Res.* 18:6771–6777.

Altermann, E., W. M. Russell, M. A. Azcarate-Peril, R. Barrangou, B. L. Buck, O. McAuliffe, N. Souther, A. Dobson, T. Duong, M. Callanan, S. Lick, A. Hamrick, R. Cano, and T. R. Klaenhammer. 2005. Complete genome sequence of the probiotic lactic acid bacterium *Lactobacillus acidophilus* NCFM. *Proc. Natl. Acad. Sci. USA* 102:3906–3912.

Anastasiou, R., P. Leverrier, I. Krestas, A. Rouault, G. Kalantzopoulos, P. Boyaval, E. Tsakalidou, and G. Jan. 2006.

Changes in protein synthesis during thermal adaptation of *Propionibacterium freudenreichii* subsp. *shermanii*. *Int. J. Food Microbiol.* 108:301–314.

Andersen, J. S., and M. Mann. 2000. Functional genomics by mass spectrometry. *FEBS Lett.* 480:25–31.

Anderson, L. B., M. Maderia, A. J. A. Ouellette, C. Putnam-Evans, L. Higgins, T. Krick, M. J. MacCoss, H. Lim, J. R. Yates III, and B. A. Barry. 2002. Posttranslational modifications in the CP43 subunit of photosystem II. *Proc. Natl. Acad. Sci. USA* 99:14676–14681.

Anglade, P., E. Demey, V. Labas, J.-P. L. Caer, and J.-F. Chich. 2000. Towards a proteomic map of *Lactococcus lactis* NCDO 763. *Electrophoresis* 21:2546–2549.

Barber, M., R. S. Bordoli, R. D. Sedgwick, and A. N. Tyler. 1981. Fast atom bombardment of solids as an ion source in mass spectrometry. *Nature* 293:270–275.

Bernstein, C., H. Bernstein, C. M. Payne, S. E. Beard, and J. Schneider. 1999. Bile salt activation of stress response promoters in *Escherichia coli*. *Curr. Microbiol.* 39:68–72.

Bonestroo, M. H., B. J. M. Kusters, J. C. De Wit, and F. M. Rombouts. 1992. Glucose and sucrose fermenting capacity of homofermentative lactic acid bacteria used as starters in fermented salads. *Int. J. Food Microbiol.* 15:365.

Bron, P. A., D. Molenaar, W. M. Vos, and M. Kleerebezem. 2006. DNA micro-array-based identification of bile-responsive genes in *Lactobacillus plantarum*. *J. Appl. Microbiol.* 100:728–738.

Budin-Verneuil, A., V. Pichereau, Y. Auffray, D. S. Ehrlich, and E. Maguin. 2005. Proteomic characterization of the acid tolerance response in *Lactococcus lactis* MG1363. *Proteomics* 5:4794–4807.

Cha, B., M. Blades, and D. J. Douglas. 2000. An interface with a linear quadrupole ion guide for an electrospray-ion trap mass spectrometer system. *Anal. Chem.* 72:5647–5654.

Chervaux, C., S. D. Ehrlich, and E. Maguin. 2000. Physiological study of *Lactobacillus delbrueckii* subsp. *bulgaricus* strains in a novel chemically defined medium. *Appl. Environ. Microbiol.* 66:5306–5311.

Cohen, D. P. A., J. Renes, F. G. Bouwman, E. G. Zoetendal, E. Mariman, W. M. de Vos, and E. E. Vaughan. 2006. Proteomic analysis of log to stationary growth phase *Lactobacillus plantarum* cells and a 2-DE database. *Proteomics* 6:6485–6493.

De Angelis, M., R. Di Cagno, C. Huet, C. Crecchio, P. F. Fox, and M. Gobbetti. 2004. Heat shock response in *Lactobacillus plantarum*. *Appl. Environ. Microbiol.* 70:1336–1346.

de Vries, M. C. 2006. *Analyzing Global Gene Expression of* Lactobacillus plantarum *in the Human Gastro-Intestinal Tract*. Laboratory of Microbiology, Wageningen University, Wageningen, The Netherlands.

Di Cagno, R., M. De Angelis, A. Limitone, P. F. Fox, and M. Gobbetti. 2006. Response of *Lactobacillus helveticus* PR4 to heat stress during propagation in cheese whey with a gradient of decreasing temperatures. *Appl. Environ. Microbiol.* 72:4503–4514.

Drews, O., G. Reil, H. Parlar, and A. Görg. 2004. Setting up standards and a reference map for the alkaline proteome of the Gram-positive bacterium *Lactococcus lactis*. *Proteomics* 4:1293–1304.

Drews, O., W. Weiss, G. Reil, H. Parlar, R. Wait, and A. Görg. 2002. High pressure effects step-wise altered protein expression in *Lactobacillus sanfranciscensis*. *Proteomics* 2:765–774.

Enan, G., A. A. El-Essawy, M. Uyttendaele, and J. Debevere. 1996. Antibacterial activity of *Lactobacillus plantarum* UG1 isolated from dry sausage: characterization, production and bactericidal action of plantaricin UG1. *Int. J. Food Microbiol.* 30:189.

Eng, J. K., A. L. McCormack, and J. R. Yates III. 1994. An approach to correlate tandem mass spectral data of peptides with amino acid sequences in a protein database. *J. Am. Soc. Mass Spectrom.* 5:976–989.

Ercolini, D., P. J. Hill, and C. E. R. Dodd. 2003. Bacterial community structure and location in Stilton cheese. *Appl. Environ. Microbiol.* 69:3540–3548.

Feder, M. E., and J.-C. Walser. 2005. The biological limitations of transcriptomics in elucidating stress and stress responses. *J. Evol. Biol.* 18:901–910.

Fenn, J. B., M. Mann, C. K. Meng, S. F. Wong, and C. M. Whitehouse. 1989. Electrospray ionization for mass spectrometry of large biomolecules. *Science* 246:64–71.

Finegold, S. M., V. L. Sutter, J. D. Boyle, and K. Shimada. 1970. The normal flora of ileostomy and transverse colostomy effluents. *J. Infect. Dis.* 122:376.

Fraenkel-Conrat, H. 1994. Early days of protein chemistry. *FASEB J.* 8:452–453.

Frees, D., F. K. Vogensen, and H. Ingmer. 2003. Identification of proteins induced at low pH in *Lactococcus lactis*. *Int. J. Food Microbiol.* 87:293–300.

Friedrich, T., and D. Scheide. 2000. The respiratory complex I of bacteria, archaea and eukarya and its module common with membrane-bound multisubunit hydrogenases. *FEBS Lett.* 479:1–5.

Gill, S. R., M. Pop, R. T. DeBoy, P. B. Eckburg, P. J. Turnbaugh, B. S. Samuel, J. I. Gordon, D. A. Relman, C. M. Fraser-Liggett, and K. E. Nelson. 2006. Metagenomic analysis of the human distal gut microbiome. *Science* 312:1355–1359.

Gitton, C., M. Meyrand, J. Wang, C. Caron, A. Trubuil, A. Guillot, and M.-Y. Mistou. 2005. Proteomic signature of *Lactococcus lactis* NCDO763 cultivated in milk. *Appl. Environ. Microbiol.* 71:7152–7163.

Graves, P. R., and T. A. J. Haystead. 2002. Molecular biologist's guide to proteomics. *Microbiol. Mol. Biol. Rev.* 66:39–63.

Grus, F. H., V. N. Podust, K. Bruns, K. Lackner, S. Fu, E. A. Dalmasso, A. Wirthlin, and N. Pfeiffer. 2005. SELDI-TOF-MS protein chip array profiling of tears from patients with dry eye. *Investig Ophthalmol. Vis. Sci.* 46:863–876.

Gygi, S. P., Y. Rochon, B. R. Franza, and R. Aebersold. 1999. Correlation between protein and mRNA abundance in yeast. *Mol. Cell. Biol.* 19:1720–1730.

Hartke, A., S. Bouché, J.-C. Giard, A. Benachour, P. Boutibonnes, and Y. Auffray. 1996. The lactic acid stress response of *Lactococcus lactis* subsp. *lactis*. *Curr. Microbiol.* 33:194–199.

Hartke, A., J. Frère, P. Boutibonnes, and Y. Auffray. 1997. Differential induction of the chaperonin GroEL and the co-chaperonin GroES by heat, acid, and UV-irradiation in *Lactococcus lactis* subsp. *lactis*. *Curr. Microbiol.* 34:23–26.

Henzel, W. J., C. Watanabe, and J. T. Stults. 2003. Protein identification: the origins of peptide mass fingerprinting. *J. Am. Soc. Mass Spectrom.* 14:931–942.

Hooper, L. V., and J. I. Gordon. 2001. Commensal host-bacterial relationships in the gut. *Science* 292:1115–1118.

Hörmann, S., C. Scheyhing, J. Behr, M. Pavlovic, M. Ehrmann, and R. F. Vogel. 2006. Comparative proteome approach to characterize the high-pressure stress response of *Lactobacillus sanfranciscensis* DSM 20451T. *Proteomics* 6:1878–1885.

Hu, Q., R. J. Noll, H. Li, A. Makarov, M. Hardman, and R. G. Cooks. 2005. The Orbitrap: a new mass spectrometer. *J. Mass Spectrom.* 40:430–443.

Inagaki, N., and K. Katsuta. 2004. Large gel two-dimensional electrophoresis: improving recovery of cellular proteome. *Curr. Proteomics* 1:35–39.

Jan, G., P. Leverrier, V. Pichereau, and P. Boyaval. 2001. Changes in protein synthesis and morphology during acid adaptation of *Propionibacterium freudenreichii*. *Appl. Environ. Microbiol.* 67:2029–2036.

Jensen, O. N. 2006. Interpreting the protein language using proteomics. *Nat. Rev. Mol. Cell Biol.* 7:391–403.

Jensen, P. R., and K. Hammer. 1993. Minimal requirements for exponential growth of *Lactococcus lactis*. *Appl. Environ. Microbiol.* 59:4363–4366.

Jin, L.-T., S.-Y. Hwang, G.-S. Yoo, and J.-K. Choi. 2006. A mass spectrometry compatible silver staining method for protein incorporating a new silver sensitizer in sodium dodecyl sulfate-polyacrylamide electrophoresis gels. *Proteomics* 6:2334–2337.

Jones, B. V., and J. R. Marchesi. 2007. Transposon-aided capture (TRACA) of plasmids resident in the human gut mobile metagenome. *Nat. Methods* 4:55–61.

Kan, J., T. E. Hanson, J. M. Ginter, K. Wang, and F. Chen. 2005. Metaproteomics analysis of Chesapeake Bay microbial communities. *Saline Syst.* 1:7.

Kanehisa, M., and S. Goto. 2000. KEGG: Kyoto Encyclopedia of Genes and Genomes. *Nucleic Acids Res.* 28:27–30.

Klaassens, E. S., W. M. De Vos, and E. E. Vaughan. 2007. Metaproteomics approach to study the functionality of the microbiota in the human infant gastrointestinal tract. *Appl. Environ. Microbiol.* 73:1388–1392.

Koistinen, K. M., C. Plumed-Ferrer, S. J. Lehesranta, S. O. Karenlampi, and A. Von Wright. 2007. Comparison of growth-phase-dependent cytosolic proteomes of two *Lactobacillus plantarum* strains used in food and feed fermentations. *FEMS Microbiol. Lett.* 273:12–21.

Krutchinsky, A. N., M. Kalkum, and B. T. Chait. 2001. Automatic identification of proteins with a MALDI-Quadrupole Ion Trap mass spectrometer. *Anal. Chem.* 73:5066–5077.

Kurokawa, K., T. Itoh, T. Kuwahara, K. Oshima, H. Toh, A. Toyoda, H. Takami, H. Morita, V. K. Sharma, T. P. Srivastava, T. D. Taylor, H. Noguchi, H. Mori, Y. Ogura, D. S. Ehrlich, K. Itoh, T. Takagi, Y. Sakaki, T. Hayashi, and M. Hattori. 2007. Comparative metagenomics revealed commonly enriched gene sets in human gut microbiomes. *DNA Res.* 14:169–181.

Lahm, H.-W., and H. Langen. 2000. Mass spectrometry: a tool for the identification of proteins separated by gels. *Electrophoresis* 21:2105–2114.

Larsen, N., M. Boye, H. Siegumfeldt, and M. Jakobsen. 2006. Differential expression of proteins and genes in the lag phase of *Lactococcus lactis* subsp. *lactis* grown in synthetic medium and reconstituted skim milk. *Appl. Environ. Microbiol.* 72:1173–1179.

Leverrier, P., D. Dimova, V. Pichereau, Y. Auffray, P. Boyaval, and G. Jan. 2003. Susceptibility and adaptive response to bile salts in *Propionibacterium freudenreichii*: physiological and proteomic analysis. *Appl. Environ. Microbiol.* 69:3809–3818.

Leverrier, P., J. P. C. Vissers, A. Rouault, P. Boyaval, and G. Jan. 2004. Mass spectrometry proteomic analysis of stress adaptation reveals both common and distinct response pathways in *Propionibacterium freudenreichii*. *Arch. Microbiol.* 181:215–230.

Lim, E. M., S. D. Ehrlich, and E. Maguin. 2000. Identification of stress-inducible proteins in *Lactobacillus delbrueckii* subsp. *bulgaricus*. *Electrophoresis* 21:2557–2561.

Makarov, A., E. Denisov, A. Kholomeev, W. Balschun, O. Lange, K. Strupat, and S. Horning. 2006. Performance evaluation of a hybrid linear ion trap/orbitrap mass spectrometer. *Anal. Chem.* 78:2113–2120.

Makarova, K., A. Slesarev, Y. Wolf, A. Sorokin, B. Mirkin, E. Koonin, A. Pavlov, N. Pavlova, V. Karamychev, N. Polouchine, V. Shakhova, I. Grigoriev, Y. Lou, D. Rohksar, S. Lucas, K. Huang, D. M. Goodstein, T. Hawkins, V. Plengvidhya, D. Welker, J. Hughes, Y. Goh, A. Benson, K. Baldwin, J. H. Lee, I. Diaz-Muniz, B. Dosti, B. Smeianov, W. Wechter, R. Barabote, G. Lorca, E. Altermann, R. Barrangou, B. Ganesan, Y. Xie, H. Rawsthorne, D. Tamir, C. Parker, F. Breidt, J. Broadbent, R. Hutkins, D. O'Sullivan, J. Steele, G. Unlu, M. Saier, T. Klaenhammer, P. Richardson, S. Kozyavkin, B. Weimer, and D. Mills. 2006. Comparative genomics of the lactic acid bacteria. *Proc. Natl. Acad. Sci. USA* 103:15611–15616.

Manichanh, C., L. Rigottier-Gois, E. Bonnaud, K. Gloux, E. Pelletier, L. Frangeul, R. Nalin, C. Jarrin, P. Chardon, P. Marteau, J. Roca, and J. Dore. 2006. Reduced diversity of faecal microbiota in Crohn's disease revealed by a metagenomic approach. *Gut* 55:205–211.

Mann, M., R. C. Hendrickson, and A. Pandey. 2001. Analysis of proteins and proteomes by mass spectrometry. *Annu. Rev. Biochem.* 70:437–473.

Marceau, A., M. Zagorec, S. Chaillou, T. Méra, and M.-C. Champomier-Vergès. 2004. Evidence for involvement of at least six proteins in adaptation of *Lactobacillus sakei* to cold temperatures and addition of NaCl. *Appl. Environ. Microbiol.* 70:7260–7268.

Marshall, A. G., C. L. Hendrickson, and G. S. Jackson. 1998. Fourier transform ion cyclotron resonance mass spectrometry: a primer. *Mass Spectrom. Rev.* 17:1–35.

Martin, S. E., J. Shabanowitz, D. F. Hunt, and J. A. Marto. 2000. Subfemtomole MS and MS/MS peptide sequence analysis using Nano-HPLC Micro-ESI Fourier Transform Ion Cyclotron Resonance mass spectrometry. *Anal. Chem.* 72:4266–4274.

Matsui, N. M., D. M. Smith, K. R. Clauser, J. Fichmann, L. E. Andrews, C. M. Sullivan, A. L. Burlingame, and L. B. Epstein. 1997. Immobilized pH gradient two-dimensional gel electrophoresis and mass spectrometric identification of cytokine-regulated proteins in ME-180 cervical carcinoma cells. *Electrophoresis* 18:409–417.

Molin, G. 2001. Probiotics in foods not containing milk or milk constituents, with special reference to *Lactobacillus plantarum* 299v. *Am. J. Clin. Nutr.* 73(2 Suppl.):380S–385S.

Nyström, T., and F. C. Neidhardt. 1994. Expression and role of the universal stress protein, UspA, of *Escherichia coli* during growth arrest. *Mol. Microbiol.* 11:537–544.

O'Farrell, P. H. 1975. High resolution two-dimensional electrophoresis of proteins. *J. Biochem.* 250:4007–4021.

O'Sullivan, E., and S. Condon. 1997. Intracellular pH is a major factor in the induction of tolerance to acid and other stresses in *Lactococcus lactis*. *Appl. Environ. Microbiol.* 63:4210–4215.

Patterson, S. D., and R. H. Aebersold. 2003. Proteomics: the first decade and beyond. *Nat. Genet.* 33:311–323.

Peng, J., and S. P. Gygi. 2001. Proteomics: the move to mixtures. *J. Mass Spectrom.* 36:1083–1091.

Pessione, E., R. Mazzoli, M. G. Giuffrida, C. Lamberti, E. Garcia-Moruno, C. Barello, A. Conti, and C. Giunta. 2005. A proteomic approach to studying biogenic amine producing lactic acid bacteria. *Proteomics* 5:687–698.

Pieterse, B., R. J. Leer, F. H. J. Schuren, and M. J. van der Werf. 2005. Unravelling the multiple effects of lactic acid stress on *Lactobacillus plantarum* by transcription profiling. *Microbiology* 151:3881–3894.

Rajilić-Stojanović, M. 2007. *Diversity of the Human Gastrointestinal Microbiota: Novel Perspectives from High Throughput Analyses*. Laboratory of Microbiology, Wageningen University, Wageningen, The Netherlands.

Ram, R. J., N. C. VerBerkmoes, M. P. Thelen, G. W. Tyson, B. J. Baker, R. C. Blake II, M. Shah, R. L. Hettich, and J. Banfield. 2005. Community proteomics of a natural microbial biofilm. *Science* 308:1915–1920.

Regula, J. T., B. Ueberle, G. Boguth, A. Görg, M. Schnölzer, R. Herrmann, and R. Frank. 2000. Towards a two-dimensional proteome map of *Mycoplasma pneumoniae*. *Electrophoresis* 21:3765–3780.

Roe, M. R., and T. J. Griffin. 2006. Gel-free mass spectrometry-based high throughput proteomics: tools for studying biological response of proteins and proteomes. *Proteomics* 6:4678–4687.

Romero, R., J. Espinoza, F. Gotsch, J. P. Kusanovic, L. A. Friel, O. Erez, S. Mazaki-Tovi, N. G. Than, S. Hassan, and G. Tromp. 2006. The use of high-dimensional biology (genomics, transcriptomics, proteomics, and metabolomics) to understand the preterm parturition syndrome. *BJOG* 113(Suppl. 3):118–135.

Schauder, S., K. Shokat, M. G. Surette, and B. L. Bassler. 2001. The LuxS family of bacterial autoinducers: biosynthesis of a novel quorum-sensing signal molecule. *Mol. Microbiol.* 41:463–476.

Singh, O. V., and N. S. Nagaraj. 2006. Transcriptomics, proteomics and interactomics: unique approaches to track the insights of bioremediation. *Brief. Funct. Genomic. Proteomic.* 4:355–362.

Spano, G., L. Beneduce, C. Perrotta, and S. Massa. 2005. Cloning and characterization of the *hsp* 18.55 gene, a new member of the small heat shock gene family isolated from wine *Lactobacillus plantarum. Res. Microbiol.* **156**:219–224.

Strange, K. 2005. The end of "naive reductionism": rise of systems biology or renaissance of physiology? *Am. J. Physiol. Cell Physiol.* **288**:C968–C974.

Takats, Z., J. M. Wiseman, B. Gologan, and R. G. Cooks. 2004. Mass spectrometry sampling under ambient conditions with desorption electrospray ionization. *Science* **306**:471–473.

Tanaka, K., H. Waki, Y. Ido, S. Akita, Y. Yoshida, T. Yoshida, and T. Matsuo. 1988. Protein and polymer analyses up to *m/z* 100 000 by laser ionization time-of-flight mass spectrometry. *Rapid Commun. Mass Spectrom.* **2**:151–153.

Tang, N., P. Tornatore, and S. R. Weinberger. 2004. Current developments in SELDI affinity technology. *Mass Spectrom. Rev.* **23**:34–44.

Tlaskalova-Hogenova, H., R. Stepankova, T. Hudcovic, L. Tuckova, B. Cukrowska, R. Lodinova-Zadnikova, H. Kozakova, P. Rossmann, J. Bartova, D. Sokol, D. Funda, D. Borovska, Z. Rehakova, J. Sinkora, J. Hofman, P. Drastich, and A. Kokesova. 2004. Commensal bacteria (normal microflora), mucosal immunity and chronic inflammatory and autoimmune diseases. *Immunol. Lett.* **15**:97–108.

Ünlü, M., M. E. Morgan, and J. S. Minden. 1997. Difference gel electrophoresis. A single gel method for detecting changes in protein extracts. *Electrophoresis* **18**:2071–2077.

van de Guchte, M., P. Serror, C. Chervaux, T. Smokvina, S. D. Ehrlich, and E. Maguin. 2002. Stress responses in lactic acid bacteria. *Antonie Leeuwenhoek* **82**:187–216.

Vaughan, E. E., M. C. de Vries, E. G. Zoetendal, K. Ben-Amor, A. D. L. Akkermans, and W. M. de Vos. 2002. The intestinal LABs. *Antonie Leeuwenhoek* **82**:341–352.

Vido, K., H. Diemer, A. Van Dorsselaer, E. Leize, V. Juillard, A. Gruss, and P. Gaudu. 2005. Roles of thioredoxin reductase during the aerobic life of *Lactococcus lactis. J. Bacteriol.* **187**:601–610.

Wayne, F. P. 2000. A thousand points of light: the application of fluorescence detection technologies to two-dimensional gel electrophoresis and proteomics. *Electrophoresis* **21**:1123–1144.

Westermeier, R., and R. Marouga. 2005. Protein detection methods in proteomics research. *Biosci. Rep.* **25**:19–32.

Wilmes, P., and P. L. Bond. 2004. The application of two-dimensional polyacrylamide gel electrophoresis and downstream analyses to mixed community of prokaryotic microorganisms. *Environ. Microbiol.* **6**:911–920.

Wollnik, H. 1993. Time-of-flight mass analyzers. *Mass Spectrom. Rev.* **12**:89–114.

Wouters, J. A., H. H. Kamphuis, J. Hugenholtz, O. P. Kuipers, W. M. de Vos, and T. Abee. 2000. Changes in glycolytic activity of *Lactococcus lactis* induced by low temperature. *Appl. Environ. Microbiol.* **66**:3686–3691.

Yoon, K. Y., E. E. Woodams, and Y. D. Hang. 2006. Production of probiotic cabbage juice by lactic acid bacteria. *Bioresour. Technol.* **97**:1427–1430.

Zhou, J., and D. K. Thompson. 2002. Challenges in applying microarrays to environmental studies. *Curr. Opin. Biotechnol.* **13**:204–207.

Therapeutic Microbiology in Human Medicine

3

Therapeutic Microbiology: Probiotics and Related Strategies
Edited by J. Versalovic and M. Wilson
© 2008 ASM Press, Washington, DC

3.1. PROBIOTICS

Jennifer K. Spinler
James Versalovic

Probiotics in Human Medicine: Overview

17

LIVING IN A MICROBIAL WORLD

The concept that specific microbial communities could substantially impact human health was pioneered by Nobel Laureate Elie Metchnikoff in the early 20th century (Metchnikoff, 1907) and, a century later, is being pursued in the international Human Microbiome Project (Turnbaugh et al., 2007). Historically, microbes have been studied individually with a lack of knowledge regarding how entire microbial communities work, thrive, and exist together within animal hosts. In fact, medical microbiology historically focused on human pathogens and infectious diseases, while research has been comparatively limited with regard to human commensal and probiotic organisms. Microbes significantly outnumber human cells in the adult body, and yet the microbial community infrastructure is mostly unknown. Even more enigmatic are the effects that these microbial communities have on human development, physiology, immunity, health, and disease (Fig. 1) (Reid, 2004).

Probiotics are defined by the World Health Organization as "live microorganisms which when administered in adequate amounts confer a health benefit on the host" (FAO/WHO, 2002). The majority of probiotic organisms studied today are lactic acid bacteria including species of the genera *Lactobacillus*, *Bifidobacterium*, and *Streptococcus*, but this group of beneficial bacteria could be expanded to include a vast array of genera with further explorations of the human microbiome. The abundance of microbes present in the human gastrointestinal tract encompasses a restricted set of bacterial phyla, suggesting that the autochthonous microbiota may be composed of a restricted set of species that possibly form a "core microbiome." The introduction of the core human microbiome concept initiates new ways of thinking about potential clinical applications of probiotics.

Is there a core human microbiome, and if so, how do alterations in this core microbial community affect human health? Do natural changes in this core microbiome

Jennifer K. Spinler and James Versalovic, Department of Pathology, Baylor College of Medicine, and Department of Pathology, Texas Children's Hospital, 6621 Fannin Street, MC 1-2261, Houston, TX 77030.

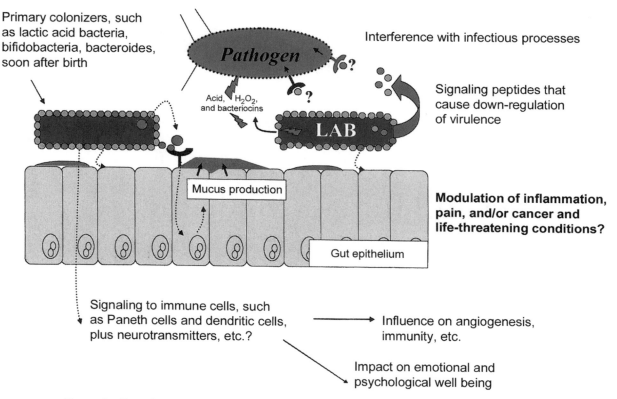

Figure 1 Complexity of microbial-host interactions. Reprinted from the *Journal of Clinical Infectious Diseases* (Reid, 2004) with permission of The University of Chicago Press. LAB, lactic acid bacteria.

occur during human development and shape physiology and immunity? Initial colonization patterns of the gastrointestinal tract during infancy may be affected by fundamental dietary issues such as whether infants consume breast or bottled milk and the timing of introduction of solid foods. Exposures to indigenous microbes in breast milk or dairy food products, in addition to antimicrobial agents, may have profound effects on the gastrointestinal microbiota, especially early in life. The relative plasticity of the intestinal microbiota in infancy may be extended to large-scale shifts occurring at other mucosal surfaces and body sites. Various fluctuations in infantile microbial populations occur in the intestine within the first year of human life, indicating that tremendous flux and opportunities for microbial population remodeling occur early in life (Palmer et al., 2007). An adultlike complex intestinal microbiota forms by the end of the first year of life, raising fundamental questions about the developmental impact of microbes on physiology and immunity.

Microbial populations associated with mammalian hosts may have beneficial or detrimental effects on

immunity and physiology. Can investigators deliberately modify the microbial community of patients in chronic disease states such that disease burden is reduced or eliminated? Do specific disease states reflect aberrations or deficiencies in aggregate microbial functions? Can disease susceptibilities be affected by remodeling the existing microbiota? The adult gut microbiota is dominated by two divisions of bacteria, *Bacteroidetes* and *Firmicutes* (Backhed et al., 2005; Eckburg et al., 2005). As an example, their relative proportions differ significantly between lean and obese subjects, and evidence suggests that modifications in microbial profiles could lead to new therapeutic options for obesity (Ley et al., 2006b).

While important characteristics of probiotics include their abilities to suppress the proliferation and virulence of pathogenic organisms, it is becoming quite clear that these organisms also have direct effects on human physiology and immunity. Studies are beginning to shed light on tangible effects of probiotics in allergic and autoimmune diseases, oral biology, diseases of the gastrointestinal and genitourinary tracts, and neurology and psychiatry.

Advances in probiotics research are resulting in implementation of probiotics as treatment and prevention strategies for a multitude of human diseases.

PROBIOTICS IN ALLERGIC AND AUTOIMMUNE DISEASES

In recent years, developed countries have experienced a striking rise in the incidence of allergic and immunological disorders including asthma, hay fever, and autoimmune diseases such as type 1 diabetes, Crohn's disease, and multiple sclerosis (Bach, 2002). Increased susceptibilities to immunological disorders may be attributed to deficient immunoregulation caused by reduced exposure to essential microorganisms, or "old friends," especially early in life (Guarner et al., 2006). The induction of immunoregulation in the intestinal tract occurs in the gut-associated lymphoid tissue and is stimulated by the presence of indigenous microbes. Mucosal immunity is underdeveloped in gnotobiotic animals, indicating that commensal microbes play an important role in immunological development. Animals reared in the absence of a complex microbiota have demonstrated relatively immature immune parameters including deficiencies in lymphoid cell compartments and circulating quantities of immunoglobulins (Wilks, 2007). The prospective use of probiotics for treatment and prevention of allergic disorders is further supported by experimental data showing that commensal populations differ between allergic and nonallergic infants (reviewed by Boyle and Tang, 2006) and that specific probiotic bacteria possess immunomodulatory properties.

PROBIOTICS IN ORAL HEALTH

Oral diseases potentially treatable by probiotics include dental caries, chronic periodontitis, *Candida albicans* infections, and halitosis (reviewed by Meurman and Stamatova, 2007). These diseases may result, at least partly, from a state of microbial imbalance in the oral cavity and may be managed by manipulating the microbial composition of the oropharynx. While much effort has been devoted to examining the potential benefits of probiotics in the gastrointestinal tract, a relative paucity of information has been generated regarding probiotics in the oral cavity. In order to confer long-term health benefits in the oral cavity, an oral probiotic must adhere to and colonize the specific surfaces of the oral cavity. While individual strains may effectively colonize mucosal surfaces in the oropharynx, the coordinated application of multiple strains may prove important as some oral strains enhance colonization of other microbes by coaggregating within this microenvironment and generating beneficial biofilms. Probiotics may reduce dental caries by decreasing pathogenic biofilms, treat periodontitis by reducing inflammation of the gingiva, and eliminate halitosis by preferentially replacing odor-causing microorganisms with probiotics.

PROBIOTICS AND THE GASTROINTESTINAL TRACT

Gastrointestinal disorders may result from aberrations in metabolic, immune, and physiologic functions, and these functions may be affected by a complex microbiota that typically resides in the gastrointestinal tract. The development of gnotobiotic animal models has helped to identify key features and functions of microbial communities. Examples of deficiencies in the germfree state include increased susceptibilities to vitamin deficiencies, enhanced vulnerabilities to enteric infections, reduced epithelial cell renewal rates, and reduced gut motility (reviewed by Boyle and Tang, 2006). Enteric disorders in humans may be associated with changes in microbial communities including, but not limited to, acute and antibiotic-associated diarrheal diseases, inflammatory bowel disease, and irritable bowel syndrome. Many probiotic investigations have focused on applications in the gastrointestinal tract. As reviewed by Guarner (Guarner, 2006), probiotics are viable options for lessening the severity of diarrheal disease, decreasing inflammation in inflammatory bowel disease, and improving gut mucosal barrier function. Another important probiotic function is the ability of beneficial microbes to form structured communities within dynamic environments. The gastrointestinal tract consists of rapid epithelial cell turnover and swift peristalsis, resulting in a dynamic environment that may be prone to fluxes in the composition of microbial populations. These microbial population fluxes may contribute to the variability of the human microbiome and may provide opportunities for intentional manipulation of intestinal microbial composition by probiotics. Beneficial microbes have evolved mechanisms for persistence despite these challenges, assembling biofilms within the mucus layer, functioning to promote digestion, enhancing intestinal fortitude, and preventing pathogen invasion (Sonnenburg et al., 2004). Further investigations of mechanisms of host recognition of beneficial microbes and, conversely, of how beneficial microbes persist in a dynamic environment to create symbiotic relationships will enable key advances in applications of probiotics in gastroenterology.

PROBIOTICS AND THE GENITOURINARY TRACT

Alterations in the natural microbial composition of the genitourinary tract may result in increased susceptibilities to disorders such as urinary tract infections, bacterial vaginosis, and vulvovaginal candidiasis. The most abundant colonizers of the healthy female urogenital tract include hydrogen peroxide-producing lactobacilli, while other microbes such as *Escherichia coli*, *Gardnerella vaginalis*, or *C. albicans* may dominate the genitourinary or vaginal microbiota in disease states (Reid and Bruce, 2003). Recent studies have included the development of genetically modified organisms, or engineered probiotics, for the prevention of human immunodeficiency virus type 1 (HIV-1) transmission (Liu et al., 2006). A *Lactobacillus* species that colonizes the healthy human vagina, *Lactobacillus jensenii*, was engineered to contain a chromosomally integrated gene encoding the HIV-1 inhibitor cyanovirin N (Liu et al., 2006). This engineered probiotic strain inhibited HIV-1 infectivity in vitro and demonstrated potential for novel applications to prevent HIV-1 transmission in the future. An improved understanding of the vaginal microbiome will result from studies of the human microbiome and may yield multiple strategies including natural and engineered probiotics. Different applications of probiotics in the genitourinary tract may include restoration of microbial balance, prevention of pathogenic biofilms by establishing and maintaining beneficial biofilms, and minimization of transmission risk of HIV-1 and other sexually transmitted diseases.

PROBIOTICS IN NEUROLOGY AND PSYCHIATRY

The use of probiotics in neurology and psychiatry is currently in its infancy, and potential applications include detoxification in autism and increased serotonin metabolism in depression. The gastrointestinal tract harbors sophisticated immune and enteric nervous systems that are linked by complex cellular interactions within the mucosa. Although the details of these interactions deserve further exploration, the proximity of a complex intestinal microbiota and the enteric nervous system provides opportunities for evaluating potential effects of beneficial microbes with respect to nociception, sensory stimulation, and neuroendocrine communication via gut hormones. Current animal studies suggest that probiotic *Lactobacillus reuteri* may diminish visceral pain via interactions with the enteric nervous system (Kamiya et al., 2006). Future research in this area will expand possible applications of probiotics for prevention and management of neurological and psychiatric

disorders and increase our understanding of host-microbe communication at a deeper level.

CONCLUDING REMARKS

Recent scientific evidence supports a paradigm shift regarding the nature of self, humanness, and the coexistence of humans and microbes. The human microbiome consists of many genes in hundreds, possibly thousands, of bacterial species, and its genetic complexity exceeds that of the human genome (Eckburg et al., 2005; Gill et al., 2006; Ley et al., 2006a). Human development and disease may be viewed through a different lens that considers microbial communities and human organ systems in intimate symbiotic relationships. The microbiome or the host's microbial composition may represent a key determinant of overall health status and disease susceptibility. Different aspects of human development rely on a complex and intricate microbiota, and deficiencies in a putative core microbiome or changes in aggregate microbial functions may result in disease susceptibilities affecting different body sites and depend partly on the host's genotype. Deliberate manipulation of the microbiome by natural or engineered probiotics could significantly advance human health and longevity as originally envisioned by Elie Metchnikoff in 1907 (Metchnikoff, 1907). The following chapters explore diverse applications of probiotics in human medicine and highlight the intricacies of human-microbe interactions in the treatment and prevention of human disease.

References

Bach, J. F. 2002. The effect of infections on susceptibility to autoimmune and allergic diseases. *N. Engl. J. Med.* 347:911–920.

Backhed, F., R. E. Ley, J. L. Sonnenburg, D. A. Peterson, and J. I. Gordon. 2005. Host-bacterial mutualism in the human intestine. *Science* 307:1915–1920.

Boyle, R. J., and M. L. Tang. 2006. The role of probiotics in the management of allergic disease. *Clin. Exp. Allergy* 36:568–576.

Eckburg, P. B., E. M. Bik, C. N. Bernstein, E. Purdom, L. Dethlefsen, M. Sargent, S. R. Gill, K. E. Nelson, and D. A. Relman. 2005. Diversity of the human intestinal microbial flora. *Science* 308:1635–1638.

FAO/WHO. 2002. *Guidelines for the Evaluation of Probiotics in Food.* FAO/WHO, London, Ontario, Canada.

Gill, S. R., M. Pop, R. T. Deboy, P. B. Eckburg, P. J. Turnbaugh, B. S. Samuel, J. I. Gordon, D. A. Relman, C. M. Fraser-Liggett, and K. E. Nelson. 2006. Metagenomic analysis of the human distal gut microbiome. *Science* 312:1355–1359.

Guarner, F. 2006. Enteric flora in health and disease. *Digestion* 73(Suppl. 1):5–12.

Guarner, F., R. Bourdet-Sicard, P. Brandtzaeg, H. S. Gill, P. McGuirk, W. van Eden, J. Versalovic, J. V. Weinstock, and G. A. Rook. 2006. Mechanisms of disease: the hygiene hypothesis revisited. *Nat. Clin. Pract. Gastroenterol. Hepatol.* 3:275–284.

Kamiya, T., L. Wang, P. Forsythe, G. Goettsche, Y. Mao, Y. Wang, G. Tougas, and J. Bienenstock. 2006. Inhibitory effects of *Lactobacillus reuteri* on visceral pain induced by colorectal distension in Sprague-Dawley rats. *Gut* 55:191–196.

Ley, R. E., D. A. Peterson, and J. I. Gordon. 2006a. Ecological and evolutionary forces shaping microbial diversity in the human intestine. *Cell* 124:837–848.

Ley, R. E., P. J. Turnbaugh, S. Klein, and J. I. Gordon. 2006b. Microbial ecology: human gut microbes associated with obesity. *Nature* 444:1022–1023.

Liu, X., L. A. Lagenaur, D. A. Simpson, K. P. Essenmacher, C. L. Frazier-Parker, Y. Liu, D. Tsai, S. S. Rao, D. H. Hamer, T. P. Parks, P. P. Lee, and Q. Xu. 2006. Engineered vaginal lactobacillus strain for mucosal delivery of the human immunodeficiency virus inhibitor cyanovirin-N. *Antimicrob. Agents Chemother.* 50:3250–3259.

Metchnikoff, E. 1907. *The Prolongation of Life: Optimistic Studies.* Heinemann, London, United Kingdom.

Meurman, J. H., and I. Stamatova. 2007. Probiotics: contributions to oral health. *Oral Dis.* 13:443–451.

Palmer, C., E. M. Bik, D. B. Digiulio, D. A. Relman, and P. O. Brown. 2007. Development of the human infant intestinal microbiota. *PLoS Biol.* 5:e177.

Reid, G. 2004. When microbe meets human. *Clin. Infect. Dis.* 39:827–830.

Reid, G., and A. W. Bruce. 2003. Urogenital infections in women: can probiotics help? *Postgrad. Med. J.* 79:428–432.

Sonnenburg, J. L., L. T. Angenent, and J. I. Gordon. 2004. Getting a grip on things: how do communities of bacterial symbionts become established in our intestine? *Nat. Immunol.* 5:569–573.

Turnbaugh, P. J., R. E. Ley, M. Hamady, C. M. Fraser-Liggett, R. Knight, and J. I. Gordon. 2007. The human microbiome project. *Nature* 449:804–810.

Wilks, M. 2007. Bacteria and early human development. *Early Hum. Dev.* 83:165–170.

Therapeutic Microbiology: Probiotics and Related Strategies
Edited by J. Versalovic and M. Wilson
© 2008 ASM Press, Washington, DC

G. A. W. Rook
N. Witt

18

Probiotics and Other Organisms in Allergy and Autoimmune Diseases

INTRODUCTION: THE HYGIENE OR "OLD FRIENDS" HYPOTHESIS

The incidences of several chronic inflammatory disorders have been increasing strikingly in the developed countries. These include allergic disorders (asthma and hay fever) and some autoimmune diseases (type 1 diabetes and multiple sclerosis [MS]) (Bach, 2002). The "Hygiene" or "Old Friends" hypothesis attributes some of these increases to a failure of immunoregulation caused by diminishing exposure to certain organisms that were part of mammalian evolutionary history. We know that a failure of immunoregulatory mechanisms can lead to simultaneous increases in diverse types of pathology, because genetic defects of Foxp3, a transcription factor that plays a crucial role in the development and function of regulatory T cells (T_{reg}), lead to a syndrome known as X-linked autoimmunity–allergic dysregulation syndrome that includes aspects of allergy, autoimmunity, and enteropathy (Hori et al., 2003; Wan and Flavell, 2007; Wildin et al., 2002).

The view that failing immunoregulation lies behind much of the increase in allergic disorders and autoimmunity in rich developed countries is supported by clear evidence that immunoregulation is indeed faulty in individuals suffering from these conditions. This situation has been demonstrated in allergic disorders (Akdis et al., 2004; Karlsson et al., 2004, Perez-Machado et al., 2003) and some autoimmune diseases (Kriegel et al., 2004; Viglietta et al., 2004). Perhaps the most striking example in autoimmunity is a recent experiment of nature. Patients in Argentina suffering from MS were monitored for up to 4.6 years. It was found that those who developed parasitic infections (which were not treated) had significantly fewer exacerbations than those who did not (Correale and Farez, 2007). Moreover, they also developed T_{reg} ($CD4^+$, $CD25^{hi}$, and $Foxp3^+$) that specifically responded to myelin basic protein. In other words, the presence of the parasite appeared to drive the development of T_{reg} that recognized the autoantigen and inhibited the disease process.

Several categories of organisms that were part of mammalian evolutionary history are now much rarer in developed countries. Helminths were almost universal and have been virtually eliminated. When humans

G. A. W. Rook and N. Witt, Centre for Infectious Diseases and International Health, Windeyer Institute of Medical Scences, Royal Free and University College Medical School, 46 Cleveland Street, London WIT 4JF, United Kingdom.

are dewormed, responses to allergens increase (Flohr et al., 2006; Yazdanbakhsh et al., 2002). Secondly, harmless organisms associated with mud and untreated water used to be abundant in the environment. Saprophytic mycobacteria were often present in a quantity of 1 mg or more per liter in untreated water supplies and were an important component of these environmental microbiotas (Rook et al., 2004; Zuany-Amorim et al., 2002b). Thirdly, organisms are associated with animals in the farming environment, to which a much smaller proportion of the population is now exposed (Riedler et al., 2001). The relevant organisms have not been identified, but the extent of protection from allergic disorders that can be derived from exposure to cowsheds in the first year of life is remarkable, and microorganisms are likely to be responsible (Riedler et al., 2001). Fourthly, organisms such as noncolonizing lactobacilli are associated with fermenting vegetable matter and primitive fermented drinks. Even in the 19th and early 20th centuries, food was often buried or kept in silos in cellars. Before the invention of refrigerators and washed packaged supermarket food, bacteria involved in fermentation were a major part of the diet. Finally, antibiotic treatment may predispose to allergies (Farooqi and Hopkin, 1998), and there is direct evidence that allergic children have

diminished numbers of colonizing lactobacilli in their intestinal microbiota (Bjorksten et al., 1999). Thus, changes in the resident microbiota are also taking place in the context of altered immunity.

Why would diminished exposure to such organisms lead to problems with immunoregulation? It is suggested that these organisms drive the development of immunoregulatory circuits, because the immune system has to tolerate them. They can be thought of as "pseudocommensals," because the external sources from which they came were so abundant that they will have been continuously present. The harmless pseudocommensals needed to be tolerated because they were constantly present in food and water throughout mammalian evolution. The helminths needed to be tolerated because, although not always harmless, once established in the host, any effort by the immune system to eliminate them tends to cause immunopathology. For instance, a futile effort to destroy *Brugia malayi* microfilariae results in lymphatic blockage and elephantiasis (Babu et al., 2006).

The mechanisms by which these organisms prime immunoregulation relevant to allergies, autoimmunity, and inflammatory bowel disease are explained in Fig. 1. Rather than provoking aggressive immune responses, these organisms cause a pattern of maturation of

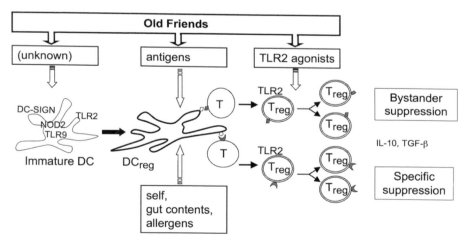

Figure 1 Immunoregulatory organisms stimulate T_{reg} responses. These organisms cause a pattern of maturation of DC such that these drive regulatory T_{reg} rather than Th1 or Th2 effector cells. TLR2, TLR9, NOD2, and DC-SIGN expressed by the DC can be involved. Moreover, the regulation-inducing materials tend to contain TLR2 agonists, and there is evidence in studies of mice and humans that TLR2 is expressed by T_{reg}, which can be directly triggered to proliferate via TLR2 ligands. Increased induction of DC_{reg} and T_{reg} leads to two mechanisms that help to control inappropriate inflammation. First, continuous exposure to Old Friends causes continuous background activation of T_{reg} specific for the Old Friends themselves. The result is a constant background of bystander suppression. Secondly, these DC_{reg} cells sample self, gut contents, and allergens and induce T_{reg} specific for target antigens, thereby suppressing inflammation.

dendritic cells (DC) (Adams et al., 2004; Smits et al., 2005; van der Kleij et al., 2002) such that these microbes drive T_{reg} rather than Th1 or Th2 effector cells. Derivatives of these microbes also may be Toll-like receptor 2 (TLR2) agonists, and evidence from studies of mice (Liu et al., 2006; Sutmuller et al., 2006) and humans (Zanin-Zhorov et al., 2006) suggests that T_{reg} may be directly triggered to proliferate via TLR2. This in turn leads to two mechanisms that help to control inappropriate inflammation. First, continuing throughput of the Old Friends causes continuous background activation of T_{reg} specific for the Old Friends themselves. The result is a constant background of bystander suppression. Secondly, DC_{reg} inevitably sample self, gut contents, and allergens and so induce T_{reg} cells specific for the illicit target antigens of the three groups of chronic inflammatory disorder. We do not understand all of the ways in which DC_{reg} and T_{reg} block or terminate inappropriate inflammatory responses, but release of anti-inflammatory cytokines interleukin-10 (IL-10) and transforming growth factor β (TGF-β) is often involved (Taylor et al., 2006b; Wilson et al., 2005; Zuany-Amorim et al., 2002b). The inhibitory mechanisms are aborted when legitimate danger signals are present and an aggressive immune response is required (Pasare and Medzhitov, 2003).

MICROORGANISMS WITH THERAPEUTIC POTENTIAL FOR ALLERGIES AND AUTOIMMUNITY

The validity of these pathways is supported by clinical trials and experimental models in which microorganisms that are depleted from the environment in rich countries have been shown to treat allergy (Wilson et al., 2005; Zuany-Amorim et al., 2002b; Ricklin-Gutzwiller et al., 2007), autoimmunity (Calcinaro et al., 2005; Kato et al., 1998; Zaccone et al., 2003), or intestinal inflammation (Di Giacinto et al., 2005; Summers et al., 2005a, 2005b).

This chapter discusses current progress in this area. We do not consider probiotics (defined as putatively beneficial bacterial strains taken by the oral route) in isolation, because it makes no biological sense to do so. All of the classes of organisms discussed above have immunoregulatory potential, and workers studying probiotics might benefit from the experience of those working with killed mycobacteria or helminths, and vice versa.

Helminths

Individuals infected by helminths are less likely to have allergic sensitization, or allergic disorders, and treating the infection tends to increase allergic sensitization

(Yazdanbakhsh et al., 2002; Yazdanbakhsh and Matricardi, 2004). This negative association has been documented in a recent study. A total of 1,601 children 6 to 18 years of age participated. In 14.4 and 27.6% of children, sensitization to dust mites and cockroaches, respectively, was present. The risk of sensitization to dust mites was reduced in those with a higher hookworm burden and with *Ascaris* infection. Nevertheless, the complexity of the situation was revealed by this study. Sensitization to house dust mites was increased in those using flush toilets. On the other hand, sensitization to cockroaches was not independently related to helminth infection but was increased in those regularly drinking piped or well water rather than from a stream (Flohr et al., 2006). It is possible that the stream water also supplied other regulation-inducing organisms such as the saprophytic mycobacteria discussed below.

The protective effects of helminths might also depend on the parasite load. High loads may drive regulatory circuits, while lower loads act as Th2 adjuvants and enhance allergic sensitization. For instance in a Costa Rican population with a low prevalence of parasitic infection but a high prevalence of parasitic exposure, sensitization to *Ascaris lumbricoides* was associated with increased severity and morbidity of asthma (Hunninghake et al., 2007). On the other hand, antibodies to *A. lumbricoides*, indicating exposure to this organism or to cross-reactive parasites, could not account for the protective effect of the farming environment in Europe (Karadag et al., 2006), nor was it associated with increased risk of allergy.

Helminths in Animal Models of Chronic Inflammatory Disorders

Animal models have confirmed the hypothesis that helminths oppose allergic manifestations by driving immunoregulation. One of the first reports involved *Strongyloides stercoralis* (Wang et al., 2001). More recently mice were infected with the gastrointestinal nematode *Heligmosomoides polygyrus* to test its influence on experimentally induced airway allergy to ovalbumin (OVA) and to the house dust mite allergen Der p1 (Wilson et al., 2005). Inflammatory cell infiltrates in the lung were suppressed in infected mice but not in uninfected controls. Suppression was reversed in mice treated with antibodies to CD25 and could be transferred with mesenteric lymph node cells. The protective cell populations contained elevated numbers of $CD4^+CD25^+Foxp3^+$ T cells and expressed TGF-β and IL-10. Interestingly, the regulatory cells could be taken from IL-10-deficient animals, so IL-10 produced by the T_{reg} themselves was not required. Other workers, using the same parasite, found IL-10 to be important (Kitagaki et al., 2006). Similar effects have been achieved using components of helminths, rather than intact worms. *Schistosoma japonicum* egg antigens were active in a murine model of asthma. This treatment increased the number and suppressive activity of CD4$^+$ CD25$^+$ T cells, which made IL-10. These cells were associated with reduced expression of Th2 cytokines and diminished antigen-induced airway inflammation (Yang et al., 2007).

Similar results have been obtained in a model of autoimmunity. In the nonobese diabetic (NOD) mouse a spontaneous Th1-mediated autoimmune response destroys the β cells in the pancreas, leading to a diabetic state analogous to human type 1 diabetes. Infection with the gastrointestinal helminths *Trichinella spiralis* or *H. polygyrus* was able to inhibit the development of diabetes (Saunders et al., 2007).

Since the parasites used in live organism infection in animal models are highly species specific, they may not be appropriate for use in humans. Two parasites are undergoing trials. *Trichuris suis*, the porcine whipworm, is undergoing trials in inflammatory bowel disease, because it fails to complete its life cycle in humans and is considered safe (Summers et al., 2005a, 2005b). Other trials are using *Necator americanus* because this human parasite is considered safe if a well-standardized low-dose infection (10 larvae) is used. In a pilot study it was well tolerated (Mortimer et al., 2006).

Mycobacteria

There has been much confusion in the literature about the relationship between exposure to mycobacteria and protection from allergic disorders. The confusion arises from the erroneous assumption that responses evoked by vaccination with *Mycobacterium bovis* bacillus Calmette-Guérin (BCG), progressive tuberculosis, latent tuberculosis, or contact with environmental mycobacteria are all functionally equivalent and that all that matters is the diameter of the tuberculin skin test response. Numerous authors have tried to relate incidence or severity of allergic disorders to tuberculin test reaction size. In view of the multiple immunologically disparate causes of tuberculin positivity, this is misleading, as extensively reviewed elsewhere (Rook et al., 2007). However, it is clear that individuals with definite latent tuberculosis (i.e., resistant to the disease, despite infection) have reduced allergic disease and reduced allergic sensitization (Obihara et al., 2005, 2006; Rook et al., 2007) and increased expression of IL-4δ2 (Demissie et al., 2004; Fletcher et al., 2004), an inhibitory splice variant of IL-4. In striking contrast, individuals with progressive tuberculosis (i.e., susceptible to the disease), particularly

if living in a developing country, have increased expression of IL-4 (Rook, 2007) and correspondingly increased immunoglobulin E (IgE) and allergic sensitization (Ellertsen et al., 2005; Rook et al., 2007; Suzuki et al., 2001). Thus, latent tuberculosis might protect from allergic disorders but is clearly not a therapeutic option.

The effects of BCG vaccination are variable and unreliable (Aaby et al., 2000; Alm et al., 1998; Gruber et al., 2002). This outcome is to be anticipated since it is also unreliable in its effects on susceptibility to tuberculosis (Fine, 1995). In animal models BCG can be effective, although this appeared to be largely due to the establishment of a Th1 pattern of response that inhibited subsequent induction of Th2 (Herz et al., 1998).

Mycobacteria in Animal Models

The mycobacterium that has received most attention is *Mycobacterium vaccae*, an environmental saprophyte that is used as a killed preparation and has repeatedly been shown to be effective in mouse models of asthma, in therapeutic as well as preventative protocols (Hopfenspirger et al., 2001; Ozdemir et al., 2003; Smit et al., 2003; Wang and Rook, 1998; Zuany-Amorim et al., 2002a, 2002b). This organism appears to work by inducing T_{reg} that inhibit Th2, rather than by inducing a Th1 bias. A single dose of *M. vaccae* given subcutaneously either before Th2-inducing immunization or after the first two of four such immunizations was able to reduce manifestations of Th2 responses elicited by a subsequent intratracheal allergen challenge (Zuany-Amorim et al., 2002a, 2002b). The mechanism was shown to be the induction of CD25$^+$ T_{reg}. These regulatory cells were enriched from crude spleen cell populations and transferred intravenously into untreated allergic recipients, where they were able to reduce the Th2-mediated pathology following airway challenge (Zuany-Amorim et al., 2002a, 2002b). The effect of the transferred T_{reg} could be blocked by simultaneously administered neutralizing antibodies to IL-10 and TGF-β, indicating that either the regulatory cells themselves secrete these cytokines or they cause their secretion by other cells in vivo. The regulatory cells were specific for antigens present during their induction, but once triggered by their specific antigen, they could exert bystander suppression of Th2 responses to unrelated antigens (Zuany-Amorim et al., 2002b). The lungs of treated allergic animals contained increased numbers of CD11c$^+$ cells that strongly expressed alpha interferon (IFN-α), IL-10, and TGF-β, suggesting that they might be plasmacytoid dendritic cells (pDC). These findings, if confirmed, would be of some interest since pDC play a major role in driving immunoregulation in the lung (De Heer et al., 2004). It is encouraging that

M. vaccae was equally effective in the mouse model when administered orally since this is a practical route of administration that avoids the scar at the injection site (Hunt et al., 2005).

In addition to these effects in the BALB/c model of allergic airway disorder, autoclaved *M. vaccae* reduced scratching (measured by a computer-linked video system) in the eczema model in NC/Nga mice (Arkwright et al., 2005). More recently, when administered as a single intradermal dose to dogs with eczema, *M. vaccae* was found to very effectively reduce all disease parameters for several months (Ricklin-Gutzwiller et al., 2007), and further regulatory level studies are now in progress with this species.

Probiotics

The idea that modulating the intestinal microbiota can modulate chronic inflammatory disorders has a long history. In 1985 Kohashi and colleagues observed that the susceptibility of rats to adjuvant arthritis depended on the nature of the gut microbiota (Kohashi et al., 1985). It was also established 10 years ago that the intestinal microbiota is required for successful induction, by the oral route, of tolerance to OVA (Sudo et al., 1997). As discussed in detail in previous sections, these effects are likely to involve maturation of immunoregulatory pathways, so it might be logical to seek strains that drive regulatory DC or T_{reg}. In practice this is not how strains have been chosen for clinical trials in the past, because a multitude of mechanisms have been proposed for various putative beneficial effects of probiotics, and these have led to selection criteria that might not always be relevant to induction of regulatory pathways (Jacobsen et al., 1999). Thus, probiotics have been used to occupy ecological niches within the gut that can otherwise be occupied by pathogenic species such as *Listeria monocytogenes*, *Escherichia coli*, or *Salmonella* spp. Thus, strains have been selected for their ability to survive acid and bile salts and to adhere to intestinal epithelial cells, and in some cases, to colonize the human gastrointestinal tract. Moreover, some strains have been selected for direct antibacterial properties mediated by secretion of inhibitory organic acids, bacteriocins, or reuterin. Strains that coaggregate with pathogens are more likely to damage the pathogen, due to proximity (Vizoso Pinto et al., 2007). Often, intestinal epithelial cell lines have been used in in vitro systems designed to show that the probiotic strain adheres to the cell line and inhibits adherence to, or invasion of the cell line by, pathogens (Rosenfeldt et al., 2003). Some workers regard the crucial property as the triggering of chemokine or cytokine release by the gut epithelium or underlying macrophages and

select probiotics based on this property in vitro (Vizoso Pinto et al., 2007). Others have considered the probiotic effect to be due to a switch from Th2 to Th1 responses and selected strains for high induction of IL-12 release in vitro (Sashihara et al., 2006). On this basis these authors selected *Lactobacillus gasseri* OLL2809 and argued that the effect was due to peptidoglycan components (Sashihara et al., 2006).

In conclusion, it seems unlikely that we have yet selected the optimal strains for restoring immunoregulation in people suffering from an increased incidence of chronic inflammatory disorders in developed northern countries. It is probable that a distinct subset of organisms will be required for this purpose. Nevertheless, some relevant results have been achieved in animal models.

Probiotics in Animal Models

Gut

In a model of dextran sulfate-induced colitis the beneficial effect of probiotics was attributed to DNA of probiotic bacteria acting via TLR9. The alleviation of colitis was unaffected by irradiating the organisms but was eliminated in TLR9 knockout mice and by DNase treatment. Moreover, the effect could be reproduced by DNA and by immunostimulatory oligonucleotides known to be TLR9 agonists. Importantly, *E. coli* DNA was also active, suggesting that the role of probiotic strains might be the appropriate presentation of the DNA or the simultaneous delivery of other signals, since probiotic DNA itself is probably not unique in terms of TLR9 agonistic effects. Further studies suggested that the active DNA might be absorbed systemically and act on the immune system in sites other than the gut (Rachmilewitz et al., 2004). Similarly *Lactobacillus salivarius* was used in the model of inflammatory bowel disease that occurs in IL-10 knockout mice. The reduction in colonic inflammatory scores following administration of the probiotic was associated with reduced production of proinflammatory (T helper 1) cytokines and increased production of TGF-β (Sheil et al., 2004). Interestingly, probiotic *L. salivarius* was effective whether delivered orally or subcutaneously (Sheil et al., 2004).

Allergy

TLR9 has also been implicated in an allergy model. Oral treatment with live *Lactobacillus reuteri*, but not *L. salivarius*, significantly attenuated the influx of eosinophils to the airway lumen and parenchyma and reduced the levels of tumor necrosis factor (TNF), monocyte chemoattractant protein-1, IL-5, and IL-13 in bronchoalveolar lavage fluid of antigen-challenged animals, but there was no change in eotaxin or IL-10. *L. reuteri*, but not *L. salivarius*, also decreased allergen-induced airway hyperresponsiveness. These responses were dependent on TLR9 and were associated with increased activity of indoleamine 2,3-dioxygenase (IDO). Killed organisms did not mimic the effects of live *L. reuteri* (Forsythe et al., 2007). Similarly an immunostimulatory oligonucleotide from the genomic DNA of *Bifidobacterium longum* BB536 prevented antigen-induced Th2 immune responses in BALB/c mice, suggesting that immunostimulatory oligonucleotides from probiotics might be useful in preventing allergic disease (Takahashi et al., 2006). These authors did not formally prove the involvement of TLR9, but it seems likely that TLR9 was involved.

Bifidobacterium bifidum and *Lactobacillus casei* were administered orally to C3H/HeJ mice before or after they were sensitized with OVA and cholera toxin. The probiotic-treated mice had decreased levels of OVA-specific IgE, total IgE, and IgG1 and decreased levels of mast cell degranulation and tail scabs (Kim et al., 2005a, 2005b). Treatment with *Bifidobacterium* before OVA sensitization suppressed the allergic response more effectively than treatment with *Bifidobacterium* after antigen sensitization (Kim et al., 2005b). A similar result was achieved in the NC/Nga mouse model of eczema. The combination of *L. casei* subsp. *casei* and dextran (administered as a prebiotic) significantly decreased clinical skin severity scores and total IgE levels in sera of NC/Nga mice (Ogawa et al., 2006).

Proof of the involvement of regulatory cells in these phenomena was obtained in a model in which newborn BALB/c mice received 10^9 CFU of either *Lactobacillus rhamnosus* GG or *Bifidobacterium lactis* orally every second day for 8 consecutive weeks and during systemic sensitization with OVA. The probiotic treatment suppressed allergen-induced proliferative responses and was associated with increased numbers of TGF-β-secreting CD4$^+$/CD3$^+$ T cells in mesenteric lymph nodes as well as a nearly twofold up-regulation of Foxp3-expressing cells in the peribronchial lymph nodes (Feleszko et al., 2007).

Autoimmunity

Kato and colleagues tested the effects of oral administration of viable bacterium *L. casei* on the development of type II collagen (CII)-induced arthritis (CIA) in DBA/1 mice. *Lactobacillus* treatment reduced the incidence and the development of CIA, and the levels of antibody to CII in serum were reduced compared with those of the control mice. The probiotic inhibited the delayed-type hypersensitivity response to CII and the CII-specific secretion of IFN-γ from splenocytes ex vivo (Kato et al.,

1998). The likely mechanism is induction of T_{reg} that release anti-inflammatory cytokines (Sheil et al., 2004). Early oral administration of VSL#3 prevented diabetes development in NOD mice. Protected mice showed reduced insulitis and a decreased rate of β-cell destruction. Prevention was associated with an increased production of IL-10 from Peyer's patches and the spleen in addition to increased IL-10 expression in the pancreas, where IL-10-positive islet-infiltrating mononuclear cells were detected (Calcinaro et al., 2005).

Recombinant Probiotic Strains, Expressing Allergens

Animals were intraperitoneally sensitized with the group-5 allergen (Der p5) of *Dermatophagoides pteronyssinus* and then treated with oral recombinant lactobacilli that did or did not contain a plasmid encoding Der p5. Twenty-one days after sensitization, mice underwent Der p5 challenge into the airways. Der p5-specific immunological responses including changes to specific IgG and IgE levels, the presence of cells in the bronchoalveolar lavage fluid, and airway hyperreactivity were assessed following this inhalational challenge (Charng et al., 2006). The authors noted that recombinant lactobacilli caused diminished IgE and airway hyperreactivity, whereas neither the wild-type organisms nor the antigen alone was able to exert these effects (Charng et al., 2006). By contrast other authors, using recombinant strains expressing Bet v 1, which is involved in birch pollen allergy, found that although the allergen-expressing strains tended to divert the response towards Th1, airway inflammation as determined by eosinophils and IL-5 in lung lavage fluids was reduced equally well using control strains not expressing Bet v 1 (Daniel et al., 2006).

INTERACTIONS WITH DC

DC are antigen-presenting cells that initiate and shape the adaptive immune response. They can influence whether naïve T cells develop Th1, Th2, or regulatory phenotypes. Therefore, several groups have studied interactions between DC and potentially immunoregulatory organisms. These studies provide strong support for the view that some such strains drive immunoregulation via effects on DC.

Probiotics and DC

Different species of lethally irradiated lactobacilli added to cultures of mouse bone marrow-derived DC showed different effects on the cytokine expression profile and on up-regulation of markers of maturation (Christensen et al., 2002; Drakes et al., 2004). For example, *L. reuteri* and *L. casei* differed in their capacity to induce IL-10 and IL-12 and expression of CD86. Interestingly, *L. reuteri*, a weak IL-12 inducer, was able to inhibit induction of IL-12, IL-6, and TNF by the strong cytokine producer *L. casei*, but IL-10 expression was unaffected. Thus, both the blend of different strains and the concentration of individual bacteria alter the DC cytokine pattern (Christensen et al., 2002).

Other authors confirmed the strain-specific interaction of lactic acid bacteria with mouse DC by using living organisms rather than irradiated ones (Foligne et al., 2007b). *L. salivarius* Ls33 and *L. rhamnosus* Lr32 on one hand and *L. acidophilus* NCFM and *L. lactis* MG1363 on the other hand showed opposite effects on DC. The first two organisms induced a regulatory DC phenotype with only low levels of cytokines and chemokines and little up-regulation of costimulation markers. In contrast to immature DC, these pretreated cells were able to reduce the colitis induced in mice by 2,4,6-trinitrobenzenesulfonic acid. This anti-inflammatory effect was accompanied by down-regulation of proinflammatory mediators and up-regulation of IFN-γ and IDO. Depletion of CD4+ CD25+ cells with an anti-CD25 antibody annulled the protective effect of probiotic-pulsed DC. This finding indicates that probiotic-treated DCs prime T_{reg} cells. The ability of Lr32 to drive immature DC into a regulatory phenotype was almost certainly connected with signaling via the pattern recognition receptors, TLR2 and NOD2, as probiotic-treated DC derived from TLR2 and NOD2 knockout mice had no anti-inflammatory properties (Foligne et al., 2007b).

These experiments performed in murine systems are probably relevant to humans. A recent study compared the immunostimulatory properties of 13 different strains of lactic acid bacteria using human peripheral blood mononuclear cells (Foligne et al., 2007a). The authors demonstrated a strain-specific pattern in IL-10 and IL-12 production after 24 h. Using the ratio of IL-10/IL-12 in the supernatants, it was possible to discriminate between pro- and anti-inflammatory strains. Interestingly, the strains that drove a high ratio of IL-10 to IL-12 production from human cells were found to be the strains that were also protective in a mouse colitis model (Foligne et al., 2007a).

Other authors have added probiotic strains to DC generated from human peripheral blood monocytes by incubation with granulocyte-macrophage colony-stimulating factor and IL-4 in vitro. The addition of the probiotics caused further maturation and specialization of the DC, which were then used to expand populations of naive CD4+ T cells. The readout was the phenotype of the expanded T-cell population. T cells driven by

DC incubated with *L. rhamnosus* were found to be hyporesponsive to stimulation with anti-CD3/CD28 and IL-2, although the authors did not implicate increased release of regulatory cytokines (Braat et al., 2004). In similar experiments *L. reuteri* and *L. casei*, but not *Lactobacillus plantarum*, were found to prime monocyte-derived DC to drive the development of T_{reg} that produced increased levels of IL-10 and inhibited the proliferation of bystander T cells in an IL-10-dependent fashion. Strikingly, both active strains (but not *L. plantarum*) were found to bind the C-type lectin DC-specific intercellular adhesion molecule 3-grabbing non-integrin (DC-SIGN), and T_{reg} were not generated if DC-SIGN was blocked (Smits et al., 2005).

Other authors are doubtful of the physiological relevance of DC derived in vitro from human peripheral blood monocytes by incubation with granulocyte-macrophase colony-stimulating factor and IL-4 and have preferred to work with naturally occurring DC enriched from human blood or from intestinal lamina propria (Hart et al., 2004). After culture with sonicates of a range of putative probiotic species, DC were identified and phenotyped in complex cell mixtures by multicolor flow cytometry. The probiotic mixture VSL#3 induced production of IL-10 in DC, and if lipopolysaccharide was also present, reduced lipopolysaccharide-driven release of IL-12. Sonicates of the individual bacterial strains present in VSL#3 provoked strain-specific responses. Only *Bifidobacterium* strains increased IL-10 expression by CD11c+ and CD11c− DC, whereas lactobacilli reduced, or had no effect on, IL-10. Similarly the number of DC expressing CD80 and CD40 was reduced by culture with bifidobacteria, while CD83 was up-regulated by *L. casei* and *L. plantarum*. Finally, T cells stimulated with VSL#3-treated DC expressed less IFN-γ. However, of the individual probiotic strains contained within VSL#3, only *B. longum* and *Bifidobacterium infantis* mimicked the IFN-γ inhibitory effect when tested as individual organisms.

A common result of all these studies is that different strains have different effects on DC. Some strains clearly induce regulatory DC that can drive T_{reg}, as indicated in Fig. 1, and appear to do so at least in part by interactions with TLR2, NOD2, or DC-SIGN. It will be important to screen for specific strains with these properties for clinical trials in the chronic inflammatory disorders.

Helminths

Infections with helminths are usually associated with a Th2 response, and several studies have shown that stimulation of murine or human DC in vitro with antigen mixtures or single molecules from helminths yields populations of DC that have the potential to drive naïve

T cells towards a Th2 type (reviewed by van Riet et al., 2007). However, as discussed earlier, chronic infection with parasitic worms can lead to an anti-inflammatory response with enhanced production of IL-10 and suppressed T-cell proliferation. Fractions of schistosomes capable of exerting such effects have been identified. Whereas a water-soluble extract of schistosome eggs modulated DC towards a Th2-driving type, the lipid lysophosphatidylserine extracted from schistosome eggs and adult worms led to the development of DC that drove IL-10-expressing T_{reg} (van der Kleij et al., 2002). As in the case of some *Lactobacillus* strains, stimulation of TLR2 on DC by lysophosphatidylserine was crucial for this effect (reviewed by van Riet et al., 2007).

Mycobacteria

All mycobacteria contain multiple ligands for pattern recognition receptors, including heat shock proteins, DNA, RNA, peptidoglycans, lipoarabinomannan, and many other complex lipids and glycolipids. Most work on *Mycobacterium*-DC interactions has been performed with *Mycobacterium tuberculosis* or BCG, which differ strikingly from *Mycobacterium leprae* in their effects on DC (Murray et al., 2007). The environmental saprophyte *M. vaccae* is likely to be different, but current data are limited. In a mouse model, data suggest that *M. vaccae* activates pDC (Adams et al., 2004), while in vitro *M. vaccae* is a potent TLR2 agonist (our unpublished observations). TLR2 stimulation may be immunomodulatory.

IMMUNOLOGICAL EFFECTS OF THERAPEUTIC MICROORGANISMS

There have been extremely few studies of the actual effects on the human immune system of the probiotics and other microbes used in clinical trials. A few studies that address the issue of immunoregulation are outlined here.

Nineteen preterm infants were divided into two groups that did or did not receive *Bifidobacterium breve* supplementation. Blood samples were collected from both groups on days 0, 14, and 28 after birth. The group that received *B. breve* had higher serum TGF-β from day 14, and by reverse transcriptase-PCR, the infants had higher Smad3 and reduced Smad7. These changes indicate increased TGF-β levels and increased TGF-β signaling (Fujii et al., 2006). In another study 72 infants consumed infant formula supplemented with *Lactobacillus* GG and *Bifidobacterium lactis* Bb-12 or a placebo during the first year of life (Rautava et al., 2006). The numbers of cow's milk-specific and total IgA-secreting

cells were measured at 3, 7, and 12 months, and serum concentrations of TGF-β and the soluble CD14 were also assayed. A modest increase in IgA-secreting cells was found in the probiotic group, possibly attributable to increased TGF-β since this cytokine drives IgA production (Rautava et al., 2006).

In a very preliminary pilot study, 10 subjects (mean age, 22.3 years) suffering from allergic rhinitis were given three vials containing spores of *Bacillus clausii* (Enterogermina; 2 billion spores/vial) every day for 4 weeks. Nasal lavage was performed in all subjects before and after the treatment. Treatment with *B. clausii* was associated with a significant reduction in quantities of IL-4 ($P = 0.004$) and a significant increase in IFN-γ, TGF-β, and IL-10, suggesting immunoregulatory effects (Ciprandi et al., 2005).

Other studies have failed to identify any evidence of increased immunoregulatory function. Babies born to allergic mothers with positive skin prick tests received either a probiotic (3×10^9 *Lactobacillus acidophilus* LAVRI-A1) or a placebo daily for the first 6 months of life (Taylor et al., 2006c). Cytokine responses (IL-5, IL-6, IL-10, IL-13, TNF, or TGF-β) to tetanus toxoid, house dust mite, OVA, beta-lactoglobulin, *Staphylococcus* enterotoxin B, and phytohemagglutinin were measured at 6 months. No significant effects of probiotics on either Th1 or Th2 responses to allergens or other stimuli were reported, although reduced TNF and IL-10 responses to house dust mite were noted. Children who received the probiotics also showed reduced production of TGF-β in response to polyclonal (*Staphylococcus* enterotoxin B) stimulation, and lower IL-10 responses to tetanus texoid compared with the placebo group (Taylor et al., 2006c). The same group also failed to find any probiotic-induced changes in responsiveness to ligands of TLR2 or TLR4 or in the levels of IL-12 or IL-10 induced by these ligands (Taylor et al., 2006a). Similarly they found that probiotics did not cause changes in expression of FOXP3 mRNA at 6 months of age (Taylor et al., 2007b).

Even fewer studies have documented the precise nature of the response evoked by *M. vaccae*. The most relevant studies might be those involving patients with tuberculosis, who in some environments have high circulating levels of IL-4. In these patients, *M. vaccae* causes a rapid fall in circulating levels of IL-4, suggesting a Th2-specific immunoregulatory effect (Dlugovitzky et al., 2006), as seen previously in mice (Zuany-Amorim et al., 2002b). However, when microarray technology was applied to blood taken from children with eczema who had received intradermal *M. vaccae*, the only significant changes were increases in mRNA encoding Th1 cytokines at 1 month, which returned to normal by 3 months (Hadley et al., 2005).

The reports of clinical trials involving helminths do not present any data on changes in parameters of immunoregulation (Summers et al., 2005a, 2005b), although the animal work discussed earlier suggests this mode of action (Saunders et al., 2007; Wilson et al., 2005).

CLINICAL TRIALS

Helminths

Trichuris suis

Trials have been performed for inflammatory bowel disease, using ova of the pig whipworm, *Trichuris suis*. One study recruited 54 patients with an ulcerative colitis disease activity index (UCDAI) of 4 or greater. Patients were randomly assigned to receive a placebo or 2,500 *T. suis* ova orally at 2-week intervals for 12 weeks. The primary end point of the trial was a reduced UCDAI. After 12 weeks of therapy, improvement was documented for 13 of 30 patients treated with the ova compared with 4 of 24 patients given a placebo ($P = 0.04$) (Summers et al., 2005b). A similar study was performed involving 29 patients with active Crohn's disease (Crohn's disease activity index [CDAI] of 220 or more). No placebo group was included in the study. All patients ingested 2,500 live *T. suis* ova every 3 weeks for 24 weeks. Remission was defined as a reduction in CDAI to less than 150, and by week 24, 70% of patients had demonstrated remission (Summers et al., 2005a).

Importantly, no adverse events in the studies above were reported. However, sporadic use of this treatment in severe cases might eventually reveal problems. One publication reported iatrogenic infection with *T. suis* in a boy with Crohn's disease (Kradin et al., 2006), although the validity of this finding is disputed by some (Summers et al., 2006) and supported by others (Van Kruiningen and West, 2007).

Hookworm

Since epidemiological studies indicated that hookworm infection producing 50 eggs/g of feces might protect against asthma, Pritchard and colleagues are arranging clinical trials using deliberate infection with this organism. These authors are also working towards trials for MS, encouraged by the new data published by Correale et al. on the apparently protective effect of naturally occurring helminth infection in this disease (Correale and Farez, 2007). The first requirement was to establish the dose of hookworm larvae needed to achieve 50 eggs/g of feces. Ten healthy subjects without asthma or airway hyperresponsiveness to inhaled methacholine received 10, 25, 50, or 100 *Necator americanus* larvae administered double blind to an area of skin on the arm.

Subjects were monitored weekly for 12 weeks. Then, they were treated with mebendazole to eliminate the parasites. A transient increase in blood eosinophils, serum IgE, and serum IgG was documented. Lung function did not change. All doses resulted in at least 50 eggs/g of feces, so the lowest dose of 10 larvae will be used in future trials. This dose was well tolerated, whereas skin itching at the entry site and gastrointestinal symptoms were common at higher doses (Mortimer et al., 2006).

Mycobacteria

The first pilot study in an allergic disorder with a single intradermal injection of heat-killed *M. vaccae* was performed for hay fever (Hopkin et al., 1998). A significant reduction in reliever drug use was reported, and post-hoc subgroup analysis showed diminished chest symptom scores calculated from diary cards. This report encouraged a small laboratory-based study with 24 male asthmatics. A bronchial allergen challenge was performed along with early and late asthmatic responses 2 weeks before and 3 weeks after a single intradermal injection of *M. vaccae* or a placebo. Serum IgE levels and in vitro production of IL-5 by peripheral blood lymphocytes were studied before and after treatment. *M. vaccae* lessened the reduction in forced expiratory volume in 1 s that occurred during the late asthmatic response, whether measured as area under the curve or as maximum reduction, although this finding failed to reach conventional statistical significance when compared with the placebo. *M. vaccae* might have caused a reduction in serum IgE and IL-5 synthesis in vitro 3 weeks posttreatment ($P = 0.07$) (Camporota et al., 2003). A large asthma study was assembled, but owing to errors in the interpretation of the inclusion criteria and in the statistical analysis plan, the study could not be assessed comprehensively. Many patients recruited had such mild disease that improvement could not be expected. Nevertheless, the results were encouraging. The primary end point was a change in symptom score to week 12. When covariate-adjusted (the adjustment was not in the original analysis plan), this effect on symptom scores was significant ($P = 0.0436$). Similarly, a significant reduction in asthma exacerbations was reported ($P = 0.0251$).

Results of eczema studies have been mixed. In the first study, 41 children aged 5 to 18 years with moderate-to-severe atopic dermatitis received a single intradermal injection of *M. vaccae* or a placebo. Changes in the skin surface area affected by dermatitis and the dermatitis severity score were assessed before treatment and at 1 and 3 months after treatment. Children treated with *M. vaccae* showed a mean 48% reduction in surface area affected by dermatitis compared to a mean 4% reduction for the placebo group ($P < 0.001$). *M. vaccae*-treated children yielded a median 68% reduction in dermatitis severity score compared with 18% for the placebo group ($P < 0.01$) at 3 months after treatment. A further study with 56 children aged 2 to 6 years showed a 38 to 54% improvement in both treated and placebo groups, with no significant difference between the two groups (Arkwright and David, 2003). It is not clear whether this result indicated lack of efficacy or merely reflected the very high rate of spontaneous remission in this younger age group. The same dilemma applies to a further study in which the placebo group showed a 30% reduction in symptom scores (Berth-Jones et al., 2006). Overall these trial results are difficult to interpret, particularly in view of the convincing effect on eczema in dogs discussed earlier (Ricklin-Gutzwiller et al., 2007). A major problem has been the local lesion caused by intradermal *M. vaccae*, which cannot be mimicked by placebo. Placebo effects are less of an issue in dogs. Local skin lesions would be unacceptable if repeated injections were needed in young people, and future studies in allergic disorders, apart from the ongoing trial in dogs, will use the oral route (Hunt et al., 2005) to avoid such potential complications.

Probiotics

Many trials of probiotics in allergic disorders have been performed, and a few trials have been arranged for chronic inflammatory conditions. These studies have been encouraged by the less stringent regulatory framework and by the fact that, even in newborn infants, probiotics appear to be safe. Probiotic administration in the first months of life was well tolerated, did not affect numbers of different types of stools, vomiting, or crying time, and did not significantly interfere with long-term composition or quantity of gut microbiota (Rinne et al., 2006). There are, however, reports of bacteremia and fungemia due to lactobacilli (certain species) and *Saccharomyces* organisms. This complication can occur in patients who are immunocompromised or have indwelling central venous catheters (Michail et al., 2006) or in patients who did not directly receive probiotics but were in the same hospital unit as individuals who did (Michail et al., 2006).

In the following paragraphs we outline 13 published studies in which probiotics have been tested in allergic disorders and 2 studies in autoimmunity, and then, we discuss the overall weight of evidence in a separate final section.

Treating Mothers with Lactobacilli

In some studies with high-risk subjects, born to mothers with a strong family history of allergy, probiotics were administered to the mother during pregnancy, as well as to the infant after birth. In one such study *Lactobacillus*

GG or a placebo was given to pregnant mothers and the infants for the first 6 months after delivery. The frequency of atopic dermatitis in the infants was significantly reduced at 2 years (Kalliomaki et al., 2001) and 4 years (Kalliomaki et al., 2003). This reduction in eczema was maintained at a further 7-year follow-up (Kalliomaki et al., 2007), but the frequency of atopic sensitization was not reduced, so the authors concluded that the effect on eczema was probably not mediated by changes in IgE production. Moreover, a trend was noted towards an increase in allergic rhinitis and asthma in the probiotic group. There were 17 cases of allergic rhinitis at 7 years among 116 subjects (15%). A total of 6 cases were reported in the placebo group, in contrast to 12 cases in the *Lactobacillus* GG group. Similarly there were 12 cases of asthma among 166 subjects (10%) at 7 years. A total of three cases were reported in the placebo group, in contrast to nine cases in the *Lactobacillus* GG group (Kalliomaki et al., 2007).

In a further analysis of a subset of these subjects, the same group concluded that a diminished frequency of atopic eczema at 2 years of age was seen in those infants whose feces contained the probiotic *Lactobacillus* strain (LGG) at 6 months (28% versus 51% in LGG-positive and LGG-negative infants, respectively; $P = 0.03$) (Gueimonde et al., 2006), although such subgroup analyses must be treated with caution. Moreover, since the organism was supposedly administered for 6 months, the presence of the organism might have merely reflected adherence to the protocol.

A larger study was undertaken in Helsinki (Kukkonen et al., 2007). Pregnant women ($n = 1,223$) carrying high-risk children were randomized to receive a probiotic preparation containing four different bacterial strains or a placebo for 2 to 4 weeks before delivery. The newborn infants then received the same probiotics plus 0.8 g of galacto-oligosaccharides (supposedly prebiotic) once daily for 6 months after birth ($n = 461$). In the placebo group, mothers and their infants ($n = 464$) took inert materials that were identical in appearance. At 2 years, cumulative incidence of allergic diseases (food allergy, eczema, asthma, and allergic rhinitis) and IgE sensitization (positive skin prick test response or antigen-specific IgE level of >0.7 kU/liter) was evaluated. Probiotic treatment compared with placebo showed no effect on the cumulative incidence of allergic diseases but tended to reduce disease (food allergy, eczema, asthma, or allergic rhinitis) associated with positive skin prick tests or raised specific IgE antibodies ($P = 0.052$). Probiotic treatment reduced eczema ($P = 0.035$) and atopic eczema ($P = 0.025$) (Kukkonen et al., 2007). No reduction in the prevalence of allergic sensitization was noted, despite the reduction in the frequency with which sensitization was associated with symptoms. In the same study fecal bacteria were analyzed during treatment and at 2 years. Lactobacilli and bifidobacteria more frequently ($P < 0.001$) colonized the guts of supplemented infants (Kukkonen et al., 2007).

Infants with Atopic Dermatitis

Probiotics have been administered to infants with atopic dermatitis. All three studies outlined below yielded, strictly speaking, negative results, although subgroup analyses resulted in some claims of efficacy. Newborns of women with allergy ($n = 231$) received either *L. acidophilus* (LAVRI-A1) or a placebo daily for the first 6 months of life. Children were assessed for atopic dermatitis (AD) and other symptoms at 6 and 12 months and had allergen skin prick tests at 12 months. A total of 178 infants completed the supplementation period. At 6 and 12 months, AD rates were similar in the probiotic and placebo groups (Taylor et al., 2007a).

Similarly 56 children aged 6 to 18 months with moderate or severe AD were recruited into a randomized double-blind placebo-controlled trial in Perth, Western Australia; 53 children completed the study. The children were given a probiotic (10^9 CFU of *Lactobacillus fermentum* VRI-033 PCC; Probiomics) or an equivalent volume of placebo, twice daily for 8 weeks. This trial did not achieve its primary outcome measure, which was a difference between test and placebo groups in severity and extent of AD at the end of the study, as measured by the objective clinical Scoring of Atopic Dermatitis index. Some interesting within-group changes were highlighted by the authors (Weston et al., 2005).

Another study with older children, aged 1 to 13 years, sought improvement in AD after a 6-week administration of *L. rhamnosus* 19070-2 and *L. reuteri* DSM 122460. Significantly more recipients of the probiotics thought their disease had improved by subjective reporting. The changes in the Scoring of Atopic Dermatitis index were not significant, except in a subgroup analysis of children with high IgE levels and one or more positive skin tests (Rosenfeldt et al., 2003).

Cow's Milk Allergy

Cow's milk allergy often has a predominant Th1 component with respect to the T-cell immune response. Evidence suggests that T_{reg} are involved in the control of this disorder, since these cells appear in children who resolve this allergy as they get older (Karlsson et al., 2004).

Infants with atopic eczema and cow's milk allergy improved symptoms more on hydrolyzed whey formula when they also received *Lactobacillus* GG in a large controlled study (Majamaa and Isolauri, 1997). Interestingly, the

fecal concentrations of α1-antitrypsin and TNF decreased significantly in the probiotic-supplemented group ($P = 0.03$) but not in the group receiving the whey formula without *Lactobacillus* GG ($P = 0.68$).

More recently a complex study with three arms (*Lactobacillus* GG, a mixture of four probiotic strains, or a placebo for 4 weeks) was performed with children with suspected cow's milk allergy. The children were also subjected at the same time to an elimination diet and to skin treatment. Four weeks after the probiotic treatments, cow's milk allergy was diagnosed by milk challenge. As often seen in studies of eczema, the eczema score decreased by 65% in the whole group, and there were no differences between treatment groups (Viljanen et al., 2005). Within-group before and after treatment comparisons yielded some evidence of efficacy in an IgE-positive subgroup, but this deduction is questionable (Viljanen et al., 2005).

Perennial Allergic Rhinitis

When *L. paracasei* 33 (LP33) was given for 30 days to 80 children with perennial rhinoconjunctivitis, the quality of life questionnaire scores significantly improved relative to those of the placebo group (Wang et al., 2004). In view of these claims, a study was set up in Taiwan to evaluate the efficacy of heat-killed LP33 in allergic rhinitis induced by house dust mite. A total of 90 patients were enrolled and assigned to groups receiving 10^{10} living or heat-killed lactobacilli or a placebo for 30 days. A questionnaire on pediatric rhinoconjunctivitis-related quality of life was administered to all subjects or their parents during each clinical visit. The authors reported that living and killed lactobacilli were equally effective ($P < 0.0001$) at improving the quality of life score (Peng and Hsu, 2005).

Japanese Cedar Pollinosis

In a very small study in Finland, *L. rhamnosus* supplementation failed to show any benefit in children allergic to birch pollen in a placebo-controlled trial (Helin et al., 2002). However, there is some evidence for efficacy of probiotics in Japan in relation to allergy to the Japanese cedar (*Cryptomeria japonica*). Xiao and colleagues tested the effect of a yogurt supplemented with *Bifidobacterium longum* BB536 in the treatment of Japanese cedar pollinosis. Subjects consumed 200 g per day for 14 weeks, in a randomized, double-blind, placebo-controlled trial. Post-hoc analyses suggested relief of eye symptoms ($P = 0.044$) but no statistically significant differences in nasal or throat symptoms (Xiao et al., 2006a). The authors then performed a second study in which patients consumed a placebo or approximately 5×10^{10} CFU of

B. longum (without yogurt) for 13 weeks, starting 4 weeks before the start of the pollen season, which peaked at week 8 of the study. Comparison of subjective symptom scores indicated significant reductions in rhinorrhea and nasal blockage and composite scores in the BB536 group compared with the placebo group (Xiao et al., 2006b). Finally, the same group designed a two-way crossover study in which patients were exposed to Japanese cedar pollen in an environmental exposure unit outside the normal pollen season. After a 1-week run-in period, subjects ($n = 24$) were randomly allocated to receive 5×10^{10} CFU of *B. longum* or a placebo twice a day for 4 weeks. After a 2-week washout period, subjects were crossed over for another 4 weeks of treatment. At the end of each treatment period, subjects received controlled pollen exposure for 4 h. In comparison with the placebo, *B. longum* intake significantly reduced the ocular symptom scores, disruption of normal activities, and medication use (Xiao et al., 2007).

Probiotics in Autoimmune Disorders

In view of the encouraging data from experiments in NOD mice, the PRODIA study was arranged in order to seek efficacy in children genetically at risk of type 1 diabetes. The probiotics were administered during the first 6 months of life (Ljungberg et al., 2006). In a pilot study of 200 subjects the protocol was safe and feasible, although the prevalence of autoantibodies among the study subjects at 6, 12, and 24 months of age was similar to the expected figures (Ljungberg et al., 2006).

Similarly, a study in rheumatoid arthritis recruited patients who were randomized to receive two capsules of *Lactobacillus* GG or a placebo twice daily in double-blind fashion for 12 months. Arthritis activity was evaluated by clinical examination, health assessment questionnaire index, and laboratory tests (e.g., tests for erythrocyte sedimentation rate, c-reactive protein, and pro- and anti-inflammatory cytokines). No statistically significant differences in the activity of the arthritis were reported (Hatakka et al., 2003).

Efficacy of Probiotics in Allergic and Autoimmune Disorders; the Debate

There is no overall agreement about the strength of the evidence for efficacy of probiotics in allergy or autoimmunity. In an optimistic review that quotes many studies in allergic disorders, Del Giudice and colleagues state that probiotics are useful for the treatment of various clinical conditions such as food allergy, atopic dermatitis, and allergic rhinitis and in primary prevention of atopy (Del Giudice et al., 2006). Another recent reviewer

was convinced of the evidence for efficacy in atopic dermatitis (Michail et al., 2006).

However, there have also been some skeptical assessments of published trials (Williams, 2006). Trials in which the primary end point was not significant are often published in such a way that a cursory scanning of the abstract leads the reader to think that the trial result was positive (Viljanen et al., 2005; Weston et al., 2005). Common defects are the use, without adequate warning, of post-hoc subgroup analyses and reliance on results that, even if statistically significant, are not clinically useful. Another misleading strategy of presentation is to emphasize within-group changes over time in a study designed to compare differences between treatments. In addition, a failure to adjust for the presence of more-severe cases in the placebo group (at baseline) may be an issue. Overall, then, we are forced to conclude that most studies of probiotics in allergic disorders are unconvincing.

On the other hand, the immunological principles behind this type of treatment are now convincing and are outlined above in the context of the Hygiene or Old Friends Hypothesis. Allergic disorders show defective immunoregulation and can almost certainly be controlled by regulatory immune cells (Akdis et al., 2004; Karlsson et al., 2004; Perez-Machado et al., 2003). We suggest that there have been three major problems. First, there is the issue of the selection of probiotic strains. Probiotics may alleviate some allergic conditions by reducing epithelial permeability, thus reducing allergen uptake. However, we suggest that probiotics, as anti-inflammatory strategies, may need to be selected on the basis of induction of DC_{reg} and T_{reg}. Few authors have used relevant selection criteria, although such studies are beginning to appear (Foligne et al., 2007b; Smits et al., 2005).

Secondly, the issue of recruitment of appropriate patients must be considered carefully. The allergic disorders are a group of disparate conditions with different underlying causes. Several studies have noted (even if only in post-hoc subgroup analyses) that the effects might be most striking in individuals with elevated IgE and skin prick test positivity. The incidence of such atopy was not altered, but the percentage of atopic individuals who developed symptoms was reduced (Kalliomaki et al., 2007; Kukkonen et al., 2007). It will be important to discover whether this tentative (post hoc) observation can be confirmed in trials in which only this atopic subgroup is recruited.

Finally, as this review tries to highlight, it is illogical to concentrate only on bacterial strains associated with intestinal microbiota or classical probiotic strains in fermented food or dairy products. For some clinical applications, other groups of organisms such as helminths or saprophytic mycobacteria might prove to be more effective, and other environmental microbes, yet to be identified, that have an equally long evolutionary relationship with the mammalian immune system and a similar ability to restore immunoregulatory circuits might prove still more effective. We remain optimistic about future developments in this field.

References

Aaby, P., S. O. Shaheen, C. B. Heyes, A. Goudiaby, A. J. Hall, A. W. Shiell, H. Jensen, and A. Marchant. 2000. Early BCG vaccination and reduction in atopy in Guinea-Bissau. *Clin. Exp. Allergy* **30:**644–650.

Adams, V. C., J. R. Hunt, R. Martinelli, R. Palmer, G. A. Rook, and L. R. Brunet. 2004. *Mycobacterium vaccae* induces a population of pulmonary CD11c+ cells with regulatory potential in allergic mice. *Eur. J. Immunol.* **34:**631–638.

Akdis, M., J. Verhagen, A. Taylor, F. Karamloo, C. Karagiannidis, R. Crameri, S. Thunberg, G. Deniz, R. Valenta, H. Fiebig, C. Kegel, R. Disch, C. B. Schmidt-Weber, K. Blaser, and C. A. Akdis. 2004. Immune responses in healthy and allergic individuals are characterized by a fine balance between allergen-specific T regulatory 1 and T helper 2 cells. *J. Exp. Med.* **199:**1567–1575.

Alm, J. S., G. Lilja, G. Pershagen, and A. Scheynius. 1998. BCG vaccination does not seem to prevent atopy in children with atopic heredity. *Allergy* **53:**537.

Arkwright, P. D., and T. J. David. 2003. Effect of *Mycobacterium vaccae* on atopic dermatitis in children of different ages. *Br. J. Dermatol.* **149:**1029–1034.

Arkwright, P. D., C. Fujisawa, A. Tanaka, and H. Matsuda. 2005. *Mycobacterium vaccae* reduces scratching behavior but not the rash in NC mice with eczema: a randomized, blinded, placebo-controlled trial. *J. Investig. Dermatol.* **124:**140–143.

Babu, S., C. P. Blauvelt, V. Kumaraswami, and T. B. Nutman. 2006. Regulatory networks induced by live parasites impair both Th1 and Th2 pathways in patent lymphatic filariasis: implications for parasite persistence. *J. Immunol.* **176:**3248–3256.

Bach, J. F. 2002. The effect of infections on susceptibility to autoimmune and allergic diseases. *N. Engl. J. Med.* **347:**911–920.

Berth-Jones, J., P. D. Arkwright, D. Marasovic, N. Savani, C. R. Aldridge, S. N. Leech, C. Morgan, S. M. Clark, S. Ogilvie, S. Chopra, J. I. Harper, C. H. Smith, G. A. Rook, and P. S. Friedmann. 2006. Killed *Mycobacterium vaccae* suspension in children with moderate-to-severe atopic dermatitis: a randomized, double-blind, placebo-controlled trial. *Clin. Exp. Allergy* **36:**1115–1121.

Bjorksten, B., P. Naaber, E. Sepp, and M. Mikelsaar. 1999. The intestinal microflora in allergic Estonian and Swedish 2-year-old children. *Clin. Exp. Allergy* **29:**342–346.

Braat, H., J. van den Brande, E. van Tol, D. Hommes, M. Peppelenbosch, and S. van Deventer. 2004. *Lactobacillus rhamnosus* induces peripheral hyporesponsiveness in stimulated CD4+ T cells via modulation of dendritic cell function. *Am. J. Clin. Nutr.* **80:**1618–1625.

Calcinaro, F., S. Dionisi, M. Marinaro, P. Candeloro, V. Bonato, S. Marzotti, R. B. Corneli, E. Ferretti, A. Gulino, F. Grasso, C. De Simone, U. Di Mario, A. Falorni, M. Boirivant, and F. Dotta. 2005. Oral probiotic administration induces interleukin-10 production and prevents spontaneous autoimmune diabetes in the non-obese diabetic mouse. *Diabetologia* **48:**1565–1575.

Camporota, L., A. Corkhill, H. Long, J. Lordan, L. Stanciu, N. Tuckwell, A. Cross, J. L. Stanford, G. A. Rook, S. T. Holgate, and R. Djukanovic. 2003. The effects of *Mycobacterium vaccae* on allergen-induced airway responses in atopic asthma. *Eur. Respir. J.* **21:**287–293.

Charng, Y. C., C. C. Lin, and C. H. Hsu. 2006. Inhibition of allergen-induced airway inflammation and hyperreactivity by recombinant lactic-acid bacteria. *Vaccine* **24:**5931–5936.

Christensen, H. R., H. Frokiaer, and J. J. Pestka. 2002. Lactobacilli differentially modulate expression of cytokines and maturation surface markers in murine dendritic cells. *J. Immunol.* **168:**171–178.

Ciprandi, G., A. Vizzaccaro, I. Cirillo, and M. A. Tosca. 2005. *Bacillus clausii* exerts immuno-modulatory activity in allergic subjects: a pilot study. *Allerg. Immunol.* (Paris) **37:**129–134.

Correale, J., and M. Farez. 2007. Association between parasite infection and immune responses in multiple sclerosis. *Ann. Neurol.* **61:**97–108.

Daniel, C., A. Repa, C. Wild, A. Pollak, B. Pot, H. Breiteneder, U. Wiedermann, and A. Mercenier. 2006. Modulation of allergic immune responses by mucosal application of recombinant lactic acid bacteria producing the major birch pollen allergen Bet v 1. *Allergy* **61:**812–819.

De Heer, H. J., H. Hammad, T. Soullie, D. Hijdra, N. Vos, M. A. Willart, H. C. Hoogsteden, and B. N. Lambrecht. 2004. Essential role of lung plasmacytoid dendritic cells in preventing asthmatic reactions to harmless inhaled antigen. *J. Exp. Med.* **200:**89–98.

Del Giudice, M. M., A. Rocco, and C. Capristo. 2006. Probiotics in the atopic march: highlights and new insights. *Dig. Liver. Dis.* **38** (Suppl. 2):S288–S290.

Demissie, A., M. Abebe, A. Aseffa, G. Rook, H. Fletcher, A. Zumla, K. Weldingh, I. Brock, P. Andersen, and T. M. Doherty. 2004. Healthy individuals that control a latent infection with *Mycobacterium tuberculosis* express high levels of Th1 cytokines and the IL-4 antagonist IL-4delta2. *J. Immunol.* **172:**6938.

Di Giacinto, C., M. Marinaro, M. Sanchez, W. Strober, and M. Boirivant. 2005. Probiotics ameliorate recurrent Th1-mediated murine colitis by inducing IL-10 and IL-10-dependent TGF-β-bearing regulatory cells. *J. Immunol.* **174:**3237–3246.

Dlugovitzky, D., G. Fiorenza, M. Farroni, C. Bogue, C. Stanford, and J. Stanford. 2006. Immunological consequences of three doses of heat-killed *Mycobacterium vaccae* in the immunotherapy of tuberculosis. *Respir. Med.* **100:**1079–1087.

Drakes, M., T. Blanchard, and S. Czinn. 2004. Bacterial probiotic modulation of dendritic cells. *Infect. Immun.* **72:**3299–3309.

Ellertsen, L. K., H. G. Wiker, N. T. Egeberg, and G. Hetland. 2005. Allergic sensitisation in tuberculosis and leprosy patients. *Int. Arch. Allergy Immunol.* **138:**217–224.

Farooqi, I. S., and J. M. Hopkin. 1998. Early childhood infection and atopic disorder. *Thorax* **53:**927–932.

Feleszko, W., J. Jaworska, R. D. Rha, S. Steinhausen, A. Avagyan, A. Jaudszus, B. Ahrens, D. A. Groneberg, U. Wahn, and E. Hamelmann. 2007. Probiotic-induced suppression of allergic sensitization and airway inflammation is associated with an increase of T regulatory-dependent mechanisms in a murine model of asthma. *Clin. Exp. Allergy* **37:**498–505.

Fine, P. E. 1995. Variation in protection by BCG: implications of and for heterologous immunity. *Lancet* **346:**1339–1345.

Fletcher, H. A., P. Owiafe, D. Jeffries, P. Hill, G. A. Rook, A. Zumla, T. M. Doherty, and R. H. Brookes. 2004. Increased expression of mRNA encoding interleukin (IL)-4 and its splice variant IL-4delta2 in cells from contacts of *Mycobacterium tuberculosis*, in the absence of *in vitro* stimulation. *Immunology* **112:**669.

Flohr, C., L. N. Tuyen, S. Lewis, R. Quinnell, T. T. Minh, H. T. Liem, J. Campbell, D. Pritchard, T. T. Hien, J. Farrar, H. Williams, and J. Britton. 2006. Poor sanitation and helminth infection protect against skin sensitization in Vietnamese children: a cross-sectional study. *J. Allergy Clin. Immunol.* **118:**1305–1311.

Foligne, B., S. Nutten, C. Grangette, V. Dennin, D. Goudercourt, S. Poiret, J. Dewulf, D. Brassart, A. Mercenier, and B. Pot. 2007a. Correlation between *in vitro* and *in vivo* immunomodulatory properties of lactic acid bacteria. *World J. Gastroenterol.* **13:**236–243.

Foligne, B., G. Zoumpopoulou, J. Dewulf, A. Ben Younes, F. Chareyre, J. C. Sirard, B. Pot, and C. Grangette. 2007b. A key role of dendritic cells in probiotic functionality. *PLoS ONE* **2:**e313.

Forsythe, P., M. D. Inman, and J. Bienenstock. 2007. Oral treatment with live *Lactobacillus reuteri* inhibits the allergic airway response in mice. *Am. J. Respir. Crit. Care Med.* **175:**561–569.

Fujii, T., Y. Ohtsuka, T. Lee, T. Kudo, H. Shoji, H. Sato, S. Nagata, T. Shimizu, and Y. Yamashiro. 2006. *Bifidobacterium breve* enhances transforming growth factor beta1 signaling by regulating Smad7 expression in preterm infants. *J. Pediatr. Gastroenterol. Nutr.* **43:**83–88.

Gruber, C., G. Meinlschmidt, R. Bergmann, U. Wahn, and K. Stark. 2002. Is early BCG vaccination associated with less atopic disease? An epidemiological study in German preschool children with different ethnic backgrounds. *Pediatr. Allergy Immunol.* **13:**177–181.

Gueimonde, M., M. Kalliomaki, E. Isolauri, and S. Salminen. 2006. Probiotic intervention in neonates—will permanent colonization ensue? *J. Pediatr. Gastroenterol. Nutr.* **42:**604–606.

Hadley, E. A., F. I. Smillie, M. A. Turner, A. Custovic, A. Woodcock, and P. D. Arkwright. 2005. Effect of *Mycobacterium vaccae* on cytokine responses in children with atopic dermatitis. *Clin. Exp. Immunol.* **140:**101–108.

Hart, A. L., K. Lammers, P. Brigidi, B. Vitali, F. Rizzello, P. Gionchetti, M. Campieri, M. A. Kamm, S. C. Knight, and A. J. Stagg. 2004. Modulation of human dendritic cell phenotype and function by probiotic bacteria. *Gut* **53:**1602–1609.

Hatakka, K., J. Martio, M. Korpela, M. Herranen, T. Poussa, T. Laasanen, M. Saxelin, H. Vapaatalo, E. Moilanen, and R. Korpela. 2003. Effects of probiotic therapy on the activity and activation of mild rheumatoid arthritis – a pilot study. *Scand. J. Rheumatol.* **32:**211–215.

Helin, T., S. Haahtela, and T. Haahtela. 2002. No effect of oral treatment with an intestinal bacterial strain, *Lactobacillus rhamnosus* (ATCC 53103), on birch-pollen allergy: a placebo-controlled double-blind study. *Allergy* **57:**243–246.

Herz, U., K. Gerhold, C. Gruber, A. Braun, U. Wahn, H. Renz, and K. Paul. 1998. BCG infection suppresses allergic sensitization and development of increased airway reactivity in an animal model. *J. Allergy Clin. Immunol.* **102:**867–874.

Hopfenspirger, M. T., S. K. Parr, R. J. Hopp, R. G. Townley, and D. K. Agrawal. 2001. Mycobacterial antigens attenuate late phase response, airway hyperresponsiveness, and bronchoalveolar lavage eosinophilia in a mouse model of bronchial asthma. *Int. Immunopharmacol.* **1:**1743–1751.

Hopkin, J. M., S. Shaldon, B. Ferry, P. Coull, P. Antrobus, T. Enomoto, T. Yamashita, F. Kurimoto, J. L. Stanford, T. Shirakawa, and G. A. W. Rook. 1998. Mycobacterial immunisation in grass pollen asthma and rhinitis. *Thorax* **53** (Suppl. 4):Abstract S63.

Hori, S., T. Nomura, and S. Sakaguchi. 2003. Control of regulatory T cell development by the transcription factor Foxp3. *Science* **299:**1057–1061.

Hunninghake, G. M., M. E. Soto-Quiros, L. Avila, N. P. Ly, C. Liang, J. S. Sylvia, B. J. Klanderman, E. K. Silverman, and J. C. Celedon. 2007. Sensitization to *Ascaris lumbricoides* and severity of childhood asthma in Costa Rica. *J. Allergy Clin. Immunol.* **119:**654–661.

Hunt, J. R., R. Martinelli, V. C. Adams, G. A. W. Rook, and L. Rosa Brunet. 2005. Intragastric administration of *Mycobacterium vaccae* inhibits severe pulmonary allergic inflammation in a mouse model. *Clin. Exp. Allergy* **35:**685–690.

Jacobsen, C. N., V. Rosenfeldt Nielsen, A. E. Hayford, P. L. Moller, K. F. Michaelsen, A. Paerregaard, B. Sandstrom, M. Tvede, and M. Jakobsen. 1999. Screening of probiotic activities of forty-seven strains of *Lactobacillus* spp. by in vitro techniques and evaluation of the colonization ability of five selected strains in humans. *Appl. Environ. Microbiol.* **65:**4949–4956.

Kalliomaki, M., S. Salminen, H. Arvilommi, P. Kero, P. Koskinen, and E. Isolauri. 2001. Probiotics in primary prevention of atopic disease: a randomised placebo-controlled trial. *Lancet* **357:**1076–1079.

Kalliomaki, M., S. Salminen, T. Poussa, H. Arvilommi, and E. Isolauri. 2003. Probiotics and prevention of atopic disease: 4-year follow-up of a randomised placebo-controlled trial. *Lancet* **361:**1869–1871.

Kalliomaki, M., S. Salminen, T. Poussa, and E. Isolauri. 2007. Probiotics during the first 7 years of life: a cumulative risk reduction of eczema in a randomized, placebo-controlled trial. *J. Allergy Clin. Immunol.* **119:**1019–1021.

Karadag, B., M. Ege, J. E. Bradley, C. Braun-Fahrlander, J. Riedler, D. Nowak, and E. von Mutius. 2006. The role of parasitic infections in atopic diseases in rural schoolchildren. *Allergy* **61:**996–1001.

Karlsson, M. R., J. Rugtveit, and P. Brandtzaeg. 2004. Allergen-responsive CD4+CD25+ regulatory T cells in children who have outgrown cow's milk allergy. *J. Exp. Med.* **199:**1679–1688.

Kato, I., K. Endo-Tanaka, and T. Yokokura. 1998. Suppressive effects of the oral administration of *Lactobacillus casei* on type II collagen-induced arthritis in DBA/1 mice. *Life Sci.* **63:**635–644.

Kim, H., K. Kwack, D. Y. Kim, and G. E. Ji. 2005a. Oral probiotic bacterial administration suppressed allergic responses in an ovalbumin-induced allergy mouse model. *FEMS Immunol. Med. Microbiol.* **45:**259–267.

Kim, H., S. Y. Lee, and G. E. Ji. 2005b. Timing of *Bifidobacterium* administration influences the development of allergy to ovalbumin in mice. *Biotechnol. Lett.* **27:**1361–1367.

Kitagaki, K., T. R. Businga, D. Racila, D. E. Elliott, J. V. Weinstock, and J. N. Kline. 2006. Intestinal helminths protect in a murine model of asthma. *J. Immunol.* **177:**1628–1635.

Kohashi, O., Y. Kohashi, T. Takahashi, A. Ozawa, and N. Shigematsu. 1985. Reverse effect of gram-positive bacteria vs. gram-negative bacteria on adjuvant-induced arthritis in germfree rats. *Microbiol. Immunol.* **29:**487–497.

Kradin, R. L., K. Badizadegan, P. Auluck, J. Korzenik, and G. Y. Lauwers. 2006. Iatrogenic *Trichuris suis* infection in a patient with Crohn's disease. *Arch. Pathol. Lab. Med.* **130:**718–720.

Kriegel, M. A., T. Lohmann, C. Gabler, N. Blank, J. R. Kalden, and H. M. Lorenz. 2004. Defective suppressor function of human CD4+ CD25+ regulatory T cells in autoimmune polyglandular syndrome type II. *J. Exp. Med.* **199:**1285–1291.

Kukkonen, K., E. Savilahti, T. Haahtela, K. Juntunen-Backman, R. Korpela, T. Poussa, T. Tuure, and M. Kuitunen. 2007. Probiotics and prebiotic galacto-oligosaccharides in the prevention of allergic diseases: a randomized, double-blind, placebo-controlled trial. *J. Allergy Clin. Immunol.* **119:**192–198.

Liu, H., M. Komai-Koma, D. Xu, and F. Y. Liew. 2006. Toll-like receptor 2 signaling modulates the functions of CD4+ CD25+ regulatory T cells. *Proc. Natl. Acad. Sci. USA* **103:**7048–7053.

Ljungberg, M., R. Korpela, J. Ilonen, J. Ludvigsson, and O. Vaarala. 2006. Probiotics for the prevention of beta cell autoimmunity in children at genetic risk of type 1 diabetes– the PRODIA study. *Ann. N. Y. Acad. Sci.* **1079:**360–364.

Majamaa, H., and E. Isolauri. 1997. Probiotics: a novel approach in the management of food allergy. *J. Allergy Clin. Immunol.* **99:**179–185.

Michail, S., F. Sylvester, G. Fuchs, and R. Issenman. 2006. Clinical efficacy of probiotics: review of the evidence with focus on children. *J. Pediatr. Gastroenterol. Nutr.* **43:**550–557.

Mortimer, K., A. Brown, J. Feary, C. Jagger, S. Lewis, M. Antoniak, D. Pritchard, and J. Britton. 2006. Dose-ranging study for trials of therapeutic infection with *Necator americanus* in humans. *Am. J. Trop. Med. Hyg.* **75:**914–920.

Murray, R. A., M. R. Siddiqui, M. Mendillo, J. Krahenbuhl, and G. Kaplan. 2007. *Mycobacterium leprae* inhibits dendritic cell activation and maturation. *J. Immunol.* **178:**338–344.

Obihara, C. C., N. Beyers, R. P. Gie, P. C. Potter, B. J. Marais, C. J. Lombard, D. A. Enarson, and J. L. Kimpen. 2005. Inverse association between *Mycobacterium tuberculosis* infection and atopic rhinitis in children. *Allergy* **60:**1121–1125.

Obihara, C. C., J. L. Kimpen, R. P. Gie, S. W. Lill, M. O. Hoekstra, B. J. Marais, H. S. Schaaf, K. Lawrence, P. C. Potter, E. D. Bateman, C. J. Lombard, and N. Beyers. 2006. *Mycobacterium tuberculosis* infection may protect against allergy in a tuberculosis endemic area. *Clin. Exp. Allergy* **36:**70–76.

Ogawa, T., S. Hashikawa, Y. Asai, H. Sakamoto, K. Yasuda, and Y. Makimura. 2006. A new synbiotic, *Lactobacillus casei* subsp. *casei* together with dextran, reduces murine and human allergic reaction. *FEMS Immunol. Med. Microbiol.* **46:**400–409.

Ozdemir, C., T. Akkoc, N. N. Bahceciler, D. Kucukercan, I. B. Barlan, and M. M. Basaran. 2003. Impact of *Mycobacterium vaccae* immunization on lung histopathology in a murine model of chronic asthma. *Clin. Exp. Allergy* **33:**266–270.

Pasare, C., and R. Medzhitov. 2003. Toll pathway-dependent blockade of CD4+CD25+ T cell-mediated suppression by dendritic cells. *Science* **299:**1033–1036.

Peng, G. C., and C. H. Hsu. 2005. The efficacy and safety of heat-killed *Lactobacillus paracasei* for treatment of perennial allergic rhinitis induced by house-dust mite. *Pediatr. Allergy Immunol.* **16:**433–438.

Perez-Machado, M. A., P. Ashwood, M. A. Thomson, F. Latcham, R. Sim, J. A. Walker-Smith, and S. H. Murch. 2003. Reduced transforming growth factor-beta1-producing T cells in the duodenal mucosa of children with food allergy. *Eur. J. Immunol.* **33:**2307–2315.

Rachmilewitz, D., K. Katakura, F. Karmeli, T. Hayashi, C. Reinus, B. Rudensky, S. Akira, K. Takeda, J. Lee, K. Takabayashi, and E. Raz. 2004. Toll-like receptor 9 signaling mediates the anti-inflammatory effects of probiotics in murine experimental colitis. *Gastroenterology* **126:**520–528.

Rautava, S., H. Arvilommi, and E. Isolauri. 2006. Specific probiotics in enhancing maturation of IgA responses in formula-fed infants. *Pediatr. Res.* **60:**221–224.

Ricklin-Gutzwiller, M. E., M. Reist, J. E. Peel, W. Seewald, L. R. Brunet, and P. J. Roosje. 2007. Intradermal injection of heat-killed *Mycobacterium vaccae* in dogs with atopic dermatitis: a multicentre pilot study. *Vet. Dermatol.* **18:**87–93.

Riedler, J., C. Braun-Fahrlander, W. Eder, M. Schreuer, M. Waser, S. Maisch, D. Carr, R. Schierl, D. Nowak, and E. von Mutius. 2001. Exposure to farming in early life and development of asthma and allergy: a cross-sectional survey. *Lancet* **358:**1129–1133.

Rinne, M., M. Kalliomaki, S. Salminen, and E. Isolauri. 2006. Probiotic intervention in the first months of life: short-term effects on gastrointestinal symptoms and long-term effects on gut microbiota. *J. Pediatr. Gastroenterol. Nutr.* **43:**200–205.

Rook, G. A. 2007. Th2 cytokines in susceptibility to tuberculosis. *Curr. Mol. Med.* **7:**327–337.

Rook, G. A., V. Adams, J. Hunt, R. Palmer, R. Martinelli, and L. R. Brunet. 2004. Mycobacteria and other environmental organisms as immunomodulators for immunoregulatory disorders. *Springer Semin. Immunopathol.* **25:**237–255.

Rook, G. A., E. Hamelmann, and L. Rosa Brunet. 2007. Mycobacteria and allergies. *Immunobiology* **212:**461–473.

Rosenfeldt, V., E. Benfeldt, S. D. Nielsen, K. F. Michaelsen, D. L. Jeppesen, N. H. Valerius, and A. Paerregaard. 2003. Effect of probiotic *Lactobacillus* strains in children with atopic dermatitis. *J. Allergy Clin. Immunol.* **111:**389–395.

Sashihara, T., N. Sueki, and S. Ikegami. 2006. An analysis of the effectiveness of heat-killed lactic acid bacteria in alleviating allergic diseases. *J. Dairy Sci.* 89:2846–2855.

Saunders, K. A., T. Raine, A. Cooke, and C. E. Lawrence. 2007. Inhibition of autoimmune type 1 diabetes by gastrointestinal helminth infection. *Infect. Immun.* 75:397–407.

Sheil, B., J. McCarthy, L. O'Mahony, M. W. Bennett, P. Ryan, J. J. Fitzgibbon, B. Kiely, J. K. Collins, and F. Shanahan. 2004. Is the mucosal route of administration essential for probiotic function? Subcutaneous administration is associated with attenuation of murine colitis and arthritis. *Gut* 53:694–700.

Smit, J. J., H. Van Loveren, M. O. Hoekstra, M. A. Schijf, G. Folkerts, and F. P. Nijkamp. 2003. *Mycobacterium vaccae* administration during allergen sensitization or challenge suppresses asthmatic features. *Clin. Exp. Allergy* 33:1083–1089.

Smits, H. H., A. Engering, D. van der Kleij, E. C. de Jong, K. Schipper, T. M. van Capel, B. A. Zaat, M. Yazdanbakhsh, E. A. Wierenga, Y. van Kooyk, and M. L. Kapsenberg. 2005. Selective probiotic bacteria induce IL-10-producing regulatory T cells *in vitro* by modulating dendritic cell function through dendritic cell-specific intercellular adhesion molecule 3-grabbing nonintegrin. *J. Allergy Clin. Immunol.* 115:1260–1267.

Sudo, N., S. Sawamura, K. Tanaka, Y. Aiba, C. Kubo, and Y. Koga. 1997. The requirement of intestinal bacterial flora for the development of an IgE production system fully susceptible to oral tolerance induction. *J. Immunol.* 159:1739–1754.

Summers, R. W., D. E. Elliott, J. F. Urban, Jr., R. Thompson, and J. V. Weinstock. 2005a. *Trichuris suis* therapy in Crohn's disease. *Gut* 54:87–90.

Summers, R. W., D. E. Elliott, J. F. Urban, Jr., R. A. Thompson, and J. V. Weinstock. 2005b. *Trichuris suis* therapy for active ulcerative colitis: a randomized controlled trial. *Gastroenterology* 128:825–832.

Summers, R. W., D. E. Elliott, and J. V. Weinstock. 2006. Therapeutic colonization with *Trichuris suis*. *Arch. Pathol. Lab. Med.* 130:1753–1754.

Sutmuller, R. P., M. H. den Brok, M. Kramer, E. J. Bennink, L. W. Toonen, B. J. Kullberg, L. A. Joosten, S. Akira, M. G. Netea, and G. J. Adema. 2006. Toll-like receptor 2 controls expansion and function of regulatory T cells. *J. Clin. Investig.* 116:485–494.

Suzuki, N., K. Kudo, Y. Sano, and K. Ito. 2001. Can *Mycobacterium tuberculosis* infection prevent asthma and other allergic disorders? *Int. Arch. Allergy Immunol.* 124:113–116.

Takahashi, N., H. Kitazawa, N. Iwabuchi, J. Z. Xiao, K. Miyaji, K. Iwatsuki, and T. Saito. 2006. Immunostimulatory oligodeoxynucleotide from *Bifidobacterium longum* suppresses Th2 immune responses in a murine model. *Clin. Exp. Immunol.* 145:130–138.

Taylor, A., J. Hale, J. Wiltschut, H. Lehmann, J. A. Dunstan, and S. L. Prescott. 2006a. Evaluation of the effects of probiotic supplementation from the neonatal period on innate immune development in infancy. *Clin. Exp. Allergy* 36:1218–1226.

Taylor, A., J. Verhagen, K. Blaser, M. Akdis, and C. A. Akdis. 2006b. Mechanisms of immune suppression by interleukin-10 and transforming growth factor-beta: the role of T regulatory cells. *Immunology* 117:433–442.

Taylor, A. L., J. A. Dunstan, and S. L. Prescott. 2007a. Probiotic supplementation for the first 6 months of life fails to reduce the risk of atopic dermatitis and increases the risk of allergen sensitization in high-risk children: a randomized controlled trial. *J. Allergy Clin. Immunol.* 119:184–191.

Taylor, A. L., J. Hale, B. J. Hales, J. A. Dunstan, W. R. Thomas, and S. L. Prescott. 2007b. FOXP3 mRNA expression at 6 months of age is higher in infants who develop atopic dermatitis, but is not affected by giving probiotics from birth. *Pediatr. Allergy Immunol.* 18:10–19.

Taylor, A. L., J. Hale, J. Wiltschut, H. Lehmann, J. A. Dunstan, and S. L. Prescott. 2006c. Effects of probiotic supplementation for the first 6 months of life on allergen- and vaccine-specific immune responses. *Clin. Exp. Allergy* 36:1227–1235.

van der Kleij, D., E. Latz, J. F. Brouwers, Y. C. Kruize, M. Schmitz, E. A. Kurt-Jones, T. Espevik, E. C. de Jong, M. L. Kapsenberg, D. T. Golenbock, A. G. Tielens, and M. Yazdanbakhsh. 2002. A novel host-parasite lipid crosstalk. Schistosomal lyso-phosphatidylserine activates Toll-like receptor 2 and affects immune polarization. *J. Biol. Chem.* 277:48122–48129.

Van Kruiningen, H. J., and A. B. West. 2007. Iatrogenic *Trichuris suis* infection. *Arch. Pathol. Lab. Med.* 131:180.

van Riet, E., F. C. Hartgers, and M. Yazdanbakhsh. 2007. Chronic helminth infections induce immunomodulation: consequences and mechanisms. *Immunobiology* 212:475–490.

Viglietta, V., C. Baecher-Allan, H. L. Weiner, and D. A. Hafler. 2004. Loss of functional suppression by CD4+CD25+ regulatory T cells in patients with multiple sclerosis. *J. Exp. Med.* 199:971–979.

Viljanen, M., E. Savilahti, T. Haahtela, K. Juntunen-Backman, R. Korpela, T. Poussa, T. Tuure, and M. Kuitunen. 2005. Probiotics in the treatment of atopic eczema/dermatitis syndrome in infants: a double-blind placebo-controlled trial. *Allergy* 60:494–500.

Vizoso Pinto, M. G., T. Schuster, K. Briviba, B. Watzl, W. H. Holzapfel, and C. M. Franz. 2007. Adhesive and chemokine stimulatory properties of potentially probiotic *Lactobacillus* strains. *J. Food Prot.* 70:125–134.

Wan, Y. Y., and R. A. Flavell. 2007. Regulatory T-cell functions are subverted and converted owing to attenuated Foxp3 expression. *Nature* 445:766–770.

Wang, C. C., T. J. Nolan, G. A. Schad, and D. Abraham. 2001. Infection of mice with the helminth *Strongyloides stercoralis* suppresses pulmonary allergic responses to ovalbumin. *Clin. Exp. Allergy* 31:495–503.

Wang, C. C., and G. A. W. Rook. 1998. Inhibition of an established allergic response to ovalbumin in Balb/c mice by killed *Mycobacterium vaccae*. *Immunology* 93:307–313.

Wang, M. F., H. C. Lin, Y. Y. Wang, and C. H. Hsu. 2004. Treatment of perennial allergic rhinitis with lactic acid bacteria. *Pediatr. Allergy Immunol.* 15:152–158.

Weston, S., A. Halbert, P. Richmond, and S. L. Prescott. 2005. Effects of probiotics on atopic dermatitis: a randomised controlled trial. *Arch. Dis. Child.* 90:892–897.

Wildin, R. S., S. Smyk-Pearson, and A. H. Filipovich. 2002. Clinical and molecular features of the immunodysregulation, polyendocrinopathy, enteropathy, X linked (IPEX) syndrome. *J. Med. Genet.* **39:**537–545.

Williams, H. C. 2006. Two "positive" studies of probiotics for atopic dermatitis: or are they? *Arch. Dermatol.* **142:**1201–1203.

Wilson, M. S., M. D. Taylor, A. Balic, C. A. Finney, J. R. Lamb, and R. M. Maizels. 2005. Suppression of allergic airway inflammation by helminth-induced regulatory T cells. *J. Exp. Med.* **202:**1199–1212.

Xiao, J. Z., S. Kondo, N. Yanagisawa, K. Miyaji, K. Enomoto, T. Sakoda, K. Iwatsuki, and T. Enomoto. 2007. Clinical efficacy of probiotic *Bifidobacterium longum* for the treatment of symptoms of Japanese cedar pollen allergy in subjects evaluated in an environmental exposure unit. *Allergol. Int.* **56:**67–75.

Xiao, J. Z., S. Kondo, N. Yanagisawa, N. Takahashi, T. Odamaki, N. Iwabuchi, K. Iwatsuki, S. Kokubo, H. Togashi, K. Enomoto, and T. Enomoto. 2006a. Effect of probiotic *Bifidobacterium longum* BB536 in relieving clinical symptoms and modulating plasma cytokine levels of Japanese cedar pollinosis during the pollen season. A randomized double-blind, placebo-controlled trial. *J. Investig. Allergol. Clin. Immunol.* **16:**86–93.

Xiao, J. Z., S. Kondo, N. Yanagisawa, N. Takahashi, T. Odamaki, N. Iwabuchi, K. Miyaji, K. Iwatsuki, H. Togashi, K. Enomoto, and T. Enomoto. 2006b. Probiotics in the treatment of Japanese cedar pollinosis: a double-blind placebo-controlled trial. *Clin. Exp. Allergy* **36:**1425–1435.

Yang, J., J. Zhao, Y. Yang, L. Zhang, X. Yang, X. Zhu, M. Ji, N. Sun, and C. Su. 2007. *Schistosoma japonicum* egg antigens stimulate CD4 CD25 T cells and modulate airway inflammation in a murine model of asthma. *Immunology* **120:**8–18.

Yazdanbakhsh, M., P. G. Kremsner, and R. van Ree. 2002. Allergy, parasites, and the hygiene hypothesis. *Science* **296:**490–494.

Yazdanbakhsh, M., and P. M. Matricardi. 2004. Parasites and the hygiene hypothesis: regulating the immune system? *Clin. Rev. Allergy Immunol.* **26:**15–24.

Zaccone, P., Z. Fehervari, F. M. Jones, S. Sidobre, M. Kronenberg, D. W. Dunne, and A. Cooke. 2003. *Schistosoma mansoni* antigens modulate the activity of the innate immune response and prevent onset of type 1 diabetes. *Eur. J. Immunol.* **33:**1439–1449.

Zanin-Zhorov, A., L. Cahalon, G. Tal, R. Margalit, O. Lider, and I. R. Cohen. 2006. Heat shock protein 60 enhances CD4+ CD25+ regulatory T cell function via innate TLR2 signaling. *J. Clin. Investig.* **116:**2022–2032.

Zuany-Amorim, C., C. Manlius, A. Trifilieff, L. R. Brunet, G. Rook, G. Bowen, G. Pay, and C. Walker. 2002a. Long-term protective and antigen-specific effect of heat-killed *Mycobacterium vaccae* in a murine model of allergic pulmonary inflammation. *J. Immunol.* **169:**1492.

Zuany-Amorim, C., E. Sawicka, C. Manlius, A. Le Moine, L. R. Brunet, D. M. Kemeny, G. Bowen, G. Rook, and C. Walker. 2002b. Suppression of airway eosinophilia by killed *Mycobacterium vaccae*-induced allergen-specific regulatory T-cells. *Nat. Med.* **8:**625–629.

Therapeutic Microbiology: Probiotics and Related Strategies
Edited by J. Versalovic and M. Wilson
© 2008 ASM Press, Washington, DC

J. H. Meurman

Probiotics in Oral Biology and Dentistry

19

The mouth, or oral cavity, is the most proximal part of the gastrointestinal tract, and it is characterized by various types of epithelium and mucosal tissue with a fairly site-specific resident microbiota. In the mouth the keratinized and nonkeratinized epithelia harbor different microbial species. The tooth and tongue surfaces harbor complex biofilm structures that include hundreds of bacterial species and other microbes such as yeasts. Saliva bathes surfaces in the oral cavity and affects the composition of oral microbial communities by immune mechanisms and buffering capacity. Patients with "dry" mouth, i.e., reduced amounts of saliva, are particularly susceptible to colonization with opportunistic and pathogenic microorganisms. For example, elderly patients taking many concomitant medications that reduce salivary secretion may be vulnerable to microbial overgrowth.

Oral microorganisms may gain access to the systemic circulation through carious teeth, inflamed periodontal tissue, and ulceration of the oral mucosa. Erupting teeth with gingival inflammation present pathology in younger individuals, mainly seen in the eruption of wisdom teeth. Bacteria of oral origin may represent potential

pathogens (Lockhart and Durack, 1999). Figure 1 depicts the systemic spread of oral infection. Classical examples of complications by oral microbes include endocarditis and glomerulonephritis caused by viridans group streptococcal bacteremia. Evidence also shows that oral bacteria may play a role in the pathogenesis of various systemic diseases, including chronic diseases such as atherosclerosis. Consequently, probiotics may be useful to control and balance the oral microbiota with subsequent improvement of oral health. In this chapter, the characteristics of the oral microbiota are discussed, and examples of potential contributions of probiotics to oral health are discussed.

ORAL MICROBIOTA AND DENTAL BIOFILMS

The first colonizers of the oral cavity are lactobacilli usually derived from the mother's vaginal microbiota at birth or from other external sources in cases of cesarean section. Viridans group streptococci are early colonizers and form the principal cultivable oral microbiota.

J. H. Meurman, Institute of Dentistry and Department of Oral and Maxillofacial Diseases, Helsinki University Central Hospital, PB 41, University of Helsinki, FI 00014 Helsinki, Finland.

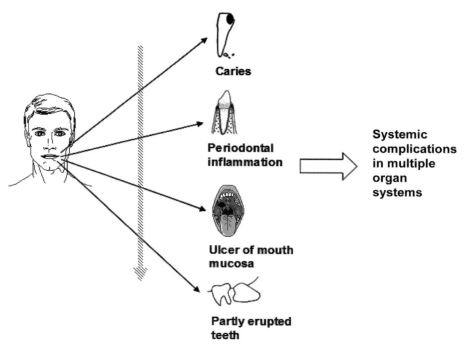

Figure 1 Schematic diagram of the potential dissemination of oral microorganisms from infectious foci in the oral cavity via hematogenous circulation. Detrimental general complications may occur in several organs. Bacteria of oral origin may trigger harmful reactions leading to pathologic processes such as atherosclerosis. Probiotic interventions (vertical arrow) may control the oral microbiota so that systemic spread of bacteria would be reduced due to improved oral health.

Streptococcus mutans, the principal etiological agent of dental caries, is not detected usually in the mouth of an infant prior to the eruption of the first teeth. The mandibular first incisors usually erupt at the age of approximately 6 months.

S. mutans requires solid surfaces for attachment and proliferation. It has highly developed cellular mechanisms for carbohydrate metabolism used for converting dietary carbohydrates to extracellular polysaccharides. These exopolysaccharides promote bacterial attachment to dental surfaces and foster accumulation of oral microorganisms in plaque that combine with saliva-derived macromolecules to form a complex biofilm. Oral microbes and biofilms are bathed in saliva with highly diverse microbial contents. Bacterial diversity in the human subgingival plaque and dorsum of the tongue is estimated to range from 200 to more than 700 species (Paster et al., 2001; Kazor et al., 2003). Of oral microbes, lactobacilli comprise approximately 1% of the cultivable oral microbiota (Marsh and Martin, 1999). In all, 1 mg of dental plaque contains 10^{11} bacteria.

Many *Lactobacillus* species have been isolated from saliva. Oral species include *L. fermentum*, *L. rhamnosus*, *L. salivarius*, *L. casei*, *L. acidophilus*, *L. plantarum*, *L. oris*, *L. paracasei*, *L. gasseri*, and *L. crispatus* (Colloca et al., 2000; Köll-Klais et al., 2005; Teanpaisan and Dahlen, 2006). Lactobacilli, as members of the resident oral microbiota, may play an important role in the microecological balance of the oral cavity. Nevertheless, few studies indicate that probiotic strains could be detected in the oral cavity and whether natural probiotic strains are prevalent in the mouth. Hence, the whole concept of "resident probiotics of the mouth" needs further investigation. Theoretically, probiotics could interfere in several steps of oral biofilm formation, the development and modification of oral microecology, and the proliferation of planktonic microorganisms in the saliva.

INTERFERENCE WITH ORAL MICROBIAL COLONIZATION

Bacterial attachment to epithelial cells or dental surfaces is the first and most essential step in colonization and development of oral biofilms. Mechanisms of adhesion to oral surfaces have been studied using model systems that mimic biofilm formation. Hydroxyapatite is the main mineral component of a tooth, and thus, hydroxyapatite assays with or without saliva, buffers, proteins, and other chemical substances have been used together with studies of bacterial attachment to epithelial cell lines (Ostengo and Nader-Macias, 2004). In a study addressing bacterial survival in saliva and adherence to oral surfaces, the colonization potential of commercially available *Lactobacillus* and *Bifidobacterium* strains was investigated. Probiotics demonstrated 24-h survival rates in saliva, but variations among the strains in their binding capacity to saliva-coated surfaces were detected. Lactobacilli showed greater adherence to saliva-coated surfaces than that of bifidobacteria. Lactobacilli may compete for the same binding sites on saliva-coated hydroxyapatite and thus affect the formation of oral biofilms. Lactobacilli have also been shown to inhibit the adherence of *S. mutans* in vitro (Haukioja et al., 2006).

Another important area of research is the coaggregation ability of probiotics with other oral bacteria known to be essential in biofilm formation and development. One of these strains is *Fusobacterium nucleatum*, which plays a role as a "bridge" organism facilitating the colonization of other bacteria by coaggregation and attachment to epithelial cells (Kolenbrander, 2000; Kang et al., 2005). Lactobacilli may interfere with such coaggregation and thus prevent colonization of pathogenic bacteria in the oral cavity (Boris et al., 1997; Reid et al., 1988). *Weissella cibaria*, a putative probiotic isolated from humans, animals, and fermented foods, was tested for its coaggregation capacity, and it appeared to efficiently coaggregate with *F. nucleatum* (Kang et al., 2005). However, this area of research is still in its cradle and more studies are needed to understand mechanisms of microbial colonization and oral biofilm development. Based on such knowledge, probiotic interference strategies can be recommended.

COLONIZATION OF PROBIOTICS IN THE ORAL CAVITY

Permanent oral colonization by established probiotics has not been reported when external strains have been administered to test subjects or patients. Yli-Knuuttila et al. (2006) assessed the colonization of *L. rhamnosus* GG in the oral cavity of healthy students. After the 14-day trial period, the occurrence of *L. rhamnosus* GG in the oral cavity decreased gradually, indicating that colonization was transient. The study confirmed earlier observations by the same group that oral colonization was temporary (Meurman et al., 1994). Long-term studies in this area have not been published. However, one person who had received probiotic *L. rhamnosus* GG-containing dairy products from early childhood remained saliva positive for this bacterium at the age of 20 years, indicating that long-term colonization is possible (data in our laboratory).

PROBIOTICS AND DENTAL CARIES

Dental caries is one of the most prevalent infectious diseases of humans, and it affects all age groups with a large socioeconomic impact. In fact, the profession of dentists principally evolved in course of history due to the special needs to treat carious teeth. If probiotics could be used to prevent or combat dental caries, new treatment modes could be developed. Earlier studies on this topic have shown promising results. Probiotics inhibited the growth of cariogenic streptococci in vitro and in clinical trials (Meurman et al., 1994; Busscher et al., 1999; Näse et al., 2001; Ahola et al., 2002; Çaglar et al., 2006). Table 1 outlines these studies, but more randomized controlled trials are needed for further recommendations.

Table 1 Effects of probiotic strains on pathogens causing dental caries

Probiotic organism tested	Type of study	Result	Reference
L. rhamnosus GG	In vitro	Inhibition of *Streptococcus sobrinus*	Meurman et al., 1994
L. casei	In vitro	Inhibition of oral streptococci	Busscher et al., 1999
L. rhamnosus GG	Randomized controlled trial	Reduction of salivary *S. mutans* counts in day care children	Näse et al., 2001
L. rhamnosus GG	Randomized controlled trial	Reduction of salivary *S. mutans* counts in young adults	Ahola et al., 2002
L. reuteri	Controlled intervention study	Reduction of oral *S. mutans* counts in clinical trial	Çaglar et al., 2006
Bifidobacterium strain DN-173 010	Randomized controlled trial	Reduction in salivary *S. mutans*	Çaglar et al., 2005

PROBIOTICS AND PERIODONTAL DISEASE

Studies on the effects of probiotics on periodontal disease are sparse. Periodontal disease affects the majority of adults throughout the developed world. The severity of the disease ranges from asymptomatic and occasional gingival bleeding to abscesses caused by severe inflammation in the oral cavity. Periodontal disease in particular has been linked with systemic consequences such as the development of atherosclerosis and poor metabolic balance of diabetic patients (Slavkin and Baum, 2007). New strategies for controlling periodontal disease might benefit overall health status. Some probiotic lactobacilli inhibit periodontal pathogens such as *Porphyromonas gingivalis*, *Prevotella intermedia* (Köll-Kleis et al., 2005), *Bacteroides* spp., *Actinomyces* spp., and *Streptococcus intermedius* (Volozhin et al., 2004). However, no randomized controlled studies have been published yet on this topic.

PROBIOTICS AND ORAL *CANDIDA* INFECTIONS

The yeast *Candida albicans* is among the most common infectious agents in the oral cavity. The incidence of yeast infections is higher in the elderly, in individuals with impaired immunity, and in patients with dry mouth. Dental prostheses further render the patient liable for yeast infections. Similar to bacterial infections of the oral cavity, the mechanisms of *Candida* colonization onto mucosal membranes and its virulence factors are poorly understood. Furthermore, *Candida* species other than *C. albicans* are emerging and may cause problems in medically compromised patients (Bagg et al., 2005). Yeasts other than *C. albicans* are often resistant to commonly used antifungal agents such as fluconazole. Therefore, new probiotic strategies would be welcome for the prevention and treatment of oral yeast infections.

One randomized controlled trial has been published regarding probiotics and oral yeast infections. The results of the trial were positive, however, in showing that a combination of probiotic *L. rhamnosus* GG and *Propionibacterium freudenreichii* subsp. *shermanii* JS reduced *Candida* counts in the saliva of elderly individuals (Hatakka et al., 2007). In an animal study, *L. acidophilus* and *L. fermentum* were investigated for enhanced clearance of *C. albicans* from the oral cavity with promising results (Elahi et al., 2005). However, more controlled human studies are needed to establish efficacy of probiotics in the context of oral fungal infections.

PROBIOTICS AND OTHER DISEASES OF THE MOUTH

The putative immunomodulatory effects of probiotic bacteria may be beneficial in the oral cavity in addition to the contiguous gastrointestinal tract (Collins et al., 1998; Fang et al., 2000). In particular, diseases of the oral mucosa such as lichen planus or manifestations of other dermatological or systemic diseases might be controlled by successful probiotic therapies. Probiotic effects may be exerted directly by inhibition of pathogenic oral microbes, or indirectly by affecting specific immune responses. In the mouth, cellular immunity at the margins of epithelium, especially at subgingival tissue, may mediate responses by translocation of blood-borne antibodies, mainly immunoglobulin G (IgG) and IgM. Saliva has its own antibodies including secretory IgA, which is synthesized by lymphatic tissue adjacent to the salivary glands. However, no studies have reported probiotic effects on immune mechanisms in the oral cavity. Nevertheless, in the intervention study of Hatakka et al. (2007), the number of subjects with low salivary buffering capacities decreased in the probiotic group. Low buffering is a sign of poor defensive or hurt response systems in the mouth. Thus, probiotics may have protective and immunomodulatory effects, but the underlying mechanisms are not known.

PROBIOTICS AND ORAL SYMPTOMATOLOGY

Xerostomia or "dry mouth" is a symptom highly prevalent in peri- and postmenopausal women and even more so in elderly populations (Närhi et al., 1999). It is a common side effect of systemic medications or due to diseases such as diabetes or rheumatic disease. In the study of Hatakka et al. (2007), the probiotic intervention resulted in less xerostomia and hyposalivation (measured low salivary output) among elderly subjects investigated. No explanation was offered, but future study plans might consider such findings. Low salivary flow renders the patient liable for oral infections, so enhanced salivary flow is beneficial for health.

Burning mouth syndrome (BMS) is another nonspecific symptom of the mouth that affects mostly elderly women. The symptom is characterized by burning, itching sensations, or pain in the oral mucosa or tongue. BMS is usually milder in the morning, but it gets worse during the course of the day. No anatomical-pathological explanation has been described for the symptoms, and its etiology is not known (Hakeberg et al., 1997). Treatment of BMS includes local ointments and analgesics if needed, but neurological drugs such as lamotrigine may be prescribed in severe cases. Hence, probiotics with

Table 2 Vision for potential future use of probiotics in oral medicine and dentistry

Indication	Expected effects (based on published findings)
Prevention and control of dental caries	Probiotic inhibition of cariogenic streptococci
Prevention and control of periodontal disease	Inhibition of periodontal pathogens such as *P. gingivalis*
Prevention and control of oral yeast infections	Inhibition of *Candida* spp.; enhancing immune system function
Ameliorating oral manifestations of skin and systemic diseases	Modulating immune system; inhibition of pathogenic microbiota
Halitosis	Inhibition of microbial production of volatile sulfur compounds
Xerostomia and burning mouth	Modulating immune system

immunomodulatory effects may ameliorate the symptoms of BMS. If probiotics are administered in milk products, the cooling effects of such preparations on the oral mucosa are often welcomed by the patients. However, no controlled studies have been published on this topic.

Halitosis or oral malodor causes subjective suffering to the patients. The reason for bad breath is poor periodontal health in the majority of cases, and the malodor is mostly due to volatile sulfur compounds (VSC) generated by anaerobic bacteria. However, for many patients the reason for halitosis cannot be found. Halitosis has recently been ameliorated by regular administration of probiotics. Kang et al. (2006) have shown an inhibitory effect on the production of VSC by *F. nucleatum* after ingestion of *W. cibaria*. A possible mechanism of VSC reduction may include generation of hydrogen peroxide by *W. cibaria* that inhibits the proliferation of *F. nucleatum*. *Streptococcus salivarius*, a possible candidate as an oral probiotic, has demonstrated inhibitory effects on VSC by competing for colonization sites with species generating VSC (Burton et al., 2005, 2006). Consequently, probiotic therapy could relieve halitosis if the preliminary observations regarding the balancing effect of probiotics on VSC-generating microbiota can be confirmed in properly controlled studies.

LACTIC ACID BACTERIA AND ORAL DISEASES

Most *Lactobacillus* species used in dairy products readily ferment dietary carbohydrates to organic acids. If such a bacterium is in close contact with tooth enamel, tissue damage may occur. The critical pH of hydroxyapatite is 5.5. Any substance with pH value lower than 5.5 may cause enamel dissolution. Subsequently, care must be taken not to promote caries or erosion by using excessively acid-producing probiotic bacteria in high amounts. Dental erosion refers to chemical dissolution of dental enamel by ingestion of sour foodstuffs or specific drinks or by gastric regurgitation. In contrast, dental caries includes an infectious component, and the acids are due to

bacterial fermentation. One of the principal safety issues for putative oral probiotic strains is the poor fermentation capacity of common dietary carbohydrates. The ubiquitous dietary sugars, such as sucrose, are important considerations in food preparations. *L. rhamnosus* GG fulfills the criterion of a candidate oral probiotic because this strain does not ferment common dietary sugars.

Whether or not probiotic interference in oral microecology can prevent or facilitate superinfections is not known. In addition, the possible transfer of antimicrobial resistance genes between probiotic strains and microorganisms of the resident microbiota also highlights the need for more studies and careful monitoring in the future. Dairy products have been used in our diet since the early history of mankind, but it is highly improbable that probiotic strains can be selected from dairy products for future oral medicine or dental purposes. Table 2 summarizes some recommendations and future visions for oral probiotics. It should be reemphasized that application of probiotics in oral biology and dentistry is still in its early stages, but rapid developments in this area bode well for the future of oral medicine.

References

Ahola, A. J., H. Yli-Knuuttila, T. Suomalainen, T. Poussa, A. Ahlström, J. H. Meurman, and R. Korpela. 2002. Short-term consumption of probiotic-containing cheese and its effect on dental caries risk factors. *Arch. Oral Biol.* 47:799–804.

Bagg, J., M. P. Sweeney, A. N. Davies, M. S. Jackson, and S. Brailsford. 2005. Voriconazole susceptibility of yeasts isolated from the mouths of patients with advanced cancer. *J. Med. Immunol.* 54:959–964.

Boris, S., J. E. Suarez, and C. Barbes. 1997. Characterization of the aggregation promoting factor from *Lactobacillus gasseri*, a vaginal isolate. *J. Appl. Microbiol.* 83:413–420.

Burton, J. P., C. N. Chilcott, and J. R. Tagg. 2005. The rationale and potential for the reduction of oral malodour using *Streptococcus salivarius* probiotics. *Oral Dis.* 11:29–31.

Burton, J. P., P. A. Wescombe, C. J. Moore, C. N. Chilcott, and J. R. Tagg. 2006. Safety assessment of the oral cavity probiotic *Streptococcus salivarius* K12. *Appl. Environ. Microbiol.* 72:3050–3053.

Busscher, H. J., A. F. Mulder, and C. H. van der Mei. 1999. *In vitro* adhesion to enamel and *in vivo* colonization of tooth surfaces by lactobacilli from a bio-yogurt. *Caries Res.* 33:403–404.

Çaglar, E., N. Sandalli, S. Twetman, S. Kavaloglu, S. Ergeneli, and S. Selvi. 2005. Effect of yogurt with *Bifidobacterium* DN-173 010 on salivary mutans streptococci and lactobacilli in young adults. *Acta Odontol. Scand.* 63:317–320.

Çaglar, E., S. K. Cilder, S. Ergeneli, N. Sandalli, and S. Twetman. 2006. Salivary mutans streptococci and lactobacilli levels after ingestion of the probiotic bacterium *Lactobacillus reuteri* ATCC 55739 by straws or tablets. *Acta Odontol. Scand.* 64:314–318.

Collins, J. K., G. Thornton, and G. O. Sullivan. 1998. Selection of probiotic strains for human applications. *Int. Dairy J.* 8:487–490.

Colloca, M. E., M. C. Ahumada, M. E. Lopez, and M. E. Nader-Macias. 2000. Surface properties of lactobacilli isolated from healthy subjects. *Oral Dis.* 6:227–233.

Elahi, S., G. Pang, A. Clancy, and R. Clancy. 2005. Enhanced clearance of *Candida albicans* from the oral cavities of mice following oral administration of *Lactobacillus acidophilus.* *Clin. Exp. Immunol.* 141:29–36.

Fang, H., E. Tuomola, H. Arvilommi, and S. Salminen. 2000. Modulation of humoral immune response through probiotic intake. *FEMS Immunol. Med. Microbiol.* 29:47–52.

Hakeberg, M., U. Beggren, C. Hägglin, and M. Ahlqwist. 1997. Reported burning mouth syndrome among middle-aged and elderly women. *Eur. J. Oral Sci.* 105:539–543.

Hatakka, K., A. J. Ahola, H. Yli-Knuuttila, M. Richardson, T. Poussa, J. H. Meurman, and R. Korpela. 2007. Probiotics reduce the prevalence of oral Candida in the elderly—a randomized controlled trial. *J. Dent. Res.* 86:125–130.

Haukioja, A., H. Yli-Knuuttila, V. Loimaranta, K. Kari, A. C. Ouwehand, J. H. Meurman, and J. Tenovuo. 2006. Oral adhesion and survival of probiotic and other lactobacilli and bifidobacteria *in vitro*. *Oral Microbiol. Immunol.* 21:326–332.

Kang, M. S., H. S. Na, and L. S. Oh. 2005. Coaggregation ability of *Weissella cibaria* isolates with *Fusobacterium nucleatum* and their adhesiveness to epithelial cells. *FEMS Microbiol. Lett.* 253:323–329.

Kang, M.-S., B.-G. Kim, H.-C. Lee, and J.-S. Oh. 2006. Inhibitory effect of *Weissella cibaria* isolates on the production of volatile sulphur compounds. *J. Clin. Periodontol.* 33:226–232.

Kazor, C. E., P. M. Mitchell, A. M. Lee, L. N. Stokes, W. J. Loesche, F. E. Dewhirst, and B. J. Paster. 2003. Diversity of bacterial populations on the tongue dorsa of patients with halitosis and healthy patients. *J. Clin. Microbiol.* 41:558–563.

Kolenbrander, P. E. 2000. Oral microbial communities: biofilms, interactions, and genetic systems. *Annu. Rev. Microbiol.* 54:413–437.

Köll-Klais, P., R. Mändar, E. Leibur, H. Marcotte, L. Hammarström, and M. Mikelsaar. 2005. Oral lactobacilli in chronic periodontitis and periodontal health: species composition and antimicrobial activity. *Oral Microbiol. Immunol.* 20:354–361.

Lockhart, P. B., and D. T. Durack. 1999. Oral microflora as a cause of endocarditis and other distant site infections. *Infect. Dis. Clin. North Am.* 13:833–850.

Marsh, P., and M. V. Martin. 1999. *Oral Microbiology*, 4th ed. Wright, Oxford, United Kingdom.

Meurman, J. H., H. Antila, and S. Salminen. 1994. Recovery of *Lactobacillus* strain GG (ATCC 53103) from saliva of healthy volunteers after consumption of yoghurt prepared with the bacterium. *Microb. Ecol. Health Dis.* 7:295–298.

Närhi, T. O., J. H. Meurman, and A. Ainamo. 1999. Xerostomia and hyposalivation: causes, consequences and treatment in the elderly. *Drugs Aging* 15:103–116.

Näse, L., K. Hatakka, E. Savilahti, M. Saxelin, A. Pönka, T. Poussa, R. Korpela, and J. H. Meurman. 2001. Effect of long-term consumption of a probiotic bacterium, *Lactobacillus rhamnosus GG*, in milk on dental caries and caries risk in children. *Caries Res.* 35:412–420.

Ostengo, M. C., and E. M. Nader-Macias. 2004. Hydroxylapatite beads as an experimental model to study adhesion of lactic acid bacteria from the oral cavity to hard tissues. *Methods Mol. Biol.* 268:447–452.

Paster, B. J., S. K. Boches, J. L. Galvin, R. E. Ericson, C. N. Lau, V. A. Levanos, A. Sahasrabudhe, and F. E. Dewhirst. 2001. Bacterial diversity in human subgingival plaque. *J. Bacteriol.* 183:3770–3783.

Reid, G., J. A. McGroarty, R. Angotti, and R. L. Cook. 1988. *Lactobacillus* inhibitor production against *Escherichia coli* and coaggregation ability with uropathogens. *Can. J. Microbiol.* 34:344–351.

Slavkin, H., and B. Baum. 2007. Relationship of dental and oral pathology to systemic illness. *J. Am. Dent. Assoc.* 284:1215–1217.

Teanpaisan, R., and G. Dahlen. 2006. Use of polymerase chain reaction techniques and sodium dodecyl sulphate-polyacrylamide get electrophoresis for differentiation of oral *Lactobacillus* species. *Oral Microbiol. Immunol.* 21:79–83.

Volozhin, A. I., V. K. Il'in, I. M. Maksimovskii, A. B. Sidorenko, L. P. Istranov, V. N. Tsarev, E. V. Istranova, and R. K. Aboiants. 2004. Development and use of periodontal dressing of collagen and *Lactobacillus casei* 37 cell suspension in combined treatment of periodontal disease of inflammatory origin (a microbiological study). *Stomatologiia* (Mosk) 83:6–8.

Yli-Knuuttila, H., J. Snäll, K. Kari, and J. H. Meurman. 2006. Colonization of *Lactobacillus rhamnosus* GG in the oral cavity. *Oral Microbiol. Immunol.* 21:129–131.

Therapeutic Microbiology: Probiotics and Related Strategies
Edited by J. Versalovic and M. Wilson
© 2008 ASM Press, Washington, DC

Francisco Guarner

Probiotics in Gastrointestinal Diseases

20

INTESTINAL MICROBIAL ECOLOGY

Human beings are associated in a symbiotic relationship with a huge population of microorganisms that live on body surfaces and in cavities connected with the external environment. The gut microbiota is a diverse and dynamic ecosystem including bacteria, archaea, and eukarya, which have adapted to live on the intestinal mucosal surface or within the gut lumen (Guarner, 2005; Ley et al., 2006). Gut microorganisms include native species that colonize the intestine permanently and a variable set of living microorganisms that transit temporarily through the gastrointestinal tract. Native species are acquired mainly at birth and during the first years of life, whereas transient microbes are continually being ingested from the environment (food, drinks, etc.).

The stomach and duodenum harbor very low numbers of microorganisms, typically $<10^3$ bacteria cells per g of contents, mainly lactobacilli and streptococci. Acid, bile, and pancreatic secretions suppress most ingested microbes, and phasic propulsive motor activity impedes stable colonization of the lumen. The numbers of bacteria progressively increase along the jejunum and ileum, from approximately 10^4 cells in the jejunum to 10^7 cells per g of contents in the distal ileum. The large intestine is heavily populated by anaerobes with approximately 10^{12} cells per g of luminal contents. In the upper gut, transit is rapid and bacterial density is low, but the impact on immune function is thought to be important because of the presence of a large number of organized lymphoid structures in the small intestinal mucosa (Peyer's patches). These structures have a specialized epithelium for uptake and sampling of antigens and contain lymphoid germinal centers for induction of adaptive immune responses (Cummings et al., 2004). In the colon, however, transit time is slow and microorganisms have the opportunity to proliferate by fermenting available substrates derived from either the diet or endogenous secretions.

Our current knowledge about the microbial composition of the intestinal ecosystem in health and disease is still very limited. Studies using classical techniques of microbiological culture can recover only a minor fraction of fecal bacteria. More than 50% of bacterial cells that are observed by microscopic examination of fecal specimens cannot be grown in culture (Suau et al., 1999).

Francisco Guarner, Digestive System Research Unit, University Hospital Vall d'Hebron, CIBEREHD, Passeig Vall d'Hebron, 119–129, 08035 Barcelona, Spain.

Molecular biological techniques based on the sequence diversity of the bacterial genome are being used to characterize noncultivable bacteria. Molecular studies of the fecal microbiota have highlighted that only 7 of the 55 known divisions or superkingdoms of the domain *Bacteria* are detected in the human gut ecosystem, and of these, 3 bacterial divisions dominate, i.e., *Bacteroidetes*, *Firmicutes*, and *Actinobacteria* (Ley et al., 2006). However, at the level of species and strains, microbial diversity between individuals is highly remarkable, so that each individual harbors his or her own distinctive pattern of bacterial composition (Eckburg et al., 2005). This pattern appears to be determined partly by the host genotype (Zoetendal et al., 2001) and by initial colonization at birth via vertical transmission (Ley et al., 2006). In healthy adults, the fecal composition is stable over time, but temporal fluctuations due to environmental factors can be detected and may involve up to 20% of the dominant groups (Zoetendal et al., 2001). Bacterial composition in the lumen varies from cecum to rectum, and fecal samples do not reflect luminal contents in proximal segments of the gastrointestinal tract. However, the community of mucosa-associated bacteria is highly stable from the terminal ileum to the large bowel in a given individual (Zoetendal et al., 2002; Lepage et al., 2005).

HOST-BACTERIA RELATIONSHIPS IN THE GUT

Some of the bacteria in the gut are pathogens or potential pathogens when the integrity of the mucosal barrier is functionally breached. However, the normal interaction between gut bacteria and their host is a symbiotic relationship, defined as mutually beneficial for both partners. The host provides a nutrient-rich habitat, and intestinal bacteria confer important benefits on the host's health (Hooper et al., 2002). Comparison of animals bred under germfree conditions with their conventionally raised counterparts (conventional microbiota) has revealed a series of anatomic characteristics and physiological functions that are associated with the presence of the microbiota (Falk et al., 1998). Organ weights (heart, lung, and liver), cardiac output, intestinal wall thickness, intestinal motor activity, serum gamma globulin levels, and lymph nodes, among other characteristics, are all reduced or atrophic in germfree animals, suggesting that gut bacteria provide important and specific functions to the host.

Functions of the gut microbiota have been assigned into three categories, i.e., metabolic, protective, and trophic functions (Guarner, 2005). Metabolic functions consist of the fermentation of nondigestible dietary substrates and endogenous mucus. Gene diversity among the microbial community provides a variety of enzymes and biochemical pathways that are distinct from the host's own constitutive resources. Fermentation of carbohydrates is a major source of energy in the colon for bacterial growth and produces short-chain fatty acids that can be absorbed by the host. These biochemical conversions result in salvage of dietary energy and favor the absorption of ions (Ca, Mg, and Fe) in the cecum. Protective functions of gut microbiota include the barrier effect that prevents invasion by pathogens. Resident bacteria represent a resistance factor to colonization by exogenous microbes or opportunistic bacteria that are present in the gut, but their growth is restricted. The equilibrium between species of resident bacteria provides stability in the microbial population, but antibiotics can disrupt the balance (for instance, overgrowth of toxigenic *Clostridium difficile*). Trophic functions include the control of epithelial cell proliferation and differentiation as well as the homeostatic regulation of the immune system. Cell differentiation is highly influenced by the interaction with resident microorganisms as shown by the expression of a variety of genes in germfree animals monoassociated with specific bacteria strains (Hooper et al., 2001). Bacteria play also an essential role in the development of a healthy immune system (Fig. 1). Animals bred in a germfree environment show low densities of lymphoid cells in the gut mucosa and low levels of serum immunoglobulins (Igs). Exposure to commensal microbes rapidly expands the number of mucosal lymphocytes and increases the size of germinal centers in lymphoid follicles (Yamanaka et al., 2003). Ig-producing cells appear in the lamina propria, and serum Ig quantities are significantly increased. Most interestingly, recent findings suggest that some commensals play a major role in the induction of regulatory T cells in gut lymphoid follicles (Mazmanian and Kasper, 2006). Control pathways mediated by regulatory T cells are essential homeostatic mechanisms by which the host can tolerate the massive burden of innocuous antigens within the gut or on other body surfaces without resulting in inflammation.

On the other hand, several disease states or disorders have been associated with changes in the composition or function of the enteric microbiota (Table 1). For instance, acute diarrhea is usually caused by pathogens that proliferate and invade or produce toxins. Antibiotic-associated diarrhea is due to imbalance in the composition and structure of the gut microbiota with overgrowth of pathogenic species, such as toxigenic *C. difficile* strains, which may cause diarrhea and colitis of variable severity. Gut bacteria may play a role in the pathogenesis of the irritable bowel syndrome (IBS) (Lin, 2004). Symptoms of

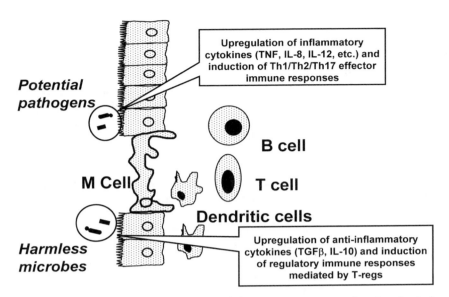

Figure 1 The specialized lymphoid follicles of the gut mucosa are major sites for induction and regulation of immune responses. Multiple and diverse interactions between microbes, epithelium, and gut lymphoid tissues are constantly reshaping local and systemic mechanisms of immunity. Gut microbes stimulate clonal expansion of lymphocytes in follicles, and the mechanisms which determine the phenotype differentiation of T-helper cells are not fully understood. However, experimental evidence indicates that innate recognition of bacteria by epithelial cells and/or antigen-presenting cells may play critical roles in the induction of either effector or regulatory pathways. Costimulatory signals (cytokines) released by these cell types dictate polarization of the adaptive immune response.

abdominal pain, bloating, and flatulence may be related to excessive production of gas by fermentations taking place in the colon. Likewise, putrefaction of proteins by bacteria within the gut lumen is associated with the pathogenesis of hepatic encephalopathy in patients with acute or chronic liver failure.

Mucosal barrier dysfunction can facilitate bacterial translocation. Translocation of viable or dead bacteria in minute amounts may constitute physiological stimulation of the immune system. However, dysfunction of

Table 1 Pathological conditions associated with dysfunction of the gut microbiota

Infectious diarrhea, antibiotic-associated diarrhea
Functional bowel disorders: diarrhea, constipation, IBS
Septic complications due to bacterial translocation in acute
   severe pancreatitis, abdominal surgery, liver failure, intestinal
   ischemia, hemorrhagic shock, multisystem organ failure, etc.
NEC
Hepatic encephalopathy
IBD
Colorectal cancer
Others: atopic and autoimmune disorders (?)

the gut mucosal barrier may result in translocation of excessive quantities of viable microorganisms, usually belonging to gram-negative genera. After crossing the epithelial barrier, bacteria may travel via the lymph to extraintestinal sites, such as mesenteric lymph nodes, liver, and spleen. Subsequently, enteric bacteria may disseminate throughout the body, producing sepsis, shock, multisystem organ failure, or death of the host. Bacterial translocation may occur in hemorrhagic shock, burn injury, trauma, intestinal ischemia, intestinal obstruction, major abdominal surgery, severe pancreatitis, acute liver failure, and cirrhosis (Lichtman, 2001).

Evidence implicates the gut microbiota as an essential factor in driving inflammation in human inflammatory bowel disease (IBD). Studies of Crohn's disease or ulcerative colitis have shown that abnormal activation of the mucosal immune system against enteric bacteria is a key event triggering inflammatory mechanisms resulting in intestinal injury (Sartor, 2004). IBD patients show increased mucosal secretion of IgG antibodies against commensal bacteria (Macpherson et al., 1996), and mucosal T lymphocytes are hyperreactive against antigens of the intestinal microbiota, suggesting that local tolerance mechanisms are inhibited (Sartor, 2004). Several factors may contribute to the pathogenesis of aberrant immune responses towards the indigenous microbiota, including genetic susceptibilities, defects in mucosal barrier function, and microbial imbalance. Several studies suggest that gut bacterial populations in patients with IBD differ from those in healthy subjects (Guarner, 2005).

In experimental models, intestinal bacteria may play a role in the initiation of colon cancer through production of carcinogens, cocarcinogens, or procarcinogens. The molecular genetic mechanisms of human colorectal cancer are well established, but epidemiological evidence suggests that environmental factors such as diet may play a major role in the development of sporadic colon cancer. Dietary fat and excessive consumption of red meat, particularly processed meat, are associated with an enhanced risk in case-control studies. In contrast, elevated intake of fruits and vegetables, whole-grain cereals, fish, and calcium has been associated with reduced cancer risk. Dietary factors and genetic factors interact in part via events taking place in the lumen of the large bowel (Rafter et al., 2004). The influence of diet on the carcinogenic process may be mediated by changes in metabolic activities and the composition of the colonic microbiota.

THERAPEUTIC MANIPULATION OF THE GUT MICROBIOTA

Symbiosis between microbiota and host can be optimized by pharmacological or nutritional intervention on the gut microbial ecosystem using probiotics or prebiotics. Administration of exogenous bacteria with known properties may improve specific functions of the gut microbiota (metabolism, protection, and trophism) or prevent dysfunction associated with disease. These bacteria are called "probiotics," a term that refers to "live micro-organisms which when administered in adequate amounts confer a health benefit on the host," as proposed by the Joint FAO/WHO Expert Consultation. This definition was also adopted by the International Scientific Association for Probiotics and Prebiotics (Reid et al., 2003). The term prebiotic refers to "a nondigestible food ingredient that beneficially affects the host by selectively stimulating growth and/or activity of one or a limited number of bacteria in the colon." A prebiotic should not be hydrolyzed by human intestinal enzymes, it should be selectively fermented by beneficial bacteria, and this selective fermentation should result in beneficial effects on health or well-being of the host (Gibson et al., 2004). The combination of probiotics and prebiotics is termed "synbiotic," and it is an exciting concept aimed at optimizing the impact of probiotics on the gut microbial ecosystem.

Human and experimental studies with probiotics have targeted specific health benefits associated with the three functional areas of the gut microbiota (metabolic effects, protective effects, and trophic effects), and worldwide research on this topic has accelerated in recent years. The scientific bases of probiosis have been reviewed in depth by a task force of the American Academy of Microbiology (Walker and Buckley, 2006). In most human studies published so far, probiotics were administered alive either by oral route (as a food component or in the form of specific preparations of viable microorganisms) or in topical preparations (skin, nasal, or vaginal applications). Synbiotics and prebiotics are administered by the oral route. Concerning the use of probiotics in human medicine, in June 2007 the Cochrane Central Register of Controlled Trials listed 109 human studies that had tested probiotic efficacy for specific indications in the field of gastroenterology and hepatology. The Cochrane Database of Systematic Reviews includes five complete reviews on the use of probiotics in gastrointestinal diseases, which are cited in the text of this chapter.

METABOLIC EFFECTS OF PROBIOTICS
Lactose Digestion
The disaccharide lactose, found mainly in milk and dairy products, is hydrolyzed to glucose and galactose by beta-galactosidase (lactase), which is present in the brush border of epithelial cells in the small intestine. After weaning, a segment of the adult population develops a progressive deficiency of lactase activity in the small intestinal mucosa. Lactose malabsorption is the result of lactase deficiency and means that a fraction of the ingested lactose is not absorbed in the small intestine and is delivered to the colon. These patients may develop gastrointestinal symptoms such as diarrhea, flatulence, abdominal bloating, and pain after ingestion of lactose-containing foods. The prevalence of lactase deficiency in adult populations is relatively high and varies between 5 and 15% in Northern European and American countries and between 50 and 100% in African, Asian, and South American countries. These subjects tend to eliminate milk and dairy products from their diet, and consequently, their calcium intake may be compromised. The bacteria used as starter cultures in yogurt (*Streptococcus thermophilus* and *Lactobacillus delbrueckii* subsp. *bulgaricus*) can improve lactose digestion and eliminate symptoms in lactase-deficient individuals (Kolars et al., 1984). The benefit is due to microbial beta-galactosidase activity that hydrolyzes lactose during its transit through the small bowel (de Vrese et al., 2001). A number of controlled studies have demonstrated lactose digestion

and absorption as well as reduction of gastrointestinal symptoms in lactase-deficient individuals consuming yogurt with live cultures (Gill and Guarner, 2004).

Hepatic Encephalopathy

Proteolytic activities of gut bacteria contribute to the generation of neurotoxins and induce hepatic encephalopathy in patients with liver failure or portosystemic shunts. Prebiotics such as lactulose are commonly used for the prevention and treatment of this complication. In a clinical trial with patients with chronic liver disease, minimal hepatic encephalopathy was reversed in 50% of the patients treated with a synbiotic preparation (four probiotic strains and four fermentable fibers, including inulin and resistant starch) for 30 days. This response was significantly higher than the frequency of reversal (13%) observed in the placebo group (Liu et al., 2004). Further evidence may support probiotic indications for hepatic encephalopathy including additional animal models and clinical studies.

Nonalcoholic Fatty Liver Disease

Nonalcoholic fatty liver disease is becoming a major public health concern, since it affects up to 30% of the adult population in developed countries. The mechanisms underlying disease development and progression are awaiting clarification, but insulin resistance and obesity-related inflammation are thought to play key roles leading to altered carbohydrate metabolism and lipid accumulation within the liver. Probiotics have been proposed as a treatment option because of the potential effects of short-chain fatty acid generated within the gut on carbohydrate and lipid metabolism in the liver (the gut-liver metabolic axis). However, a recent systematic review by the working group appointed by Cochrane concluded that the lack of randomized clinical trials made it difficult to support or refute the use of probiotics for patients with nonalcoholic fatty liver disease (Lirussi et al., 2007).

Production of Intestinal Gas: IBS

Colonic fermentations result in the generation of variable gas volumes in the intestine. However, some gut bacteria degrade metabolic substrates without producing gas, and some microbial species may consume gas, particularly hydrogen. Symptoms of abdominal pain, bloating, and flatulence are commonly seen in patients with IBS. Hypothetically, administration of appropriate bacterial strains could reduce gas accumulation within the bowel in these patients and induce symptomatic improvement.

Table 2 shows data from double-blind controlled clinical trials testing probiotics in patients with IBS. In most studies, both probiotic and placebo treatments decreased scores of abdominal pain to some extent. Such equivocal findings are common observations in trials of patients with IBS, which respond to placebo formulations at variable rates. However, several studies have demonstrated significant therapeutic gains by probiotics when compared to placebo, as assessed by increased response rates to probiotic treatments or enhanced relief in symptom scores. A consistent finding in published studies is a reduction of abdominal bloating and flatulence by probiotic treatments. Bifidobacterial strains appear to contribute to higher rates of therapeutic success in adult patients with IBS. In addition, a recent trial with 90 breast-fed babies with infantile colic has shown that probiotic *Lactobacillus reuteri* may improve colicky symptoms within 1 week of treatment (Savino et al., 2007). Disordered bowel habits (diarrhea, constipation, or alternating episodes of constipation and diarrhea) are common in subjects with IBS, but consistent efficacy of probiotics with respect to improved bowel habits in IBS has not been demonstrated. Probiotics need to be evaluated further, but beneficial microbes may be useful for control of symptoms related to the altered handling or perception of intestinal gas.

PROTECTIVE EFFECTS OF PROBIOTICS

Prevention of Diarrhea

Clinical trials have tested the efficacy of probiotics in the prevention of acute diarrheal conditions, including antibiotic-associated diarrhea, nosocomial and community-acquired infectious enteritis, and traveler's diarrhea (Sazawal et al., 2006). Different probiotics show promise as effective therapies for the prevention of antibiotic-associated diarrhea. Both the short- and long-term use of antibiotics can result in diarrhea, particularly during regimens with multiple drugs. In placebo-controlled studies, diarrhea occurred at a rate of 15 to 26% in the placebo arms but only in 3 to 7% of patients receiving a probiotic. Different strains have been tested including *Lactobacillus rhamnosus* strain GG, *Lactobacillus acidophilus*, *Lactobacillus casei*, *Bacillus clausii*, the yeast "*Saccharomyces boulardii*," and others (Fig. 2). One study has shown efficacy of *L. casei* for the prevention of diarrhea induced by overgrowth of *C. difficile* during antibiotic therapy (Hickson et al., 2007). Several published meta-analyses of controlled trials and the Cochrane systematic review concluded that some probiotics can be used to prevent antibiotic-associated diarrhea in children and adults (Cremonini et al., 2002; D'Souza et al., 2002; Szajewska and Mrukowicz, 2005; Johnston et al., 2007).

Table 2 Clinical studies investigating the efficacy of probiotics in the treatment of IBS[a]

Study	n	Probiotic(s)	Duration (wk)	End point	Response rate (%)		
					Test group	Control group	P
Nobaek et al., 2000	60	L. plantarum	4	Pain response rate	36	18	NS
				Flatulence response rate	44	18	<0.05
Kim et al., 2003	25	Probiotic mix (VSL#3)	8	Overall response rate	33	38	NS
Kajander et al., 2005	103	Probiotic mix: L. rhamnosus GG, L. rhamnosus, Propionibacterium freudenreichii, and Bifidobacterium breve	24	Bloating score[d]	−13.7	−1.7	<0.05
				Symptom score[d]	−42	−6	<0.05
O'Mahony et al., 2005	77	Two intervention arms: Lactobacillus salivarius and Bifidobacterium infantis	8	Symptom score[d]	−13 (L. salivarius); −46 (B. infantis)	−16	NS; <0.05
Niv et al., 2005	50	L. reuteri	24	Symptom score[d]	—[e]	—[e]	NS
Bausserman and Michail, 2005[b]	117	L. rhamnosus GG	6	Overall response rate	44	40	NS
Kim et al., 2005	48	Probiotic mix (VSL#3)	8	Flatulence score[d]	−21	−9	<0.05
Whorwell et al., 2006[c]	362	B. infantis	4	Pain score[d]	−89	−58	<0.05
Gawronska et al., 2007[b]	37	L. rhamnosus GG	4	Overall response rate	33	5	<0.05
Guyonnet et al., 2007	274	Bifidobacterium animalis	6	QoL response rate	65	48	<0.05

[a]Abbreviations: NS, not significant; QoL, health-related quality of life.
[b]Children.
[c]Women.
[d]Change versus score at entry.
[e]—, not quantified, but showed improvement.

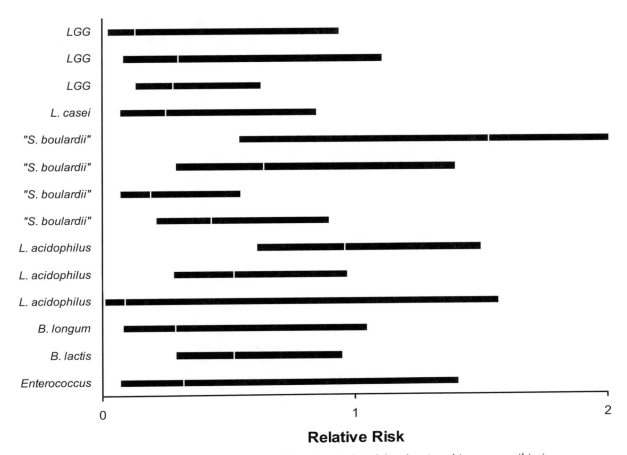

Figure 2 Relative risks (and 95% confidence intervals) of diarrhea in subjects on antibiotics and probiotics as normalized by the incidence of diarrhea in control subjects on antibiotics and placebo in 14 controlled clinical trials. Twelve studies estimated a relative risk lower than 1, and in seven of these studies the upper limit of the 95% confidence interval was also below 1. Overall, the combined relative risk is significantly reduced, as determined in published meta-analyses (Cremonini et al., 2002; D'Souza et al., 2002; Szajewska and Mrukowicz, 2005; Sazawal et al., 2006). LGG, *L. rhamnosus* GG.

Prophylactic use of probiotics has proven useful for the prevention of acute diarrhea in infants admitted into the hospital ward for a chronic disease condition (Saavedra et al., 1994; Szajewska et al., 2001). Supplementation of an infant formula with *Bifidobacterium bifidum* and *S. thermophilus* significantly prevented the incidence of diarrhea in hospitalized infants aged 5 to 24 months (31% in placebo versus 7% in probiotic group). A placebo-controlled double-blind study with infants (1 to 36 months old) tested the *L. rhamnosus* strain GG and reported similar findings. Probiotics may also be useful in the prevention of community-acquired diarrhea, despite a lack of data from community-based

trials evaluating the effect on acute diarrhea unrelated to antibiotic usage (Sazawal et al., 2006).

Several studies have investigated the efficacy of probiotics in the prevention of traveler's diarrhea in adults, but methodological deficiencies, such as reduced treatment compliance and patient follow-up issues, limit the validity of their conclusions. A recent meta-analysis suggested that probiotics may offer a safe and effective method to prevent traveler's diarrhea (McFarland, 2007).

The efficacy of the probiotic mixture VSL#3 in the prevention of acute diarrhea induced by radiation in cancer patients has been tested in a double-blind study with 490 patients. The probiotic significantly reduced the incidence and severity of radiation-induced diarrhea (Delia et al., 2007).

Treatment of Acute Diarrhea

Probiotics are useful as treatment of acute infectious diarrhea in children. Different strains, including *L. reuteri*, *L. rhamnosus* GG, *L. casei*, and "*S. boulardii*," have been tested in controlled clinical trials and were proven useful in reducing the severity and duration of diarrhea. Oral administration of probiotics shortens the duration of acute diarrheal illness in children by approximately 1 day. Several meta-analyses of controlled clinical trials have been published (Huang et al., 2002; Van Niel et al., 2002; Allen et al., 2004; Szajewska et al., 2007). The results of the systematic reviews are consistent and suggest that probiotics are safe and effective.

Eradication of *Helicobacter pylori*

Probiotics have been tested as a strategy for eradication of *H. pylori* infection of the gastric mucosa in humans. Some strains of lactic acid bacteria are known to inhibit the growth of *H. pylori* in vitro. However, administration of one of these strains in a specially designed yogurt was not effective for the eradication of *H. pylori* infection (Wendakoon et al., 2002). On the other hand, several clinical studies have tested the efficacies of different probiotic strains in combination with standard therapies of antibiotics. Adding probiotics can increase eradication rates after triple or quadruple anti-*H. pylori* antibiotic regimens (Tong et al., 2007). Several lactobacillus and bifidobacterial strains as well as *B. clausii* appeared to reduce side effects of antibiotic therapies and improved patient compliance. A recent meta-analysis of 14 randomized trials suggests that supplementation of anti-*H. pylori* regimens with probiotics can be effective in increasing eradication rates and may be considered helpful for patients with eradication failure (Tong et al., 2007).

Prevention of Systemic Infections

Bacterial translocation of gut bacteria can produce systemic infections and sepsis. These complications have been shown to occur in some pathologic conditions associated with mucosal barrier dysfunction such as postoperative sepsis, severe acute pancreatitis, multisystem organ failure, and necrotizing enterocolitis.

Probiotics have been used to prevent sepsis in patients with severe acute pancreatitis. In a randomized double-blind trial, patients were treated with either *Lactobacillus plantarum* or a placebo. Pancreatic abscesses occurred at a significantly lower rate in *L. plantarum*-treated patients than in controls (Olah et al., 2002). A large double-blind multicenter study (PROPATRIA) is currently testing a multispecies probiotic preparation in adult patients with a first episode of predicted severe acute pancreatitis. The researchers are investigating the effects of probiotics on several factors including total numbers of infectious complications, mortality, use of antibiotics, total costs, and bacterial resistance. This information is needed to confirm the efficacy of probiotic therapy in severe acute pancreatitis.

A randomized study involving 95 liver transplant patients compared the incidences of infections among three groups of patients undergoing different prophylaxis procedures: selective bowel decontamination with antibiotics, administration of live *L. plantarum* supplemented with fermentable fiber (synbiotic), and administration of heat-killed *L. plantarum* with the fiber supplement (Rayes et al., 2002). Postoperative infections were recorded in 15 of 32 patients (48%) in the antibiotics group, 4 of 31 patients (13%) in the live *L. plantarum* group, and 11 of 32 patients (34%) in the heat-killed *L. plantarum* group. The difference in postoperative infections was significant only between antibiotics and live *L. plantarum* groups. In a second study by the same group, patients were randomized to receive a synbiotic preparation (including four probiotic strains and four fermentable fibers) or a placebo consisting of four fibers only (Rayes et al., 2005). Postoperative infections occurred in only 1 patient in the treatment group ($n = 33$), in contrast to 17 of 33 patients in the placebo group. The difference between the synbiotic-treated and control groups was highly significant. However, another clinical study performed with patients undergoing elective abdominal surgery found no effect of synbiotic treatment (four bacteria strains plus oligofructose) with respect to prevention of postoperative infections (Anderson et al., 2004). In this trial, synbiotic treatment after surgery was delayed until patients were able to tolerate oral nutrition. In contrast, the liver transplant studies introduced synbiotic therapy by nasogastric tube immediately after surgery. Another clinical study with surgical patients has recently confirmed that pre- and postoperative enteral feeding with a synbiotic preparation is significantly more effective in preventing infectious complications than postoperative synbiotic treatment only (Sugawara et al., 2006). These data suggest that early administration of live probiotics may become a useful and effective therapy to prevent postoperative infections. Probiotics and synbiotics are being tested in adult intensive care unit patients. While some studies have shown benefits (Alberda et al., 2007), evidence is insufficient to support the use of probiotics and synbiotics in critically ill patients in intensive care units (Watkinson et al., 2007).

Necrotizing enterocolitis (NEC) is a severe clinical condition that may occur in low-birth-weight neonates due to relative immaturity and dysfunction of the gut mucosal barrier. Several controlled studies have demonstrated that the use of probiotic mixtures in low-birth-weight infants significantly reduces the incidence and severity of NEC and may prevent mortality by NEC. A meta-analysis of the published trials suggests that probiotics reduced the risk of developing NEC by two-thirds and the risk of death by one-half (Deshpande et al., 2007). These data are impressive since very few other strategies have proven effective in decreasing the incidence of NEC in preterm infants.

TROPHIC EFFECTS OF PROBIOTICS ON MUCOSAL IMMUNITY AND EPITHELIAL CELL GROWTH

IBD

Although the etiologies of Crohn's disease and ulcerative colitis are unknown, substantial experimental and clinical evidence suggests that uncontrolled T-lymphocyte activation in individuals with genetic susceptibilities is a central mechanism in the pathophysiology of chronic intestinal inflammation (Sartor, 2004). Cell-mediated immunity against luminal bacteria appears to be a key event in driving the inflammatory process that generates intestinal lesions and impairs resolution of lesions leading to chronic intestinal disease. The role of aberrant mucosal immune responses to luminal bacteria in IBD pathogenesis has been confirmed by clinical studies. Fecal stream diversion prevents recurrence of Crohn's disease, whereas infusion of intestinal contents to excluded intestinal segments reactivated the mucosal lesions (D'Haens et al., 1998). In ulcerative colitis (Casellas et al., 1998),

short-term treatment with an enteric-coated preparation of broad-spectrum antibiotics rapidly reduced mucosal inflammation as assessed by marked reduction in the luminal release of interleukin-8, a potent chemokine. In experimental settings, some commensal bacteria activate mucosal proinflammatory responses but other bacteria are able to downregulate intestinal inflammation (Borruel et al., 2002). Thus, a favorable local microecology could restore homeostasis of the mucosal immune system and lead to resolution of intestinal inflammation. This hypothesis is currently being investigated by experimental and clinical approaches.

Several probiotic strains have been tested in controlled clinical trials with patients with IBD, including ulcerative colitis, Crohn's disease, and pouchitis. For ulcerative colitis, three randomized controlled trials investigated the effectiveness of an orally administered enteric-coated preparation of viable *Escherichia coli* strain Nissle 1917 and compared it with mesalazine, the standard treatment for maintenance of remission (Table 3). These studies concluded that this strain has an effect equivalent to that of mesalazine in maintaining remission. Zocco et al. (2006) randomized 187 patients to three open-label arms (*L. rhamnosus* GG, *L. rhamnosus* GG plus mesalazine, and mesalazine only) and demonstrated that both *Lactobacillus* arms experienced a prolonged relapse-free period, similar to that achieved with mesalazine treatment only. Finally, a study with 21 ulcerative colitis patients in remission and on standard medication (mesalazine and others) tested a *Bifidobacterium*-fermented milk in a nonblinded design. Patients receiving supplements of bifidobacteria had fewer relapses during the 12-month follow-up period (Ishikawa et al., 2003).

Table 3 Clinical studies investigating the efficacy of probiotics in maintenance of remission in ulcerative colitis[a]

Study	n	Intervention Test group	Intervention Control group	Duration (mo)	Relapse rate (%) Test group	Relapse rate (%) Control group	P
Kruis et al., 1997	120	*E. coli* Nissle	Mesalazine	3	14	12	NS
Rembacken et al., 1999	116	*E. coli* Nissle	Mesalazine	12	33	27	NS
Ishikawa et al., 2003	21	*B. breve, B. bifidum,* *L. acidophilus*	None	12	27	90	<0.01
Kruis et al., 2004	327	*E. coli* Nissle	Mesalazine	12	36	34	SE
Zocco et al., 2006	187	*L. rhamnosus* GG	Mesalazine	12	15	20	NS
		L. rhamnosus GG + mesalazine			17		NS

[a]Abbreviations: NS, not significant; SE, significant equivalence.

Table 4 Clinical studies investigating the efficacy of probiotics in maintenance of remission in Crohn's disease

Study	n	Intervention		Duration (mo)	Relapse rate (%)		
		Test group	Control group		Test group	Control group	P
Prantera et al., 2002	45	*L. rhamnosus* GG	Placebo	12	16	11	NS[a]
Schultz et al., 2004	11	*L. rhamnosus* GG	Placebo	6	60	67	NS
Bousvaros et al., 2005	75	*L. rhamnosus* GG	Placebo	24	31	17	NS
Marteau et al., 2006	98	*L. johnsonii*	Placebo	6	49	64	NS
Van Gossum et al., 2007	70	*L. johnsonii*	Placebo	3	15	14	NS
Chermesh et al., 2007	30	Synbiotic 2000	Placebo	24	25	20	NS

[a]NS, not significant.

Probiotic therapies may have equivalent efficacy when compared to conventional drug therapies for maintenance of remission in ulcerative colitis. In contrast, the efficacy of probiotics to treat active ulcerative colitis has not been demonstrated, but two small pilot studies suggest that some bifidobacterial strains added to standard drug therapy may be beneficial for treatment of mild to moderately active ulcerative colitis (Kato et al., 2004; Furrie et al., 2005).

The efficacy of *L. rhamnosus* GG to maintain remission of Crohn's disease was tested in a randomized, double-blind trial with patients undergoing curative surgery (Table 4). The probiotic showed no effect in the prevention of clinical and endoscopic recurrence compared with the placebo (Prantera et al., 2002). Two other clinical trials confirmed the lack of efficacy of this strain to maintain remission of Crohn's disease. Likewise, postoperative recurrence of Crohn's disease could not be prevented by *Lactobacillus johnsonii* or a synbiotic preparation (Table 4). Two small studies have evaluated the use of probiotics for treating patients with active Crohn's disease, but neither demonstrated convincing efficacy. Thus, there is no evidence to support the use of probiotics as therapy for Crohn's disease.

The VSL#3 mixture has been proven highly effective for maintenance of remission of chronic relapsing pouchitis, after induction of remission with antibiotics (Gionchetti et al., 2000; Mimura et al., 2004). In the first study, a relapse occurred in only 3 of 20 patients of the VSL#3 group and in all 20 patients of the placebo group. Of interest, all patients on remission in the probiotic arm had relapses within 4 months after stopping probiotic treatment at the conclusion of the trial. In the second study, the probiotic mixture was administered in a once-a-day schedule, and similar efficacy was demonstrated (Mimura et al., 2004). Treatment with VSL#3 was also effective for the prevention of the onset of pouchitis after ileal pouch-anal anastomosis (Gionchetti et al., 2003). In contrast, *L. rhamnosus* strain GG was ineffective as a primary therapy for induction of clinical or endoscopic responses in patients with chronic pouchitis (Kuisma et al., 2003).

The therapeutic manipulation of the luminal microecology with probiotics and prebiotics has attracted high expectations as a strategic area for the control and prevention of IBD. The evidence for the use of probiotics in IBD is strongest in the case of pouchitis and, in particular, for the use of the probiotic mixture VSL#3. In addition, the *E. coli* strain Nissle appears to be equivalent to mesalazine in maintaining remission of ulcerative colitis. However, studies of probiotics in Crohn's disease have been disappointing, and a recent Cochrane systematic review concluded that there is no evidence to suggest that probiotics are beneficial for maintenance of remission in Crohn's disease (Rolfe et al., 2006). Further research is needed to explore potential applications of probiotics or prebiotics for this indication.

Food Allergy

The prevalence of allergic diseases in Western societies is increasing at an alarming rate, whereas such disorders remain uncommon in the developing world. It has been suggested that food allergies may result from inappropriate microbial stimuli during infancy as a result of improved hygienic conditions. Some epidemiological and experimental studies have indicated that stimulation of the immune system by certain microbes or microbial products may be effective in the prevention and management of allergic diseases. The effectiveness of probiotic therapy in the prevention of atopic eczema has been clearly demonstrated in randomized controlled trials (Kalliomaki et al., 2001). Likewise, well-designed studies have provided evidence that specific probiotic strains can be effective for treatment of a subset of patients with atopic eczema (Viljanen et al., 2005). A single study has reported efficacy of a formula supplemented with *Lactobacillus* strain GG in infants with cow's milk allergy (Majamaa and Isolauri, 1997). Infants receiving the probiotic showed significant improvement in both clinical symptoms and markers of intestinal inflammation compared with the placebo group. However, little is known about the efficacy of probiotics in preventing other types of food allergy.

Colon Cancer

Experimental studies clearly demonstrate a protective effect of probiotics such as *Lactobacillus* and *Bifidobacterium* strains, or the combination of prebiotics and probiotics, against colon cancer. Beneficial bacteria can prevent the establishment, growth, and metastasis of transplantable and chemically induced tumors. Several possible mechanisms of cancer protection and reduction of cancer risk have been identified (Rafter et al., 2004).

Human intervention trials to corroborate the evidence obtained in experimental studies have intrinsic difficulties due to the natural history of the disease (difficulty in selection of subjects at high risk and requirement of long-term follow-up). Such studies require the validation of intermediate end points that can be used as valid biomarkers of colon cancer risk (Rafter et al., 2004). A Japanese study including 398 subjects with previous histories of colonic polyps, who were monitored for 4 years, found that oral administration of *L. casei* reduced the degree of atypia in the recurrent polyps (Ishikawa et al., 2005). The SYNCAN study is another human intervention trial, which tested a synbiotic (oligofructose plus two probiotic strains) in patients at risk of developing colonic cancer and examined intermediate end points that were used as biomarkers of cancer risk. This study found a reduction in epithelial cell proliferation in subjects undergoing treatment with the synbiotic preparation, but the changes were not observed in subjects taking the placebo (Rafter et al., 2007). Likewise, genotoxicity assays of colonic biopsy samples indicated decreased exposure to genotoxins in the synbiotic-treated subjects (Fig. 3). Epithelial cell hyperproliferation and a high level of genetic damage in intestinal epithelial cells are recognized as markers of risk for colon cancer. Thus, the SYNCAN study suggests that a synbiotic preparation can decrease the expression of biomarkers for colorectal cancer. Further clinical studies are needed to translate the experimental findings of these colorectal cancer studies to practical human applications.

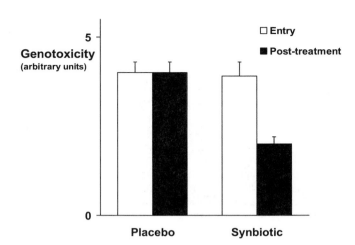

Figure 3 Colorectal cancer is induced by a series of mutational events in a number of critical genes of epithelial stem cells in the mucosa. The presence in the colonic lumen of DNA-damaging agents could represent an important risk factor for colonic cancer. Diet and gut bacteria are likely to play a role in the production and/or elimination of genotoxic compounds in the colonic lumen. The SYNCAN study found a decrease in genotoxicity indexes in colonic mucosal biopsy samples from patients taking a synbiotic (prebiotic plus two probiotic strains), whereas this change was not observed in subjects taking a placebo (data from Rafter et al., 2007). This finding suggests a decreased mucosal exposure to genotoxins associated with the consumption of the synbiotic.

SUMMARY AND FUTURE DIRECTIONS

A large and diverse community of commensal bacteria is harbored in the human gut, in a symbiotic arrangement that influences both the physiology and pathology of the host. Microbial ecology in the gut can be modulated by pharmacological and nutritional interventions with probiotics and prebiotics, and a balanced microbial environment would likely promote symbiotic functions of bacteria and enhance human health. In controlled human studies, probiotics and prebiotics have been used, safely and successfully, for improving certain metabolic functions of the microbiota (lactose digestion, reduction of gas-related symptoms, and prevention of hepatic encephalopathy), for protection against infections (prevention and treatment of acute enteritis and prevention of bacterial translocation), and for modulation of the immune system (prevention and treatment of atopic diseases and chronic pouchitis).

Table 5 summarizes the recommendation grades for the use of probiotics in gastroenterology according to the criteria of evidence-based medicine. Grade A recommendations should be implemented in patient care and are

Table 5 Probiotics in evidence-based medicine

Grade A recommendation (level 1 evidence)
  Treatment of lactose maldigestion
  Treatment of acute infectious diarrhea in children
  Prevention of antibiotic-associated diarrhea in children and
    adults
  Prevention of nosocomial diarrhea in children
  Prevention of pouchitis and maintenance of remission
  Maintenance of remission of ulcerative colitis (*E. coli* strain
    Nissle)
  Symptomatic improvement of IBS
  Prevention of NEC in preterm infants
Grade B recommendation (level 2 evidence)
  Prevention of traveler's diarrhea
  Prevention of sepsis associated with severe acute
    pancreatitis (synbiotics)
  Prevention of postoperative infections (synbiotics)

supported by level 1 evidence (high-quality randomized controlled trials with statistically significant results and few limitations in their design, or by conclusions from systematic reviews of trials). Grade B recommendations favor a therapeutic option that is supported by level 2 evidence (randomized controlled trials that have limitations in study methodology or results showing wide confidence intervals, or conflicting results between randomized controlled trials of methodological quality without systematic reviews supporting clear conclusions). Grade B recommendations may change in the future if level 1 evidence from negative or positive studies becomes available.

Current clinical research is focused mainly at establishing the role and efficacy of probiotics and prebiotics in the prevention and control of IBD and colon cancer. Experimental studies have yielded convincing evidence of their potential utility for these indications. However, human studies have failed in some attempts to provide effective therapeutic strategies with probiotics and prebiotics. It is likely that the development of improved tools to investigate gut colonization will provide a more complete picture of the actual scenario in inflammatory disorders and colon cancer. As a consequence, new interventions will aim towards more robust modifications or remodeling of intestinal microbial populations with applications for improving gut health.

References

Alberda, C., L. Gramlich, J. Meddings, C. Field, L. McCargar, D. Kutsogiannis, R. Fedorak, and K. Madsen. 2007. Effects of probiotic therapy in critically ill patients: a randomized, double-blind, placebo-controlled trial. *Am. J. Clin. Nutr.* 85:816–823.

Allen, S. J., B. Okoko, E. Martinez, G. Gregorio, and L. F. Dans. 2004. Probiotics for treating infectious diarrhoea. *Cochrane Database Syst. Rev.* 2:CD003048.

Anderson, A. D., C. E. McNaught, P. K. Jain, and J. MacFie. 2004. Randomised clinical trial of synbiotic therapy in elective surgical patients. *Gut* 53:241–245.

Bausserman, M., and S. Michail. 2005. The use of *Lactobacillus GG* in irritable bowel syndrome in children: a double-blind randomized control trial. *J. Pediatr.* 147:197–201.

Borruel, N., M. Carol, F. Casellas, M. Antolín, F. de Lara, E. Espín, J. Naval, F. Guarner, and J. R. Malagelada. 2002. Increased mucosal TNFα production in Crohn's disease can be downregulated *ex vivo* by probiotic bacteria. *Gut* 51:659–664.

Bousvaros, A., S. Guandalini, R. N. Baldassano, C. Botelho, J. Evans, G. D. Ferry, B. Goldin, L. Hartigan, S. Kugathasan, J. Levy, K. F. Murray, M. Oliva-Hemker, J. R. Rosh, V. Tolia, A. Zholudev, J. A.Vanderhoof, and P. L. Hibberd. 2005. A randomized, double-blind trial of *Lactobacillus GG* versus placebo in addition to standard maintenance therapy for children with Crohn's disease. *Inflamm. Bowel Dis.* 11:833–839.

Casellas, F., N. Borruel, M. Papo, F. Guarner, M. Antolín, S. Videla, and J. R. Malagelada. 1998. Antiinflammatory effects of enterically coated amoxicillin-clavulanic acid in active ulcerative colitis. *Inflamm. Bowel Dis.* 4:1–5.

Chermesh, I., A. Tamir, R. Reshef, S. Chowers, A. Suissa, D. Katz, M. Gelber, Z. Halpern, S. Bengmark, and R. Eliakim. 2007. Failure of Synbiotic 2000 to prevent postoperative recurrence of Crohn's disease. *Dig. Dis. Sci.* 52:385–389.

Cremonini, F., S. Di Caro, E. C. Nista, F. Bartolozzi, G. Capelli, G. Gasbarrini, and A. Gasbarrini. 2002. Meta-analysis: the effect of probiotic administration on antibiotic-associated diarrhoea. *Aliment. Pharmacol. Ther.* 16:1461–1467.

Cummings, J. H., J. M. Antoine, F. Azpiroz, R. Bourdet-Sicard, P. Brandtzaeg, P. C. Calder, G. R. Gibson, F. Guarner, E. Isolauri, D. Pannemans, C. Shortt, S. Tuijtelaars, and B. Watzl. 2004. PASSCLAIM--gut health and immunity. *Eur. J. Nutr.* 43(Suppl. 2):118–173.

Delia, P., G. Sansotta, V. Donato, P. Frosina, G. Messina, C. De Renzis, and G. Famularo. 2007. Use of probiotics for prevention of radiation-induced diarrhea. *World J. Gastroenterol.* 13:912–915.

Deshpande, G., S. Rao, and S. Patole. 2007. Probiotics for prevention of necrotising enterocolitis in preterm neonates with very low birth weight: a systematic review of randomised controlled trials. *Lancet* 369:1614–1620.

de Vrese, M., A. Stegelmann, B. Richter, S. Fenselau, C. Laue, and J. Shrezenmeir. 2001. Probiotics—compensation for lactase insufficiency. *Am. J. Clin. Nutr.* 73(Suppl):421S–429S.

D'Haens, G. R., K. Geboes, M. Peeters, F. Baert, F. Penninckx, and P. Rutgeerts. 1998. Early lesions of recurrent Crohn's disease caused by infusion of intestinal contents in excluded ileum. *Gastroenterology* 114:262–267.

D'Souza, A. L., C. Rajkumar, J. Cooke, and C. J. Bulpitt. 2002. Probiotics in prevention of antibiotic associated diarrhoea: meta-analysis. *Br. Med. J.* 324:1361–1366.

Eckburg, P. B., E. M. Bik, C. N. Bernstein, E. Purdom, L. Dethlefsen, M. Sargent, S. R. Gill, K. E. Nelson, and

D. A. Relman. 2005. Diversity of the human intestinal microbial flora. *Science* 308:1635–1638.

Falk, P. G., L. V. Hooper, T. Midtvedt, and J. I. Gordon. 1998. Creating and maintaining the gastrointestinal ecosystem: what we know and need to know from gnotobiology. *Microbiol. Mol. Biol. Rev.* 62:1157–1170.

Furrie, E., S. Macfarlane, A. Kennedy, J. H. Cummings, S. V. Walsh, D. A. O'Neil, and G. T. Macfarlane. 2005. Synbiotic therapy (*Bifidobacterium longum*/Synergy 1) initiates resolution of inflammation in patients with active ulcerative colitis: a randomised controlled pilot trial. *Gut* 54:242–249.

Gawronska, A., P. Dziechciarz, A. Horvath, and H. Szajewska. 2007. A randomized double-blind placebo-controlled trial of *Lactobacillus* GG for abdominal pain disorders in children. *Aliment. Pharmacol. Ther.* 25:177–184.

Gibson, G. R., H. M. Probert, J. Van Loo, R. A. Rastall, and M. B. Roberfroid. 2004. Dietary modulation of the human colonic microbiota: updating the concept of prebiotics. *Nutr. Res. Rev.* 17:259–275.

Gill, H. S., and F. Guarner. 2004. Probiotics and human health: a clinical perspective. *Postgrad. Med. J.* 80:516–526.

Gionchetti, P., F. Rizzello, A. Venturi, P. Brigidi, D. Matteuzzi, G. Bazzocchi, G. Poggioli, M. Miglioli, and M. Campieri. 2000. Oral bacteriotherapy as maintenance treatment in patients with chronic pouchitis: a double-blind, placebo-controlled trial. *Gastroenterology* 119:305–309.

Gionchetti, P., F. Rizzello, U. Helwig, A. Venturi, K. M. Lammers, P. Brigidi, B. Vitali, G. Poggioli, M. Miglioli, and M. Campieri. 2003. Prophylaxis of pouchitis onset with probiotic therapy: a double-blind, placebo-controlled trial. *Gastroenterology* 124:1202–1209.

Guarner, F. 2005. The intestinal flora in inflammatory bowel disease: normal or abnormal? *Curr. Opin. Gastroenterol.* 21:414–418.

Guyonnet, D., O. Chassany, P. Ducrotte, C. Picard, M. Mouret, C. H. Mercier, and C. Matuchansky. 2007. Effect of a fermented milk containing *Bifidobacterium animalis* DN-173 010 on the health-related quality of life and symptoms in irritable bowel syndrome in adults in primary care: a multicentre, randomized, double-blind, controlled trial. *Aliment. Pharmacol. Ther.* 26:475–486.

Hickson, M., A. L. D'Souza, N. Muthu, T. R. Rogers, S. Want, C. Rajkumar, and C. J. Bulpitt. 2007. Use of probiotic *Lactobacillus* preparation to prevent diarrhoea associated with antibiotics: randomised double blind placebo controlled trial. *BMJ.* 335:80.

Hooper, L. V., M. H. Wong, A. Thelin, L. Hansson, P. G. Falk, and J. I. Gordon. 2001. Molecular analysis of commensal host-microbial relationships in the intestine. *Science* 291:881–884.

Hooper, L. V., T. Midtvedt, and J. I. Gordon. 2002. How host-microbial interactions shape the nutrient environment of the mammalian intestine. *Annu. Rev. Nutr.* 22:283–307.

Huang, J. S., A. Bousvaros, J. W. Lee, A. Diaz, and E. J. Davidson. 2002. Efficacy of probiotic use in acute diarrhea in children: a meta-analysis. *Dig. Dis. Sci.* 47:2625–2634.

Ishikawa, H., I. Akedo, Y. Umesaki, R. Tanaka, A. Imaoka, and T. Otani. 2003. Randomized controlled trial of the effect of bifidobacteria-fermented milk on ulcerative colitis. *J. Am. Coll. Nutr.* 22:56–63.

Ishikawa, H., I. Akedo, T. Otani, T. Suzuki, T. Nakamura, I. Takeyama, S. Ishiguro, E. Miyaoka, T. Sobue, and T. Kakizoe. 2005. Randomized trial of dietary fiber and *Lactobacillus casei* administration for prevention of colorectal tumors. *Int. J. Cancer* 116:762–767.

Johnston, B. C., A. L. Supina, M. Ospina, and S. Vohra. 2007. Probiotics for the prevention of pediatric antibiotic-associated diarrhea. *Cochrane Database Syst. Rev.* 2:CD004827.

Kajander, K., K. Hatakka, T. Poussa, M. Farkkila, and R. Korpela. 2005. A probiotic mixture alleviates symptoms in irritable bowel syndrome patients: a controlled 6-month intervention. *Aliment. Pharmacol. Ther.* 22:387–394.

Kalliomaki, M., S. Salminen, H. Arvilommi, P. Kero, P. Koskinen, and E. Isolauri. 2001. Probiotics in primary prevention of atopic disease: a randomised placebo-controlled trial. *Lancet* 357:1076–1079.

Kato, K., S. Mizuno, Y. Umesaki, Y. Ishii, M. Sugitani, A. Imaoka, M. Otsuka, O. Hasunuma, R. Kurihara, A. Iwasaki, and Y. Arakawa. 2004. Randomized placebo-controlled trial assessing the effect of bifidobacteria-fermented milk on active ulcerative colitis. *Aliment. Pharmacol. Ther.* 20:1133–1141.

Kim, H. J., M. Camilleri, S. McKinzie, M. B. Lempke, D. D. Burton, G. M. Thomforde, and A. R. Zinsmeister. 2003. A randomized controlled trial of a probiotic, VSL#3, on gut transit and symptoms in diarrhoea-predominant irritable bowel syndrome. *Aliment. Pharmacol. Ther.* 17:895–904.

Kim, H. J., M. I. Vazquez Roque, M. Camilleri, D. Stephens, D. D. Burton, K. Baxter, G. Thomforde, and A. R. Zinsmeister. 2005. A randomized controlled trial of a probiotic combination VSL# 3 and placebo in irritable bowel syndrome with bloating. *Neurogastroenterol Motil.* 17:687–696.

Kolars, J. C., M. D. Levitt, M. Aouji, and D. A. Savaiano. 1984. Yogurt—an autodigesting source of lactose. *N. Engl. J. Med.* 310:1–3.

Kruis, W., E. Schutz, P. Fric, B. Fixa, G. Judmaier, and M. Stolte. 1997. Double-blind comparison of an oral *Escherichia coli* preparation and mesalazine in maintaining remission of ulcerative colitis. *Aliment. Pharmacol. Ther.* 11:853–858.

Kruis, W., P. Fric, J. Pokrotnieks, M. Lukas, B. Fixa, M. Kascak, M. A. Kamm, J. Weismueller, C. Beglinger, M. Stolte, C. Wolff, and J. Schulze. 2004. Maintaining remission of ulcerative colitis with the probiotic *Escherichia coli* Nissle 1917 is as effective as with standard mesalazine. *Gut* 53:1617–1623.

Kuisma, J., S. Mentula, H. Jarvinen, A. Kahri, M. Saxelin, and M. Farkkila. 2003. Effect of *Lactobacillus rhamnosus* GG on ileal pouch inflammation and microbial flora. *Aliment. Pharmacol. Ther.* 17:509–515.

Lepage, P., P. Seksik, M. Sutren, M. F. de la Cochetiere, R. Jian, P. Marteau, and J. Dore. 2005. Biodiversity of the mucosa-associated microbiota is stable along the distal digestive tract in healthy individuals and patients with IBD. *Inflamm. Bowel Dis.* 11:473–480.

Ley, R. E., D. A. Peterson, and J. I. Gordon. 2006. Ecological and evolutionary forces shaping microbial diversity in the human intestine. *Cell* 124:837–848.

Lichtman, S. M. 2001. Baterial translocation in humans. *J. Pediatr. Gastroenterol. Nutr.* 33:1–10.

Lin, H. C. 2004. Small intestinal bacterial overgrowth: a framework for understanding irritable bowel syndrome. *JAMA* **292**:852–858.

Lirussi, F., E. Mastropasqua, S. Orando, and R. Orlando. 2007. Probiotics for non-alcoholic fatty liver disease and/or steatohepatitis. *Cochrane Database Syst. Rev.* 1:CD005165.

Liu, Q., Z. P. Duan, D. K. Ha, S. Bengmark, J. Kurtovic, and S. M. Riordan. 2004. Synbiotic modulation of gut flora: effect on minimal hepatic encephalopathy in patients with cirrhosis. *Hepatology* **39**:1441–1449.

Macpherson, A., U. Y. Khoo, I. Forgacs, J. Philpott-Howard, and I. Bjarnason. 1996. Mucosal antibodies in inflammatory bowel disease are directed against intestinal bacteria. *Gut* **38**:365–375.

Majamaa, H., and E. Isolauri. 1997. Probiotics: a novel approach in the management of food allergy. *J. Allergy Clin. Immunol.* **99**:179–185.

Marteau, P., M. Lemann, P. Seksik, D. Laharie, J. F. Colombel, Y. Bouhnik, G. Cadiot, J. C. Soule, A. Bourreille, E. Metman, E. Lerebours, F. Carbonnel, J. L. Dupas, M. Veyrac, B. Coffin, J. Moreau, V. Abitbol, S. Blum-Sperisen, and J. Y. Mary. 2006. Ineffectiveness of *Lactobacillus johnsonii* LA1 for prophylaxis of postoperative recurrence in Crohn's disease: a randomised, double blind, placebo controlled GETAID trial. *Gut* **55**:842–847.

Mazmanian, S. K., and D. L. Kasper. 2006. The love-hate relationship between bacterial polysaccharides and the host immune system. *Nat. Rev. Immunol.* **6**:849–858.

McFarland, L. V. 2007. Meta-analysis of probiotics for the prevention of traveler's diarrhea. *Travel Med. Infect. Dis.* **5**:97–105.

Mimura, T., F. Rizzello, U. Helwig, G. Poggioli, S. Schreiber, I. C. Talbot, R. J. Nicholls, P. Gionchetti, M. Campieri, and M. A. Kamm. 2004. Once daily high dose probiotic therapy (VSL#3) for maintaining remission in recurrent or refractory pouchitis. *Gut* **53**:108–114.

Niv, E., T. Naftali, R. Hallak, and N. Vaisman. 2005. The efficacy of *Lactobacillus reuteri* ATCC 55730 in the treatment of patients with irritable bowel syndrome-a double blind, placebo-controlled, randomized study. *Clin. Nutr.* **24**:925–931.

Nobaek, S., M. L. Johansson, G. Molin, S. Ahrne, and B. Jeppsson. 2000. Alteration of intestinal microflora is associated with reduction in abdominal bloating and pain in patients with irritable bowel syndrome. *Am. J. Gastroenterol.* **95**:1231–1238.

Olah, A., T. Belagyi, A. Issekutz, M. E. Gamal, and S. Bengmark. 2002. Randomized clinical trial of specific lactobacillus and fibre supplement to early enteral nutrition in patients with acute pancreatitis. *Br. J. Surg.* **89**:1103–1107.

O'Mahony, L., J. McCarthy, P. Kelly, G. Hurley, F. Luo, K. Chen, G. C. O'Sullivan, B. Kiely, J. K. Collins, F. Shanahan, and E. M. Quigley. 2005. Lactobacillus and bifidobacterium in irritable bowel syndrome: symptom responses and relationship to cytokine profiles. *Gastroenterology* **128**:541–551.

Prantera, C., M. L. Scribano, G. Falasco, A. Andreoli, and C. Luzi. 2002. Ineffectiveness of probiotics in preventing recurrence after curative resection for Crohn's disease: a randomised controlled trial with *Lactobacillus GG. Gut* **51**:405–409.

Rafter, J., M. Govers, P. Martel, D. Pannemans, B. Pool-Zobel, G. Rechkemmer, I. Rowland, S. Tuijtelaars, and J. van Loo. 2004. PASSCLAIM—diet-related cancer. *Eur. J. Nutr.* **43**(Suppl. 2):1147–1184.

Rafter, J., M. Bennett, G. Caderni, Y. Clune, R. Hughes, P. C. Karlsson, A. Klinder, M. O'Riordan, G. C. O'Sullivan, B. Pool-Zobel, G. Rechkemmer, M. Roller, I. Rowland, M. Salvadori, H. Thijs, J. Van Loo, B. Watzl, and J. K. Collins. 2007. Dietary synbiotics reduce cancer risk factors in polypectomized and colon cancer patients. *Am. J. Clin. Nutr.* **85**:488–496.

Rayes, N., D. Seehofer, S. Hansen, K. Boucsein, A. R. Muller, S. Serke, S. Bengmark, and P. Neuhaus. 2002. Early enteral supply of lactobacillus and fiber versus selective bowel decontamination: a controlled trial in liver transplant recipients. *Transplantation* **74**:123–127.

Rayes, N., D. Seehofer, T. Theruvath, R. A. Schiller, J. M. Langrehr, S. Jonas, S. Bengmark, and P. Neuhaus. 2005. Supply of pre- and probiotics reduces bacterial infection rates after liver transplantation—a randomized, double-blind trial. *Am. J. Transplant.* **5**:125–130.

Reid, G., M. E. Sanders, H. R. Gaskins, G. R. Gibson, A. Mercenier, R. Rastall, M. Roberfroid, I. Rowland, C. Cherbut, and T. R. Klaenhammer. 2003. New scientific paradigms for probiotics and prebiotics. *J. Clin. Gastroenterol.* **37**:105–118.

Rembacken, B. J., A. M. Snelling, P. M. Hawkey, D. M. Chalmers, and A. T. Axon. 1999. Non-pathogenic *Escherichia coli* versus mesalazine for the treatment of ulcerative colitis: a randomised trial. *Lancet* **354**:635–639.

Rolfe, V. E., P. J. Fortun, C. J. Hawkey, and F. Bath-Hextall. 2006. Probiotics for maintenance of remission in Crohn's disease. *Cochrane Database Syst. Rev.* 4:CD004826.

Saavedra, J. M., N. A. Bauman, I. Oung, J. A. Perman, and R. H. Yolken. 1994. Feeding of *Bifidobacterium bifidum* and *Streptococcus thermophilus* to infants in hospital for prevention of diarrhoea and shedding of rotavirus. *Lancet* **334**:1046–1049.

Sartor, R. B. 2004. Therapeutic manipulation of the enteric microflora in inflammatory bowel diseases: antibiotics, probiotics, and prebiotics. *Gastroenterology* **126**:1620–1633.

Savino, F., E. Pelle, E. Palumeri, R. Oggero, and R. Miniero. 2007. *Lactobacillus reuteri* (American Type Culture Collection Strain 55730) versus simethicone in the treatment of infantile colic: a prospective randomized study. *Pediatrics* **119**:e124–e130.

Sazawal, S., G. Hiremath, U. Dhingra, P. Malik, S. Deb, and R. E. Black. 2006. Efficacy of probiotics in prevention of acute diarrhoea: a meta-analysis of masked, randomised, placebo-controlled trials. *Lancet Infect. Dis.* **6**:374–382.

Schultz, M., A. Timmer, H. H. Herfarth, R. B. Sartor, J. A. Vanderhoof, and H. C. Rath. 2004. *Lactobacillus GG* in inducing and maintaining remission of Crohn's disease. *BMC Gastroenterol.* **4**:5.

Suau, A., R. Bonnet, M. Sutren, J. J. Godon, G. Gibson, M. D. Collins, and J. Dore. 1999. Direct rDNA community analysis reveals a myriad of novel bacterial lineages within the human gut. *Appl. Environ. Microbiol.* **65**:4799–4807.

Sugawara, G., M. Nagino, H. Nishio, T. Ebata, K. Takagi, T. Asahara, K. Nomoto, and Y. Nimura. 2006. Perioperative synbiotic treatment to prevent postoperative infectious complications in biliary cancer surgery: a randomized controlled trial. *Ann. Surg.* 244:706–714.

Szajewska, H., M. Kotowska, J. Z. Mrukowicz, M. Armanska, and W. Mikolajczyk. 2001. Efficacy of *Lactobacillus GG* in prevention of nosocomial diarrhea in infants. *J. Pediatr.* 138:361–365.

Szajewska, H., and J. Mrukowicz. 2005. Meta-analysis: nonpathogenic yeast *Saccharomyces boulardii* in the prevention of antibiotic-associated diarrhoea. *Aliment. Pharmacol. Ther.* 22:365–372.

Szajewska, H., A. Skorka, and M. Dylag. 2007. Meta-analysis: *Saccharomyces boulardii* for treating acute diarrhoea in children. *Aliment. Pharmacol. Ther.* 25:257–264.

Tong, J. L., Z. H. Ran, J. Shen, C. X. Zhang, and S. D. Xiao. 2007. Meta-analysis: the effect of supplementation with probiotics on eradication rates and adverse events during *Helicobacter pylori* eradication therapy. *Aliment. Pharmacol. Ther.* 25:155–168.

Van Gossum, A., O. Dewit, E. Louis, G. de Hertogh, F. Baert, F. Fontaine, M. DeVos, M. Enslen, M. Paintin, and D. Franchimont. 2007. Multicenter randomized-controlled clinical trial of probiotics (*Lactobacillus johnsonii*, LA1) on early endoscopic recurrence of Crohn's disease after ileo-caecal resection. *Inflamm. Bowel Dis.* 13:135–142.

Van Niel, C. W., C. Feudtner, M. M. Garrison, and D. A. Christakis. 2002. Lactobacillus therapy for acute infectious diarrhea in children: a meta-analysis. *Pediatrics* 109:678–684.

Viljanen, M., E. Savilahti, T. Haahtela, K. Juntunen-Backman, R. Korpela, T. Poussa, T. Tuure, and M. Kuitunen. 2005. Probiotics in the treatment of atopic eczema/dermatitis syndrome in infants: a double-blind placebo-controlled trial. *Allergy* 60:494–500.

Walker, R., and M. Buckley. 2006. *Probiotic Microbes: the Scientific Basis.* American Academy of Microbiology, American Society for Microbiology, Washington, DC. http://www.asm.org/Academy/index.asp.

Watkinson, P. J., V. S. Barber, P. Dark, and J. D. Young. 2007. The use of pre-, pro- and synbiotics in adult intensive care unit patients: systematic review. *Clin. Nutr.* 26:182–192.

Wendakoon, C. N., A. B. Thomson, and L. Ozimeki. 2002. Lack of therapeutic effect of a specially designed yogurt for the eradication of *Helicobacter pylori* infection. *Digestion* 65:16–20.

Whorwell, P. J., L. Altringer, J. Morel, Y. Bond, D. Charbonneau, L. O'Mahony, B. Kiely, F. Shanahan, and E. M. Quigley. 2006. Efficacy of an encapsulated probiotic *Bifidobacterium infantis* 35624 in women with irritable bowel syndrome. *Am. J. Gastroenterol.* 101:1581–1590.

Yamanaka, T., L. Helgeland, I. N. Farstad, H. Fukushima, T. Midtvedt, and P. Brandtzaeg. 2003. Microbial colonization drives lymphocyte accumulation and differentiation in the follicle-associated epithelium of Peyer's patches. *J. Immunol.* 170:816–822.

Zocco, M. A., L. Z. dal Verme, F. Cremonini, A. C. Piscaglia, E. C. Nista, M. Candeli, M. Novi, D. Rigante, I. A. Cazzato, V. Ojetti, A. Armuzzi, G. Gasbarrini, and A. Gasbarrini. 2006. Efficacy of *Lactobacillus GG* in maintaining remission of ulcerative colitis. *Aliment. Pharmacol. Ther.* 23:1567–1574.

Zoetendal, E. G., A. D. Akkermans, W. M. Akkermans-van Vliet, J. A. de Visser, and W. M. de Vos. 2001. The host genotype affects the bacterial community in the human gastrointestinal tract. *Microb. Ecol. Health Dis.* 13:129–134.

Zoetendal, E. G., A. vom Wright, T. Vilpponen-Salmela, K. Ben-Amor, A. D. L. Akkermans, and W. M. de Vos. 2002. Mucosa-associated bacteria in the human gastrointestinal tract are uniformly distributed along the colon and differ from the community recovered from feces. *Appl. Environ. Microbiol.* 68:3401–3407.

Therapeutic Microbiology: Probiotics and Related Strategies
Edited by J. Versalovic and M. Wilson
© 2008 ASM Press, Washington, DC

Gregor Reid

Probiotics and Diseases of the Genitourinary Tract

21

PROBIOTICS

Over the past 5 years, probiotic research and the business of selling probiotic products have been on a rapid growth spurt. This has been spawned by consumer interest in natural products, dissatisfaction with side effects or failures of pharmaceutical agents, and mounting scientific and clinical evidence on the efficacy of probiotics. In 2001, the government of Argentina expressed concern about the lack of a global regulatory framework and definition of probiotics and requested assistance from the Food and Agriculture Organization of the United Nations (FAO) and World Health Organization (WHO). The FAO/WHO responded by forming an Expert Panel of leading figures in the area and asking them to prepare a Consultation Report. This was duly accomplished, and it includes a definition that for the first time was inclusive of all probiotic applications, not just those designed for intestinal use. The definition has since been widely adopted, including by the International Scientific Association for Probiotics and Prebiotics, the International Probiotics Association, the Polish Probiotics Society, Yogurt & Live Fermented milks Association–International, and the International

Dairy Foundation, to name but a few. The following definition is the one used here: "Live microorganisms which when administered in adequate amounts confer a health benefit on the host" (FAO/WHO, 2001).

HISTORICAL PERSPECTIVE ON PROBIOTICS FOR THE UROGENITAL TRACT

The rationale for using lactic acid bacteria to provide tangible health benefits dates back to Biblical times, but Elie Metchnikoff is credited more recently with observing an association between long life and regular intake of fermented foods. While his Nobel Prize in 1908 was for research in immunology, his legacy in probiotics is arguably more widely remembered. In 1915, perhaps influenced by Metchnikoff's work, Newman in the United Kingdom reported the first known insertion of lactic acid bacteria into the bladder with the intent to treat infection (Newman, 1915). Although the details of his work are sketchy and it is difficult to trace what happened beyond the published studies, the concept was not widely pursued. It was almost 60 years later that a

---

Gregor Reid, Canadian R&D Centre for Probiotics, Lawson Health Research Institute, F2–116, 268 Grosvenor Street, London, Ontario, N6A 4V2, Canada.

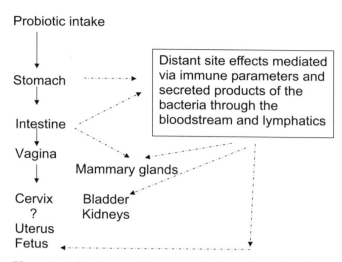

Figure 1 This diagram illustrates that ingestion of probiotic organisms has the potential to affect other parts of the host, either through direct passage to the genitourinary tract or through indirect effects on the host.

clinical observation by Bruce et al. (1973) showed that lactobacilli were predominant in the vagina of healthy women, whereas uropathogens dominated the vagina of subjects with a history of urinary tract infections (UTI). These important clinical findings reignited an interest, at least for Bruce, in exploring the reimplantation of lactobacilli into the vagina as a means to stop ascension of pathogens into the bladder.

Much later, it was shown that ingestion of probiotics can have effects on the urogenital tract through different channels. The obvious route is by transfer of the probiotic organisms through the intestine along the outer skin from the anus to the perineum and then to the vagina and cervix, and possibly ascension to the upper reproductive tract (Fig. 1). In addition, it has been discovered that the organisms or their by-products can mediate various effects in the urogenital tract, for example through systemic or local immune modulation, through intestinal and local anticarcinogenic effects, and through release of by-products that have different functions, including signaling activities. In this chapter, the development of probiotics for the urogenital tract and the various applications, whether tested or in developmental stages, are discussed.

THE RATIONALE FOR PROBIOTICS IN PREVENTION OR TREATMENT OF DISEASES OF THE GENITOURINARY TRACT

Numerous diseases occur in the genitourinary tract of men, women, and children. These disorders cover the gamut of infection, incontinence, cancer, inflammatory

problems, and anatomical malfunctions in the urethra, bladder, kidney, prostate, vulva, vagina, cervix, and uterus. The potential for probiotics to counter these ailments is not restricted to infection, as shall be discussed, but it is in this area that most of the research to date has been done (Table 1). The present discussion begins with conditions under which there is somewhat of a rationale for probiotics to affect the urogenital tract, but for which actual data are sparse.

Sexually Transmitted Infections

The ability of lactobacilli or other indigenous organisms to interfere with the process of sexual transmission of organisms such as herpes simplex virus, *Neisseria gonorrhoeae*, *Chlamydia trachomatis*, *Trichomonas* spp., and human immunodeficiency virus (HIV) is far from proven. However, the rationale has developed from clinical observations that have shown that an absence of lactobacilli significantly increases the risk of these infections (Sewankambo et al., 1997; Cherpes et al., 2003; Ness et al., 2005). The concept is that an acidic pH or perhaps hydrogen peroxide produced by lactobacilli suppresses the pathogens or reduces their exposure to T cells, macrophages, or epithelial cells which these intracellular organisms might invade. However, to test the theory would require a large clinical trial in a cohort of women at high risk of acquiring HIV, and such a study would be expensive and difficult to justify to an ethics committee.

Table 1 Diseases of the urogenital tract for which there is a rationale for probiotics or evidence that probiotics are effective

Disease/condition	Evidence of effect has been reported	Rationale for an effect but data are sparse
UTI	x	
BV	x	
Yeast vaginitis	x	
Urolithiasis	x	
Bladder and/or cervical cancer	x	
Sexually transmitted infections including HIV, gonorrhea, herpes, and chlamydia		x
Group B streptococcal colonization during pregnancy		x
Prostatitis		x
Interstitial cystitis		x

Group B Streptococcal Colonization

Group B streptococci (*Streptococcus agalactiae*) are commonly found in the vagina and usually do not cause symptomatic infections. However, the organisms are dangerous if passed to newborns during vaginal delivery, and thus antibiotics are prescribed in female carriers just prior to birthing. Some lactobacilli can inhibit growth of Group B streptococci in vitro (Zarate and Nader-Macias, 2006), but data on clinical efficacy are not yet available.

Prostatitis

The infectious process in the urogenital tract of men occurs through pathogens ascending the urethra, and in some cases passing into the epididymis and prostate, where they can survive and form biofilms that are invariably recalcitrant to treatment. The urethra can harbor lactobacilli, but probiotic therapy has not yet been designed for intraurethral application in men.

Numerous website postings ostensibly promote the use of probiotics for men with recurrent prostatitis. The only logical way that oral probiotics could impact prostatitis would be through systemic immune modulation, as delivery into the tissue would not be easy or ethically appropriate. Some researchers are investigating the systemic effects in animals, but such studies will not assess the impact on symptoms and quality of life, two hallmarks of chronic prostatitis.

Interstitial Cystitis

The most common and puzzling condition associated with inflammation in the urogenital tract is interstitial cystitis. This bladder syndrome has no known etiology and presents as severe pressure and pain in the bladder area or lower pelvis that is frequently or typically relieved by voiding, along with urgency or frequency of urination in the absence of infection (Theoharides, 2007). It is often characterized by cystoscopic visualization of ulcerations of the bladder mucosa, or submucosal petechial hemorrhages following hydrodistension under anesthesia. The condition can coincide with allergies, endometriosis, fibromyalgia, irritable bowel syndrome, and panic syndrome, all of which are affected by stress. Treatment is varied and includes intravesical dimethyl sulfoxide, amitriptyline, and pentosan polysulfate. The last drug is supposed to replace a presumably defective bladder glycosaminoglycan layer, but it may function as an inhibitor of mast cell histamine release or neutralizing toxic substances (Mayer, 2007).

Probiotics might interfere with interstitial cystitis in two ways. The first mechanism includes modulation of inflammatory processes by probiotic production of anti-inflammatory factors in the intestine, vagina, then indirectly to the bladder. This process might have some remediation effects, but given the degree of discomfort suffered by patients, it seems doubtful that this anti-inflammatory activity would be the definitive clinical breakthrough. The second mechanism could be through prevention of pathogenic involvement in interstitial cystitis. Although controversial because current concepts assume that the bladder is sterile before interstitial cystitis is diagnosed, advances in molecular diagnosis have resulted in identification of bacteria in bladders of patients with interstitial cystitis, and some patients have responded to antibiotic treatment (Theoharides, 2007; Mayer, 2007).

Cancer

Urinary and vaginal cancers remain a common cause of morbidity and mortality. Bladder and kidney cancers together account for 5% of cancers worldwide and represent the 9th and 14th most common cancers in absolute numbers (Pelucchi et al., 2006; Scelo and Brennan, 2007). Bladder cancer can be induced by chronic infection, making it feasible to reduce the incidence through probiotic instillation into the bladder or prevention of ascension of pathogens from the urethra and vagina. If the carcinogens are produced in the intestine, oral probiotic use might play a role in interfering with their production and adsorption into the bloodstream to the kidneys and bladder, or stimulating an immune response that could counter the carcinogenic process. Infections and urinary stones have also been found to increase bladder cancer risk, thus making it feasible for benefits to accrue from probiotic interventions.

Cervical cancer caused by human papillomavirus is common, but a new vaccine holds promise for its prevention (Wheeler, 2007). Treatment for Stage III cervical cancer often includes radiation, but failure rates are quite high, raising interest in the use of lactobacilli as biological response modifiers. In one study of 228 patients, a substance prepared from heat-killed *Lactobacillus casei* (YIT9018) enhanced tumor regression ($P < 0.1$) by radiation both after 30 Gy of external radiation and at the completion of radiation therapy (Okawa et al., 1993). The combination therapy also prolonged survival and the relapse-free interval ($P < 0.05$) compared to radiation alone. The results suggested that this probiotic derivative might help to prevent leukopenia during radiation therapy.

Calculi

Urolithiasis, or calculus formation in the urinary tract, is common especially in men. While infection-associated stones can occur, idiopathic calcium oxalate urolithiasis is the most frequent and recurrent problem. The intraluminal oxalate-degrading capacity of bacteria such as *Oxalobacter* has been proposed as an important means of reducing the risk of urinary calculi. These organisms have been shown to interact physiologically with colonic mucosa by inducing enteric oxalate secretion, leading to reduced urinary excretion (Hatch et al., 2006). Evidence suggests that lactic acid bacteria can also reduce the risk of renal calculi by reducing renal excretion of oxalate and prevalence of oxaluria, as shown in a small human study where people were treated with the probiotics combination VSL#3 (Lieske et al., 2005).

Bacterial Vaginosis

Although sexual intercourse or female-to-female sexual activities have been known to transfer bacterial vaginosis (BV) and UTI pathogens (Foxman et al., 2002; Marrazzo et al., 2002), the gastrointestinal tract is the most common origin of microbes infecting the female genitourinary tract. Pathogens emerge from the anus, ascend along the perineal skin in women, enter the vagina and urethra and cause an estimated 1 billion infections worldwide each year. This staggering number is more easily envisaged given that the prevalence of BV has recently been reported to be 29% (Allsworth and Peipert, 2007), sales of over-the-counter antifungal agents used for vaginal candidiasis exceeded $300 million in the United States, and at least 11 million cases of UTI each year have been reported in the United States alone (11 million women of 120 million women in the population, extrapolated to 3 billion females worldwide equals 300 million women with UTI). Because of the involvement of the gut and vagina in these disease processes, it was hypothesized by our group in the early 1980s that vaginal lactobacilli might interfere with urogenital pathogenesis. Healthy women are colonized with lactobacilli in the vagina, and these organisms are severely depleted in diseased patients, especially those with BV (Spiegel, 1991).

In recent times, interest has risen in BV, in parallel with an enhanced understanding of this disorder. Described by Gardner and Dukes in 1954 (Gardner and Duke, 1954), BV has generally been diagnosed by the Amsel criteria, based on pH values of >4.5, fishy amine odors in vaginal discharge, and findings of biofilms covering vaginal cells (Amsel et al., 1983). While this method has merit, as our understanding of BV evolves, it is not sufficient to use the Amsel test alone for diagnosis (Sha et al., 2005). A study of 2,888 women showed that 75% of patients with BV and 82% of individuals without BV never noted any vaginal odor in the preceding 6 months, while vaginal "wetness," discharge, irritation, itching, or dysuria yielded no differences between BV and non-BV groups (Klebanoff et al., 2004). If vaginal

discharge and odor are not reliable clinical signs, perhaps elevated inflammatory levels of interleukin-1β might facilitate the diagnosis of BV (Cauci et al., 2003). However, the role of inflammation in BV has not been clearly defined.

A Gram stain method was developed by Nugent et al. (1991) as a means of identifying patients with BV. The absence of lactobacilli in favor of densely packed gram-negative anaerobes adherent to vaginal cells and visible by bright-field microscopy is an indicative feature of BV, as is the presence of aerobic pathogens in biofilms (Donder et al., 2002). However, clue cells with adherent biofilms are not always visible by microscopy. This microbiological method has been verified as effective in many studies, but the vagina is not always dominated by lactobacilli (Forney et al., 2006), and the discovery that gram-positive *Atopobium* spp. are a primary cause of BV (Burton et al., 2004) makes it difficult to diagnose this condition by using microscopy alone.

A diagnostic system, the BV Blue kit, has been developed to detect BV by the presence of sialidase, an enzyme produced by a number of gram-negative anaerobes (Cauci et al., 2002), and it has been verified in clinical studies (Thanavuth et al., 2007). However, based on measurement of sialidase concentrations, it has been reported that sialidase alone is not sufficient to diagnose BV (Ombrella et al., 2006). The lack of sialidase in *Atopobium* means that a mixed infection is required for sialidase to be used as a diagnostic test (Sumeksri et al., 2005). This issue might explain a study which showed that sialidase is not a good marker for BV (Ombrella et al., 2006). A DNA-hybridization kit (Affirm VPIII) has been introduced to assist with diagnosis of BV. Although apparently used widely in the United States, it is expensive and lacks specificity as it only detects *Gardnerella vaginalis*, *Candida* spp., and *Trichomonas vaginalis* (Schwiertz et al., 2006). The last two microbes are not indicative of BV, and *G. vaginalis* is often associated with a healthy vaginal microbiota.

One factor that appears consistent with BV, and particularly with the association of *Atopobium* spp., is the elevation of vaginal pH above 4.5. Vaginal pH measurements have merit in clinical settings and may be superior to other more sophisticated diagnostic strategies. A conclusive diagnosis of BV usually requires detection of elevated pH and symptoms or signs of disease. The issue is further complicated by the existence of aerobic BV whereby pathogens such as enterococci can survive in low pH. Of 90 subjects studied in Bosnia, *Enterococcus faecalis* was found in 24.05% of cases with vaginal pH values of ≤4.0, but enterococci were isolated in 52.78% of patients with BV and pH values of >4.0

(Jahic et al., 2006). Enterococci in BV may deplete lactobacilli via bacteriocin production (Kelly et al., 2003), by aggregation and overgrowth (Tendolkar et al., 2003), or by coaggregating with other organisms to colonize or infect the host (von Graevenitz, 1982).

Interesting studies of pregnant women, which have shown the existence of lactobacilli in the mammary ducts (Martin et al., 2005), suggest that intestinal sampling by host defense cells can result in transfer of pathogens to external sites. A recent study claims that intestinally derived bacterial components may be transported to the lactating breast within mononuclear cells (Perez et al., 2007), but these results are preliminary as others have not identified lactobacilli in the mammary duct. In terms of vaginal colonization by lactobacilli resulting from intestinal translocation, little is currently known and further studies are needed.

Urinary Tract Infections

The primary cause of UTI is *Escherichia coli*, followed by other pathogens including other gram-negative enteric bacteria and enterococci. Interestingly, the high density of *E. coli* often found in the vagina of patients with UTI does not appear to cause infection in that niche. This finding is somewhat puzzling because of the presence of pathogenicity islands and virulence factors in *E. coli* and the known potency of these organisms when interacting with the bladder epithelium (Lloyd et al., 2007). *E. coli* adheres to squamous epithelial cells in the trigone of the bladder as well as cells lining the vagina. Why do pathogens not infect the vagina in many individuals? The painful symptoms that occur in the urethra upon micturition and the frequency and urgency accompanying UTI represent the main reasons that women seek medical attention. Disruption of the mucopolysaccharide layer in the bladder may be one factor associated with development of UTI, while such damage to the epithelial lining in the vagina has not been reported. Asymptomatic bacteriuria remains a poorly understood phenomenon. Studies are needed to examine this condition, as well as to investigate whether the vagina is infected when *E. coli* is present in large numbers despite a lack of symptoms. Often patients will complain of suprapubic discomfort and pain, as well as fatigue that could originate in an infected vagina.

In two patients seen in our clinic, dense enterococcal populations were found in the vagina, and upon their displacement and eradication by lactobacilli, the symptoms of UTI ceased. This treatment outcome implied a continual seeding of the bladder by the vaginal enterococcal population. More studies are warranted to investigate this possibility. Not many studies have tested whether lactobacillus probiotics can prevent UTI. The use of *Lactobacillus rhamnosus* GG orally did not prevent UTI in preterm infants, although the therapy was only given for 7 days (Dani et al., 2002). A study of adults showed that time to recurrent UTI did not increase with a beverage of *L. rhamnosus* GG (4×10^{10} CFU of *L. rhamnosus* GG/100 ml per day) consumed 5 days per week for 1 year (Kontiokari et al., 2001). Vaginal instillation of a nondocumented *Lactobacillus acidophilus* strain also failed to lower the recurrence of UTI (Baerheim et al., 1994). However, intravaginal instillation of *L. rhamnosus* GR-1 combined with *Lactobacillus fermentum* B-54 once weekly for 1 year significantly reduced infections compared to the previous year (Reid et al., 1995). More recently, a prospective randomized controlled study of 120 children with persistent primary vesicoureteral reflux after antibiotic prophylaxis for 1 year showed equivalent rates of UTI with *L. acidophilus* (18.3% [11/60] UTI with 10^8 CFU/g twice a day) and trimethoprim-sulfamethoxazole (21.6% [13/60] UTI with 2/10 mg/kg of body weight at bedtime) (Lee et al., 2007). In summary, evidence supports potential applications of lactobacilli to prevent UTI, but more studies are needed with well-characterized strains, involving adults that are monitored for a sufficient time period.

Yeast Vaginitis

Yeast vaginitis, caused by *Candida albicans* in most cases, is common in adolescent and adult females. Many cases are misdiagnosed and treated with antifungal agents when in fact they are due to BV. The occurrence of yeast vaginitis following antibiotic use depends on the antibiotic, the duration of treatment, and how the yeast infection was diagnosed. In a study of 24 women treated with antibiotics and randomly assigned to take oral probiotic *L. rhamnosus* GR-1 and *Lactobacillus reuteri* RC-14, no yeast infections occurred, but 25% of the controls developed BV within 3 weeks after cessation of antibiotic therapy (Reid et al., 2003b). The primary rationale for probiotic use in recurrent yeast infections is not for treatment, as lactobacilli and *Candida* organisms can coexist within the acidic vaginal ecosystem. Rather, the main goal of probiotics applications is to prevent genitourinary tract infections by populating the vagina with lactobacilli after antifungal agents have reduced the yeast count. Another potential role for probiotics in the context of vaginitis could be to enhance eradication of yeasts through combined antifungal and probiotic therapies. This effect has been achieved successfully using *L. rhamnosus* GR-1 and *L. reuteri* RC-14 in a study performed in Brazil which is being prepared for publication.

In terms of mechanisms of probiosis, it has been shown that *L. rhamnosus* GR-1 can significantly reduce biofilm formation by *C. albicans* (Koehler and Reid, 2006).

SELECTION OF LACTOBACILLI OR OTHER PROBIOTICS FOR APPLICATIONS IN THE HUMAN UROGENITAL TRACT

Clear guidelines have not been defined for the selection of probiotics in specific medical applications. The host origin of the probiotic species has been recommended to match the host species (i.e., humans) for medical applications. However, one could argue that humans inherit these strains from food sources, and such stipulations may be unnecessary. The species of organism has been chosen because of dominance in a particular niche, such as *Lactobacillus* organisms in the vagina. In fact, this concept is evolving, as some species like *E. coli*, in an avirulent form, could compete for particular ecologic niches more effectively and interfere with pathogens infecting the host. Indeed, avirulent *E. coli* 83972 has been shown to colonize the bladder of spinal cord injury patients in pilot studies and prolong the time interval to subsequent infections (Darouiche et al., 2005). As our understanding of the microbial composition of the healthy urogenital tract improves, it is highly likely that different probiotic formulations will include different species that, although not necessarily the most commonly found organisms, may possess an array of properties suitable for remediation or prevention of disease.

In the past, acid tolerance and bile resistance were viewed as prerequisite features for successful probiotics. However, both properties can be addressed by current delivery systems, and neither characteristic is needed for vaginal, skin, or mouth applications. Likewise, high levels of adherence to cells in vitro have been used to select probiotic strains, but few studies have compared these in vitro studies with in vivo adhesion levels. In addition, adhesion may not be a necessary probiotic feature or in some instances may not provide the ideal means for probiotics to interfere with pathogens or perform other desirable tasks. In the vagina, adhesion likely aids persistence, but if the strain does not produce other beneficial factors, it could be a poor choice for probiotic applications. Likewise, a poorly adherent strain in vitro may have other factors that make it able to displace infectious agents or inhibit pathogenesis. Production of substances that inhibit pathogen growth, such as hydrogen peroxide, bacteriocins, and lactic acid, appears to play a role in preventing infections, but animal studies have only recently provided proof for the importance of bacteriocins in the gut (Corr et al., 2007), and more in vivo studies are needed to determine the key protective components in the vagina. Twenty-five years after using in vitro assays to select probiotics for urogenital health, it appears that the most important functionality of probiotics in preventing genitourinary tract infections is through interference with pathogen ascension from the anus into the vagina and urethra, something that could not be predicted from in vitro data. Thus, the mechanisms of interference are multifactorial.

In the early 1980s, lactobacilli were selected as probiotics for the human genitourinary tract because these organisms were the most common species associated with a healthy urogenital tract, and they could block adhesion of pathogens and inhibit their growth (Chan et al., 1984, 1985; Reid et al., 1987). Using this selection process, three lactobacillus strains were pursued with the central goal of preventing pathogen ascension to the urogenital tract.

The first strain, isolated from the distal urethra of a healthy woman, was originally classified as *Lactobacillus casei* but subsequently was reclassified as *L. rhamnosus* GR-1. It was selected for its robust adherence to uroepithelial cells and inhibition of the growth of gram-negative pathogens, particularly uropathogenic *E. coli* (Chan et al., 1984; Reid et al., 1987; McGroarty and Reid, 1988a). As more investigations of this strain were performed, it was found to have a range of properties and attributes including a hydrophobic capsule that could mediate adhesion (Cook et al., 1988), lactic acid production that could adversely affect the outer membrane of *E. coli* (Cadieux et al., unpublished data), coaggregation properties believed to bind potential pathogens and reduce their ability to infect the host (Reid et al., 1990), an ability to resist the killing action of spermicide nonoxyl-9 (Tomeczek et al., 1992), biosurfactant production capacity that is believed to produce an area of epithelial cells less conducive to pathogen adhesion (Velraeds et al., 1996), an ability to reduce *Salmonella* gut translocation and enhance the phagocytic killing of these enteropathogens (Reid et al., 2002), signaling factors that have anti-inflammatory properties (Kim et al., 2006) and potentially reduce the risk of preterm labor by down-regulating COX-2 (cyclooxygenase 2) and tumor necrosis factor as well as up-regulation of PGDH (prostaglandin dehydrogenase) (Yeganegi et al., 2007), an ability to displace and suppress biofilms of *G. vaginalis* (Saunders et al., 2007) and *C. albicans* (Koehler and Reid, 2006), quorum-sensing signals that may interfere with urogenital bacterial pathogenesis (Elwood et al., 2006), and the ability to reduce fungal infections and diarrhea and increase perceived energy levels in HIV/AIDS patients (Anukam et al., 2008; J. Hemsworth, G. Reid, and S. Hekmat, unpublished data).

With such diverse features, *L. rhamnosus* GR-1 clearly has a multitude of properties that can influence outcomes in the host. Probiotics, commensal bacteria, and bacterial pathogens may share some traits. For example, uropathogenic *E. coli* strains harbor genes for adhesion, biofilm formation, hemolysin expression, and other virulence factors. Sometimes these factors appear to induce symptomatic infections, while on other occasions, the organisms multiply without inducing symptoms and signs of infection (Reid et al., 1984; Marrs et al., 2005). The gene pool in bacteria, such as *L. rhamnosus* GR-1, has likely evolved to facilitate adaptation to its host environment. The organism's origin and survival in the gut (Morelli et al., 2004) include many challenges such as constant changes in nutrient availability, variable transit times, host immune factors, and infection followed by rapid excretion of the organisms. The adaptation of *L. rhamnosus* to the distal urethra and vagina (Chan et al., 1984) includes the ability to utilize its gene pool for survival and competition on surfaces exposed to numerous microbes, and therefore it is not surprising that *L. rhamnosus* GR-1 can induce different host responses. The pending genomic sequence of *L. rhamnosus* GG will help to understand the innate properties of this species, while future sequencing and genomic functionality studies of strain GR-1 will hopefully elucidate its array of mechanisms in response to microbes and the host, particularly in the urogenital tract of women. Preliminary human microarray studies suggest that *L. rhamnosus* GR-1 can up-regulate host defenses in the vagina when instilled directly into the genitourinary tract (Kirjavainen et al., in press).

The combination of *L. reuteri* RC-14 and *L. rhamnosus* GR-1 for human medical applications resulted from a series of studies pertaining to the functions of *L. reuteri* RC-14. These findings provide insights into the process of strain selection for human applications. Selection of probiotics can be influenced by the intended use of the product. Isolated in 1985 and classified as *L. acidophilus* RC-14 by a series of biochemical tests, the strain had antipathogenic properties (Reid et al., 1987) but was not pursued further as its adhesiveness in vitro was not perceived to be sufficient for colonization of the vagina. Adhesiveness was a property deemed to be critical for success in 1987. Probiotics repopulate the genitourinary tract, compete with other bacteria, and are flushed from the host, necessitating regular, repeated administration. Furthermore, adhesiveness is not necessarily critical for persistence or performance of probiotic activities, and excessive adhesion and long-term colonization might be intentionally avoided if persistence deters replenishment of the host's own lactobacilli.

Following a clinical study in 1988 (Bruce and Reid, 1988) in which intravaginal instillation of *L. rhamnosus* GR-1 alone did not appear to displace enterococci, a search for a second probiotic strain began. Several candidates were considered, but *L. fermentum* B-54 was initially chosen because it inhibited the growth of gram-positive bacteria that colonize the genitourinary tract (Reid et al., 1987; McGroarty and Reid, 1988b). Added to *L. rhamnosus* GR-1, *L. fermentum* B-54 was effective at reducing the risk of recurrent UTI by direct vaginal instillation (Bruce et al., 1992; Reid et al., 1992a, 1995).

In the early 1990s, it was believed that vaginal lactobacilli needed to produce hydrogen peroxide for efficacy, even if such strains were susceptible to killing by spermicide (McGroarty et al., 1992). In addition, physicochemical studies clarified the role of cell surface components with respect to adhesion of bacteria on hydrophilic (human cells) and hydrophobic (biopolymers such as catheters or intrauterine devices) surfaces (Busscher and van der Mei, 1997). As *L. rhamnosus* GR-1 was hydrophilic (Reid et al., 1992b), it was theorized that adding a hydrophobic, hydrogen peroxide-producing strain that was active against gram-positive bacteria could provide robust coverage of pathogens that infect the urogenital tract. While *L. fermentum* B-54 had some of these properties, the discovery of highly active anti-gram-positive coccal biosurfactant in *L. reuteri* RC-14 (known then as *L. acidophilus*) (Velraeds et al., 1996) led to the development of this strain for human use. Not only were biosurfactants believed to be important in reducing pathogen colonization, but also these compounds have broad-spectrum antimicrobial activity including effects against *C. albicans* (Busscher et al., 1997; Velraeds et al., 1998). Further studies identified unique amino acid sequences among the biosurfactant mixtures (Howard et al., 2000) and a collagen-binding protein (Heinemann et al., 2000) that was an important factor in reducing infectivity of *Staphylococcus aureus* (Gan et al., 2002).

In 1998, ribosomal typing identified the strain as *L. fermentum* RC-14, making it a relatively easy replacement for *L. fermentum* B-54 in the probiotic preparations for human trials (Zhong et al., 1998). More recently, DNA-DNA hybridization would classify the RC-14 strain as *L. reuteri*, even though it does not produce the reuterin antibiotic, which is a principal trait of this species. In time, it is possible that *L. reuteri* strains lacking evidence of reuterin production, including *L. reuteri* RC-14, will be reclassified. For now, the strain identified in 1985 and described in studies as *L. acidophilus* or *L. fermentum* is known today as *L. reuteri* RC-14.

The net outcome of these studies is that two probiotic strains were selected by a combination of bacterial attributes perceived to be important for clinical efficacy and experience gained by clinical studies. If strains are to be termed probiotic organisms for human patients, benefits for humans must be demonstrated. The development of this combination therapy shows the importance of linking clinical observations with a scientific understanding of bacterial properties. Of note, animal studies were not a key component of the development of this probiotic strategy partly because useful animal models are sparse for UTIs and BV, and human probiotics research (in contrast to probiotics for agriculture or animal health) may require information beyond cell culture studies using human cells in the laboratory and information gained from animal studies. The knowledge acquired in this development process and by other scientists who had used in vitro assays for probiotics research led the FAO/WHO Expert Panel in 2001 to state that "The currently available (*in vitro*) tests are not adequate to predict the functionality of probiotic microorganisms in the intestine."

In 2000–2001, the idea of simulating natural vaginal colonization by passive transfer from the anal skin to perineum and vagina was conceived, and two proof-of-principle studies were undertaken. To show that *Lactobacillus* strains GR-1 and RC-14 could traverse the gut, subjects ingested them in milk and provided fecal samples for analyses. The organisms were indeed recovered from fecal specimens (Gardiner et al., 2002). Then, 10 women ingested the probiotics-containing milk for 2 weeks, and vaginal swabs were tested and found to contain the probiotic organisms within 1 week of oral intake (Reid et al., 2001b). Using technology developed by Chr. Hansen A/S (Horsholm, Denmark) to protect the lactobacilli in the stomach and bile ducts (even though both strains are acid and bile tolerant), clinical studies were performed to test the abilities of the organisms to prevent, and improve treatment of, urogenital infections, particularly BV.

EFFICACY OF PROBIOTICS FOR UROGENITAL HEALTH

The first study using oral capsules was one of only a few studies to have tested different dosages of probiotics in human patients. Three concentrations of lactobacilli were administered orally to adult women (mostly Caucasian) in London, Canada, and capsules containing *L. rhamnosus* GG were used as the control probiotic formulation. The 44-subject study indicated that a minimum dose of 10^9 CFU per day could maintain a normal *Lactobacillus* vaginal microbiota and, in 50% of cases, the BV-associated microbiota reverted to a microbial

composition similar to that of control individuals (Reid et al., 2001a). This pilot study was followed by a series of trials to better understand the benefits and limitations of probiotic therapies.

A study was designed to examine whether healthy women could benefit from lactobacilli in daily capsules. The issue is whether healthy individuals benefit from probiotic supplements. Implications for other probiotic applications emerged from this study. While disease is well understood and relatively easily diagnosed by our health care professionals, the term "health" is not clearly defined. According to the World Health Organization, the definition of health is "a state of complete physical, mental and social well-being and not merely the absence of disease or infirmity" (WHO, 1946). In practice, medical examinations are designed to exclude disease rather than to diagnose overall health status. In a clinical study, 64 women were referred by their family physicians as being healthy, and all reported feeling well. However, an examination of their vaginal microbiota showed that 25% of subjects had evidence of BV (Reid et al., 2003a). At the time, such a diagnosis was known as asymptomatic BV. However, as more studies of this condition have been performed, it appears that many BV patients do not express the classic signs of vaginal discharge and fishy odor (Klebanoff et al., 2004). As BV is a condition that can lead to complications in pregnancy as well as increased risks of symptomatic and sexually transmitted infections, new treatment strategies may have important consequences for female patients.

The daily oral intake of the *L. rhamnosus* GR-1 and *L. reuteri* RC-14 capsules resulted in a significant reduction of the transfer of uropathogenic bacteria and yeasts from the anus to the vagina, as detected by blinded analyses of vaginal swabs (Reid et al., 2003a). The apparent ability to cure BV in 7 of 8 subjects compared to 0 of 7 patients in the placebo group (Reid et al., 2004) was noteworthy despite the fact that this outcome was not the central aim of the study. The key finding was that healthy women could obtain health benefits in the vagina from daily ingestion of lactobacilli.

A study was performed to examine the ability of probiotics to prevent BV and yeast vaginitis in patients receiving antibiotic therapy. The sample size was small, mostly due to a reduction in antibiotic-prescribing patterns in London, Ontario. Nevertheless, two intriguing outcomes resulted from this study. The hypothesis, and widely held perception among patients and doctors, that yeast vaginitis is a predictable outcome of 10 days of antibiotic therapy was nullified. None of the 24 subjects who received antibiotics plus probiotics or placebo had yeast infections at 30 days of follow-up (Reid et al., 2003b). However, 25%

of individuals in the placebo group developed BV. This finding could have occurred by chance, given the small sample size, but further studies are warranted. The true prevalence of BV compared to yeast vaginitis remains an open issue. BV may be difficult to diagnose and can yield symptoms and signs similar to those of yeast infections. As women can purchase over-the-counter antiyeast medications, many do not seek medical confirmation of their condition and simply self-treat based on the assumption that yeasts are the etiological agents for their conditions. Unfortunately, many patient self-treatment decisions are misguided, and a high proportion of women are wrongly self-treating with antiyeast products (Ferris et al., 1996; Sihvo et al., 2000). Evidence suggests that self-treatment can result in a disturbed genitourinary microbiota, chronic symptomatology, and psychosocial problems (Lowe and Ryan-Wenger, 2003; Patel et al., 2006; Ernst et al., 2005).

Another problem facing women is the growing dissatisfaction with pharmaceutical remedies for urogenital infections. These challenges include nuisance side effects such as diarrhea, nausea, superinfections, and major complications such as Stevens Johnson syndrome (Iannini et al., 2006), anaphylactic shock (Rafal'skii, 2000), and other serious adverse events (Onrust et al., 1998; Arundel and Lewis, 2007). In some cases, antibiotics like temafloxacin and grepafloxacin have been removed from the market due to severe adverse effects. Of the agents that do cure infection, antibiotics may be ineffective due to antimicrobial resistance as well as an inability of drugs to disrupt biofilms associated with many infections (Lima et al., 2001; Dasgupta, 2002; Yoon and Hassett, 2004; Klotz et al., 2007) and intracellular subversion of biofilms (Anderson et al., 2004). Since probiotic *L. rhamnosus* GR-1 and *L. reuteri* RC-14 have anti-biofilm effects, three clinical studies were undertaken in an effort to improve the efficacy of currently approved antimicrobial agents.

In the first study, 106 women were enrolled only if BV was diagnosed by the standard Amsel criteria, Nugent Gram stain, and BV Blue kit. Subjects were treated with 1 g of metronidazole plus lactobacilli or placebo. The cure rate of the metronidazole and placebo group was only 40% compared to 88% for the metronidazole and lactobacilli group (Anukam et al., 2006b). Critics might argue that this metronidazole cure rate is surprisingly low. Still, if a secondary analysis of the data included "intermediate" BV cure, this rate only reaches 70% and is still significantly lower than the 100% cure rate for the group using metronidazole plus probiotic. One criticism was that the study was performed in Nigeria and that women in Africa may somehow be different

from women in different geographic regions. Nevertheless, the vaginal microbiota of Nigerian women, when assessed by molecular methods, is similar to that of women in Bulgaria, Germany, Canada, Sweden, the United States, and other parts of Africa (Vasquez et al., 2002; Fredricks et al., 2005; Hill et al., 2005; Anukam et al., 2006a; Stoyancheva et al., 2006; Thies et al., 2007; Jin et al., 2007), with *Lactobacillus iners*, *L. crispatus*, and *L. jensenii* being the predominant species in healthy women. One difference among BV patients was that the prevalence of *Mycoplasma hominis* seemed to be higher in Nigerian subjects than in North American or European cohort groups (Anukam et al., 2005). However, since metronidazole can cure *Mycoplasma* infections (Austin et al., 2005), this difference does not explain the findings. To further explore differences between human populations, a study was performed in Brazil using a similar protocol with tinidazole instead of metronidazole. The outcome of the study ($n = 64$ patients) was very similar to the Nigerian one described above.

The ability of probiotics to treat BV was reported in a randomized, placebo-controlled study of 40 subjects (Anukam et al., 2006b). The cure rate of intravaginal therapy with *L. rhamnosus* GR-1 and *L. reuteri* RC-14 administered for 5 days was 90% (18 of 20 patients) compared to 60% (12 of 20 patients) with metronidazole. So far, no trials have been done to examine whether probiotics can cure BV plus diminish the risk of sexually transmitted infections. The successful reduction in cases of *Chlamydia* infections with intravaginal metronidazole (Schwebke and Desmond, 2007) suggests that probiotics may potentially do the same.

The availability of clinically documented, efficacious products for women's health remains restricted (Fallagas et al., 2007), and companies are promoting untested products or products lacking clinical or scientific data. Without appropriate clinical studies, it is a grave disservice to women to sell and promote products that have not been sufficiently tested in humans and proven to provide benefits. At the very least, all probiotic products should meet FAO/WHO guidelines (FAO/WHO, 2002).

CONCLUSIONS AND FUTURE DIRECTIONS

Widespread and growing interest in the use of probiotics for urogenital health has served as an impetus for numerous research studies. While some of the research is market driven, it is only through scientific studies that we can understand the factors involved in maintaining and restoring vaginal health, and therefore producing appropriate probiotic interventions for the genitourinary tract. Applications with *L. rhamnosus* and *L. reuteri* strains are an initial step to provide novel alternatives to women whose only options to date have been antimicrobial washes and pharmaceutical anti-infectives with broad-spectrum activities and multiple side effects. Probiotics will not replace antimicrobial agents in the foreseeable future, but recombinant strains may be developed to target disease treatment. Probiotic strains might augment the effectiveness of antimicrobial agents, and the high prevalence of conditions such as BV suggests that modulation of the urogenital microbiota may help prevent disease.

Future advances may result from studies with new clinically proven strains such as *L. crispatus* (Marrazzo et al., 2006; Uehara et al., 2006) as well as species other than lactobacilli or even organisms outside the lactic acid bacterial group. New product formulations may take account of fluctuating conditions in the vagina and yield by-products from probiotic strains that modulate pathogenesis and inflammation. Progress will be faster if granting agencies become more open to studying the microbial ecology of the gut and urogenital tract and if food and pharmaceutical companies invest in comprehensive clinical studies. The recent launch of the International Human Microbiome Project includes the female genitourinary tract as a primary study region, and it is expected that new organisms and microbial ecology features will be unraveled in the next decade. While many urogenital tract problems are not life threatening, the adverse cumulative impact on morbidity and the quality of life of women by these disorders demands that new approaches to the enhancement of human health be seriously considered.

Our research is supported by grants from AFMnet, OMAF, NSERC, and CIHR. I declare ownership of patents associated with L. rhamnosus GR-1 and L. reuteri RC-14.

References

Allsworth, J. E., and J. F. Peipert. 2007. Prevalence of bacterial vaginosis: 2001–2004 National Health and Nutrition Examination Survey data. *Obstet. Gynecol.* **109:**114–120.

Amsel, R., P. A. Totten, C. A. Spiegel, K. C. Chen, D. Eschenbach, and K. K. Holmes. 1983. Nonspecific vaginitis. Diagnostic criteria and microbial and epidemiologic associations. *Am. J. Med.* **74:**14–22.

Anderson, G. G., S. M. Martin, and S. J. Hultgren. 2004. Host subversion by formation of intracellular bacterial communities in the urinary tract. *Microbes Infect.* **6:**1094–1101.

Anukam, K. C., E. O. Osazuwa, I. Ahonkhai, and G. Reid. 2006a. *Lactobacillus* vaginal microbiota of women attending a reproductive health care service in Benin city, Nigeria. *Sex. Transm. Dis.* **33:**59–62.

Anukam, K. C., E. O. Osazuwa, I. Ahonkhai, and G. Reid. 2005. Association between absence of vaginal lactobacilli PCR products and Nugent scores interpreted as bacterial vaginosis. *Trop. J. Obstet. Gynaecol.* **22:**103–107.

Anukam, K. C., E. Osazuwa, G. I. Osemene, F. Ehigiagbe, A. W. Bruce, and G. Reid. 2006b. Clinical study comparing probiotic *Lactobacillus* GR-1 and RC-14 with metronidazole vaginal gel to treat symptomatic bacterial vaginosis. *Microbes Infect.* **8:**2772–2776.

Anukam, K. C., E. O. Osazuwa, B. E. Osadolor, A. W. Bruce, and G. Reid. 2008. Yogurt containing probiotic *Lactobacillus rhamnosus* GR-1 and *L. reuteri* RC-14 helps resolve moderate diarrhea and increases CD4 count in HIV/AIDS patients. *J. Clin. Gastroenterol.* **42:**239–243.

Arundel, C., and J. H. Lewis. 2007. Drug-induced liver disease in 2006. *Curr. Opin. Gastroenterol.* **23:**244–254.

Austin, M. N., R. H. Beigi, L. A. Meyn, and S. L. Hillier. 2005. Microbiologic response to treatment of bacterial vaginosis with topical clindamycin or metronidazole. *J. Clin. Microbiol.* **43:**4492–4497.

Baerheim, A., E. Larsen, and A. Digranes. 1994. Vaginal application of lactobacilli in the prophylaxis of recurrent lower urinary tract infection in women. *Scand. J. Prim. Health Care* **12:**239–243.

Bruce, A. W., P. Chadwick, A. Hassan, and G. F. VanCott. 1973. Recurrent urethritis in women. *Can. Med. Assoc. J.* **108:**973–976.

Bruce, A. W., G. Reid, J. A. McGroarty, M. Taylor, and C. Preston. 1992. Preliminary study on the prevention of recurrent urinary tract infections in ten adult women using intravaginal lactobacilli. *Int. Urogynecol. J.* **3:**22–25.

Bruce, A. W., and G. Reid. 1988. Intravaginal instillation of lactobacilli for prevention of recurrent urinary tract infections. *Can. J. Microbiol.* **34:**339–343.

Burton, J. P., E. Devillard, P. A. Cadieux, J.-A. Hammond, and G. Reid. 2004. Detection of *Atopobium vaginae* in postmenopausal women by cultivation-independent methods warrants further investigation. *J. Clin. Microbiol.* **42:**1829–1831.

Busscher, H. J., and H. C. van der Mei. 1997. Physico-chemical interactions in initial microbial adhesion and relevance for biofilm formation. *Adv. Dent. Res.* **11:**24–32.

Busscher, H. J., C. G. van Hoogmoed, G. I. Geertsema-Doornbusch, M. van der Kuijl-Booij, and H. C. van der Mei. 1997. *Streptococcus thermophilus* and its biosurfactants inhibit adhesion by *Candida* spp. on silicone rubber. *Appl. Environ. Microbiol.* **63:**3810–3817.

Cauci, S., S. Guaschino, D. De Aloysio, S. Driussi, D. De Santo, P. Penacchioni, and F. Quadrifoglio. 2003. Interrelationships of interleukin-8 with interleukin-1beta and neutrophils in vaginal fluid of healthy and bacterial vaginosis positive women. *Mol. Hum. Reprod.* **9:**53–58.

Cauci, S., J. Hitti, C. Noonan, K. Agnew, F. Quadrifoglio, S. L. Hillier, and D. A. Eschenbach. 2002. Vaginal hydrolytic enzymes, immunoglobulin A against *Gardnerella vaginalis* toxin, and risk of early preterm birth among women in preterm labor with bacterial vaginosis or intermediate flora. *Am. J. Obstet. Gynecol.* **187:**877–881.

Chan, R. C. Y., A. W. Bruce, and G. Reid. 1984. Adherence of cervical, vaginal and distal urethral normal microbial flora to human uroepithelial cells and the inhibition of adherence of uropathogens by competitive exclusion. *J. Urol.* **131:**596–601.

Chan, R. C. Y., G. Reid, R. T. Irvin, A. W. Bruce, and J. W. Costerton. 1985. Competitive exclusion of uropathogens from uroepithelial cells by *Lactobacillus* whole cells and cell wall fragments. *Infect. Immun.* **47:**84–89.

Cherpes, T. L., L. A. Meyn, M. A. Krohn, and S. L. Hillier. 2003. Risk factors for infection with herpes simplex virus type 2: role of smoking, douching, uncircumcised males, and vaginal flora. *Sex. Transm. Dis.* **30:**405–410.

Cook, R. L., R. J. Harris, and G. Reid. 1988. Effect of culture media and growth phase on the morphology of lactobacilli and on their ability to adhere to epithelial cells. *Curr. Microbiol.* **17:**159–166.

Corr, S. C., Y. Li, C. U. Riedel, P. W. O'Toole, C. Hill, and C. G. Gahan. 2007. Bacteriocin production as a mechanism for the antiinfective activity of *Lactobacillus salivarius* UCC118. *Proc. Natl. Acad. Sci. USA* **104:**7617–7621.

Dani, C., R. Biadaioli, G. Bertini, E. Martelli, and F. F. Rubaltelli. 2002. Probiotics feeding in prevention of urinary tract infection, bacterial sepsis and necrotizing enterocolitis in preterm infants. A prospective double-blind study. *Biol. Neonate* **82:**103–108.

Darouiche, R. O., J. I. Thornby, C. Cerra-Stewart, W. H. Donovan, and R. A. Hull. 2005. Bacterial interference for prevention of urinary tract infection: a prospective, randomized, placebo-controlled, double-blind pilot trial. *Clin. Infect. Dis.* **41:**1531–1534.

Dasgupta, M. K. 2002. Biofilms and infection in dialysis patients. *Semin. Dial.* **15:**338–346.

Donder, G. G., A. Vereecken, E. Bosmans, A. Dekeersmaecker, G. Salembier, and B. Spitz. 2002. Definition of a type of abnormal vaginal flora that is distinct from bacterial vaginosis: aerobic vaginitis. *BJOG* **109:**34–43.

Elwood, C., G. Reid, and J. Jass. 2006. Characterization of the interaction between uropathogenic *E. coli* and probiotic *Lactobacillus* through auto-inducer-2 signaling. MSc thesis. University of Western Ontario, London, Ontario, Canada.

Ernst, E. J., M. E. Ernst, J. D. Hoehns, and G. R. Bergus. 2005. Women's quality of life is decreased by acute cystitis and antibiotic adverse effects associated with treatment. *Health Qual. Life Outcomes* **3:**45.

Fallagas, M. E., G. I. Betsi, and S. Athanasiou. 2007. Probiotics for the treatment of women with bacterial vaginosis. *Clin. Microbiol. Infect.* **13:**657–664.

FAO/WHO. 2001. *Evaluation of Health and Nutritional Properties of Powder Milk and Live Lactic Acid Bacteria. Food and Agriculture Organization of the United Nations and World Health Organization Expert Consultation Report.* ftp://ftp.fao.org/docrep/fao/009/a0512e/a0512e00.pdf. (Accessed 6 May 2008.)

FAO/WHO. 2002. *Guidelines for the Evaluation of Probiotics in Food. Food and Agriculture Organization of the United Nations and World Health Organization Working Group Report.* ftp://ftp.fao.org/docrep/fao/009/a0512e/a0512e00.pdf. (Accessed 6 May 2008.)

Ferris, D. G., C. Dekle, and M. S. Litaker. 1996. Women's use of over-the-counter antifungal medications for gynecologic symptoms. *J. Fam. Pract.* **42:**595–600.

Forney, L. J., J. A. Foster, and W. Ledger. 2006. The vaginal flora of healthy women is not always dominated by *Lactobacillus* species. *J. Infect. Dis.* **194:**1468–1469.

Foxman, B., S. D. Manning, P. Tallman, R. Bauer, L. Zhang, J. S. Koopman, B. Gillespie, J. D. Sobel, and C. F. Marrs. 2002. Uropathogenic *Escherichia coli* are more likely than commensal *E. coli* to be shared between heterosexual sex partners. *Am. J. Epidemiol.* **156:**1133–1140.

Fredricks, D. N., T. L. Fiedler, and J. M. Marrazzo. 2005. Molecular identification of bacteria associated with bacterial vaginosis. *N. Engl. J. Med.* **353:**1899–1911.

Gan, B. S., J. Kim., G. Reid, P. Cadieux, and J. C. Howard. 2002. *Lactobacillus fermentum* RC-14 inhibits *Staphylococcus aureus* infection of surgical implants in rats. *J. Infect. Dis.* **185:**1369–1372.

Gardiner, G., C. Heinemann, M. L. Baroja, A. W. Bruce, D. Beuerman, J. Madrenas, and G. Reid. 2002. Oral administration of the probiotic combination *Lactobacillus rhamnosus* GR-1 and *L. fermentum* RC-14 for human intestinal applications. *Int. Dairy J.* **12:**191–196.

Gardner, H. L., and C. D. Dukes. 1954. New etiologic agent in nonspecific bacterial vaginitis. *Science* **120:**853.

Hatch, M., J. Cornelius, M. Allison, H. Sidhu, A. Peck, and R. W. Freel. 2006. *Oxalobacter* sp. reduces urinary oxalate excretion by promoting enteric oxalate secretion. *Kidney Int.* **69:**691–698.

Heinemann, C., J. E. van Hylckama Vlieg, D. B. Janssen, H. J. Busscher, H. C. van der Mei, and G. Reid. 2000. Purification and characterization of a surface-binding protein from *Lactobacillus fermentum* RC-14 inhibiting *Enterococcus faecalis* 1131 adhesion. *FEMS Microbiol. Lett.* **190:**177–180.

Hill, J. E., S. H. Goh, D. M. Money, M. Doyle, A. Li, W. L. Crosby, M. Links, A. Leung, D. Chan, and S. M. Hemmingsen. 2005. Characterization of vaginal microflora of healthy, nonpregnant women by chaperonin-60 sequence-based methods. *Am. J. Obstet. Gynecol.* **193**(3 Pt 1):682–692.

Howard, J., C. Heinemann, B. J. Thatcher, B. Martin, B. S. Gan, and G. Reid. 2000. Identification of collagen-binding proteins in *Lactobacillus* spp. with surface-enhanced laser desorption/ionization-time of flight ProteinChip technology. *Appl. Environ. Microbiol.* **66:**4396–4400.

Iannini, P., L. Mandell, J. Felmingham, G. Patou, and G. S. Tillotson. 2006. Adverse cutaneous reactions and drugs: a focus on antimicrobials. *J. Chemother.* **18:**127–139.

Jahic, M., M. Nurkic, and Z. Fatusic. 2006. Association of the pH change of vaginal environment in bacterial vaginosis with presence of *Enterococcus faecalis* in vagina. *Med. Arh.* **60:**364–368.

Jin, L., L. Tao, S. I. Pavlova, J. S. So, N. Kiwanuka, Z. Namukwaya, B. A. Saberbein, and M. Wawer. 2007. Species diversity and relative abundance of vaginal lactic acid bacteria from women in Uganda and Korea. *J. Appl. Microbiol.* **102:**1107–1115.

Kelly, M. C., M. J. Mequio, and V. Pybus. 2003. Inhibition of vaginal lactobacilli by a bacteriocin-like inhibitor produced by *Enterococcus faecium* 62–6: potential significance for bacterial vaginosis. *Infect. Dis. Obstet. Gynecol.* **11**:147–156.

Kim, S. O., H. I. Sheik, S.-D. Ha, A. Martins, and G. Reid. 2006. G-CSF mediated inhibition of JNK is a key mechanism for *Lactobacillus rhamnosus*-induced anti-inflammatory effects in macrophages. *Cell. Microbiol.* **8**:1958–1971.

Kirjavainen, P. K., R. M. Laine, D. Carter, J.-A. Hammond, and G. Reid. Expression of anti-microbial defense factors in vaginal mucosa following exposure to *Lactobacillus rhamnosus* GR-1. *Int. J. Probiot.*, in press.

Klebanoff, M. A., J. R. Schwebke, J. Zhang, T. R. Nansel, K. F. Yu, and W. W. Andrews. 2004. Vulvovaginal symptoms in women with bacterial vaginosis. *Obstet. Gynecol.* **104**:267–272.

Klotz, S. A., N. K. Gaur, R. De Armond, D. Sheppard, N. Khardori, J. E. Edwards, Jr., P. N. Lipke, and M. El-Azizi. 2007. *Candida albicans* Als proteins mediate aggregation with bacteria and yeasts. *Med. Mycol.* **45**:363–370.

Koehler, G., and G. Reid. 2006. Mechanisms of probiotic interference with *Candida albicans*, abstr. C126. Abstr. 8th *ASM Conf. Candida Candidiasis.* American Society for Microbiology, Washington, DC.

Kontiokari, T., K. Sundqvist, M. Nuutinen, T. Pokka, M. Koskela, and M. Uhari. 2001. Randomised trial of cranberry-lingonberry juice and *Lactobacillus* GG drink for the prevention of urinary tract infections in women. *BMJ* **322**:1571.

Lee, S. J., Y. H. Shim, S. J. Cho, and J. W. Lee. 2007. Probiotics prophylaxis in children with persistent primary vesicoureteral reflux. *Pediatr. Nephrol.* **22**:1315–1320.

Lieske, J. C., D. S. Goldfarb, C. De Simone, and C. Regnier. 2005. Use of a probiotic to decrease enteric hyperoxaluria. *Kidney Int.* **68**:1244–1249.

Lima, K. C., L. R. Fava, and J. F. Siqueira, Jr. 2001. Susceptibilities of *Enterococcus faecalis* biofilms to some antimicrobial medications. *J. Endod.* **27**:616–619.

Lloyd, A. L., D. A. Rasko, and H. L. Mobley. 2007. Defining genomic islands and uropathogen-specific genes in uropathogenic *Escherichia coli. J. Bacteriol.* **189**:3532–3546.

Lowe, N. K., and N. A. Ryan-Wenger. 2003. Military women's risk factors for and symptoms of genitourinary infections during deployment. *Mil. Med.* **168**:569–574.

Marrazzo, J. M., R. L. Cook, H. C. Wiesenfeld, P. J. Murray, B. Busse, M. Krohn, and S. L. Hillier. 2006. Women's satisfaction with an intravaginal *Lactobacillus* capsule for the treatment of bacterial vaginosis. *J. Womens Health (Larchmt)* **15**:1053–1060.

Marrazzo, J. M., L. A. Koutsky, D. A. Eschenbach, K. Agnew, K. Stine, and S. L. Hillier. 2002. Characterization of vaginal flora and bacterial vaginosis in women who have sex with women. *J. Infect. Dis.* **185**:1307–1313.

Marrs, C. F., L. Zhang, and B. Foxman. 2005. *Escherichia coli* mediated urinary tract infections: are there distinct uropathogenic *E. coli* (UPEC) pathotypes? *FEMS Microbiol. Lett.* **252**:183–190.

Martin, R., M. Olivares, M. L. Marin, L. Fernandez, J. Xaus, and J. M. Rodriguez. 2005. Probiotic potential of 3 lactobacilli strains isolated from breast milk. *J. Hum. Lact.* **21**:8–17.

Mayer, R. 2007. Interstitial cystitis pathogenesis and treatment. *Curr. Opin. Infect. Dis.* **20**:77–82.

McGroarty, J. A., and G. Reid. 1988a. Detection of a lactobacillus substance which inhibits *Escherichia coli. Can. J. Microbiol.* **34**:974–978.

McGroarty, J. A., and G. Reid. 1988b. Inhibition of enterococci by *Lactobacillus* species *in vitro. Microb. Ecol. Health Dis.* **1**:215–219.

McGroarty, J. A., L. Tomeczek, D. G. Pond, G. Reid, and A. W. Bruce. 1992. Hydrogen peroxide production by *Lactobacillus* species, correlation with susceptibility to the spermicidal compound nonoxynol-9. *J. Infect. Dis.* **165**: 1142–1144.

Morelli, L., D. Zonenenschain, M. Del Piano, and P. Cognein. 2004. Utilization of the intestinal tract as a delivery system for urogenital probiotics. *J. Clin. Gastroenterol.* **38** (6 Suppl.):S107–S110.

Ness, R. B., K. E. Kip, D. E. Soper, S. Hillier, C. A. Stamm, R. L. Sweet, P. Rice, and H. E. Richter. 2005. Bacterial vaginosis (BV) and the risk of incident gonococcal or chlamydial genital infection in a predominantly black population. *Sex. Transm. Dis.* **32**:413–417.

Newman, D. 1915. The treatment of cystitis by intravesical injections of lactic *Bacillus* cultures. *Lancet* **August 14**:330–332.

Nugent, R. P., M. A. Krohn, and S. L. Hillier. 1991. Reliability of diagnosing bacterial vaginosis is improved by a standardized method of gram stain interpretation. *J. Clin. Microbiol.* **29**:297–301.

Okawa, T., H. Niibe, T. Arai, K. Sekiba, K. Noda, S. Takeuchi, S. Hashimoto, and N. Ogawa. 1993. Effect of LC9018 combined with radiation therapy on carcinoma of the uterine cervix. A phase III, multicenter, randomized, controlled study. *Cancer* **72**:1949–1954.

Ombrella, A. M., A. Belmonte, M. G. Nogueras, I. R. Abad, E. G. Sutich, and D. G. Dlugovitzky. 2006. Sialidase activity in women with bacterial vaginosis. *Medicina (Buenos Aires)* **66**:131–134.

Onrust, S. V., H. M. Lamb, and J. A. Balfour. 1998. Ofloxacin. A reappraisal of its use in the management of genitourinary tract infections. *Drugs* **56**:895–928.

Patel, V., H. A. Weiss, B. R. Kirkwood, S. Pednekar, P. Nevrekar, S. Gupte, and D. Mabey. 2006. Common genital complaints in women: the contribution of psychosocial and infectious factors in a population-based cohort study in Goa, India. *Int. J. Epidemiol.* **35**:1478–1485.

Pelucchi, C., C. Bosetti, E. Negri, M. Malvezzi, and C. La Vecchia. 2006. Mechanisms of disease: the epidemiology of bladder cancer. *Nat. Clin. Pract. Urol.* **3**:327–340.

Perez, P. F., J. Dorè, M. Leclerc, F. Levenez, J. Benyacoub, P. Serrant, I. Segura-Roggero, E. J. Schiffrin, and A. Donnet-Hughes. 2007. Bacterial imprinting of the neonatal immune system: lessons from maternal cells? *Pediatrics* **119**:e724–e732.

Rafal'skii, V. V. 2000. Drug reactions on antibiotics used in the treatment of urinary tract infections. *Urologiia* **6**:51–55.

Reid, G., D. Beuerman, C. Heinemann, and A. W. Bruce. 2001a. Probiotic *Lactobacillus* dose required to restore and maintain a normal vaginal flora. *FEMS Immunol. Med. Microbiol.* **32**:37–41.

Reid, G., A. W. Bruce, N. Fraser, C. Heinemann, J. Owen, and B. Henning. 2001b. Oral probiotics can resolve urogenital infections. *FEMS Immunol. Med. Microbiol.* **30**:49–52.

Reid, G., A. W. Bruce, and M. Taylor. 1992a. Influence of three day antimicrobial therapy and *Lactobacillus* suppositories on recurrence of urinary tract infection. *Clin. Ther.* **14:**11–16.

Reid, G., A. W. Bruce, and M. Taylor. 1995. Instillation of *Lactobacillus* and stimulation of indigenous organisms to prevent recurrence of urinary tract infections. *Microecol. Ther.* **23:**32–45.

Reid, G., J. Burton, J.-A. Hammond, and A. W. Bruce. 2004. Nucleic acid based diagnosis of bacterial vaginosis and improved management using probiotic lactobacilli. *J. Med. Food* **7:**223–228.

Reid, G., D. Charbonneau, J. Erb, B. Kochanowski, D. Beuerman, R. Poehner, and A. W. Bruce. 2003a. Oral use of *Lactobacillus rhamnosus* GR-1 and *L. fermentum* RC-14 significantly alters vaginal flora: randomized, placebo-controlled trial in 64 healthy women. *FEMS Immunol. Med. Microbiol.* **35:**131–134.

Reid, G., D. Charbonneau, S. Gonzalez, G. Gardiner, J. Erb, and A. W. Bruce. 2002. Ability of *Lactobacillus* GR-1 and RC-14 to stimulate host defences and reduce gut translocation and infectivity of *Salmonella typhimurium*. *Nutraceut. Food* **7:**168–173.

Reid, G., R. L. Cook, and A. W. Bruce. 1987. Examination of strains of lactobacilli for properties which may influence bacterial interference in the urinary tract. *J. Urol.* **138:**330–335.

Reid, G., P. L. Cuperus, A. W. Bruce, L. Tomeczek, H. C. van der Mei, A. H. Khoury, and H. J. Busscher. 1992b. Comparison of contact angles and adhesion to hexadecane of urogenital, dairy and poultry lactobacilli: effect of serial culture passages. *Appl. Environ. Microbiol.* **58:**1549–1553.

Reid, G., J.-A. Hammond, and A. W. Bruce. 2003b. Effect of lactobacilli oral supplement on the vaginal microflora of antibiotic treated patients: randomized, placebo-controlled study. *Nutraceut. Food* **8:**145–148.

Reid, G., J. A. McGroarty, P. A. G. Domingue, A. W. Chow, A. W. Bruce, A. Eisen, and J. W. Costerton. 1990. Coaggregation of urogenital bacteria *in vitro* and *in vivo*. *Curr. Microbiol.* **20:**47–52.

Reid, G., M. L. Zorzitto, A. W. Bruce, M. A. S. Jewett, R. C. Y. Chan, and J. W. Costerton. 1984. The pathogenesis of urinary tract infection in the elderly: the role of bacterial adherence to uroepithelial cells. *Curr. Microbiol.* **11:**67–72.

Saunders, S. G., A. Bocking, J. Challis, and G. Reid. 2007. Disruption of *Gardnerella vaginalis* biofilms by *Lactobacillus*. *Coll. Surf. B* **55:**138–142.

Scelo, G., and P. Brennan. 2007. The epidemiology of bladder and kidney cancer. *Nat. Clin. Pract. Urol.* **4:**205–217.

Schwebke, J. R., and R. Desmond. 2007. A randomized trial of metronidazole in asymptomatic bacterial vaginosis to prevent the acquisition of sexually transmitted diseases. *Am. J. Obstet. Gynecol.* **196:**517.e1–6.

Schwiertz, A., D. Taras, K. Rusch, and V. Rusch. 2006. Throwing the dice for the diagnosis of vaginal complaints? *Ann. Clin. Microbiol. Antimicrob.* **5:**4.

Sewankambo, N., R. H. Gray, M. J. Wawer, L. Paxton, D. McNaim, F. Wabwire-Mangen, D. Serwadda, C. Li, N. Kiwanuka, S. L. Hillier, L. Rabe, C. A. Gaydos, T. C.

Quinn, and J. Konde-Lule. 1997. HIV-1 infection associated with abnormal vaginal flora morphology and bacterial vaginosis. *Lancet* **350:**546–550.

Sha, B. E., H. Y. Chen, Q. J. Wang, M. R. Zariffard, M. H. Cohen, and G. T. Spear. 2005. Utility of Amsel criteria, Nugent score, and quantitative PCR for *Gardnerella vaginalis*, *Mycoplasma hominis*, and *Lactobacillus* spp. for diagnosis of bacterial vaginosis in human immunodeficiency virus-infected women. *J. Clin. Microbiol.* **43:**4607–4612.

Sihvo, S., R. Ahonen, H. Mikander, and E. Hemminki. 2000. Self-medication with vaginal antifungal drugs: physicians' experiences and women's utilization patterns. *Fam. Pract.* **17:**145–149.

Spiegel, C. A. 1991. Bacterial vaginosis. *Clin. Microbiol. Rev.* **4:**485–502.

Stoyancheva, G. D., S. T. Danova, and I. Y. Boudakov. 2006. Molecular identification of vaginal lactobacilli isolated from Bulgarian women. *Antonie Leeuwenhoek* **90:**201–210.

Sumeksri, P., C. Koprasert, and S. Panichkul. 2005. BVBLUE test for diagnosis of bacterial vaginosis in pregnant women attending antenatal care at Phramongkutklao Hospital. *J. Med. Assoc. Thai.* **88**(Suppl. 3):S7–S13.

Tendolkar, P. M., A. S. Baghdayan, and N. Shankar. 2003. Pathogenic enterococci: new developments in the 21st century. *Cell. Mol. Life Sci.* **60:**2622–2636.

Thanavuth, A., A. Chalermchockcharoenkit, D. Boriboonhirunsarn, R. Sirisomboon, and K. Pimol. 2007. Prevalence of bacterial vaginosis in Thai pregnant women with preterm labor in Siriraj hospital. *J. Med. Assoc. Thai.* **90:**437–441.

Theoharides, T. C. 2007. Treatment approaches for painful bladder syndrome/interstitial cystitis. *Drugs* **67:**215–235.

Thies, F. L., W. Konig, and B. Konig. 2007. Rapid characterization of the normal and disturbed vaginal microbiota by application of 16S rRNA gene terminal RFLP fingerprinting. *J. Med. Microbiol.* **56**(Pt. 6):755–761.

Tomeczek, L., G. Reid, P. L. Cuperus, J. A. McGroarty, H. C. van der Mei, A. W. Bruce, A. H. Khoury, and H. J. Busscher. 1992. Correlation between hydrophobicity and resistance to nonoxynol-9 and vancomycin for urogenital isolates of lactobacilli. *FEMS Microbiol. Lett.* **94:**101–104.

Uehara, S., K. Monden, K. Nomoto, Y. Seno, R. Kariyama, and H. Kumon. 2006. A pilot study evaluating the safety and effectiveness of *Lactobacillus* vaginal suppositories in patients with recurrent urinary tract infection. *Int. J. Antimicrob. Agents* **28**(Suppl. 1):S30–S34.

Vasquez, A., T. Jakobsson, S. Ahrne, U. Forsum, and G. Molin. 2002. Vaginal *Lactobacillus* flora of healthy Swedish women. *J. Clin. Microbiol.* **40:**2746–2749.

Velraeds, M. M., van de Belt-Gritter, H. C. van der Mei, G. Reid, and H. J. Busscher. 1998. Interference in initial adhesion of uropathogenic bacteria and yeasts to silicone rubber by a *Lactobacillus acidophilus* biosurfactant. *J. Med. Microbiol.* **47:**1081–1085.

Velraeds, M. M., H. C. van der Mei, G. Reid, and H. J. Busscher. 1996. Inhibition of initial adhesion of uropathogenic *Enterococcus faecalis* by biosurfactants from *Lactobacillus* isolates. *Appl. Environ. Microbiol.* **62:**1958–1963.

von Graevenitz, A. 1982. Pathogenicity of enterococci outside of urinary tract and blood stream. *Klin. Wochenschr.* 60:696–698.

Wheeler, C. M. 2007. Advances in primary and secondary interventions for cervical cancer: human papillomavirus prophylactic vaccines and testing. *Nat. Clin. Pract. Oncol.* 4:224–235.

WHO. 1946. Constitution of the World Health Organization, Geneva, 1946. http://www.who.int/about/definition/en/print.html. Accessed 30 October 2006.

Yeganegi, M., G. Reid, J. R. G. Challis, and A. Bocking. 2007. Lactobacilli supernatant inhibits TNFα production and COX2 expression in LPS-activated placental trophoblasts, abstr. 55, p. 20. Abstr. 2007 *SGI Annu. Sci. Mtg.*

Yoon, S. S., and D. J. Hassett. 2004. Chronic *Pseudomonas aeruginosa* infection in cystic fibrosis airway disease: metabolic changes that unravel novel drug targets. *Expert Rev. Anti Infect. Ther.* 2:611–623.

Zarate, G., and M. E. Nader-Macias. 2006. Influence of probiotic vaginal lactobacilli on *in vitro* adhesion of urogenital pathogens to vaginal epithelial cells. *Lett. Appl. Microbiol.* 43:174–180.

Zhong, W., K. Millsap, H. Bialkowska-Hobrzanska, and G. Reid. 1998. Differentiation of *Lactobacillus* species by molecular typing. *Appl. Environ. Microbiol.* 64:2418–2423.

Therapeutic Microbiology: Probiotics and Related Strategies
Edited by J. Versalovic and M. Wilson
© 2008 ASM Press, Washington, DC

Paul Forsythe
John Bienenstock

22

Probiotics in Neurology and Psychiatry

Probiotics are live nonpathogenic organisms that promote beneficial health effects when ingested (Reid et al., 2003). Organisms used as probiotics are generally commensal bacteria that exist naturally in the gut and are most frequently of the *Lactobacillus* or *Bifidobacterium* species. Strong evidence supports a therapeutic role for probiotics in the treatment of inflammatory bowel disease. Randomized controlled trials of probiotics have proved successful in patients with chronic pouchitis and irritable bowel syndrome (IBS) (Gionchetti et al., 2003; McCarthy et al., 2003). Increasing numbers of reports indicate that probiotics may have therapeutic potential in disorders ranging from atopic dermatitis to arthritis (Baharav et al., 2004; Kalliomaki et al., 2001, 2003), highlighting the systemic impact of these organisms. While probiotics have been proposed as adjuvant therapy for depression (Logan and Katzman, 2005), to date little is known of the ability of probiotic treatment to modulate brain function. However, as is outlined below, pathways do exist that allow microorganisms in the gut to communicate with the central nervous system (CNS).

BRAIN-GUT-MICROBIOTA AXIS

The brain and the gut are engaged in constant bidirectional communication. Such communication becomes apparent when alterations in gastrointestinal (GI) function are communicated to the brain, bringing about the perception of visceral events such as nausea, satiety, and pain or when, in turn, stressful experiences lead to altered GI secretions and motility (Drossman, 1998). This communication system involves neural pathways as well as immune and endocrine mechanisms.

It is becoming increasingly clear that when considering the gut and its interactions with other body systems, including the brain, we must also consider the contribution of the intestinal microbiota. The human intestine is more densely populated with microbes than any other organ, with 10^{14} bacteria inhabiting the GI tract of adult humans (Borrielo, 2002). The metabolic capacity of the gut microbiota is greater than that of the liver, and the collective microbial genome, termed the microbiome, has coding capacity that vastly exceeds that of the human genome (Backhed et al., 2005). It is therefore not surprising that the gut microbiota impacts a range of

Paul Forsythe and John Bienenstock, The Brain-Body Institute and Department of Pathology and Molecular Medicine, McMaster University, and St. Joseph's Healthcare Hamilton, Ontario, Canada.

host physiological systems and plays a principal role in postnatal maturation of the mammalian immune system (Hooper et al., 2001). The GI tract is thus a point of interaction between microorganisms, the body's largest concentration of immune cells, and a vast network of over 100 million neurons. It is clear that, in addition to bidirectional communication between the brain and GI tract, cross talk likely occurs between the brain and the gut microbiota (Fig. 1).

In this respect, *Lactobacillus* and *Bifidobacterium* seem particularly sensitive to signals from the CNS. Lower levels of lactobacilli have been correlated with the display of stress-indicative behaviors in animals. Studies with nonhuman primates have shown that maternal stress during pregnancy can result in a reduction of both lactobacilli and bifidobacteria in offspring relative to controls (Bailey and Coe, 1999; Bailey et al., 2004), and measures of infant independence are correlated with concentrations of total anaerobes, lactobacilli, and *Bifidobacterium* (Bailey and Coe, 1999). Restraint stress and excessive physical demands can also lead to decreases in these organisms in the GI tract (Lizko, 1987). Evidence from human studies indicates that stress can negatively affect the gut microbiota (Holdeman et al., 1976; Lizko, 1991; Moore et al., 1978). Emotional stress can result in acute and long-term reductions in lactobacilli and bifidobacteria (Holdeman et al., 1976; Moore et al., 1978). These changes in the GI microbiota may be a result of changes in gut motility or GI acidity and/or the direct effects of neurochemicals such as norepinephrine.

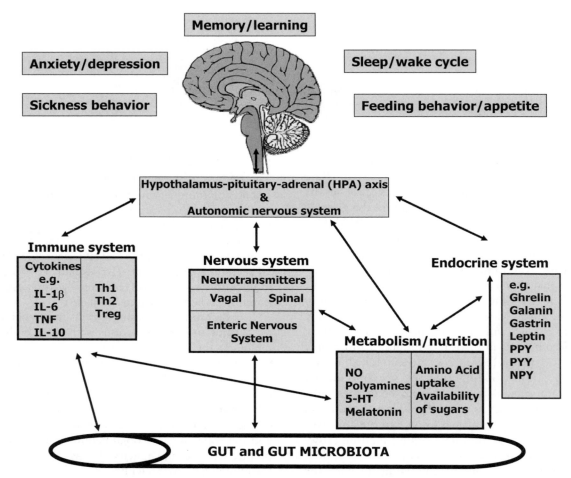

Figure 1 The brain-gut-microbiota axis. Gut microbiota organisms are in intimate contact with the immune and nervous systems of the host. Microorganisms alter the metabolic profiles and nutrient content of the gut, which may influence neuroendocrine responses. Commensal organisms, pathogens, and probiotics have the potential to influence major communication routes between the gut and brain. See the text for details.

For example, in *Escherichia coli* O157:H7, the QseC sensor kinase is a bacterial receptor for the host epinephrine/norepinephrine. This signaling activates transcription of virulence genes in the bacteria and can be blocked specifically by adrenergic antagonists (Clarke et al., 2006).

Just as microorganisms are responsive to the host's neuroendocrine environment, conversely, bacteria can influence the neuroendocrine environment by the production of various biologically active peptides and neurotransmitters such as nitric oxide (NO), melatonin, gamma-aminobutyric acid, and serotonin (Iyer et al., 2004). For example, lactobacilli converted nitrate to NO, a potent regulator of both the immune and nervous systems (Sobko et al., 2006). NO levels in the small intestine and the cecum were three- to eightfold higher in rats that had been fed live lactobacilli and nitrate than in controls. In addition, hydrogen sulfide (H_2S) that is produced by constituents of the gut microbiota has been shown to modulate gut motility through action at the vanilloid receptor TRPV1 in capsaicin-sensitive nerve fibers (Schicho et al., 2006).

THE IMMUNE SYSTEM AND MOOD DISORDERS

Consistent observations have suggested that patients with major depression who are otherwise healthy have activated inflammatory pathways, as indicated by increased proinflammatory cytokines, increased acute-phase proteins, and greater expression of chemokines and adhesion molecules (Alesci et al., 2005; Kahl et al., 2005; Maes et al., 1997; Maes, 1999; Miller et al., 2002; Musselman et al., 2001; Sluzewska et al., 1995). The most common observations are increased serum and/or plasma concentrations of interleukin (IL)-6, C-reactive protein, IL-1β, and tumor necrosis factor (TNF). In addition, positive correlations between concentrations of various inflammatory mediators in plasma and depressive symptom severity have been reported (Alesci et al., 2005; Miller et al., 2002).

Anti-inflammatory cytokines (IL-1, IL-4, IL-10, and transforming growth factor β1 [TGF-β1]) can antagonize the actions of proinflammatory cytokines. All major classes of antidepressants can increase the release of anti-inflammatory cytokines while suppressing proinflammatory cytokine production, and such actions may contribute to the therapeutic efficacy of these drugs (Maes, 2001). Indeed, recent data indicate that the antidepressant-like effects of desipramine in the forced swim test (FST) (an animal model frequently used to evaluate antidepressant efficacy) depend on the ability of the drug to inhibit production of TNF in the CNS (Reynolds et al., 2004).

In humans, a variety of antidepressant strategies (including medication, electroconvulsive shock therapy, and psychotherapy) also appear to attenuate inflammatory activity in concert with improvements in depressive symptoms, suggesting that reductions in inflammation might contribute to treatment response (Frommberger et al., 1997; Hestad et al., 2003; Tuglu et al., 2003). Interestingly, a recent study (O'Brien et al., 2007) demonstrated that proinflammatory cytokine levels are not suppressed in depressed patients who are resistant to selective serotonin reuptake inhibitor treatment, suggesting that this may be an important component of clinical recovery.

Certain cytokines (alpha interferon [IFN-α], IFN-β, IFN-γ, and IL-2) are commonly used in the treatment of medical conditions including hepatitis C, multiple sclerosis, and leukemia. Each of these cytokines has been reported to produce side effects such as fatigue and confusion. Similarly, endotoxin and IL-1 administration to animals results in so-called sickness behaviors such as hypomotility, hypophagia, hyperalgesia, and a diminished interest in exploring the environment (Capuron and Dantzer, 2003; Schiepers et al., 2005). These cytokine-induced behavioral changes are associated with alterations in brain chemistry consistent with the pathophysiology of depression. In depression, the metabolism of serotonin, norepinephrine, and dopamine is altered in brain regions essential to the regulation of emotion, including the limbic system (amygdala, hippocampus, and nucleus accumbens), as well as the regulation of psychomotor function and reward, including the basal ganglia (Dunn et al., 1999; Gao et al., 2002).

In addition to the effects of inflammatory cytokines on mood and behavior, a number of studies have found that the ability to cope with neurodegenerative conditions depends on autoreactive CD4$^+$ T-cell function, indicating a link between brain maintenance and peripheral adaptive immunity (Moalem et al., 1999; Kipnis et al., 2001; Yoles et al., 2001). Recently, it was demonstrated that a deficit in peripheral T cells in mice can lead to cognitive and behavioral impairments that were repaired by T-cell restoration (Kipnis et al., 2004). Furthermore, in mice with an intact immune system, boosting autoreactive T-cell function could attenuate the behavioral and cognitive abnormalities that accompanied the neurotransmitter imbalance induced by psychotomimetic drugs. These studies highlight the importance of properly functioning adaptive immunity in the maintenance of mental activity and in coping with conditions leading to cognitive deficits. Such findings may also explain why the elderly, who are known to suffer from declining immune function (Linton and Dorshkind, 2004), also have an increased burden of dementia (Wick et al., 2003).

Commensal bacteria profoundly influence the development of humoral components of the gut mucosal immune system (Weinstein and Cebra, 1991) and also modulate the fine-tuning of T-cell repertoires and T-helper (Th)-cell type 1 or type 2 cytokine profiles (Cebra, 1999; Shanahan, 2002). Thus, it is possible that the composition of the colonizing microbiota influences interindividual variation in immunity.

The immunomodulatory actions of probiotics are well documented (Braat et al., 2004; Ghosh et al., 2004; Hart et al., 2004), and given the potentially important role of cytokines in mood disorders, it is possible that they may influence brain function by their effects on the immune system. While most of the research on probiotics and cytokine production has focused on local GI effects, evidence of systemic effects has been documented and various strains of probiotics have been shown to attenuate IL-1β, TNF, IL-6, and IFN-γ in the periphery (Braat et al., 2004). Oral administration of a *Lactobacillus* species can inhibit allergic inflammation of the airway, highlighting the abilities of these organisms to induce systemic immunomodulation.

However, evidence suggests that probiotics play a paradoxical role in immune regulation and, dependent on the strain of organism, can mediate general immunostimulatory responses or tolerogenic responses. In an extensive study of this issue, Maassen et al. (Maassen et al., 1998) analyzed eight different common *Lactobacillus* strains with respect to gut mucosal induction of pro- and anti-inflammatory cytokines in mice in response to a parenterally administered antigen. *Lactobacillus casei* tended to induce the production of IL-10 and TGF-β. IL-10 and TGF-β have immunosuppressive effects on Th1 cells and are thought to be involved in oral tolerance. In contrast, individual strains of species *Lactobacillus reuteri* and *Lactobacillus brevis* induced several proinflammatory and/or Th1 cytokines IL-1β, IL-2, and TNF but not anti-inflammatory or Th2 cytokines such as IL-10 and IL-4. These same strains were able to significantly enhance systemic antibody responses to the antigen. In addition, the capacity of lactobacilli to variably induce maturation and the cytokine profile expressed by dendritic cells (Christensen et al., 2002; Smits et al., 2005) indicates that species of probiotics may differentially determine whether dendritic cells drive Th1, Th2, or regulatory T-cell responses. These findings also open the possibility that the ability of probiotics to influence T-cell development and function is another mechanism through which these microbes could contribute to behavioral or mood changes. It is clear that realizing the true potential of probiotic-induced immunomodulation to treat mood and/or cognitive disorders will require both a greater understanding of the nature of immune disturbances that contribute to such disorders and the mechanisms behind the quantitative and qualitative differences in immune regulation that exist among probiotic organisms.

STRESS RESPONSE SYSTEMS

Psychological stress is a common risk factor for the development of major depression and an identifiable stressor precedes most initial episodes of major depression (Kendler et al., 2000). Furthermore, hyperactivity of one of the body's major stress response systems, the hypothalamic-pituitary-adrenal (HPA) axis, has been found in some psychiatric disorders, especially in older patients with severe depression. This hyperactivity may be due to altered feedback inhibition, as demonstrated by increased circulating cortisol and nonsuppression of cortisol following administration of dexamethasone. Two glucocorticoid receptors control the HPA axis, the mineralocorticoid receptor (MR) and the glucocorticoid receptor (GR). MR regulates normal HPA fluctuations, and the GR regulates in times of stress. Long-term antidepressant treatment in humans has been shown to up-regulate both GR and MR in the brain. Chronic antidepressant treatment in rodents has been shown to reduce HPA activity, even in the absence of GR or MR up-regulation. Such studies suggest that the relationship between the state of the HPA axis and depression may, at least in part, be causal.

As discussed previously, psychological stress is known to alter the gut microbial composition of both animals and humans and, in particular, induces a reduction in *Lactobacillus* and *Bifidobacterium* populations (Bailey and Coe, 1999; Bailey et al., 2004; Holdeman et al., 1976; Lizko, 1991; Moore et al., 1978). Conversely, while there have been no reports of the action of probiotics on physiological stress responses in conventional animals, commensal microbiota are known to regulate postnatal development of the HPA axis (Sudo et al., 2004). Germfree animals have an exaggerated HPA activation in response to stress. This hyperresponsiveness can be reversed by reconstitution with feces from animals kept in a pathogen-free environment or with *Bifidobacterium infantis* (Sudo et al., 2004). In contrast, monoassociation with an enteropathogenic *E. coli* strain further enhances the response to stress. Moreover, GF mice also exhibited reduced brain-derived neurotrophic factor expression levels in the cortex and hippocampus relative to conventional mice (Sudo et al., 2004). This finding is of particular interest because several reports demonstrated that levels of brain-derived neurotrophic factor in serum were significantly decreased in the plasma of depressed patients (Karege et al., 2002; Shimizu et al., 2003) and in the postmortem hippocampal tissue of individuals who committed depression-related suicide (Chen et al., 2001;

Dwivedi et al., 2003; Karege et al., 2005). It is therefore plausible that changes in the gut microbiota or exposure to probiotic commensals may alter the HPA axis or other stress response systems and, in turn, modulate stress-related mood or behavioral disorders. In support of this concept, Lowry et al. (Lowry et al., 2007) recently demonstrated that peripheral immune activation with the nonpathogenic bacterium *Mycobacterium vaccae* activated a specific subset of serotonergic neurons in the dorsal raphe nucleus of mice. These effects were associated with increases in serotonin metabolism within the ventromedial prefrontal cortex, suggesting immune activation of the mesolimbocortical serotonergic system thought to play a role in coping with stressors. In keeping with this finding, *M. vaccae* administration was also associated with decreased immobility in the FST, indicating a change in stress-related behavior similar to that observed following treatment with established antidepressants.

THE VAGUS NERVE AND PARASYMPATHETIC NERVOUS SYSTEM

Neural information from the heart, lungs, pancreas, liver, stomach, and intestines is delivered tonically to the brain via sensory fibers in the vagus nerve (Browning and Mendelowitz, 2003; Chang et al., 2003). Sensory vagal inputs arrive in the nucleus of the solitary tract, from where they are transmitted to widespread areas of the CNS, ranging from the medulla oblongata to the cerebral cortex. Neurons of the rostral ventrolateral medulla oblongata provide one of two major sources of afferent inputs to the locus ceruleus (Aston-Jones et al., 1986), which in turn has projections to widespread areas of the cortex that are associated with stress-related behavior and affective disorders. The locus ceruleus is also considered to be one of the main sites for integrating stress responses (Aston-Jones et al., 1996). During repeated activation, a powerful feed-forward system between the noradrenergic locus ceruleus neurons and areas of the forebrain that produce corticotropin-releasing factor can lead to generation of augmented behavioral responses (Ziegler et al., 1999). Sustained activation of this system induces changes in neuronal activity that underlie anxiety, panic disorders, and chronic depression (Arborelius et al., 1999). The role of visceral sensory input in physiological or pathological modulation of perception was only recently recognized. Previous studies have concentrated on the modulation of responses directly relevant to a given sensory input (e.g., hunger to feeding, stomach movements to nausea), but visceral sensory inputs have now been linked to long-term and possible pathological modulation of behavioral patterns (Zagon, 2001).

Some experimental data suggest that changes in visceral sensation can affect the perception and interpretation of external inputs (Crucian et al., 2000), leading to the suggestion that altered sensory vagal inputs can influence our attitude to the outside world and that pathological changes in sensory vagal inputs may increase the risk of affective behavioral disorders. It has been proposed that chronic sensory vagal inputs could act as natural breaks for augmentation of stress-related behavioral responses via tonic modulation of the neuronal activity in the locus ceruleus and the forebrain (Zagon, 2001).

Vagal stimulation is accepted by the FDA in the United States as an alternative treatment for intractable depression and has also been used successfully in the treatment of refractory epilepsy, demonstrating clear behavioral effects of modulating afferent signals (Walsh and Kling, 2004). Evidence from animal studies suggests that gut microorganisms can directly activate the vagus and other neural pathways. Subdiaphragmatic vagotomy attenuates c-fos expression in the paraventricular nucleus of the hypothalamus in rats inoculated with *Salmonella enterica* serovar Typhimurium (Wang et al., 2002), and studies indicate that GI microorganisms can directly activate neural pathways even in the absence of a detectable immune response (Goehler et al., 2005). Orally administered *Campylobacter jejuni*, in subclinical doses too low to elicit immune activation, can result in anxiety-provoking effects in mice. In addition, *C. jejuni* can activate visceral sensory nuclei in the brain stem when bacterial counts are too low to activate an immune response. Areas of brain stem activation, the nucleus of the solitary tract and lateral parabrachial nucleus, participate in neural information processing that ultimately leads to autonomic neuroendocrine and behavioral responses (Goehler et al., 2005).

Evidence of neurophysiological effects of probiotics has been reported, as treatment with *L. reuteri* can inhibit the constitutive cardioautonomic response to colorectal distension in rats through effects on enteric nerves (Kamiya et al., 2006). These bacteria also significantly decreased dorsal root ganglion single unit activity to distension. More recently the ability of this *L. reuteri* strain to inhibit a specific ion channel in enteric neurons has been identified (Kunze et al., 2007). Therefore, in addition to modulating the immunoendocrine environment, probiotics may communicate with the brain through direct interactions with the nervous system.

GUT ENDOCRINOLOGY

In addition to direct neural pathways, the gut also communicates to the brain utilizing hormonal signaling pathways that involve the release of gut peptides from enteroendocrine cells which can act directly on the brain at the area postrema, one of the circumventricular organs that lie outside the blood-brain barrier. These gut peptides include orexin, galanin, ghrelin, gastrin, and leptin. While these gut peptides are primarily identified for their role in modulating feeding behavior and energy homeostasis, they have also been linked with changes in the sleep-wake cycle, sexual behavior, arousal, and anxiety (Cameron and Doucet, 2007; Wren and Bloom, 2007).

Galanin stimulates the activity of the central branch of the HPA axis (i.e., the release of corticotropin-releasing hormone and adrenocorticotropin), thereby enhancing glucocorticoid secretion from the adrenal cortex. This peptide can also directly stimulate glucocorticoid secretion from adrenocortical cells and norepinephrine release from adrenal medulla (Tortorella et al., 2007; Wrenn and Holmes, 2006). Evidence suggests that galanin plays a role in the modulation of the HPA axis response to stress and, considering the well-established deleterious effects of galanin on cognitive function, may act as a novel link between stress, anxiety, and memory (Robinson, 2004; Rustay et al., 2005; Wrenn et al., 2004). This potential link has led to suggestions that drugs targeting the galaninergic system could provide a novel therapeutic option for psychopathologies, such as posttraumatic stress syndrome (Wrenn and Holmes, 2006). Similarly, ghrelin, which acts in the brain to mediate anxiogenesis and increase memory retention (Carlini et al., 2004), possesses a marked adrenocorticotropin/cortisol-releasing effect in humans and is probably involved in the modulation of the HPA response to stress and nutritional/metabolic variation (Giordano et al., 2004, 2006; Jaszberenyi et al., 2006). Studies with mice deficient in another gut hormone, gastrin, found that mutant animals displayed increased anxiety-like behavior compared to wild-type mice, indicating that normal circulating levels of gastrin may play a role in the regulation of locomotor activity and anxiety-like behavior (Wada et al., 1997; Yamada et al., 2000, 2001).

Neurotensin is an endogenous brain-gut peptide, with a close functional relationship with the mesocorticolimbic and neostriatal dopamine system. Dysregulation of neurotensin-mediated neurotransmission in this system has been hypothesized to be involved in the pathogenesis of schizophrenia. Additionally, neurotensin-containing circuits have been demonstrated to mediate mechanisms of action of antipsychotic drugs, as well as the rewarding and/or sensitizing properties of drugs of abuse (Holsboer, 2003). Similarly, recent behavioral studies have found that activation of the orexin system may be integral to motivation for drugs of abuse (Boutrel et al., 2005; Harris et al., 2005; Borgland et al., 2006), as well as natural food rewards (Thorpe et al., 2005).

The pancreatic polypeptide fold family includes pancreatic polypeptide (PP) and peptide YY (PYY) and neuropeptide Y (NPY). These peptides have broad peripheral actions on a number of organs. Both NPY and PYY have anxiolytic effects in rats, and NPY has been implicated in feeding and obesity, neuronal excitability, memory retention, anxiety, and depression (Berglund et al., 2003). NPY is reduced in the cerebrospinal fluid of depressed patients (Hou et al., 2006) while antidepressive treatments (lithium, selective serotonin reuptake inhibitors, and electroconvulsive stimuli) increase NPY selectively in rat hippocampus and in human cerebrospinal fluid (Bjornebekk et al., 2006; Ishida et al., 2005; Makino et al., 2000; Mathe et al., 2007). Moreover, intracerebroventricular injection of NPY to rats has antidepressive effects that are antagonized by NPY receptor blockers (Ishida et al., 2007).

Leptin, a hormone secreted from adipose tissue, was originally discovered to regulate body weight. Leptin receptors can be found in limbic structures, suggesting a potential role for this hormone in emotional processes. Lu et al. (2006) demonstrated that rats exposed to chronic unpredictable stress and chronic social defeat exhibit low leptin levels in plasma. Systemic treatment with leptin reversed the hedonic-like deficit induced by chronic unpredictable stress and decreased immobility in the FST, indicative of antidepressant-like activity. The behavioral effects of leptin in the FST were accompanied by increased neuronal activation in limbic structures, particularly in the hippocampus. Similar antidepressant-like effects of leptin have also been observed in diabetic mice (Hirano et al., 2007). Studies with germfree animals suggest that the gut microbiota influences the release of biologically active peptides and participates in the regulation of GI endocrine cells (Uribe et al., 1994). However, little is known about the effects of changes in the gut microbiota and, in particular, probiotic treatment on the expression and release of hormonal components of gut-brain communication. However, given the ability of the gut microbiota to alter nutrient bioavailability and the relationship between nutrient sensing and peptide secretion by enteroendocrine cells, it seems plausible that probiotics may modulate hormonal signaling by the gut. A study by Lesniewska et al. (2006) demonstrated that treatment with a mixture of *Lactobacillus rhamnosus* GG, *Bifidobacterium lactis*, and inulin increased the portal plasma concentrations of NPY and PYY in adult rats, whereas in elderly animals, the PYY concentration was unchanged and NPY levels were decreased by probiotic treatment. This study supports the idea that changes in composition of the gut microbiota can alter gut hormone release and that effects are age dependent and may be gut physiology and microbiome status dependent. This is clearly an area of research that demands more attention.

PROBIOTICS, NUTRITION, AND CNS FUNCTION

Healthy humans have up to 1,000 microbial species in their large bowel that can directly deliver compounds from the microbial metabolome and contribute to human metabolism (such as amino acids, vitamins, and energy substrates). Partly via the production of short-chain fatty acids, resident bacteria positively influence intestinal epithelial cell differentiation and proliferation and mediate metabolic effects on host GI physiology (Shanahan, 2002). Together, complex metabolic activities of the microbiota recover valuable energy and absorbable substrates for the host and provide energy and nutrients for bacterial growth and proliferation. Colonization increases the uptake of glucose in the intestine, and compared with colonized mice, germfree mice require a greater caloric intake to sustain a normal body weight (Backhed et al., 2004). This finding implicates gut bacteria as modulators of fat deposition in the host. Recent genetic analyses have determined that our microbiome provides us with abilities for enhanced metabolism of glycans, amino acids, and xenobiotics; methanogenesis; and 2-methyl-D-erythritol 4-phosphate pathway-mediated biosynthesis of vitamins and isoprenoids (Gill et al., 2006). Thus, human metabolism represents a fusion of microbial and human attributes.

Metabolomic studies of rat urine have shown marked differences between rats with a germfree status and rats with a conventional status fed the same diet (Coburn et al., 1989; Elmer and Remmel, 1984; George et al., 1994). Whereas large differences between the total absence of a gut microbiota and its presence might be expected, exactly how diet-related changes in the composition of the gut microbiota of humans influence the metabolomic profiles remains to be determined. However, studies have indicated that probiotic treatment can alter uptake or production of nutrients that have been linked to mood disorders.

Lactose malabsorption is a very common condition characterized by lactase deficiency, an enzyme occurring in the brush border membrane of the intestinal mucosa that hydrolyzes lactose to its components, galactose and glucose. Lactose malabsorption has been associated with early signs of major depressive disorders in women (Ledochowski et al., 1998). It has been suggested that high intestinal lactose concentrations may interfere with L-tryptophan metabolism and thus alter serotonin

bioavailability. Probiotics and yogurt have been shown to improve lactose digestion, an ability primarily attributed to bacterial β-galactosidase activity (Montalto et al., 2006). Mental depression could also be aggravated by micronutrient deficiencies since lactose and fructose malabsorption are often associated with decreased orocecal transit time, thus decreasing the mucosal contact time of micronutrients. Such altered transit times could result in vitamin or other nutrient deficiencies. Interestingly, an increased frequency of signs of depression was found in subjects with fructose malabsorption (Ledochowski et al., 2001).

Patients with depression have low levels of folic acid, vitamin B_{12}, and vitamin B_6. Accumulating evidence suggests that elevated homocysteine levels, potentially resulting from low B-complex vitamin levels, are associated with depression and cognitive deficiencies. The relationship of the homocysteine-methyl donor pathway to depression was noted first by Reynolds and colleagues in the 1970s. Subsequent clinical and population-based studies have noted elevated homocysteine levels in depression (Bottiglieri et al., 2000). However, much of the evidence comes from case-control and cross-sectional studies. Cohort studies and definitive randomized-controlled trials are needed to test the therapeutic benefit of folate and its possible association with depression. A plausible hypothesis for such a causal relationship is that cerebrovascular disease induced by elevated homocysteine levels results in neurotransmitter deficiencies that, in turn, lead to depression of mood or cognitive dysfunction. Folate synthesized by the gut microbiota can be incorporated into liver and kidney tissue of rats (Rong et al., 1991). In addition, data indicate that probiotic treatment can reduce homocysteine levels in humans. Oral administration of *Bifidobacterium longum* to hemodialysis patients was effective in decreasing the prehemodialysis levels of homocysteine, indoxyl sulfate, and triglycerides in serum. The reduction in serum homocysteine was mainly attributable to the supply of folate produced by *B. longum* in the human intestine (Taki et al., 2005).

Clinical studies have demonstrated beneficial effects of omega-3 fatty acids in various psychiatric disorders and, in particular, eicosapentaenoic acid (EPA) and docosahexaenoic acid have favorable effects on major depressive and bipolar disorders (Freeman et al., 2006; Horrobin, 2002). Dietary fats have differential effects on the intestinal microbiota. Mice on a diet containing fish oil had a threefold increase in quantities of bifidobacteria and reduced quantities of *Bacteroides* when compared to mice fed corn oil or beef fat-containing diets (Kuda et al., 2000). In vitro, omega-6-rich oil and linoleic acid can specifically inhibit the growth of bifidobacteria while, in contrast, EPA inhibits the growth of *Bacteroides* (Thompson and Spiller, 1995). Seal oil, which is high in EPA, increased the adhesion of *Lactobacillus paracasei* to the intestinal mucosa of piglets (Bomba et al., 2002). The relationship between omega-3 fatty acids and probiotics appears to be bidirectional. Treating atopic infants with *Bifidobacterium* for 7 months resulted in increased amounts of alpha-linolenic acid in plasma phospholipids (Kankaanpaa et al., 2002). Overall, it is clear that the apparent bidirectional relationship between probiotics and dietary fatty acids and the potential impact of these factors on mental health warrant further investigation.

DYSBIOSIS AND NEUROPSYCHIATRIC DISEASE

No studies of the composition of gut microbiota in patients suffering from psychiatric disorders have been published. However, evidence suggests that disturbances in the microbial balance, termed dysbiosis, may contribute to conditions such as mood-associated disorders or cognitive deficits. Chronic fatigue syndrome and fibromyalgia are conditions frequently associated with symptoms of depression. Researchers have documented lower levels of *Bifidobacterium* and higher levels of *Enterococcus* in these patients. The *Enterococcus* count in chronic fatigue syndrome and fibromyalgia patients correlated with neurological and cognitive deficits (Logan and Katzman, 2005). Many autistic children experience severe dietary and GI problems (including abdominal pain, constipation, diarrhea, and bloating) and symptoms that may be due to a disruption of the indigenous gut microbiota. Studies have correlated gut dysfunction with autistic spectrum disorders (ASD) and suggest a role of the GI microbiota in the development and severity of symptoms in autistic children (Bolte, 1998; Finegold et al., 2002). Interestingly, restricted diets (such as gluten-free or casein-free diets) have been associated with reduced GI disorders and improved behavior in ASD individuals (Knivsberg et al., 2002). Food intolerance is suspected to play a role in ASD, but the underlying cause of GI symptoms remains unclear.

One recent study by Parracho et al. (2005) utilized the culture-independent technique fluorescence in situ hybridization to assess the predominant components of the gut microbiota in children with ASD, their healthy siblings, and unrelated healthy controls. The fecal microbiota of ASD patients contained elevated quantities of the *Clostridium histolyticum* group of bacteria, compared to healthy children. However, the nonautistic sibling group had an intermediate level of the *C. histolyticum* group, which was not significantly different from either of the other subject groups. Members of the *C. histolyticum* group produce toxins including neurotoxins, and these toxins may contribute to gut dysfunction and systemic effects including aspects of autism.

Based on such data, it has been suggested that modulation of the gut microbiota of ASD patients by reducing the numbers of certain clostridia while stimulating beneficial gut bacteria may help alleviate some of the neurological symptoms. The majority of autistic patients in the study by Parracho et al. were taking probiotics, but probiotics did not seem to affect the relative quantities of *Clostridium* spp. in these patients. This study indicates that clostridial populations may not be affected by certain probiotic formulations (Parracho et al., 2005). However, this study lacked recorded standardization of probiotic strains or formulations administered to patients.

High rates of associated psychiatric disorders have been reported among patients with functional GI disorders. In the case of IBS, 50 to 90% of individuals seeking treatment have comorbid psychiatric disorders, especially depressive and anxiety disorders (Lydiard and Falsetti, 1999). IBS patients have decreased *Lactobacillus* and *Bifidobacterium* counts and a reduction of anaerobe-to-aerobe ratios (Madden and Hunter, 2002; Nobaek et al., 2000). Abnormal cytokine production found in association with IBS (O'Mahony et al., 2005) and major depression (Madden and Hunter, 2002; Nobaek et al., 2000) is a potential unifying mechanism connecting events in the nervous system (central or enteric) with symptoms such as fatigue, myalgia, and sleep disturbances.

Several lines of evidence suggest an association between depression and atopic allergies (i.e., asthma, atopic eczema, and allergic rhinitis) (Bell et al., 1991; Centanni et al., 2000; Goethe et al., 2001). An excess of immunoglobulin E-mediated allergies has been reported in patients with depression (Bell et al., 1991), and increased amounts of depressive symptoms have been reported in patients suffering from atopic disorders (Centanni et al., 2000; Goethe et al., 2001). Numerous studies indicate that the GI microbiota is different in atopic versus nonatopic individuals (Bjorksten et al., 1999, 2001; Kirjavainen et al., 2001). Sweden has a high incidence of allergic disease, while Estonia has a low incidence of such disorders. In a series of studies, it was shown that the microbial composition of atopic children differs from that of nonatopic children in both countries. Atopy was associated with increased levels of aerobic microbes and decreased levels of anaerobic microbes, particularly lactobacilli, in fecal samples (Bjorksten et al., 1999). A prospective study reported that infants who developed allergies had decreased levels of bifidobacteria and *Enterococcus* species but increased levels of *Clostridium* species (Bjorksten et al., 2001). These findings are consistent with reports of decreased levels of bifidobacteria and gram-positive organisms in infants with atopic eczema (Kirjavainen et al., 2001). Studies of a population who was living an anthroposophic lifestyle, abstaining from antibiotic use and ingesting fermented foods containing probiotic organisms (Alm et al., 1999), noted a decreased incidence of atopy compared with individuals in surrounding areas and increased quantities of lactic acid bacteria in fecal samples. Such findings have resulted in the hygiene hypothesis, which proposes that a more sterile environment in industrialized countries has disrupted the normal microbiota-mediated mechanisms of immunological tolerance in the mucosa, leading to an increased incidence of allergic disease in specific geographic regions (Noverr and Huffnagle, 2005). In addition to increased incidence of allergic diseases, the developed world is also experiencing a steady increase in the prevalence of autoimmune diseases (e.g., multiple sclerosis and type 1 diabetes) and inflammatory bowel disease (Crohn's disease and ulcerative colitis). Both Th1- and Th2-mediated immune diseases are increasing in prevalence, suggesting an overall rise in immune dysregulation. Alterations in the gut microbiota due to diet and antibiotic utilization may contribute to immune disorders, and these changes may have a relationship with the parallel increase in the incidence of depression and psychiatric disorders.

While associations between an altered gut microbiota and psychiatric disorders have been noted, causality and potential therapeutic benefits of probiotic treatment warrant further investigation. While early life treatment with probiotics reduced the incidence of atopic diseases (Kalliomaki et al., 2001, 2003) and improved symptom scores in women with IBS (O'Mahony et al., 2005), no such studies have been published addressing psychiatric disorders or symptoms. Few studies have addressed the impact of the human microbiota or probiotic therapies on mood or cognitive function in either animals or humans.

Gruenwald et al. (2002) evaluated a probiotic and multivitamin preparation given to 42 adult men and women assessed by a questionnaire as suffering from stress or exhaustion. The preparation was taken daily with breakfast during a 6-month period. At the end of the study, an overall reduction in self-perceived stress was noted. In addition, decreased frequencies of established stress indicators (rates of infection and GI discomfort) were recorded. More recently, Benton et al. (2007) conducted a double-blind placebo-controlled trial with 124 healthy volunteers. These volunteers consumed a probiotic-containing milk drink or a placebo daily for a 3-week period. Mood and cognition were measured at baseline and after 10 and 20 days of consumption of probiotic beverages. When those subjects in the bottom third of the depressed/elated dimension at baseline were considered, they selectively responded by reporting themselves as happy, rather than depressed, after taking the probiotic for 20 days. Unexpectedly the study also found that the consumption of probiotics resulted in slightly poorer performance with respect to two measures of memory. The effects were small and necessitate follow-up studies before conclusions can be formulated. However, this study is the first report to indicate that probiotic treatment can alter mood and cognitive function in healthy subjects.

CONCLUSIONS

A series of intricate interactions between the gut microbiota and the immune and nervous systems are necessary for optimal development of the physiological functions of the host. Commensal microorganisms have access to major channels of communication between the gut and the CNS, particularly between the gut and areas of the brain involved in processing of stress and emotional responses. Changes in the gut microbial composition are associated with physiological disorders that have psychiatric symptoms or demonstrate significant comorbidity with depression. While such associations are intriguing, the nature of a causal relationship between changes in the gut microbiota and mood or cognitive function has yet to be established. Overall, evidence warrants further investigation of the benefits of probiotic therapy in the treatment of mood and behavioral disorders. Future research should be aimed at determining specific mechanisms involved in linking the human microbiota in general with CNS homeostasis and function.

References

Alesci, S., P. E. Martinez, S. Kelkar, I. Ilias, D. S. Ronsaville, S. J. Listwak, A. R. Ayala, J. Licinio, H. K. Gold, M. A. Kling, G. P. Chrousos, and P. W. Gold. 2005. Major depression is associated with significant diurnal elevations in plasma interleukin-6 levels, a shift of its circadian rhythm, and loss of physiological complexity in its secretion: clinical implications. *J. Clin. Endocrinol. Metab.* **90:**2522–2530.

Alm, J. S., J. Swartz, G. Lilja, A. Scheynius, and G. Pershagen. 1999. Atopy in children of families with an anthroposophic lifestyle. *Lancet* **353:**1485–1488.

Arborelius, L., M. J. Owens, P. M. Plotsky, and C. B. Nemeroff. 1999. The role of corticotropin-releasing factor in depression and anxiety disorders. *J. Endocrinol.* **160:**1–12.

Aston-Jones, G., M. Ennis, V. A. Pieribone, W. T. Nickell, and M. T. Shipley. 1986. The brain nucleus locus coeruleus:

restricted afferent control of a broad efferent network. *Science* **234**:734–737.

Aston-Jones, G., J. Rajkowski, P. Kubiak, R. J. Valentino, and M. T. Shipley. 1996. Role of the locus coeruleus in emotional activation. *Prog. Brain Res.* **107**:379–402.

Backhed, F., H. Ding, T. Wang, L. V. Hooper, G. Y. Koh, A. Nagy, C. F. Semenkovich, and J. I. Gordon. 2004. The gut microbiota as an environmental factor that regulates fat storage. *Proc. Natl. Acad. Sci. USA* **101**:15718–15723.

Backhed, F., R. E. Ley, J. L. Sonnenburg, D. A. Peterson, and J. I. Gordon. 2005. Host-bacterial mutualism in the human intestine. *Science* **307**:1915–1920.

Baharav, E., F. Mor, M. Halpern, and A. Weinberger. 2004. *Lactobacillus* GG bacteria ameliorate arthritis in Lewis rats. *J. Nutr.* **134**:1964–1969.

Bailey, M. T., and C. L. Coe. 1999. Maternal separation disrupts the integrity of the intestinal microflora in infant rhesus monkeys. *Dev. Psychobiol.* **35**:146–155.

Bailey, M. T., G. R. Lubach, and C. L. Coe. 2004. Prenatal stress alters bacterial colonization of the gut in infant monkeys. *J. Pediatr. Gastroenterol. Nutr.* **38**:414–421.

Bell, I. R., M. L. Jasnoski, J. Kagan, and D. S. King. 1991. Depression and allergies: survey of a nonclinical population. *Psychother. Psychosom.* **55**:24–31.

Benton, D., C. Williams, and A. Brown. 2007. Impact of consuming a milk drink containing a probiotic on mood and cognition. *Eur. J. Clin. Nutr.* **61**:355–361.

Berglund, M. M., P. A. Hipskind, and D. R. Gehlert. 2003. Recent developments in our understanding of the physiological role of PP-fold peptide receptor subtypes. *Exp. Biol. Med.* (Maywood) **228**:217–244.

Bjorksten, B., P. Naaber, E. Sepp, and M. Mikelsaar. 1999. The intestinal microflora in allergic Estonian and Swedish 2-year-old children. *Clin. Exp. Allergy* **29**:342–346.

Bjorksten, B., E. Sepp, K. Julge, T. Voor, and M. Mikelsaar. 2001. Allergy development and the intestinal microflora during the first year of life. *J. Allergy Clin. Immunol.* **108**:516–520.

Bjornebekk, A., A. A. Mathe, and S. Brene. 2006. Running has differential effects on NPY, opiates, and cell proliferation in an animal model of depression and controls. *Neuropsychopharmacology* **31**:256–264.

Bolte, E. R. 1998. Autism and *Clostridium tetani*. *Med. Hypotheses* **51**:133–144.

Bomba, A., R. Nemcova, S. Gancarcikova, R. Herich, P. Guba, and D. Mudronova. 2002. Improvement of the probiotic effect of micro-organisms by their combination with maltodextrins, fructo-oligosaccharides and polyunsaturated fatty acids. *Br. J. Nutr.* **88**(Suppl. 1):S95–S99.

Borgland, S. L., S. A. Taha, F. Sarti, H. L. Fields, and A. Bonci. 2006. Orexin A in the VTA is critical for the induction of synaptic plasticity and behavioral sensitization to cocaine. *Neuron* **49**:589–601.

Borrielo, S. P. 2002. The normal flora of the gastrointestinal tract, p. 1–24. *In* A. L. Hart, A. J. Stagg, H. Graffner, H. Glise, P. Falk, and N. A. Kamm (ed.), *Gut Ecology*. Cromwell Press, Trowbridge, United Kingdom.

Bottiglieri, T., M. Laundy, R. Crellin, B. K. Toone, M. W. Carney, and E. H. Reynolds. 2000. Homocysteine, folate, methylation, and monoamine metabolism in depression. *J. Neurol. Neurosurg. Psychiatry* **69**:228–232.

Boutrel, B., P. J. Kenny, S. E. Specio, R. Martin-Fardon, A. Markou, G. F. Koob, and L. de Lecea. 2005. Role for hypocretin in mediating stress-induced reinstatement of cocaine-seeking behavior. *Proc. Natl. Acad. Sci. USA* **102**:19168–19173.

Braat, H., J. van den Brande, E. van Tol, D. Hommes, M. Peppelenbosch, and S. van Deventer. 2004. *Lactobacillus rhamnosus* induces peripheral hyporesponsiveness in stimulated CD4+ T cells via modulation of dendritic cell function. *Am. J. Clin. Nutr.* **80**:1618–1625.

Browning, K. N., and D. Mendelowitz. 2003. Musings on the wanderer: what's new in our understanding of vago-vagal reflexes? II. Integration of afferent signaling from the viscera by the nodose ganglia. *Am. J. Physiol. Gastrointest. Liver Physiol.* **284**:G8–G14.

Cameron, J., and E. Doucet. 2007. Getting to the bottom of feeding behaviour: who's on top? *Appl. Physiol. Nutr. Metab.* **32**:177–189.

Capuron, L., and R. Dantzer. 2003. Cytokines and depression: the need for a new paradigm. *Brain Behav. Immun.* **17**(Suppl 1):S119–S124.

Carlini, V. P., M. M. Varas, A. B. Cragnolini, H. B. Schioth, T. N. Scimonelli, and S. R. de Barioglio. 2004. Differential role of the hippocampus, amygdala, and dorsal raphe nucleus in regulating feeding, memory, and anxiety-like behavioral responses to ghrelin. *Biochem. Biophys. Res. Commun.* **313**:635–641.

Cebra, J. J. 1999. Influences of microbiota on intestinal immune system development. *Am. J. Clin. Nutr.* **69**:1046S–1051S.

Centanni, S., F. Di Marco, F. Castagna, B. Boveri, F. Casanova, and A. Piazzini. 2000. Psychological issues in the treatment of asthmatic patients. *Respir. Med.* **94**:742–749.

Chang, H. Y., H. Mashimo, and R. K. Goyal. 2003. Musings on the wanderer: what's new in our understanding of vago-vagal reflex? IV. Current concepts of vagal efferent projections to the gut. *Am. J. Physiol. Gastrointest. Liver Physiol.* **284**:G357–G366.

Chen, B., D. Dowlatshahi, G. M. MacQueen, J. F. Wang, and L. T. Young. 2001. Increased hippocampal BDNF immunoreactivity in subjects treated with antidepressant medication. *Biol. Psychiatry* **50**:260–265.

Christensen, H. R., H. Frokiaer, and J. J. Pestka. 2002. Lactobacilli differentially modulate expression of cytokines and maturation surface markers in murine dendritic cells. *J. Immunol.* **168**:171–178.

Clarke, M. B., D. T. Hughes, C. Zhu, E. C. Boedeker, and V. Sperandio. 2006. The QseC sensor kinase: a bacterial adrenergic receptor. *Proc. Natl. Acad. Sci. USA* **103**:10420–10425.

Coburn, S. P., J. D. Mahuren, B. S. Wostmann, D. L. Snyder, and D. W. Townsend. 1989. Role of intestinal microflora in the metabolism of vitamin B-6 and 4′-deoxypyridoxine examined using germfree guinea pigs and rats. *J. Nutr.* **119**:181–188.

Crucian, G. P., J. D. Hughes, A. M. Barrett, D. J. Williamson, R. M. Bauer, D. Bowers, and K. M. Heilman. 2000. Emotional and physiological responses to false feedback. *Cortex* **36**:623–647.

Drossman, D. A. 1998. Presidential address: gastrointestinal illness and the biopsychosocial model. *Psychosom. Med.* 60:258–267.

Dunn, A. J., J. Wang, and T. Ando. 1999. Effects of cytokines on cerebral neurotransmission. Comparison with the effects of stress. *Adv. Exp. Med. Biol.* 461:117–127.

Dwivedi, Y., H. S. Rizavi, R. R. Conley, R. C. Roberts, C. A. Tamminga, and G. N. Pandey. 2003. Altered gene expression of brain-derived neurotrophic factor and receptor tyrosine kinase B in postmortem brain of suicide subjects. *Arch. Gen. Psychiatry* 60:804–815.

Elmer, G. W., and R. P. Remmel. 1984. Role of the intestinal microflora in clonazepam metabolism in the rat. *Xenobiotica* 14:829–840.

Finegold, S. M., D. Molitoris, Y. Song, C. Liu, M. L. Vaisanen, E. Bolte, M. McTeague, R. Sandler, H. Wexler, E. M. Marlowe, M. D. Collins, P. A. Lawson, P. Summanen, M. Baysallar, T. J. Tomzynski, E. Read, E. Johnson, R. Rolfe, P. Nasir, H. Shah, D. A. Haake, P. Manning, and A. Kaul. 2002. Gastrointestinal microflora studies in late-onset autism. *Clin. Infect. Dis.* 35(Suppl. 1):S6–S16.

Freeman, M. P., J. R. Hibbeln, K. L. Wisner, J. M. Davis, D. Mischoulon, M. Peet, P. E. Keck Jr., L. B. Marangell, A. J. Richardson, J. Lake, and A. L. Stoll. 2006. Omega-3 fatty acids: evidence basis for treatment and future research in psychiatry. *J. Clin. Psychiatry* 67:1954–1967.

Frommberger, U. H., J. Bauer, P. Haselbauer, A. Fraulin, D. Riemann, and M. Berger. 1997. Interleukin-6-(IL-6) plasma levels in depression and schizophrenia: comparison between the acute state and after remission. *Eur. Arch. Psychiatry Clin. Neurosci.* 247:228–233.

Gao, H. M., J. Jiang, B. Wilson, W. Zhang, J. S. Hong, and B. Liu. 2002. Microglial activation-mediated delayed and progressive degeneration of rat nigral dopaminergic neurons: relevance to Parkinson's disease. *J. Neurochem.* 81:1285–1297.

George, S. E., R. W. Chadwick, M. J. Kohan, J. C. Allison, R. W. Williams, and J. Chang. 1994. Role of the intestinal microbiota in the activation of the promutagen 2,6-dinitrotoluene to mutagenic urine metabolites and comparison of GI enzyme activities in germ-free and conventionalized male Fischer 344 rats. *Cancer Lett.* 79:181–187.

Ghosh, S., D. van Heel, and R. J. Playford. 2004. Probiotics in inflammatory bowel disease: is it all gut flora modulation? *Gut* 53:620–622.

Gill, S. R., M. Pop, R. T. Deboy, P. B. Eckburg, P. J. Turnbaugh, B. S. Samuel, J. I. Gordon, D. A. Relman, C. M. Fraser-Liggett, and K. E. Nelson. 2006. Metagenomic analysis of the human distal gut microbiome. *Science* 312:1355–1359.

Gionchetti, P., F. Rizzello, U. Helwig, A. Venturi, K. M. Lammers, P. Brigidi, B. Vitali, G. Poggioli, M. Miglioli, and M. Campieri. 2003. Prophylaxis of pouchitis onset with probiotic therapy: a double-blind, placebo-controlled trial. *Gastroenterology* 124:1202–1209.

Giordano, R., A. Picu, F. Broglio, L. Bonelli, M. Baldi, R. Berardelli, E. Ghigo, and E. Arvat. 2004. Ghrelin, hypothalamus-pituitary-adrenal (HPA) axis and Cushing's syndrome. *Pituitary* 7:243–248.

Giordano, R., M. Pellegrino, A. Picu, L. Bonelli, M. Balbo, R. Berardelli, F. Lanfranco, E. Ghigo, and E. Arvat. 2006. Neuroregulation of the hypothalamus-pituitary-adrenal (HPA) axis in humans: effects of GABA-, mineralocorticoid-, and GH-Secretagogue-receptor modulation. *Scientific World-Journal* 6:1–11.

Goehler, L. E., R. P. Gaykema, N. Opitz, R. Reddaway, N. Badr, and M. Lyte. 2005. Activation in vagal afferents and central autonomic pathways: early responses to intestinal infection with *Campylobacter jejuni*. *Brain Behav. Immun.* 19:334–344.

Goethe, J. W., R. Maljanian, S. Wolf, P. Hernandez, and Y. Cabrera. 2001. The impact of depressive symptoms on the functional status of inner-city patients with asthma. *Ann. Allergy Asthma Immunol.* 87:205–210.

Gruenwald, J., H. J. Graubaum, and A. Harde. 2002. Effect of a probiotic multivitamin compound on stress and exhaustion. *Adv. Ther.* 19:141–150.

Harris, G. C., M. Wimmer, and G. Aston-Jones. 2005. A role for lateral hypothalamic orexin neurons in reward seeking. *Nature* 437:556–559.

Hart, A. L., K. Lammers, P. Brigidi, B. Vitali, F. Rizzello, P. Gionchetti, M. Campieri, M. A. Kamm, S. C. Knight, and A. J. Stagg. 2004. Modulation of human dendritic cell phenotype and function by probiotic bacteria. *Gut* 53:1602–1609.

Hestad, K. A., S. Tonseth, C. D. Stoen, T. Ueland, and P. Aukrust. 2003. Raised plasma levels of tumor necrosis factor alpha in patients with depression: normalization during electroconvulsive therapy. *J. ECT* 19:183–188.

Hirano, S., S. Miyata, and J. Kamei. 2007. Antidepressant-like effect of leptin in streptozotocin-induced diabetic mice. *Pharmacol. Biochem. Behav.* 86:27–31.

Holdeman, L. V., I. J. Good, and W. E. Moore. 1976. Human fecal flora: variation in bacterial composition within individuals and a possible effect of emotional stress. *Appl. Environ. Microbiol.* 31:359–375.

Holsboer, F. 2003. The role of peptides in treatment of psychiatric disorders. *J. Neural Transm. Suppl.* 2003:17–34.

Hooper, L. V., M. H. Wong, A. Thelin, L. Hansson, P. G. Falk, and J. I. Gordon. 2001. Molecular analysis of commensal host-microbial relationships in the intestine. *Science* 291:881–884.

Horrobin, D. F. 2002. Food, micronutrients, and psychiatry. *Int. Psychogeriatr.* 14:331–334.

Hou, C., F. Jia, Y. Liu, and L. Li. 2006. CSF serotonin, 5-hydroxyindolacetic acid and neuropeptide Y levels in severe major depressive disorder. *Brain Res.* 1095:154–158.

Ishida, H., Y. Shirayama, M. Iwata, and R. Kawahara. 2005. Subchronic treatment with imipramine ameliorates the decreased number in neuropeptide Y-positive cells in the hippocampus of learned helplessness rats. *Brain Res.* 1046:239–243.

Ishida, H., Y. Shirayama, M. Iwata, S. Katayama, A. Yamamoto, R. Kawahara, and K. Nakagome. 2007. Infusion of neuropeptide Y into CA3 region of hippocampus produces antidepressant-like effect via Y1 receptor. *Hippocampus* 17:271–280.

Iyer, L. M., L. Aravind, S. L. Coon, D. C. Klein, and E. V. Koonin. 2004. Evolution of cell-cell signaling in animals: did late horizontal gene transfer from bacteria have a role? *Trends Genet.* 20:292–299.

Jaszberenyi, M., E. Bujdoso, Z. Bagosi, and G. Telegdy. 2006. Mediation of the behavioral, endocrine and thermoregulatory actions of ghrelin. *Horm. Behav.* 50:266–273.

Kahl, K. G., S. Rudolf, B. M. Stoeckelhuber, L. Dibbelt, H. B. Gehl, K. Markhof, F. Hohagen, and U. Schweiger. 2005. Bone mineral density, markers of bone turnover, and cytokines in young women with borderline personality disorder with and without comorbid major depressive disorder. *Am. J. Psychiatry* 162:168–174.

Kalliomaki, M., S. Salminen, H. Arvilommi, P. Kero, P. Koskinen, and E. Isolauri. 2001. Probiotics in primary prevention of atopic disease: a randomised placebo-controlled trial. *Lancet* 357:1076–1079.

Kalliomaki, M., S. Salminen, T. Poussa, H. Arvilommi, and E. Isolauri. 2003. Probiotics and prevention of atopic disease: 4-year follow-up of a randomised placebo-controlled trial. *Lancet* 361:1869–1871.

Kamiya, T., L. Wang, P. Forsythe, G. Goettsche, Y. Mao, Y. Wang, G. Tougas, and J. Bienenstock. 2006. Inhibitory effects of *Lactobacillus reuteri* on visceral pain induced by colorectal distension in Sprague-Dawley rats. *Gut* 55:191–196.

Kankaanpaa, P. E., B. Yang, H. P. Kallio, E. Isolauri, and S. J. Salminen. 2002. Influence of probiotic supplemented infant formula on composition of plasma lipids in atopic infants. *J. Nutr. Biochem.* 13:364–369.

Karege, F., G. Perret, G. Bondolfi, M. Schwald, G. Bertschy, and J. M. Aubry. 2002. Decreased serum brain-derived neurotrophic factor levels in major depressed patients. *Psychiatry Res.* 109:143–148.

Karege, F., G. Vaudan, M. Schwald, N. Perroud, and R. La Harpe. 2005. Neurotrophin levels in postmortem brains of suicide victims and the effects of antemortem diagnosis and psychotropic drugs. *Brain Res. Mol. Brain Res.* 136:29–37.

Kendler, K. S., L. M. Thornton, and C. O. Gardner. 2000. Stressful life events and previous episodes in the etiology of major depression in women: an evaluation of the "kindling" hypothesis. *Am. J. Psychiatry* 157:1243–1251.

Kipnis, J., E. Yoles, H. Schori, E. Hauben, I. Shaked, and M. Schwartz. 2001. Neuronal survival after CNS insult is determined by a genetically encoded autoimmune response. *J. Neurosci.* 21:4564–4571.

Kipnis, J., H. Cohen, M. Cardon, Y. Ziv, and M. Schwartz. 2004. T cell deficiency leads to cognitive dysfunction: implications for therapeutic vaccination for schizophrenia and other psychiatric conditions. *Proc. Natl. Acad. Sci. USA* 101:8180–8185.

Kirjavainen, P. V., E. Apostolou, T. Arvola, S. J. Salminen, G. R. Gibson, and E. Isolauri. 2001. Characterizing the composition of intestinal microflora as a prospective treatment target in infant allergic disease. *FEMS Immunol. Med. Microbiol.* 32:1–7.

Knivsberg, A. M., K. L. Reichelt, T. Hoien, and M. Nodland. 2002. A randomised, controlled study of dietary intervention in autistic syndromes. *Nutr. Neurosci.* 5:251–261.

Kuda, T., T. Enomoto, T. Yano, and T. Fujii. 2000. Cecal environment and TBARS level in mice fed corn oil, beef tallow and menhaden fish oil. *J. Nutr. Sci. Vitaminol.* (Tokyo) 46:65–70.

Kunze, W., Y. K. Mao, P. Forsythe, and J. Bienenstock. 2007. Effect of *Lactobacillus* sp. (Lb) probiotic ingestion on membrane properties of intrinsic sensory neurons in rat colon. *Gastroenterology* 132:A–401.

Ledochowski, M., B. Sperner-Unterweger, and D. Fuchs. 1998. Lactose malabsorption is associated with early signs of mental depression in females: a preliminary report. *Dig. Dis. Sci.* 43:2513–2517.

Ledochowski, M., B. Widner, C. Murr, B. Sperner-Unterweger, and D. Fuchs. 2001. Fructose malabsorption is associated with decreased plasma tryptophan. *Scand. J. Gastroenterol.* 36:367–371.

Lesniewska, V., I. Rowland, P. D. Cani, A. M. Neyrinck, N. M. Delzenne, and P. J. Naughton. 2006. Effect on components of the intestinal microflora and plasma neuropeptide levels of feeding *Lactobacillus delbrueckii*, *Bifidobacterium lactis*, and inulin to adult and elderly rats. *Appl. Environ. Microbiol.* 72:6533–6538.

Linton, P. J., and K. Dorshkind. 2004. Age-related changes in lymphocyte development and function. *Nat. Immunol.* 5:133–139.

Lizko, N. N. 1987. Stress and intestinal microflora. *Nahrung* 31:443–447.

Lizko, N. N. 1991. Problems of microbial ecology in man space mission. *Acta Astronaut.* 23:163–169.

Logan, A. C., and M. Katzman. 2005. Major depressive disorder: probiotics may be an adjuvant therapy. *Med. Hypotheses* 64:533–538.

Lowry, C. A., J. H. Hollis, A. de Vries, B. Pan, L. R. Brunet, J. R. Hunt, J. F. Paton, E. van Kampen, D. M. Knight, A. K. Evans, G. A. Rook, and S. L. Lightman. 2007. Identification of an immune-responsive mesolimbocortical serotonergic system: potential role in regulation of emotional behavior. *Neuroscience* 146:756–772.

Lu, X. Y., C. S. Kim, A. Frazer, and W. Zhang. 2006. Leptin: a potential novel antidepressant. *Proc. Natl. Acad. Sci. USA* 103:1593–1598.

Lydiard, R. B., and S. A. Falsetti. 1999. Experience with anxiety and depression treatment studies: implications for designing irritable bowel syndrome clinical trials. *Am. J. Med.* 107:65S–73S.

Maassen, C. B., J. C. van Holten, F. Balk, M. J. Heijne den Bak-Glashouwer, R. Leer, J. D. Laman, W. J. Boersma, and E. Claassen. 1998. Orally administered *Lactobacillus* strains differentially affect the direction and efficacy of the immune response. *Vet. Q.* 20:S81–S83.

Madden, J. A., and J. O. Hunter. 2002. A review of the role of the gut microflora in irritable bowel syndrome and the effects of probiotics. *Br. J. Nutr.* 88:S67–S72.

Maes, M., E. Bosmans, R. De Jongh, G. Kenis, E. Vandoolaeghe, and H. Neels. 1997. Increased serum IL-6 and IL-1 receptor antagonist concentrations in major depression and treatment resistant depression. *Cytokine* 9:853–858.

Maes, M. 1999. Major depression and activation of the inflammatory response system. *Adv. Exp. Med. Biol.* 461:25–46.

Maes, M. 2001. The immunoregulatory effects of antidepressants. *Hum. Psychopharmacol.* 16:95–103.

Makino, S., R. A. Baker, M. A. Smith, and P. W. Gold. 2000. Differential regulation of neuropeptide Y mRNA expression in the arcuate nucleus and locus coeruleus by stress and anti-depressants. *J. Neuroendocrinol.* 12:387–395.

Mathe, A. A., H. Husum, A. El Khoury, P. Jimenez-Vasquez, S. H. Gruber, G. Wortwein, G. Nikisch, P. Baumann, H. Agren, W. Andersson, A. Sodergren, and F. Angelucci. 2007. Search for biological correlates of depression and mechanisms of action of antidepressant treatment modalities. Do neuropeptides play a role? *Physiol. Behav.* 92:226–231.

McCarthy, J., L. O'Mahony, L. O'Callaghan, B. Sheil, E. E. Vaughan, N. Fitzsimons, J. Fitzgibbon, G. C. O'Sullivan, B. Kiely, J. K. Collins, and F. Shanahan. 2003. Double blind, placebo controlled trial of two probiotic strains in interleu-kin 10 knockout mice and mechanistic link with cytokine balance. *Gut* 52:975–980.

Miller, G. E., C. A. Stetler, R. M. Carney, K. E. Freedland, and W. A. Banks. 2002. Clinical depression and inflammatory risk markers for coronary heart disease. *Am. J. Cardiol.* 90:1279–1283.

Moalem, G., R. Leibowitz-Amit, E. Yoles, F. Mor, I. R. Cohen, and M. Schwartz. 1999. Autoimmune T cells protect neu-rons from secondary degeneration after central nervous sys-tem axotomy. *Nat. Med.* 5:49–55.

Montalto, M., V. Curigliano, L. Santoro, M. Vastola, G. Cam-marota, R. Manna, A. Gasbarrini, and G. Gasbarrini. 2006. Management and treatment of lactose malabsorption. *World J. Gastroenterol.* 12:187–191.

Moore, W. E., E. P. Cato, and L. V. Holdeman. 1978. Some current concepts in intestinal bacteriology. *Am. J. Clin. Nutr.* 31:S33–S42.

Musselman, D. L., A. H. Miller, M. R. Porter, A. Manatunga, F. Gao, S. Penna, B. D. Pearce, J. Landry, S. Glover, J. S. McDaniel, and C. B. Nemeroff. 2001. Higher than nor-mal plasma interleukin-6 concentrations in cancer patients with depression: preliminary findings. *Am. J. Psychiatry* 158:1252–1257.

Nobaek, S., M. L. Johansson, G. Molin, S. Ahrne, and B. Jeppsson. 2000. Alteration of intestinal microflora is associated with reduction in abdominal bloating and pain in patients with irritable bowel syndrome. *Am. J. Gastro-enterol.* 95:1231–1238.

Noverr, M. C., and G. B. Huffnagle. 2005. The 'microflora hypothesis' of allergic diseases. *Clin. Exp. Allergy* 35:1511–1520.

O'Brien, S. M., P. Scully, P. Fitzgerald, L. V. Scott, and T. G. Dinan. 2007. Plasma cytokine profiles in depressed patients who fail to respond to selective serotonin reuptake inhibitor therapy. *J. Psychiatr. Res.* 41:326–331.

O'Mahony, L., J. McCarthy, P. Kelly, G. Hurley, F. Luo, K. Chen, G. C. O'Sullivan, B. Kiely, J. K. Collins, F. Shanahan, and E. M. Quigley. 2005. *Lactobacillus* and *Bifidobacterium* in irritable bowel syndrome: symptom responses and rela-tionship to cytokine profiles. *Gastroenterology* 128:541–551.

Parracho, H. M., M. O. Bingham, G. R. Gibson, and A. L. McCartney. 2005. Differences between the gut microflora of children with autistic spectrum disorders and that of healthy children. *J. Med. Microbiol.* 54:987–991.

Reid, G., J. Jass, M. T. Sebulsky, and J. K. McCormick. 2003. Potential uses of probiotics in clinical practice. *Clin. Micro-biol. Rev.* 16:658–672.

Reynolds, J. L., T. A. Ignatowski, R. Sud, and R. N. Spen-gler. 2004. Brain-derived tumor necrosis factor-alpha and its involvement in noradrenergic neuron functioning involved in the mechanism of action of an antidepressant. *J. Pharma-col. Exp. Ther.* 310:1216–1225.

Robinson, J. K. 2004. Galanin and cognition. *Behav. Cogn. Neurosci. Rev.* 3:222–242.

Rong, N., J. Selhub, B. R. Goldin, and I. H. Rosenberg. 1991. Bacterially synthesized folate in rat large intestine is incorporated into host tissue folyl polyglutamates. *J. Nutr.* 121:1955–1959.

Rustay, N. R., C. C. Wrenn, J. W. Kinney, A. Holmes, K. R. Bai-ley, T. L. Sullivan, A. P. Harris, K. C. Long, M. C. Saavedra, G. Starosta, C. E. Innerfield, R. J. Yang, J. L. Dreiling, and J. N. Crawley. 2005. Galanin impairs performance on learn-ing and memory tasks: findings from galanin transgenic and GAL-R1 knockout mice. *Neuropeptides* 39:239–243.

Schicho, R., D. Krueger, F. Zeller, C. W. Von Weyhern, T. Friel-ing, H. Kimura, I. Ishii, R. De Giorgio, B. Campi, and M. Schemann. 2006. Hydrogen sulfide is a novel prosecre-tory neuromodulator in the Guinea-pig and human colon. *Gastroenterology* 131:1542–1552.

Schiepers, O. J., M. C. Wichers, and M. Maes. 2005. Cytokines and major depression. *Prog. Neuropsychopharmacol. Biol. Psychiatry* 29:201–217.

Shanahan, F. 2002. The host-microbe interface within the gut. *Best Pract. Res. Clin. Gastroenterol.* 16:915–931.

Shimizu, E., K. Hashimoto, N. Okamura, K. Koike, N. Kom-atsu, C. Kumakiri, M. Nakazato, H. Watanabe, N. Shinoda, S. Okada, and M. Iyo. 2003. Alterations of serum levels of brain-derived neurotrophic factor (BDNF) in depressed patients with or without antidepressants. *Biol. Psychiatry* 54:70–75.

Sluzewska, A., J. K. Rybakowski, M. Laciak, A. Mackiewicz, M. Sobieska, and K. Wiktorowicz. 1995. Interleukin-6 serum levels in depressed patients before and after treatment with fluoxetine. *Ann. N. Y. Acad. Sci.* 762:474–476.

Smits, H. H., A. Engering, D. van der Kleij, E. C. de Jong, K. Schipper, T. M. van Capel, B. A. Zaat, M. Yazdanbakhsh, E. A. Wierenga, Y. van Kooyk, and M. L. Kapsenberg. 2005. Selective probiotic bacteria induce IL-10-producing regula-tory T cells *in vitro* by modulating dendritic cell function through dendritic cell-specific intercellular adhesion mol-ecule 3-grabbing nonintegrin. *J. Allergy Clin. Immunol.* 115:1260–1267.

Sobko, T., L. Huang, T. Midtvedt, E. Norin, L. E. Gustafsson, M. Norman, E. A. Jansson, and J. O. Lundberg. 2006. Gen-eration of NO by probiotic bacteria in the gastrointestinal tract. *Free Radic. Biol. Med.* 41:985–991.

Sudo, N., Y. Chida, Y. Aiba, J. Sonoda, N. Oyama, X. N. Yu, C. Kubo, and Y. Koga. 2004. Postnatal microbial coloniza-tion programs the hypothalamic-pituitary-adrenal system for stress response in mice. *J. Physiol.* 558:263–275.

Taki, K., F. Takayama, and T. Niwa. 2005. Beneficial effects of Bifidobacteria in a gastroresistant seamless capsule on hyperhomocysteinemia in hemodialysis patients. *J. Ren. Nutr.* 15:77–80.

Thompson, L., and R. C. Spiller. 1995. Impact of polyunsatu-rated fatty acids on human colonic bacterial metabolism: an *in vitro* and *in vivo* study. *Br. J. Nutr.* 74:733–741.

Thorpe, A. J., J. P. Cleary, A. S. Levine, and C. M. Kotz. 2005. Centrally administered orexin A increases motivation for sweet pellets in rats. *Psychopharmacology* (Berlin) **182:** 75–83.

Tortorella, C., G. Neri, and G. G. Nussdorfer. 2007. Galanin in the regulation of the hypothalamic-pituitary-adrenal axis. *Int. J. Mol. Med.* **19:**639–647.

Tuglu, C., S. H. Kara, O. Caliyurt, E. Vardar, and E. Abay. 2003. Increased serum tumor necrosis factor-alpha levels and treatment response in major depressive disorder. *Psychopharmacology* (Berlin) **170:**429–433.

Uribe, A., M. Alam, O. Johansson, T. Midtvedt, and E. Theodorsson. 1994. Microflora modulates endocrine cells in the gastrointestinal mucosa of the rat. *Gastroenterology* **107:**1259–1269.

Wada, E., K. Watase, K. Yamada, H. Ogura, M. Yamano, Y. Inomata, J. Eguchi, K. Yamamoto, M. E. Sunday, H. Maeno, K. Mikoshiba, H. Ohki-Hamazaki, and K. Wada. 1997. Generation and characterization of mice lacking gastrin-releasing peptide receptor. *Biochem. Biophys. Res. Commun.* **239:**28–33.

Walsh, S. P., and M. A. Kling. 2004. VNS and depression: current status and future directions. *Expert Rev. Med. Devices* **1:**155–160.

Wang, X., B. R. Wang, X. J. Zhang, Z. Xu, Y. Q. Ding, and G. Ju. 2002. Evidences for vagus nerve in maintenance of immune balance and transmission of immune information from gut to brain in STM-infected rats. *World J. Gastroenterol.* **8:**540–545.

Weinstein, P. D., and J. J. Cebra. 1991. The preference for switching to IgA expression by Peyer's patch germinal center B cells is likely due to the intrinsic influence of their microenvironment. *J. Immunol.* **147:**4126–4135.

Wick, G., P. Berger, P. Jansen-Durr, and B. Grubeck-Loebenstein. 2003. A Darwinian-evolutionary concept of age-related diseases. *Exp. Gerontol.* **38:**13–25.

Wren, A. M., and S. R. Bloom. 2007. Gut hormones and appetite control. *Gastroenterology* **132:**2116–2130.

Wrenn, C. C., J. W. Kinney, L. K. Marriott, A. Holmes, A. P. Harris, M. C. Saavedra, G. Starosta, C. E. Innerfield, A. S. Jacoby, J. Shine, T. P. Iismaa, G. L. Wenk, and J. N. Crawley. 2004. Learning and memory performance in mice lacking the GAL-R1 subtype of galanin receptor. *Eur. J. Neurosci.* **19:**1384–1396.

Wrenn, C. C., and A. Holmes. 2006. The role of galanin in modulating stress-related neural pathways. *Drug News Perspect.* **19:**461–467.

Yamada, K., E. Wada, and K. Wada. 2000. Male mice lacking the gastrin-releasing peptide receptor (GRP-R) display elevated preference for conspecific odors and increased social investigatory behaviors. *Brain Res.* **870:**20–26.

Yamada, K., E. Wada, and K. Wada. 2001. Female gastrin-releasing peptide receptor (GRP-R)-deficient mice exhibit altered social preference for male conspecifics: implications for GRP/GRP-R modulation of GABAergic function. *Brain Res.* **894:**281–287.

Yoles, E., E. Hauben, O. Palgi, E. Agranov, A. Gothilf, A. Cohen, V. Kuchroo, I. R. Cohen, H. Weiner, and M. Schwartz. 2001. Protective autoimmunity is a physiological response to CNS trauma. *J. Neurosci.* **21:**3740–3748.

Zagon, A. 2001. Does the vagus nerve mediate the sixth sense? *Trends Neurosci.* **24:**671–673.

Ziegler, D. R., W. A. Cass, and J. P. Herman. 1999. Excitatory influence of the locus coeruleus in hypothalamic-pituitary-adrenocortical axis responses to stress. *J. Neuroendocrinol.* **11:**361–369.

Therapeutic Microbiology: Probiotics and Related Strategies
Edited by J. Versalovic and M. Wilson
© 2008 ASM Press, Washington, DC

3.2. PREBIOTICS

Ian Rowland

Prebiotics in Human Medicine

23

Prebiotics are generally considered to be food ingredients, and unlike probiotics, which have been extensively investigated in patient groups with a variety of clinical disorders and diseases, testing for health benefits of prebiotics has focused more on healthy subjects with the aim of improving general health status and reducing disease risk.

The clinical studies on prebiotics that have been reported have generally used small numbers of subjects, but some have shown promising results that will need confirmation in larger-scale interventions. The tendency to use combinations of pre- and probiotics (so-called synbiotics) may impede the complete understanding of the contribution of prebiotics to beneficial health effects. The main areas that are reviewed in this chapter include constipation, diarrhea, irritable bowel syndrome, inflammatory bowel disease (ulcerative colitis and Crohn's disease), and colorectal cancer.

CONSTIPATION

Constipation is a common bowel dysfunction, particularly prevalent in older people, that is defined usually by the occurrence of fewer than three bowel movements per week (Whitehead et al., 1989). However, constipation manifests itself as a wide range of reported symptoms including hard stools, pain, straining, and incomplete evacuation, even though the number of bowel movements may be within the normal range (Potter, 2003). The prevalence of constipation varies considerably, between 2 and 34% in different groups (Garrigues et al., 2004; Higgins and Johanson, 2004), possibly because of inconsistencies in the application of specific diagnostic criteria to constipation. A recent systematic review of studies conducted in the United States revealed that the majority of reports documented an increase in the prevalence of constipation with age (Higgins and Johanson, 2004), although a cross-sectional survey in Spain found no such relationship (Garrigues et al., 2004). Constipation has a complex and varied etiology, particularly in the elderly, including alterations in neural innervation, smooth muscle activity, and neuroendrocrine function (Potter, 2003). Constipation may also be a side effect of medication intake, in particular, antidepressants, antihistamines, opioids, and diuretics (Talley et al., 2003). This variation in the underlying pathophysiology of constipation suggests that nutritional solutions such as prebiotics

Ian Rowland, Department of Food Biosciences, University of Reading, PO Box 226, Whiteknights, Reading RG6 6AP, United Kingdom.

may be a simplistic approach. However, dietary remedies represent a less invasive strategy than enemas and laxatives, they have minimal side effects, and some evidence indicates that prebiotics and probiotics may be effective.

Evidence suggests that changes in the composition of the intestinal microbiota can alter intestinal motility (Husebye et al., 2001; Lesniewska et al., 2006) and short-chain fatty acids produced by bacteria in the gut can influence transit time (Scheppach, 1994). A potential approach to relieving constipation is, therefore, to modify intestinal microbial composition by using prebiotics. The disaccharide lactulose is a widely used laxative that has prebiotic effects, in that it is not digested in the upper gastrointestinal tract and stimulates bifidobacterial proliferation in the colon. Short-chain fatty acids generated by fermentation of lactulose create osmotic effects that may promote laxation (Kot and Pettit-Young, 1992). Other prebiotics such as inulin, fructo-oligosaccharides (FOS), and galacto-oligosaccharides (GOS) have also been reported to exert laxative effects, although the effects are usually mild and do not reach statistical significance partly due to the degree of interindividual variation in dietary responses (reviewed by Macfarlane et al., 2006). For example, Teuri and Korpela (1998) conducted a small double-blind, crossover study with 14 female volunteers aged 69 to 87 with constipation. The subjects consumed either two control yogurts or two yogurts containing GOS, providing a daily GOS dose of 9 g per day for 2 weeks. During the GOS intake period, the defecation frequency was higher (7.1 per week) than during the control period (5.9 per week), and the subjects reported that defecation was easier during the GOS intervention period, although this finding did not reach statistical significance. Furthermore, GOS had no statistically significant effect on the consistency of feces, and the authors reported considerable interindividual variation. Similar between-subject variation was noted by Kleessen et al. (1997) in a study comparing lactose and inulin in elderly subjects (15 and 10 subjects, respectively). Inulin, in doses of 20 g increasing to 40 g/day for 19 days, had the more effective laxative action of the two carbohydrates.

One approach to evaluating the effect of prebiotics and other nondigestible carbohydrates on laxation is to compare effects on fecal bulking. Wheat bran (insoluble fiber) increased stool weight in healthy volunteers by 5 g/g of ingested carbohydrate (Cummings et al., 1992), whereas soluble fiber such as that in pectin and guar gum had relatively minor effects (1- to 2-g increase in fecal weight/g of carbohydrate) (Cummings et al., 1976). For nondigestible oligosaccharides, increased stool weight

by 1.5 to 2.2 g/g of ingested carbohydrate and modest stool bulking effects have been reported (Cummings et al., 1992; Gibson and Roberfroid, 1995).

DIARRHEA AND ACUTE GASTROENTERITIS

Diarrhea is an important problem worldwide, especially for young children and elderly individuals. For example, approximately 85% of mortality associated with diarrhea in the developed world involves the elderly (Gangarosa et al., 1992). Diarrhea can be acute (less than 14 days duration and usually caused by enteric infections), persistent (lasting more than 14 days), or chronic (lasting 30 days or more).

AAD

Antibiotic-associated diarrhea (AAD) is a common complication of antibiotic use. Although relatively rare in nonhospitalized patients, AAD is much more common in hospitals, nursing homes, and other types of chronic care facilities, where the frequency of disease can range from 3 to 60% (McFarland, 1993, 1998). AAD usually occurs 2 to 8 weeks after treatment with antibiotics, especially broad-spectrum antimicrobial agents. This disorder is probably due to disruption of the intestinal microbiota with concomitant reduction of colonization resistance to opportunistic intestinal pathogens. One such pathogen, *Clostridium difficile*, has been implicated as a cause of AAD in 10 to 26% of patients, including fatal infections (McFarland, 1998). The incidence of nosocomial *C. difficile* infections has increased markedly in the past 10 years in many developed countries.

Probiotics, particularly "*Saccharomyces boulardii*" and *Lactobacillus rhamnosus* GG, have demonstrated potential as therapeutic and preventative treatments for AAD and *C. difficile* infections (Macfarlane et al., 2006). It seems reasonable to hypothesize that prebiotics might be similarly effective by elevating bifidobacterial concentrations in the gut and increasing colonization resistance. This hypothesis has been tested in two large-scale interventions with varying results. In one placebo-controlled, randomized, double-blind trial (Lewis et al., 2005a), 435 hospitalized patients more than 65 years of age who had been prescribed a broad-spectrum antibiotic in the preceding 24 h were allocated to either the FOS (from Orafti, Inc.) or sucrose (12 g/day) groups. Carbohydrates were consumed for the duration of the antibiotic treatment (variable time) and for 1 week after antibiotic treatment. Subjects were monitored for an additional week because *C. difficile*-associated diarrhea occurs within 14 days of antibiotic treatment. The end points were based on stool form, defecation frequency, and fecal microbiology.

Of the 435 subjects, 116 (27%) individuals developed diarrhea, and 49 (11%) patients had positive samples for *C. difficile* toxin. No significant differences were uncovered between FOS and placebo groups for any of the end points despite significant increases in fecal bifidobacterial counts in the FOS group, indicating effective compliance within the group. In summary, FOS did not protect elderly patients treated with broad-spectrum antibiotics from AAD, whether associated with *C. difficile* or not (Lewis et al., 2005a).

In a second study, the same authors investigated the effect of FOS on relapse of treated *C. difficile* diarrhea (Lewis et al., 2005b). About 10 to 20% of patients relapse with AAD despite successful treatment for *C. difficile*-associated diarrhea (Kelly et al., 1994). This study included a randomized double-blind, placebo-controlled design in which 142 patients (>18 years) with *C. difficile*-associated diarrhea (treated with metronidazole and vancomycin) were allocated to FOS or sucrose (12 g/day) groups. The supplemental carbohydrates were ingested as soon as possible after a diagnosis of AAD until 30 days after cessation of diarrhea, with a 30-day follow-up. Relapses occurred in 30 patients after approximately 18 days and were more common in the placebo group (34.3%) than the FOS group (8.3%; $P < 0.001$). The mean length of hospital stay was reduced for individuals ingesting supplemental FOS.

Effects of prebiotic and synbiotic treatments on the composition of fecal microbiota and *C. difficile* carriage were compared by Orrhage et al. (2000) in a placebo-controlled, parallel design intervention. Three groups of 10 healthy subjects (21 to 50 years) were given oral cefpodoxime proxetil for 7 days. One group was given a placebo (milk), a second group received the same milk plus FOS (15 g/day), and a third group received a synbiotic composed of FOS (15 g/day) with fermented milk providing *Bifidobacterium longum* BB536 (2.5×10^{10} to 10×10^{10} CFU/day) plus *Lactobacillus acidophilus* NCFB 1748 (10×10^{10} to 15×10^{10} CFU/day). The dietary treatments were consumed for 21 days and initiated at the time that antibiotic treatment was started. In all three groups, the numbers of aerobic organisms, especially *Escherichia coli*, declined during antibiotic treatment followed by relative proliferation of enterococci. Anaerobe numbers (bifidobacteria, *Bacteroides*, and lactobacilli) also decreased markedly in all groups during antibiotic treatment. Among the placebo and prebiotics-treated volunteers, 6 of 10 subjects in each group were colonized by *C. difficile*, and 3 of 6 colonized patients yielded cytotoxin-positive specimens. In contrast, in the synbiotic group, only one subject yielded detectable numbers of *C. difficile* on one sampling occasion.

In summary, a combination of probiotics and prebiotics, but not prebiotics alone, diminished *C. difficile* carriage with antibiotic treatment.

Traveler's Diarrhea

Only one study of the effect of prebiotics consumption on prevention of traveler's diarrhea has been published. In this study (Cummings et al., 2001), 244 healthy subjects who were traveling to destinations at high or medium risk for traveler's diarrhea were randomized to groups receiving either FOS (10 g/day) or a placebo orally for 2 weeks prior to and during a 2-week excursion. Differences in the incidence of diarrhea (as determined in a poststudy questionnaire) did not reach statistical significance ($P = 0.08$) when both groups were compared, but diarrhea occurred less frequently in the FOS group (11.2%) than in the placebo group (19.5%). Furthermore, diarrheal episodes were reported by subjects in the FOS group as being less severe ($P < 0.05$), and no significant differences were apparent between the two groups with respect to bowel frequency or consistency. Such equivocal results are similar to findings obtained in studies of probiotics in patients with traveler's diarrhea and may reflect the diversity of microbes that may cause gastroenteritis. Pathogens may target the small intestine rather than the colon, circumventing effects of prebiotics and probiotics active in the large intestine.

IBS

Irritable bowel syndrome (IBS) is a very common gastrointestinal disorder associated with a wide range of symptoms, including abdominal pain or discomfort, loose or hard stools, bloating, and flatulence. Generally, treatment of IBS is focused on medications rather than nutritional approaches. A number of investigations of the potentially ameliorative effects of probiotics on IBS symptoms have been published. In total, nine randomized placebo-controlled trials, during periods of up to 6 months, have been reported, with variable results. Three trials including different beneficial microbes such as *L. acidophilus* (Halpern et al., 1996), *Lactobacillus plantarum* 299V (Niedzielin et al., 2001), and *Bifidobacterium infantis* 35624 (Whorwell et al., 2006) demonstrated significant improvements in a wide range of symptoms. Other studies reported improvements in only one or a few symptoms, and one study (with *Lactobacillus reuteri*) showed no effect (Niv et al., 2005). Overall these studies indicate that modification of components of the lactic acid bacterial microbiota may influence IBS symptoms. In contrast to probiotics, however, studies of prebiotics in the context of IBS are much more limited.

Hunter et al. (1999) conducted a double-blind, placebo-controlled, crossover trial with 21 subjects (14 patients with diarrhea and 7 patients with constipation) given, for 4 weeks, short-chain FOS or sucrose (3 times 2 g per day). No significant changes were noted for any of the end points including fecal weight, fecal pH, transit time, and breath hydrogen concentration. Colecchia et al. (2006) reported an open, multicenter trial (approximately 36 days) on a synbiotic preparation comprising short-chain FOS plus *B. longum* W11. The study used a large number of male and female patients (636 in total, aged 18 to 80 years) with constipation-type IBS (Rome II criteria). Unfortunately, the study design did not include a placebo. The synbiotic dose was low (3 g per day), but improvements in stool frequencies were detected, increasing from 2.9 ± 1.6 times/week to 4.1 ± 1.6 times/week in the synbiotic-treated group. However, in the group initially classified as having no symptoms, significant increases in frequencies of abdominal pain (8 to 44%) and bloating (3 to 27%) were reported. In contrast, in the group initially classified as having moderate-to-severe symptoms, symptom frequencies dropped significantly in the synbiotic group (from 38.8 to 4.1% for abdominal pain and 62.9 to 9.6% for bloating).

IBD

The term inflammatory bowel disease (IBD) encompasses two important chronic intestinal disorders, ulcerative colitis and Crohn's disease. Both diseases are characterized as chronic intestinal disorders of unknown etiology in which the mucosal immune system in genetically susceptible individuals demonstrates an aberrant response towards commensal bacteria in the gut (Strober et al., 2007).

Reports of reduced amounts of bifidobacteria in IBD and reported immunomodulatory functions of lactobacilli and bifidobacteria have resulted in clinical trials of probiotics for therapy and maintenance of remission after treatment of patients with Crohn's disease, ulcerative colitis, or pouchitis. Probiotics appear to yield a consistent benefit in a small number of studies, particularly pouchitis (see chapter 20). Studies of prebiotics applications in the context of IBD are limited.

Furrie et al. (2005) conducted a small double-blind, parallel-design, and randomized pilot study with 18 patients (aged 24 to 67 years) with active ulcerative colitis. The test treatment was a combination of probiotic *B. longum*, isolated from healthy rectal epithelium, and prebiotic fructans (Beneo Synergy 1; Orafti Inc.). Subjects in the treatment group consumed a capsule containing freeze-dried viable *B. longum* (2×10^{11} CFU/capsule) and prebiotic fructans (6 g) twice per day for 4 weeks. The control group received maltodextrin (6 g/day) instead of the prebiotic and a capsule of potato starch instead of the probiotic. Clinical status was scored, and rectal biopsy specimens were collected before and after treatment (1 month) for measurement of histology and inflammatory markers. Fourteen patients completed the study (eight treated patients and six controls). Sigmoidoscopy scores (evaluated on a scale of 0 to 6) were reduced in the test group ($n = 8$) by a mean of 1.3 points during the 4-week study period. Five patients demonstrated improvement by sigmoidoscopy, two patients were unchanged, and one patient showed evidence of more severe disease. The placebo group ($n = 6$) yielded a mean increase of 0.58 in sigmoidoscopy scores during the same period (three patients with increased scores and three patients with decreased scores). When compared with the placebo, the increased scores for the synbiotic group were borderline significant ($P = 0.06$). Histological examination of biopsy specimens revealed similar effects. Biopsy specimens obtained from seven patients in the synbiotic group showed an overall reduction in histology scores (1.7 at the start and 1.1 after treatment), whereas mean scores in the placebo group (five biopsy specimens) were increased. The biopsy samples in the test group exhibited reduced inflammation and showed evidence of epithelial regeneration. Proinflammatory cytokines, tumor necrosis factor, and interleukin-1 (IL-1) were significantly reduced after synbiotic treatment (Furrie et al., 2005). Quantities of mRNA for human beta-defensins 2, 3, and 4, which are strongly upregulated in active ulcerative colitis, were also reduced in the synbiotic treatment group.

Welters et al. (2002) investigated effects of prebiotic treatment (inulin) in patients with pouchitis. Pouchitis refers to inflammation of the ileal pouch-anal anastomosis formed after resection of the colon in patients with ulcerative colitis. Twenty patients were given inulin (24 g/day) or a placebo for 3 weeks in a randomized, double-blind, crossover study. Stools were analyzed after each test period for pH, short-chain fatty acids, microbial composition, and bile acids. Inflammation was assessed by endoscopy and by histological examination of biopsy material. The endoscopy scores indicated an improvement in symptoms following prebiotic treatment, and mucosal inflammation in the ileal reservoir was reduced. These two small studies indicate that prebiotic or synbiotic treatment of patients with active ulcerative colitis or pouchitis was associated with improvement of clinical outcomes and inflammation in IBD and strongly suggest that more comprehensive studies are warranted.

Studies of prebiotics and synbiotics in patients with Crohn's disease have been less convincing. Lindsay et al. (2006) conducted a small, open-label trial with 10 patients (8 males and 2 females; age range, 29 to 46 years) with active ileocolonic or colonic Crohn's disease. The trial consisted of a 1-week baseline period followed by a 3-week intervention with fructan prebiotics, which comprised a mixture of FOS (70%) and inulin (30%). Disease activity, as measured by the Harvey Bradshaw index (HBI), diminished significantly from a mean of 9.8 (standard deviation, 3.1) at baseline to 6.9 (3.4) after fructan administration ($P = 0.01$). Four patients went into remission, as defined by a reduction in HBI to 5 or less. The mean reduction in HBI of those patients entering clinical remission was 4.5 (range, 1 to 7), compared with the overall mean reduction in HBI of 3 (range, 0 to 7). C-reactive protein was not reduced during the intervention, and the mean percentages of IL-10-positive mucosal dendritic cells measured by flow cytometry of dissociated rectal biopsy specimens increased from 30.1 to 53.3 ($P = 0.06$).

Two published studies using synbiotic mixtures in patients with Crohn's disease yielded negative results. In the first study (Rutgeerts et al., 2004), a double-blind, placebo-controlled parallel trial with 63 patients with Crohn's disease on anti-inflammatory medications included 31 patients in the placebo group and 32 patients in the treatment group (lactobacilli strains [4×10^{10} CFU/day] plus beta-glucan, inulin, pectin, and resistant starch). The end point, or time to relapse, was unaffected by synbiotic treatment. A similarly negative result was obtained in a second study (Chermesh et al., 2007). This prospective multicenter, randomized study of 30 patients with Crohn's disease included placebo and synbiotic groups (which received four probiotic species and four prebiotics). No significant effects on endoscopic or clinical postoperative relapse rates were reported.

COLORECTAL CANCER

Within Europe, North America, Australia, and New Zealand, the incidence of colorectal cancer is exceeded only by that of lung and prostate cancer in men and breast cancer in women (Boyle and Langman, 2000). Epidemiological evidence suggests that diet plays a significant role in the etiology of colorectal cancer. However, identification of specific risk factors in the diet has been problematic owing to inconsistent data (reviewed by Heavey et al., 2004). Considerable evidence suggests that the gut microbiota plays a role in the etiology of colorectal cancer. The evidence is based on the fact that certain gut bacteria are capable of synthesizing or activating carcinogens from dietary precursors, such as N-nitroso-compounds (Rowland and Gangolli, 1999; Hughes and Rowland, 2003). In addition, Venturi et al. (1997) detected the presence of DNA-damaging activity in fecal samples from human volunteers. The postulated involvement of the gut microbiota in causation of colorectal cancer suggests that prebiotics, by altering the intestinal microbial composition, may modify cancer risk.

Studies in animal models provide evidence that probiotics, prebiotics, and synbiotics can beneficially influence various stages in the initiation and development of colon cancer (Commane et al., 2005). Limited evidence from epidemiological studies supports the protective effects of products containing probiotics and prebiotics in humans, but a recent randomized, double-blind, placebo-controlled dietary intervention study with a synbiotic preparation yielded promising results on the basis of biomarkers of cancer risk (Rafter et al., 2007) (Table 1). Patients who had polyps or adenocarcinomas removed previously were randomized to placebo or synbiotic (*Lactobacillus delbrueckii* subsp. *rhamnosus* GG [10^{10} CFU/day] plus *Bifidobacterium lactis* strain Bb12 [10^{10} CFU/day] together with a sachet of an inulin-FOS mixture [12 g/day]) treatment groups for 12 weeks.

The synbiotic intervention reduced epithelial cell proliferation in rectal biopsy specimens from the polypectomized patients, a change indicative of reduced cancer risk. Genotoxicity assays of rectal biopsy specimens and fecal water indicated a reduced exposure to genotoxins in both patient groups receiving synbiotics. The intervention also decreased the capacity of fecal water to induce necrosis in colonic cells and yielded beneficial effects on fecal water modulation of epithelial barrier function in polypectomized patients. Both end points are indicative of antiproliferative potential in the intestine. Thus, several colorectal cancer biomarkers were altered favorably by the synbiotic intervention and reflected results with the same synbiotic formulation in experimental animal models (Femia et al., 2002).

IMMUNE FUNCTION

Aging is associated with deterioration and dysregulation of immunity in the elderly (Pawelec and Solana, 1997). The decline in immune function is associated mainly with changes in T-cell populations, although other components of the immune system are also affected (Pawelec et al., 1999). Chronic inflammation may also contribute to immune dysfunction in the elderly (Franceschi et al., 2000). Aging is also characterized by chronic inflammation due to increased amounts of proinflammatory cytokines (Franceschi et al., 2000). Considerable

Table 1 Effect of synbiotic treatment on colon cancer-related biomarkers in polypectomized patients[a]

Biomarker	Placebo group		Synbiotic group		P
	Day 0	6 wk	Day 0	6 wk	
Proliferative activity in biopsy sample (no. of labeled cells/crypt)	7.12 ± 2.94	7.62 ± 2.50	7.16 ± 2.22	6.19 ± 1.64	0.067
Epithelial barrier function (% transepithelial resistance)	133 ± 3	124 ± 4.6	126 ± 4.9	128 ± 5	0.025
Cytotoxicity (%)	7.56 ± 8.00	11.8 ± 11.2	17.59 ± 13.90	11.90 ± 9.8	0.033

[a]Polypectomy patients consumed either synbiotic (*L. rhamnosus* GG, *B. lactis* Bb12 + FOS-synergy 1) or placebo for 12 weeks. Effects on epithelial barrier function and cell toxicity were determined on fecal water samples in vitro. Values shown are means ± SD for 17 to 21 subjects. Data from Rafter et al. (2007).

interindividual variability in immune function in the elderly is a likely consequence of genetic, environmental, general health status, and nutritional factors.

A number of studies have reported that probiotics stimulate the immune system in elderly subjects. For example, Gill et al. (2001) showed that 3-week supplementation with *B. lactis* HN019 in elderly healthy volunteers significantly increased total lymphocyte counts, CD4[+] and CD25[+] cell counts, and NK cell activities.

Studies of the effects of prebiotics on immune function in elderly populations are limited and have yielded inconsistent results. Guigoz et al. (2002) conducted a 3-week intervention with short-chain FOS (8 g of Actilight per day) in 19 elderly nursing home patients. Blood and fecal samples were obtained before, immediately after, and 3 weeks following FOS supplementation, but no concurrent placebo control group was included. Fecal bifidobacterial counts increased after 3 weeks of FOS supplementation, and these changes were associated with significantly increased percentages of peripheral T lymphocytes and T-lymphocyte subsets (CD4[+] and CD8[+] T cells). Total numbers of white blood cells, activated T lymphocytes, and natural killer (NK) cells were not affected by the ingestion of FOS. Unexpectedly, changes in innate immune responses included decreased phagocytic activities of granulocytes and monocytes and decreased expression of IL-6 mRNA in peripheral blood monocytes. These results suggest a possible amelioration of inflammation in elderly subjects after FOS supplementation.

Bunout et al. (2002) investigated the effects of a prebiotic mixture on the immune response in healthy elderly people (70 years and older). The subjects (*n* = 66) were randomly assigned to the prebiotic mixture (6 g/day of a mixture of 70% short-chain [Raftilose] and 30% long-chain [Raftiline] FOS) or a placebo (6 g of maltodextrin powder). Two weeks after the start of the study, all subjects were vaccinated with influenza and pneumococcal vaccines. No changes in serum proteins, albumin, immunoglobulins, and secretory immunoglobulin A were observed at 8 weeks. Antibodies against influenza B and *Streptococcus pneumoniae* increased significantly from weeks 0 to 8, but no significant differences between groups were seen. Antibodies against influenza A did not increase in either group. No effects of prebiotics on IL-4 and gamma interferon secretion by cultured monocytes were observed.

OTHER EFFECTS

Barrier Function in Patients with Burn Injuries

Burn injury is associated with dramatic alterations of the intestinal microbiota and concomitant changes in gastrointestinal barrier function and permeability (Deitch, 1990). The evidence that consumption of probiotics can stabilize gut barrier function (Gotteland et al., 2001) led Olguin et al. (2005) to investigate whether prebiotics may be similarly effective. The study was a randomized double-blind, controlled clinical trial with 31 burn patients who ingested FOS (6 g/day) or sucrose (6 g/day) as a placebo for 15 days. Gastrointestinal permeability to sucrose and lactulose/mannitol was evaluated before, during, and after (day 21) treatment. By comparison to healthy subjects, sucrose excretion and lactose:mannitol ratios initially increased four- to fivefold in patients with burn injuries, and these high levels of marker excretion decreased significantly during the study, indicating a gradual recovery in barrier function. However, no significant differences were noted between the FOS and placebo groups, indicating that the normalization of gastrointestinal permeability was not accelerated by prebiotic consumption.

CONCLUSIONS

Clinical studies of applications of prebiotics in human medicine are limited compared to the numbers of reports regarding probiotics. Small numbers of patients have been included in many studies, which limits the nature and number of definitive conclusions that can be drawn. However, some studies, particularly in the areas of ulcerative colitis and acute gastroenteritis, have demonstrated promising results that may be confirmed in larger-scale intervention studies. Studies on the influence of prebiotics on immune function have focused on elderly subjects and have failed to yield consistent beneficial effects. However, in the area of colorectal cancer, more promising results of prebiotics in combination with probiotics (synbiotics) on biomarkers of cancer risk have been obtained, and these data are consistent with extensive studies in animal models showing protective effects of probiotics and prebiotics on tumor initiation and development.

References

Boyle, P., and J. S. Langman. 2000. ABC of colorectal cancer: epidemiology. *Br. Med. J.* 321:805–808.

Bunout, D., S. Hirsch, M. Pia de la Maza, C. Munoz, F. Haschke, P. Steenhout, P. Klassen, G. Barrera, V. Gattas, and M. Petermann. 2002. Effects of prebiotics on the immune response to vaccination in the elderly. *J. Parenteral Enteral Nutr.* 26:372–376.

Chermesh, I., A. Tamir, R. Reshef, Y. Chowers, A. Suissa, D. Katz, M. Gelber, Z. Halpern, S. Bengmark, and S. R. Eliakim. 2007. Failure of Synbiotic 2000 to prevent postoperative recurrence of Crohn's disease. *Dig. Dis. Sci.* 52:385–389.

Colecchia, A., A. Vestito, A. La Rocca, F. Pasqui, A. Nikiforaki, D. Festi, and the Symbiotic Study Group. 2006. Effect of a symbiotic preparation on the clinical manifestations of irritable bowel syndrome, constipation-variant. Results of an open, uncontrolled multicenter study. *Minerva Gastroenterol. Dietol.* 52:349–358.

Commane, D., R. Hughes, C. Shortt, and I. Rowland. 2005. The potential mechanisms involved in the anti-carcinogenic action of probiotics. *Mutat. Res.* 591:278–289.

Cummings, J. H., S. A. Bingham, K. W. Heaton, and M. A. Eastwood. 1992. Fecal weight, colon cancer risk, and dietary intake of nonstarch polysaccharides (dietary fiber). *Gastroenterology* 103:1783–1789.

Cummings, J. H., S. Christie, and T. J. Cole. 2001. A study of fructo oligosaccharides in the prevention of travellers' diarrhoea. *Aliment. Pharmacol. Ther.* 15:1139–1145.

Cummings, J. H., M. J. Hill, D. J. Jenkins, J. R. Pearson, and H. W. Wiggins. 1976. Changes in fecal composition and colonic function due to cereal fiber. *Am. J Clin. Nutr.* 29:1468–1473.

Deitch, E. A. 1990. Intestinal permeability is increased in burn patients shortly after injury. *Surgery* 107:411–416.

Femia, A. P., C. Luceri, P. Dolara, A. Giannini, A. Biggeri, M. Salvadori, Y. Clune, K. J. Collins, M. Paglierani, and

G. Caderni. 2002. Antitumorigenic activity of the prebiotic inulin enriched with oligofructose in combination with the probiotics *Lactobacillus rhamnosus* and *Bifidobacterium lactis* on azoxymethane-induced colon carcinogenesis in rats. *Carcinogenesis* 23:1953–1960.

Franceschi, C., M. Bonafe, S. Valensin, F. Olivieri, M. De Luca, E. Ottaviani, and G. De Benedictis. 2000. Inflamm-aging. An evolutionary perspective on immunosenescence. *Ann. N. Y. Acad. Sci.* 908:244–254.

Furrie, E., S. Macfarlane, A. Kennedy, J. H. Cummings, S. V. Walsh, D. A. O'Neil, and G. T. Macfarlane. 2005. Synbiotic therapy (*Bifidobacterium longum*/Synergy 1) initiates resolution of inflammation in patients with active ulcerative colitis: a randomised controlled pilot trial. *Gut* 54:242–249.

Gangarosa, R. E., R. I. Glass, J. F. Lew, and J. R. Boring. 1992. Hospitalizations involving gastroenteritis in the United States 1985: the special burden of the disease in the elderly. *Am. J. Epidemiol.* 135:281–290.

Garrigues, V., C. Galvez, V. Ortiz, M. Ponce, P. Nos, and J. Ponce. 2004. Prevalence of constipation: agreement among several criteria and evaluation of the diagnostic accuracy of qualifying symptoms and self-reported definition in a population-based survey in Spain. *Am. J. Epidemiol.* 159:520–526.

Gibson, G. R., and M. B. Roberfroid. 1995. Dietary modulation of the human colonic microbiota: introducing the concept of prebiotics. *J. Nutr.* 125:1401–1412.

Gill, H. S., K. J. Rutherfurd, and M. L. Cross. 2001. Enhancement of immunity in the elderly by dietary supplementation with the probiotic *Bifidobacterium lactis* HNO19. *Am. J. Clin. Nutr.* 74:833–839.

Gotteland, M., S. Cruchet, and S. Verbeke. 2001. Effect of *Lactobacillus* ingestion on the gastrointestinal mucosal barrier alterations induced by indomethacin in humans. *Aliment. Pharmacol. Ther.* 15:11–17.

Halpern, G. M., T. Prindiville, M. Blankenburg, T. Hsia, and M. E. Gershwin. 1996. Treatment of irritable bowel syndrome with Lacteol Fort: a randomized, double-blind, crossover trial. *Am. J. Gastroenterol.* 91:579–585.

Heavey, P. M., D. McKenna, and I. R. Rowland. 2004. Colorectal cancer and the relationship between genes and environment. *Nutr. Cancer* 48:124–141.

Guigoz, Y., F. Rochat, G. Perruisseau-Carrier, I. Rochat, and E. J. Schiffrin. 2002. Effects of oligosaccharide on the faecal flora and non-specific immune system in elderly people. *Nutr. Res.* 22:3–25.

Higgins, P. D., and J. F. Johanson. 2004. Epidemiology of constipation in North America: a systematic review. *Am. J. Gastroenterol.* 99:750–759.

Hughes, R., and I. Rowland. 2003. Nutritional and microbial modification of carcinogenesis, pp. 208–236. *In* R. Fuller and G. Perdigon (ed.), *Gut Flora, Nutrition, Immunity and Health*. Blackwell Publishing, Oxford, United Kingdom.

Hunter, J. O., Q. Tuffnell, and A. J. Lee. 1999. Controlled trial of oligofructose in the management of irritable bowel syndrome. *J. Nutr.* 129:1451S–1453S.

Husebye, E., P. M. Hellstrom, F. Sundler, J. Chen, and T. Midtvedt. 2001. Influence of microbial species on small intestinal myoelectric activity and transit in germ-free rats. *Am. J. Physiol. Gastroenterol. Liver Physiol.* 280:G368–G380.

Kelly, C. P., C. Pothoulakis, and J. T. LaMont. 1994. *Clostridium difficile* colitis. *N. Engl. J. Med.* 330:257–262.

Kleessen, B., B. Sykura, H.-J. Zunft, and M. Blaut. 1997. Effects of inulin and lactose on fecal microflora, microbial activity and bowel habit in elderly constipated persons. *Am. J. Clin. Nutr.* 65:1397–1402.

Kot, T. V., and N. A. Pettit-Young. 1992. Lactulose in the management of constipation: a current review. *Ann. Pharmacother.* 26:1277–1282.

Lesniewska, V., I. Rowland, H. N. Laerke, G. Grant, and P. J. Naughton. 2006. Relationship between dietary induced changes in intestinal commensal microflora and duodenojejunal myoelectric activity monitored by radiotelemetry in the rat in vivo. *Exp. Physiol.* 91:229–237.

Lewis, S., S. Burmeister, S. Cohen, J. Brazier, and A. Awasthi. 2005a. Failure of dietary oligofructose to prevent antibiotic-associated diarrhea. *Aliment. Pharmacol. Ther.* 21:469–477.

Lewis, S., S. Burmeister, and J. Brazier. 2005b. Effect of prebiotic oligofructose on relapse of *Clostridium difficile*-associated diarrhea: a randomized, controlled study. *Clin. Gastroenterol. Hepatol.* 3:442–448.

Lindsay, J. O., K. Whelan, A. J. Stagg, P. Gobin, H. O. Al-Hassi, N. Rayment, M. A. Kamm, S. C. Knight, and A. Forbes. 2006. Clinical, microbiological, and immunological effects of fructo-oligosaccharide in patients with Crohn's disease. *Gut* 55:348–355.

Macfarlane, S., G. T. Macfarlane, and J. H. Cummings. 2006. Review article: prebiotics in the gastrointestinal tract. *Aliment. Pharmacol. Ther.* 24:701–714.

McFarland, L. V. 1993. Diarrhoea acquired in the hospital. *Gastroenterol. Clin. North Am.* 22:563–577.

McFarland, L. V. 1998. Epidemiology, risk factors and treatments for antibiotic-associated diarrhea. *Dig. Dis.* 16:292–307.

Niedzielin, K., H. Kordecki, and B. Birkenfeld. 2001. A controlled, double-blind, randomized study on the efficacy of *Lactobacillus plantarum* 299V in patients with irritable bowel syndrome. *Eur. J. Gastroenterol. Hepatol.* 13:1135–1136.

Niv, E., T. Naftali, R. Hallak, and N. Vaisman. 2005. The efficacy of *Lactobacillus reuteri* ATCC 55730 in the treatment of patients with irritable bowel syndrome—a double blind, placebo-controlled, randomized study. *Clin. Nutr.* 24:925–931.

Olguin, F., M. Araya, S. Hirsch, O. Brunser, V. Ayala, R. Rivera, and M. Gotteland. 2005. Prebiotic ingestion does not improve gastrointestinal barrier function in burn patients. *Burns* 31:482–488.

Orrhage, K., S. Sjostedt, and C. E. Nord. 2000. Effect of supplements with lactic acid bacteria and oligofructose on the intestinal microflora during administration of cefpodoxime proxetil *J. Antimicrob. Chemother.* 46:603–612.

Pawelec, G., and R. Solana. 1997. Immunosenescence. *Immunol. Today* 18:514–516.

Pawelec, G., R. B. Effros, C. Caruso, E. Remarque, Y. Barnett, and R. Solana. 1999. T cells and aging. *Front. Biosci.* 4: D216–D269.

Potter, J. 2003. Bowel care in older people. *Clin. Med.* 3:48–51.

Rafter, J., M. Bennett, G. Caderni, Y. Clune, R. Hughes, P. C. Karlsson, A. Klinder, M. O'Riordan, G. O'Sullivan, B. Pool-Zobel, G. Rechkemmer, M. Roller, I. Rowland, M. Salvadori, H. Thijs, J. Van Loo, B. Watzl, and J. K. Collins. 2007. Dietary synbiotics reduce cancer risk factors in polypectomised and colon cancer patients. *Am. J. Clin. Nutr.* 85:488–496.

Rowland, I. R., and S. D. Gangolli. 1999. Role of gastrointestinal flora in the metabolic and toxicological activities of xenobiotics, p. 561–576. *In* B. Ballantyne, T. C. Marrs, and T. Syverson (ed.), *General and Applied Toxicology*, 2nd ed. Macmillan Publishers Ltd, London, United Kingdom.

Rutgeerts, P., G. Van Assche, and S. Vermeire. 2004. Optimizing anti-TNF treatment in inflammatory bowel disease. *Gastroenterology* 126:1593–1610.

Scheppach, W. 1994. Effects of short chain fatty acids on gut morphology and function. *Gut* 35:S35–S38.

Strober, W., I. Fuss, and P. Mannon. 2007. The fundamental basis of inflammatory bowel disease. *J. Clin. Investig.* 117:514–521.

Talley, N. J., M. Jones, G. Nuyts, and D. Dubois. 2003. Risk factors for chronic constipation based on a general practice sample. *Am. J. Clin. Gastroenterol.* 98:1107–1111.

Teuri, U., and R. Korpela. 1998. Galacto-oligosaccharides relieve constipation in elderly people. *Ann. Nutr. Metab.* 42:319–327.

Venturi, M., R. J. Hambly, B. Glinghammar, J. J. Rafter, and I. R. Rowland. 1997. Genotoxic activity in human faecal water and the role of bile acids: a study using the Comet assay. *Carcinogenesis* 18:2353–2359.

Whitehead, W. E., D. Drinkwater, L. J. Cheskin, B. R. Heller, and M. M. Schuster. 1989. Constipation in the elderly living at home. Definition, prevalence, and relationship to lifestyle and health status, *J. Am. Geriatr. Soc.* 37:423–429.

Whorwell, P. J., L. Altringer, J. Morel, Y. Bond, D. Charbonneau, L. O'Mahony, B. Kiely, F. Shanahan, and E. M. Quigley. 2006. Efficacy of an encapsulated probiotic *Bifidobacterium infantis* 35624 in women with irritable bowel syndrome. *Am. J. Gastroenterol.* 101:1581–1590.

Therapeutic Microbiology: Probiotics and Related Strategies
Edited by J. Versalovic and M. Wilson
© 2008 ASM Press, Washington, DC

3.3. SYNBIOTICS

Stig Bengmark

Synbiotics in Human Medicine

24

Thirty years have passed since Gilliland and Speck reported that patients with inflammatory bowel disease (IBD) had a significantly different microbiota from that of healthy individuals (Gilliland and Speck, 1977). Finegold and Sutter reported in the following year an altered microbiota in 75% of healthy omnivorous and 35% of vegetarian Americans (Finegold and Sutter, 1978). Similar observations were later made for European populations (Ahrne et al., 1998).

Numerous attempts during the last 30 years to reconstitute or remodel the microbiota in order to prevent or treat diseases were repeatedly made. However, these often produced dissatisfying results. One obvious explanation suggested by recent reviews (Sartor, 2004; Marteau, 2006) is that the majority of clinical studies thus far have been underpowered.

FACTORS INFLUENCING CLINICAL STUDY OUTCOMES

Several factors might contribute to differences in the outcome of interventions with probiotics and prebiotics.

Regenerative Capacity

The spontaneous regenerative capacity of the gastrointestinal tract is much greater in young experimental animals and in animals with induced disease. Regenerative capacity is greater in humans with acute disease than in humans with chronic disease.

Differences in Daily Doses

The daily dose related to body weight or to the gastrointestinal mucosal surface is generally much larger in experimental animals and in pediatric cases. In the majority of studies, the daily dose used in humans has been 1 billion lactic acid bacteria (LAB) once or twice per day, up to 10 billion organisms/day. Larger doses delivered more impressive results. Large-scale doses in liver transplantation (Rayes et al., 2005) and trauma (Spindler-Vesel et al., 2007) with Synbiotic 2000 and Synbiotic 2000 Forte (see below) included 40 and 400 billion LAB per day. In IBD, VSL#3 was administered at a dosage of 1,200 billion LAB per day (Venturi et al., 1999). A total of 80 billion LAB of Synbiotic 2000 per day were administered to patients with chronic liver disease, according

Stig Bengmark, Departments of Hepatology and Surgery, Institute of Hepatology, University College London Medical School, 69-75 Chenies Mews, London WC1E 6HX, United Kingdom.

to recent reviews (Liu et al., 2004; Riordan et al., 2007). Large differences in the relative abilities of various LAB to survive the harsh environment of the upper gastrointestinal tract explain why supplemented LAB may reach the lower gastrointestinal tract in concentrations too low to generate clinical effects (Miettinen et al., 1998). Some of the strains tested (*Lactobacillus plantarum*) demonstrated, however, an increased ability to influence cytokine production and modulate inflammation.

Variability of Probiotic Strains

Probiotic strains vary with respect to efficacy or potency. Studies using LAB have focused on LAB commonly used by the dairy industry and have failed to demonstrate positive effects either in connection with elective surgery (Woodcock et al., 2004) or with intensive care unit (ICU) patients (Jain et al., 2004). In these studies a composition of LABs consisting of *Lactobacillus acidophilus* LA5, *Bifidobacterium lactis* BP12, *Streptococcus thermophilus*, and *Lactobacillus bulgaricus* (TREVIS; Chr. Hansen, Hørsholm, Denmark) was used. Although the treatments in both studies favorably influenced the microbial composition of the upper gastrointestinal tract, probiotics did not influence intestinal permeability, nor were they associated with measurable clinical benefits. Other studies have demonstrated the inability of *Lactobacillus rhamnosus* GG to affect human antibiotic-associated diarrhea caused by *Clostridium difficile* (Thomas et al., 2001) and *Helicobacter pylori* infections (Armuzzi et al., 2001a, 2001b).

LAB and probiotics derived from LAB differ with respect to relative abilities to modulate the innate immune system and to control disease. The strains with the greatest capacity to induce interleukin-12 (IL-12) seem to be the most effective probiotics to up-regulate major histocompatibility complex class II and B7-2 (CD86), indicative of immune cell maturation (Armuzzi et al., 2001b). Striking differences in lactobacillus production of IL-12 and tumor necrosis factor (TNF) were reported, with production ranging in descending order from strong (*Lactobacillus casei*) to somewhat strong *L. plantarum* Lb1 to weak (*L. fermentum* Lb20, *L. johnsonii* La1, and *L. plantarum* 299v) to none (*L. reuteri*). The ability to control various pathogens is also strain specific and seems to be limited to a few strains. For example, when the ability of 50 different LAB to control 23 different pathogenic *C. difficile* strains was tested, only 5 probiotics (LABs) proved effective against all *C. difficile* isolates and 18 strains were antagonistic versus a subset of *C. difficile* strains, but as many as 27 candidate probiotics were totally ineffective (Naaber et al., 2004). The five most effective strains demonstrating potent inhibition against *C. difficile* were *L. paracasei* subsp. paracasei (two strains) and *L. plantarum* (three strains). *L. paracasei* subsp. *paracasei* proved to be the most potent inducer of

Th1 cytokines and potently repressed Th2 cytokines when more than 100 LAB organisms were compared with each other (Fujiwara et al., 2004).

Multispecies Communities

A combination of several probiotic bacteria may be necessary as probiotic bacteria function in vivo as multispecies communities. The microbiota consists of approximately 800 or more different bacterial species with at least 40 predominant species. The human microbiota functions like an organ, and different bacterial species interact as a microbial consortium with the host mucosa. The microbiota constitutes a good example of both symbiosis (living together for mutual benefit) and synergy (increased potency that exceeds additive effects). As the knowledge about the mammalian microbiota expands, the scientific community can progress from a probiotic soloist (single-strain) strategy to a "chamber orchestra" of probiotics (multistrain) to a full probiotic or synbiotic "symphony orchestra." Solo or multiprobiotic strategies may be relevant for different health promotion or disease prevention strategies. Such multistrain formulations might benefit from the addition of prebiotics, micronutrients, or other plant-derived products.

The effects of treatment may vary depending on the application of single-strain or multistrain probiotics. Total microbiota replacement may include the transfer of donated microbiota (feces) from one individual to another. Such an approach will most likely never become widely accepted therapy, but dramatic effects have been reported (Borody et al., 2003, 2004). Multistrain probiotics have been reported to reduce antibiotic-associated diarrhea, prevent enteric infections (*Salmonella enterica* serovar Typhimurium), and reduce pathogenic colonization (*Escherichia coli*) (Timmerman et al., 2004). However, limited knowledge and experience have restricted efforts to construct formulas for supplementation of microbiota to more than a handful of LAB. In my experience, multistrain formulations, including more than four or five strains, may at present not provide additional value.

Suboptimal Supply of Nutrients

The supply of substrate/nutrients for growth and function of LAB might not be optimal. The colonic mucosa has a limited ability to derive nourishment from the circulation and depends on specific nutrients, especially short-chain fatty acids (SCFAs) and plant-derived antioxidants produced by microbial enzymes. The microbiota receives its nutrition from sloughed gastrointestinal epithelia, gastrointestinal secretions, and dietary components. A well-functioning microbiota is key to the body's ability to spare nitrogen, and large amounts of nitrogen are absorbed and reused by the body's protein synthesis machinery. The feeding formulas commonly given to critically ill and other patient groups usually contain relatively small amounts of fiber. Furthermore, processing of foods reduces the ingestion of plant-associated probiotic microbes naturally supplied by eating of raw plants. The degree of milling of grains and mastication strongly influences the proportion of plant food and fiber reaching the colon. Large particles travel more rapidly through the gut. A reduced degree of milling and less mastication will reduce the degree of digestibility by eukaryotic enzymes and increase the amount of food left for fermentation in the colon.

The Influence of Diet

Diet may aggravate systemic inflammation and poses challenges for probiotics/synbiotics. The modern Western diet is based on nutrients received from only a small number of plants, with 80% of the nutrients derived from 17 plants and 50% of the calories from eight grains. Furthermore, foods in the developed world may be extensively processed, which can potentially reduce their nutritional value. Examples of nutrients and antioxidants that do not resist heating and drying are important amino acids such as glutamine, fuel for intestinal epithelial cells, and the "master antioxidant" glutathione. In addition, manipulation of food, especially heating to extreme temperatures, increases the content of unwanted proinflammatory ingredients such as oxidized or *trans*-fatty acids. Heating, ionization, and irradiation of food result in increased production of proinflammatory proteins called Maillard products, otherwise known as advanced glycation or advanced lipoxidation end products. Foods rich in these end products include dairy products such as powdered milk (frequently used in enteral nutrition, infant formulas, and ice cream), cheeses, bakery products (bread crusts, crisp breads, pretzels, and biscotti) and cereals, overheated (especially deep-fried and oven-fried) meat, poultry, and fish, caffeinated drinks including coffee and soda, Chinese soy and balsamic products, and smoked foods in general (Goldberg et al., 2004; Bengmark, 2007). The consumption of such highly processed foods has increased dramatically in recent decades, in parallel to the rise of endemic chronic diseases. The antiinflammatory effects of beneficial bacteria may counteract dietary influences on immune responses.

CLINICAL EXPERIENCE WITH SUPPLEMENTED PREBIOTICS

Prebiotics in Constipation

Chronic constipation is a common disorder in the developed world. Its etiology remains unclear despite numerous clinical, pathophysiologic, and epidemiologic studies, but a high intake of dairy products and plant fibers may play a significant role in its pathogenesis. A randomized case-control study compared 291 children with idiopathic chronic constipation and 1,602 healthy controls (Kaplan and Hutkins, 2000). Constipation was negatively correlated with a low intake of cellulose and pentose fiber ($P < 0.001$). Fructo-oligosaccharides (FOS) may have potential benefits in constipation due to their soluble dietary fiber-like properties. In a recent study, a total of 56 healthy infants (ages 16 to 46 weeks; mean age, 32 weeks) were randomly assigned to receive either FOS (0.75 g) or a placebo added to one serving of cereal per day for 28 days (Roma et al., 1999). The mean number ($\pm$ standard deviation [SD]) of stools per infant was 1.99 ± 0.62 per day in the FOS-supplemented group compared with 1.58 ± 0.66 in the control group ($P = 0.02$).

Prebiotics To Prevent and Treat Diarrhea

In a large randomized study with acutely ill medical and surgical patients, some individuals requiring enteral nutrition received a supplementation of hydrolyzed guar gum for 5 days and were compared with individuals receiving fiber-free enteral nutrition. The incidence of diarrhea was 9% in the group receiving fiber supplementation, compared with 32% in the group treated with fiber-free nutrition ($P > 0.05$) (Moore et al., 2003). One effect of fiber, especially oligosaccharides, is increased bioavailability and absorption of zinc. In a randomized study including children 3 to 59 months of age in Bangladesh, zinc supplementation was proven to be effective for reducing the incidence and duration of diarrhea (Rushdi et al., 2004). In another study in Bangladesh, unripe banana (250 g/liter; equivalent to two fruits) or pectin (2 g/kg of food) was supplemented to a rice diet given to children suffering from persistent diarrhea (Baqui et al., 2002). The amounts and frequency of stools, the duration of diarrhea, vomiting frequency, and utilization of oral and intravenous rehydration solutions were significantly reduced with supplementation of either unripe banana or pure pectin. Recovery by 3 days was observed in 59% of children in the unripe banana group and in 55% of children in the pectin group, compared with 15% of children in the control group, receiving only rice.

Prebiotics To Support Mineral Absorption

Recent studies suggest that increased intake of plant fibers, fruits, and vegetables is associated with increased bone mineral density in male and female elderly subjects (Tucker et al., 1999; Rabbani et al., 2001). Calcium absorption, bone calcium content, bone mineral density, bone balance, and bone formation/bone absorption index were significantly increased following 3 weeks of supplementation of a mixture of inulin and FOS (Tucker et al., 2002).

Prebiotics To Control Weight

The effects of dietary fiber on hunger and weight loss were studied approximately 20 years ago. One hundred eight of 135 members completed the trial including 23 controls, 45 individuals consuming ispaghula granulate, and 40 persons ingesting bran sachets (Hylander and Rossner, 1983). Both fiber preparations reduced hunger at all meals. The mean ($\pm$SD) weight reductions during the trial were 4.6 ± 2.7 kg for the controls, 4.2 ± 3.2 kg for the ispaghula group, and 4.6 ± 2.3 kg for the bran group ($P > 0.05$ for both groups). Although supply of dietary fiber immediately before meals did reduce the feeling of hunger, this intervention did not provide any additional benefits for weight reduction. A recent crossover study compared the effects on satiety with dietary supplementation of fermentable fiber (pectin, beta-glucan; 27 ± 0.6 g/day) versus similar amounts of nonfermentable fiber (methylcellulose). Daily satiety was significantly greater with nonfermentable (methylcellulose) than with fermentable fibers (beta-glucan, pectin; $P = 0.01$), but no differences were observed in daily energy intake or loss of body weight or body fat (Howarth et al., 2003).

Prebiotics in IBD

Although both patients with IBD and patients with irritable bowel syndrome (IBS) may consume insufficient amounts of dietary fiber, little evidence exists that lack of dietary fiber contributes to the pathogenesis of IBD or IBS. The ability of maintaining remission in patients with ulcerative colitis by a daily supply of *Plantago ovata* seeds (10 g per day; also called psyllium or ispaghula husk) was compared with daily treatment of mesalamine (500 mg/day) and a combination of mesalamine and *P. ovata* seeds (Fernandez-Banares et al., 1999). Twelve months of treatment failed to demonstrate any difference in clinical benefits among the three groups. Germinated barley foodstuff, a by-product from breweries that is rich in hemicellulose and glutamine, was administered to 39 patients with mild-to-moderately active ulcerative colitis (Kanauchi et al., 2001). Daily supply of germinated barley foodstuff (30 g/day) significantly reduced disease activity, increased SCFA concentrations, and increased the numbers of *Bifidobacterium* and *Eubacterium* isolated from stool specimens. Observed effects were probably due to the increased supply of glutamine and other antioxidants such as B complex vitamins rather than the fiber. Glutamine and other antioxidants attenuated proinflammatory cytokines such as TNF and enhanced release of heat shock proteins (HSP-72)

(Wischmeyer et al., 2003). A controlled study using oat bran as a fiber source was recently reported, involving 22 patients and 10 controls with quiescent ulcerative colitis. Daily supply with as much as 60 g of oat bran (equivalent to 20 g of dietary fiber) for 3 months resulted in significantly increased quantities of fecal butyrate and diminished abdominal pain. Most patients tolerated elevated quantities of dietary fiber, and signs of disease relapse were not seen in any patients with colitis (Hallert et al., 2003). Butyrate inhibited nuclear factor (NF) κB activation of lamina propria macrophages, reduced the number of neutrophils in crypts and the epithelium, and reduced the density of lamina propria lymphocytes/plasma cells in patients with ulcerative colitis (Luhrs et al., 2002), correlating findings with observed reductions in disease activity. Twenty patients with ileal pouch-anal anastomosis received inulin daily for 2 weeks (24 g/day). Significant reductions in inflammation were observed by endoscopy and histology. In addition to histology, significantly increased fecal concentrations of butyrate, reduced fecal pH, reduced fecal content of secondary bile acids, and diminished growth of *Bacteroides fragilis* were observed with prebiotic inulin supplementation (Welters et al., 2002).

Prebiotics in IBS

Some evidence suggests that various dysmotility disorders including gastroesophageal reflux problems, infantile colic, and constipation manifest food-related features and may be due to intolerance of proteins in cow's milk (Murch, 2000). IBS is a clinical diagnosis based on the occurrence of abdominal distension, abdominal cramps, more frequent stools, and relief of pain on defecation. The prevalence of the syndrome varies between 7 and 22%, making IBS the most common functional gastrointestinal disorder (Bommelaer et al., 2002). A study published in 1990 reported that supplementation of diet with corn (20 g of fiber per day) would significantly improve IBS, ameliorate pain, and increase frequency of stools and may reduce rectosigmoid pressure (Cook et al., 1990). A recent meta-analysis based on 17 studies did conclude that fiber supplementation is generally effective for relief of global symptoms of IBS (relative risk, 1.33; 95% confidence interval [CI], 1.19 to 1.50) (Bijkerk et al., 2004). Patients with constipation-predominant IBS appeared to receive benefit from fiber intake (relative risk, 1.56; 95% CI, 1.21 to 2.02), while fiber seemed to be ineffective for relief of IBS-associated abdominal pain. Clinical improvement was observed only with soluble fiber (psyllium, ispaghula, and calcium polycarbophil) (relative risk, 1.55; 95% CI, 1.35 to 1.78), whereas insoluble fiber (corn and wheat bran) occasionally worsened clinical outcome. Beneficial effects of supplementation with soluble fiber (guar gum) were also observed in a recent study of 188 adult patients with IBS (Parisi et al., 2002).

Prebiotics To Control Infections

In an effort to prevent nosocomial pneumonia and sepsis, patients with severe multiple trauma were treated with beta 1-3 polyglucose (glucan), a component of cell walls of plants and microbes (de Felippe Junior et al., 1993). Pneumonia occurred in 2 of 21 glucan-treated patients and 11 of 20 control patients ($P < 0.01$). Infectious complications (pneumonia or general sepsis) occurred in 14% of glucan-supplemented patients versus 65% of individuals in the control group ($P < 0.001$). Another study compared the effects of a high-protein formula enriched with fiber, arginine, and antioxidants with those of a standard high-protein formula given as early enteral nutrition to critically ill patients (Caparros et al., 2001). The supplemented group had, in comparison to nonsupplemented controls, a lower incidence of catheter-related sepsis (0.4 episodes/1,000 ICU days) than the control group (5.5 episodes/1,000 ICU days) ($P < 0.001$), but no differences were observed between the groups in incidence of ventilator-associated pneumonia, surgical infections, bacteremia, urinary tract infections, mortality, or long-term survival.

LAB AND VITAMINS/ANTIOXIDANTS

LAB produce important vitamins and antioxidants. One important example is the essential B vitamin folate, which is known to reduce homocysteine quantities and may prevent some chronic diseases. Folate is synthesized by LAB such as *Lactococcus lactis* and *L. plantarum*. Other LAB, however, such as *Lactobacillus gasseri*, are net consumers of folate. A recent publication describes the successful transfer of five genes essential for folate biosynthesis from *L. lactis* to *L. gasseri*, converting *L. gasseri* into a net producer of folate (Wegkamp et al., 2004). Anemia, iron deficiency, and folate deficiency are common among patients with IBD (Pironi et al., 1988; Gasche et al., 2004). Plasma total homocysteine (tHcy) concentrations were examined in a pediatric study of 43 patients and 46 controls and shown to be significantly higher in children with IBD than in control subjects ($P < 0.05$). Furthermore, the level of plasma tHcy correlated well with observed reductions in plasma 5-methyltetrahydrofolate ($P < 0.0005$) (Nakano et al., 2003). A similar study with 108 adult patients with IBD and 74 adult healthy controls yielded significantly lower levels of folate in patients with IBD ($P < 0.05$)

(Koutroubakis et al., 2000). The mean concentration of tHcy in serum was significantly higher in patient groups with ulcerative colitis (15.9 ± 10.3 mmol/liter) and patients with Crohn's disease (13.6 ± 6.5 mmol/liter) than in controls (9.6 ± 3.4 mmol/liter) ($P < 0.05$).

COMBINING PREBIOTICS AND PROBIOTICS

Prebiotics and LAB (probiotics) have demonstrated beneficial effects with respect to the function of innate immunity, intestinal barrier function, and increased resistance to disease. The gut mucosa and microbiota are intimately linked in the maintenance of a functional interface between the host and the external environment (Henke and Bassler, 2004; Sansonetti, 2004). The hope is that a combined supply of prebiotics and probiotics (synbiotics) shall have synergistic effects in enhancing immunity and facilitating intestinal barrier function.

The term "defense by diversity" was coined in 1999 (Hill, 1999) and seems applicable to synbiotic treatment. Natural foods may contain both LAB, fiber, and prebiotic components. A recent study concluded that combining fiber has more than additive effects on the functions of microbial ecosystems and host immune responses (Peuranen et al., 2004). A recent review suggests that multispecies probiotics may be superior to single-species probiotics in reducing antibiotic-associated diarrhea, preventing infections (*S. enterica* serovar Typhimurium), and reducing pathogenic colonization (*E. coli*) (Timmerman et al., 2004). The choice of prebiotics and probiotics must be based on scientific evidence, and LAB may have variable effects on immune function and outcome. One consideration is that most LAB have limited abilities to ferment bioactive fibers such as inulin or phlein, variable abilities to adhere to human mucus, low antioxidant capacity, and differences with respect to survival in acid conditions or presence of bile in the gastrointestinal tract. LAB selected for synbiotic studies should be selected for functional activities in the context of a specific combination formulation with prebiotics. Unfortunately, few studies have closely examined potentially synergistic effects of simultaneous administration of synbiotics containing LAB (or other probiotics) and prebiotics.

Synbiotic 2000 consists of a mixture of 10^{10} CFU (or Synbiotic Forte with 10^{11} CFU) of each of four LAB species, including *Pediacoccus pentosaceus*, *Leuconostoc mesenteroides*, *L. paracasei* subsp. *paracasei*, and *L. plantarum*, and 2.5 g of each of the four fermentable fibers or prebiotics including beta-glucan, inulin, pectin, and resistant starch (Medipharm AB, Kågeröd, Sweden, and Des Moines, IA).

Microbiologists Åsa Ljungh and Torkel Wadström at Lund University developed this multicomponent synbiotic formula, which has been extensively used in clinical trials. The choice of LAB for the formulation was finalized after extensive studies of >350 human microbial strains (Kruszewska et al., 2002) and >180 plant microbial strains (Ljungh et al., 2002). Strain selection was based on the ability of LAB to produce bioactive proteins, induce NF-κB signaling, stimulate pro- and anti-inflammatory cytokines, enhance antioxidants, and functionally complement each other. In recent studies both the Synbiotic 2000 Forte and a Probiotic 2000 Forte (no fiber added), containing 10^{11} CFU of each of the four LAB (e.g., 400 billion LAB per dose), have been tested clinically.

Synbiotics and Pancreatitis

Sixty-two patients with severe acute pancreatitis (mean ± SD Apache II scores: Synbiotic 2000-treated, 11.7 ± 1.9; controls, 10.4 ± 1.5) received either two sachets per day of Synbiotic 2000 (80 billion LAB/day) and 20 g of fiber/day or the same amounts of fiber (20 g per day) as in Synbiotic 2000 during the first 14 days after hospital admission (Olah et al., 2007). Notably, 9 of 33 patients (27%) in the Synbiotic 2000-treated group and 15 of 29 patients (52%) in the fiber-only-treated group developed subsequent infections. Consistent with infection data, 8 of 33 (24%) Synbiotic 2000-treated and 14 of 29 (48%) of the fiber-only-treated patients developed systemic inflammatory response syndrome, multiorgan failure, or both ($P < 0.005$) (Olah et al., 2007). Seven pathogenic

microorganisms were cultivated in the synbiotic-treated group compared to 17 in the fiber-only group (Table 1).

Synbiotics and Trauma

Two prospective randomized trials involving polytrauma patients, the study using Synbiotic 2000 and the other using Synbiotic 2000 Forte, have been concluded. The first study compared diets including either Synbiotic 2000 (40 billion LAB/day), soluble fiber, a peptide diet, or supplementation with glutamine for patients with acute extensive trauma. Treatment with Synbiotic 2000 resulted in a highly significant reduction in the number of chest infections (4 of 26 or 15% of patients), compared to patients on the peptide diet (11 of 26 or 42% of patients, $P < 0.04$), glutamine diet (11 of 32 or 34% of patients, $P < 0.03$), or fiber-only diet (12 of 29 or 41% of patients, $P < 0.002$) (Spindler-Vesel et al., 2007). The total number of infections was significantly decreased in the Synbiotic 2000 with only 5 of 26 patients developing infections (19%) versus 17 of 29 patients (59%) in the fiber-only group, 13 of 26 patients (50%) on a peptide diet, and 16 of 32 patients (50%) receiving glutamine.

In another study, 65 polytrauma patients were randomized to receive one dose daily of Synbiotic 2000 Forte (400 billion LAB + 10 g of fiber, see above) for 15 days or maltodextrin as a placebo. Significant reductions were observed in patient mortality (5 of 35 versus 9 of 30, $P < 0.02$), severe sepsis (6 of 35 versus 13 of 30, $P < 0.02$), chest infections (19 of 35 versus 24 of 30,

Table 1 Pathogens isolated from acute pancreatitis patients receiving synbiotic treatment or fiber-only treatment[a]

Microorganism(s) isolated	No. of patients infected	
	Synbiotic 2000 group	Fiber-only group
Pseudomonas aeruginosa	1	4
E. faecalis	1	2
Enterobacter spp.	1	1
Streptococcus spp.	2	
S. aureus	1	1
E. faecium	1	
Candida spp.		2
Staphylococcus haemolyticus		1
Serratia spp.		2
Klebsiella spp.		1
E. coli		1
Stenotrophomonas maltophilia		1
Citrobacter freundii		1
Total	7	17

[a]Data from Olah et al., 2007.

Table 2 Pathogens isolated from polytrauma patients receiving synbiotic treatment or fiber-only treatment[a]

	No. of patients infected	
Microorganism(s) isolated	Synbiotic 2000 group	Fiber-only group
Acinetobacter baumannii	21	35
Candida albicans	7	17
Pseudomonas aeruginosa	15	14
Staphylococcus epidermidis	2	10
S. aureus	4	7
Staphylococcus hominis		2
Enterobacter aerogenes		2
Staphylococcus haemolyticus		1
Serratia spp.		2
Klebsiella spp.	5	12
Proteus spp.		1
Total	54	103

[a]Data from Kotzampassi et al., 2006.

$P < 0.03$), central line infections (13 of 32 versus 20 of 30, $P < 0.02$), and ventilation days (average, 15 versus 26 days). Pathogenic microorganisms were cultivated from 54 individuals in the synbiotic-treated group compared with 103 individuals in the fiber-only group (Table 2) (Kotzampassi et al., 2006).

Synbiotics and Surgical Patients

In a randomized controlled study, 45 patients undergoing major surgery for abdominal cancer were divided into three treatment groups including patients receiving enteral nutrition (EN) plus Synbiotic 2000 (LEN), EN plus fiber (FEN) in the same amount (20 g per day), or standard parenteral nutrition (PN). Synbiotic treatment lasted for two preoperative and seven postoperative days. The incidence of postoperative bacterial infections was 47% with PN, 20% with FEN, and 6.7% with LEN ($P < 0.05$) (H. Chunmao, R. Martindale, H. Huang, and S. Bengmark, in preparation). A total of 34 pathogenic microorganisms were cultivated in the synbiotic-treated group compared with 54 pathogens in the fiber-only group (Table 3). Significant improvements were also documented in prealbumin (LEN and FEN), C-reactive protein (LEN and FEN), serum cholesterol (LEN and FEN), peripheral leukocyte count (LEN), serum endotoxin (LEN and FEN), and serum immunoglobulin A (LEN).

In another prospective randomized double-blind trial, 80 patients subjected to pylorus-preserving pancreatoduodenectomy received either Synbiotic 2000 (40 billion LAB twice per day) or fiber only twice daily beginning on the day before surgery and continuing for the first seven postoperative days (Rayes et al., 2007). A highly significant difference in infection rate ($P = 0.005$) was observed,

as only 5 of 40 (12.5%) patients in the Synbiotic 2000-treated group suffered infections (four wound infections and one urinary tract infection) versus 16 of 40 (40%) patients in the fiber-only group (six wound infections, five cases of peritonitis, four chest infections, two cases of sepsis, and either urinary tract infection, cholangitis, or empyema). The infecting microorganisms in the synbiotic-treated group were *Klebsiella pneumoniae* (two patients), *Enterobacter cloacae* (two patients), *Proteus mirabilis* (one patient), and *Enterococcus faecalis/faecium* (one patient). In the fiber-only group, pathogens included *E. cloacae* (eight patients), *E. faecalis/faecium* (seven patients), *E. coli* (seven patients), *K. pneumoniae* (two patients), *Staphylococcus aureus* (two patients), and *P. mirabilis* (one patient) (Table 4). Statistically significant differences between the groups were observed in the duration of antibiotic utilization (mean ± SD for the Synbiotic 2000 group, 2 ± 5 days; for the fiber-only group, 10 ± 14 days).

Synbiotics and Liver Disease

Fifty-eight patients with hepatic cirrhosis diagnosed with minimal encephalopathy were randomized into three treatment groups. Group 1 (20 patients) received Synbiotic 2000 (40 billion LAB), group 2 (20 patients) received the same amount of prebiotic/fiber component as in Synbiotic 2000 only, and group 3 (15 patients) received a placebo (nonfermentable, nonabsorbable fiber [crystalline cellulose]) (Liu et al., 2004). A significant increase in intestinal LAB was observed after 1 month of supplementation in the synbiotic-treated group, in contrast to the other two groups. Intestinal pH was significantly reduced in both treatment groups, but pH was not reduced in the placebo-treated group. Significant

Table 3 Pathogens recovered from synbiotic-treated patients versus patients receiving only fiber and undergoing surgery for abdominal cancer[a]

Microorganism(s) isolated	No. of patients infected	
	Synbiotic 2000 group	Fiber-only group
Pseudomonas aeruginosa	17	24
S. aureus	8	11
Staphylococcus epidermidis	1	1
Staphylococcus faecalis		1
E. cloacae	4	
Acinetobacter spp.	2	3
Staphylococcus haemolyticus		1
Serratia spp.		2
Klebsiella spp.		1
P. mirabilis		2
Candida albicans	2	6
Aspergillus spp.		
Bacillus subtilis		1
Klebsiella spp.		1
Total	34	54

[a]Data from Chunmao et al., in preparation.

reductions in fecal counts of *E. coli*, *Staphylococcus* spp., and *Fusobacterium* spp. but not of *Pseudomonas* spp. or *Enterococcus* spp. were reported in the synbiotic-treated group. Significant reductions in ammonia, endotoxin, alanine aminotransferase, and bilirubin levels were observed in the synbiotic-treated group compared to the fiber-only and placebo groups. The improvements in liver function were accompanied by significant improvements in performance of psychometric tests and degree of encephalopathy.

In a follow-up study, 30 patients with hepatic cirrhosis were randomized to receive either Synbiotic 2000 or a placebo (crystalline cellulose) for 7 days (Riordan et al., 2007). Viable fecal counts of *Lactobacillus* species, stage

Table 4 Pathogens isolated from patients treated with synbiotics versus patients receiving only fiber and undergoing pancreatectomy[a]

Microorganism isolated	No. of patients infected	
	Synbiotic 2000 group	Fiber-only group
E. cloacae	2	8
E. faecalis/faecium	1	7
E. coli	0	7
K. pneumoniae	2	2
P. mirabilis	1	1
S. aureus	0	2
Total	6	27

[a]Data from Rayes et al., 2007.

of liver disease (Child-Pugh classification), plasma retention rate of indocyanine green (ICG_{R15}), whole-blood TNF and IL-6 mRNA, serum TNF, soluble TNF receptor I (sTNFRI), soluble TNF receptor II (sTNFRII), and plasma endotoxin levels were evaluated pre- and posttreatment. Synbiotic treatment was associated with significantly increased fecal lactobacilli counts and significant improvements in ICG_{R15} and Child-Pugh classification. No significant changes in any study parameter followed the placebo treatment, but significant elevations in whole-blood TNF and IL-6 mRNA, in addition to concentrations of soluble sTNFRI and sTNFRII in serum, were observed in synbiotic-treated patients. TNF and IL-6 levels correlated significantly with each other, both at baseline and after the synbiotic treatment. Synbiotic-related improvements in ICG_{R15} were significantly associated with changes in IL-6 and unrelated to plasma endotoxin values. Short-term synbiotic treatment may significantly modulate gut microbial function and improve hepatic function in patients with cirrhosis. The observed benefits seemed unrelated to a reduction in endotoxemia but could be mediated, at least in part, by treatment-related induction of IL-6 synthesis by TNF. These results offer hope that synbiotic treatment administered to patients awaiting liver transplantation might prevent septic episodes, improve liver function, and promote patient outcomes.

Sixty-six patients were randomized to receive either Synbiotic 2000 or fiber only in connection with human orthotopic liver transplantation. The treatment started

Table 5 Pathogens isolated from patients treated with synbiotics versus patients receiving only fiber and undergoing liver transplantation[a]

Bacterium isolated	No. of patients infected	
	Synbiotic 2000 group	Fiber-only group
E. faecalis	1	11
E. coli	0	3
E. cloacae	0	2
Pseudomonas aeruginosa	0	2
S. aureus	0	1
Total	1	18

[a]Data from Rayes et al., 2005.

on the day before surgery and continued for 14 days after surgery. During the first postoperative month, only one patient in the synbiotic-treated group (3%) showed signs of infection (urinary tract infection) compared to 17 of 33 (51%) patients supplemented with multiple fiber components (Rayes et al., 2005). A single pathogenic microorganism (E. faecalis) was cultivated in the synbiotic-treated group compared with 18 pathogens in the fiber-only group (Table 5). The duration of antibiotic utilization was only 0.1 day (± 0.1 day) in synbiotic-treated patients compared with 3.8 days (± 0.9 day) in the fiber-only group.

Synbiotics and IBD
Daily rectal instillations with Synbiotic 2000 reconstituted in saline were administered to 10 patients with distal colitis during 2 weeks. Synbiotic-treated patients demonstrated dramatic improvements in various disease scores, such as episodes of diarrhea (initially 2.4, decreased to 0.8), visible blood in stool (2.2 to 0.8), nightly diarrhea (0.5 to 0), urgency (1.9 to 1.0), and stool consistency (1.1 to 0.8) (Pathmakanthan et al., 2002). Two patients reported significant bloating, but other adverse or side effects were not reported. In a pilot study (Furrie et al., 2005), nine patients with active ulcerative colitis received a synbiotic composed of freeze-dried *Bifidobacterium longum* (4×10^{11} CFU) and a prebiotic FOS/inulin mixture (6 g) daily for 4 weeks. Nine patients received a placebo consisting of powdered maltodextrose (6 g per day). The quantities of intestinal bifidobacteria were increased 42-fold compared to 4.6-fold in the placebo group. The sigmoidoscopy score, based on clinical assessment of disease activity (Baron et al., 1964), decreased by an average of 1.3 units compared to an increase of 0.58 units in the placebo group ($P = 0.06$). The mean histology score was diminished in the

synbiotic group and increased in the placebo group. However, the total number of patients was small ($n = 8$), and the results were not statistically significant. The bowel habit index scores decreased by 20.4% in the synbiotic group, and the scores increased by 70.4% in the placebo group. Human beta-defensin 2, 3, and 4, TNF, and IL-1 were reduced after synbiotic treatment but remained unchanged in the placebo group ($P = 0.05$). As stated by Aberra (Aberra, 2005), "slowly, the links of diet to the intestinal environment and the association of the intestinal environment to IBD are becoming evident. The prebiotic and probiotic trials reveal the importance of the intestinal environment as a potent regulator of IBD activity." Seven malnourished patients with short bowel syndrome and refractory enterocolitis were treated for more than 1 year with a synbiotic formulation consisting of *Bifidobacterium breve*, *L. casei*, and galacto-oligosaccharides. Synbiotic treatment reportedly enhanced the function and composition of the intestinal bacterial microbiota and increased the content of SCFAs in feces (from 27.8 to 65.09 μmol/g of wet feces) (Kanamori et al., 2004).

Synbiotics and IBS
The effects of twice-daily consumption of a probiotic fruit drink, ProViva (Skånemejerier, Malmo, Sweden), containing *L. plantarum* 299v (6×10^7 CFU/drink) or a placebo for 4 weeks were studied in a controlled study including 40 patients (Nobaek et al., 2000). The vast majority (95% of LAB-treated versus 15% of the placebo-treated patients) of individuals in the probiotic consumption group reported general improvement. A total of 20 of 20 patients in the LAB-supplemented group and 11 of 20 patients in the placebo group ($P = 0.0012$) reported resolution of abdominal pain. A similar study, using the same formula, was performed with patients who received the treatment for 4 weeks. A significant enhancement of LAB composition in probiotics-supplemented patients was described. Flatulence was rapidly and significantly reduced in the LAB-treated group, but no difference in bloating was reported between the groups (Sen et al., 2001). The same formula was applied in a crossover trial of 4 weeks of duration involving 12 patients. A significant reduction in breath hydrogen was registered after 2 h of ingestion, without a change in total hydrogen production or any symptomatic improvement (Madden and Hunter, 2002). Several studies have been performed with probiotics including one trial with synbiotics (for further details, see Young and Cash, 2006). Sixty-eight patients with IBS were treated for 12 weeks with a vitamin- and plant fiber-enriched diet containing either live or heat-inactivated LAB including 10^9 each

of *L. acidophilus*, *L. helveticus*, and *Bifidobacterium* spp. (Tsuchiya et al., 2004). Eighty percent and 40% of the patients, respectively, reported significant improvements in pain, bloating, constipation, and bowel habits ($P < 0.01$).

Synbiotics and Short Bowel Syndrome

Seven malnourished patients (aged 2.5 to 24 years) with short bowel syndrome and refractory enterocolitis received a synbiotic formulation consisting of *B. breve* and *L. casei* (approximately 10^9 CFU) and galacto-oligosaccharides (approximately 3 g) three times daily for a period of 15 to 55 months (Kanamori et al., 2004). Alterations in microbial composition (increased amounts of anaerobic bacteria and suppression of pathogenic microbes) and increased fecal content of SCFAs (from an average of 27.8 to 65.09 μmol/g of wet feces) were described in the synbiotics-treated group. Six of seven patients demonstrated increased body weight from 1.0 to 4.2 kg/year, and prealbumin concentrations were increased in synbiotic-treated patients ($P = 0.05$).

Synbiotics and *H. pylori* Infection

Synbiotics have been applied in the context of *H. pylori* gastritis. A clinical trial was performed in a school from a low socioeconomic area of Santiago, Chile. *H. pylori*-positive children were randomly distributed into four groups. Children received daily antibiotic treatment (lansoprazole, clarithromycin, and amoxicillin) (Ab) for 8 days, "*Saccharomyces boulardii*" (250 mg) plus inulin (5 g) (SbI) daily for 8 weeks, *L. acidophilus* LB (10^9 CFU per day) (LB), or no treatment (Gotteland et al., 2005). A ^{13}C-urea breath test (^{13}C-UBT) was performed before and after the study, and differences in $^{13}CO_2$ quantities were calculated (DDOB). *H. pylori* was eradicated in 66, 12, or 6.5% of the children in the Ab, SbI, or LB groups, respectively, while no spontaneous clearance was observed in children not receiving treatment. A moderate but significant difference in DDOB was detected in children receiving SbI (76.31; 95% CI, 711.84 to 70.79), but not LB (+0.70; 95% CI, 75.84 to +7.24). *H. pylori* infection was eradicated in 12% of synbiotic-treated and 6.5% of probiotic-treated children. Different species of LAB, doses of synbiotics, and combinations of antibiotics and synbiotics may yield a wider spectrum of beneficial effects in different disorders.

Synbiotics and Allergy

A synbiotic combination of *L. casei* subsp. *casei* and dextran prevented cedar-pollen-induced onset of nasal and ocular symptoms, cedar pollen-specific immunoglobulin E responses, and elevation of eosinophil counts (Ogawa et al., 2006). In a recent randomized study, children >2 years of age with atopic dermatitis received either a combination of potato starch and *L. rhamnosus* or potato starch alone three times per day for 3 months. Disease scores were reduced with synbiotic treatment from 39.1 to 20.7 ($P < 0.0001$). No differences were observed after 3 months of treatment ($P = 0.535$) (Passeron et al., 2006).

Synbiotics and Cancer

A synbiotic preparation, consisting of oligofructose-enriched inulin (12 g) (SYN1) and *L. rhamnosus* GG and *B. lactis* Bb12 (BB12) (10^{10} CFU), was recently administered in a 12-week randomized, double-blind, placebo-controlled trial including 37 patients with colon cancer and 43 polypectomized patients (Rafter et al., 2007). The intervention resulted in significant changes in the fecal microbiota, including increases in *Bifidobacterium* spp. and *Lactobacillus* spp. and reductions of *Clostridium perfringens*. The intervention reduced colorectal proliferation and the capacity of fecal water to induce necrosis in colonic cells and improved epithelial barrier function in polypectomized patients. Genotoxicity assays of colonic biopsy samples at the end of the intervention period indicated a decreased exposure to genotoxins in the polypectomized patients. Synbiotic consumption prevented an increased secretion of IL-2 by peripheral blood mononuclear cells in the polypectomized patients and increased the production of gamma interferon in the patients with colon cancer. It was concluded that several colorectal cancer biomarkers may be favorably altered by synbiotic intervention.

LIMITATIONS OF SYNBIOTICS

Two studies with Synbiotic 2000 have resulted in negative outcomes in the context of IBD. After an initial treatment with infliximab, 63 patients were randomized to daily administration of either Synbiotic 2000 or crystalline cellulose as a placebo (Rutgeerts et al., 2004). Median times to relapse for synbiotic or placebo groups were 9.8 and 10.1 months, respectively. In a second study, patients following surgery were supplemented with either Synbiotic 2000 or crystalline cellulose as a placebo. Seven patients in the synbiotic-treated group and two patients in the placebo group completed the scheduled 24-month treatment (Chermesh et al., 2007). No significant differences were observed between the two groups either in endoscopic findings or in rate of clinical relapse. The Rutgeerts disease scores were calculated as 0.6 (SD, ±0.8) in the synbiotic-treated group and 0.8 (SD, ±1) in the placebo group after 3 months of treatment.

SYNBIOTICS AND SEPSIS?

Two large studies have been performed involving ICU groups treated with synbiotics. Synbiotic 2000 (40 billion LAB) was administered to 162 patients. No significant differences were observed in patient mortality or multiorgan dysfunction (C. D. Gomersall, G. M. Joynt, P. Tan, P. Leung, and S. Bengmark, presented at the Australian and New Zealand College of Anaesthetists Annual Scientific Meeting, 2006). In another study, Synbiotic 2000 Forte was administered to 130 patients twice daily during ICU stays (2 × 400 billion LAB), and the results were compared with those of 129 patients supplemented with a cellulose-based placebo. No statistical differences were demonstrated between the groups with respect to the incidence of ventilator-associated pneumonia, the rate of ventilator-associated pneumonia per 1,000 ventilator days, and hospital mortality (Knight et al., 2004).

CHALLENGING INFORMATION FROM RECENT ANIMAL STUDIES

Prevention of Lung Inflammation and Tissue Destruction

Experimental animals subjected to cecal ligation and puncture and subsequent stress-induced neutrophil infiltration of the lung can be treated prophylactically by oral supplementation of a synbiotic cocktail. Synbiotic 2000 Forte was administered orally during 3 days before the trauma (Tok et al., 2007), and the four LAB species in the cocktail were injected subcutaneously at the time of trauma (Ilkgul et al., 2005). Both treatments effectively prevented neutrophil accumulation and tissue destruction in the lungs. The average neutrophil counts in the lungs of the groups were as follows (average of five fields and SD): mixture of LAB and mixture of bioactive fibers containing inulin, beta-glucan, pectin, and resistant starch (group 1), 9.00 ± 0.44; LAB only (group 2), 8.40 ± 0.42; mixture of bioactive fibers containing inulin, beta-glucan, pectin, and resistant starch (group 3), 31.20 ± 0.98; and placebo (nonfermentable fiber/crystalline cellulose) (group 4), 51.10 ± 0.70 (Tok et al., 2007). The corresponding values of myeloperoxidase were 25.62 ± 2.19 (group 1), 26.75 ± 2.61 (group 2), 56.59 ± 1.73 (group 3), and 145.53 ± 7.53 (group 4). The values for nitric oxide were 17.16 ± 2.03 (group 1), 18.91 ± 2.24 (group 2), 47.71 ± 3.20 (group 3), and 66.22 ± 5.92 (group 4) (Tok et al., 2007). All differences between treatment groups and placebo were statistically significant ($P > 0.05$). The results were similar for animals treated with subcutaneous injections of viable LAB (Ilkgul et al., 2005).

Prevention of Colonic Cancer

Male Sprague-Dawley rats were subjected to a single injection of the genotoxic compound azoxymethane and supplemented for 4 weeks with *L. acidophilus* or *B. lactis* (10^{10} CFU/g) plus or minus resistant starch (10% Hi-Maize) (Le Leu et al., 2005). The administration of resistant starch significantly increased the numbers of bifidobacteria and lactobacilli in the intestine ($P \approx 0.001$) and reduced pH levels and total numbers of coliforms ($P \approx 0.001$). Compared to animals supplemented with resistant starch only, rats fed *B. lactis* and supplemented with resistant starch demonstrated a significantly greater apoptotic deletion of carcinogen-damaged cells, increased cell proliferation, increased crypt column heights ($P \approx 0.001$), and increased levels of SCFAs in the colon.

Influence on Circulatory Neuropeptides

Circulatory levels of neuropeptides like neuropeptide Y (NPY) and peptide YY (PYY) have profound inhibitory effects on gastric acid secretion, gastric emptying, gut motility, and exocrine pancreatic secretions (Yang, 2002). Adult and elderly rats were supplemented with a mixture of *Lactobacillus delbrueckii* GG, *B. lactis* Bb12, and inulin for 3 weeks (Lesniewska et al., 2006). Synbiotic treatment elevated plasma PYY in adult rats, but the same treatment did not affect portal plasma PYY in elderly rats. Furthermore, portal plasma concentrations of NPY were decreased by synbiotics in the elderly, while NPY levels were elevated for adult animals. The results indicate that the results of synbiotic treatment on gastrointestinal function might be dependent on the age of the animal or human individual.

Influence on Plasma Lipid Profiles and Erythrocyte Membrane Properties

A synbiotic formulation containing *L. acidophilus* ATCC 4962, FOS, inulin, and mannitol was administered to hypercholesterolemic pigs on high- and low-fat diets. The aims of this study included assessments of effects of synbiotics on plasma lipid profiles and erythrocyte membrane properties (Liong et al., 2007). The supplementation of synbiotics reduced, irrespective of fat content in the feed, total plasma cholesterol ($P = 0.001$), triacylglycerol ($P = 0.002$), and low-density lipoprotein cholesterol ($P = 0.045$). Synbiotic supplementation also improved membrane fluidity, reduced membrane rigidity, and decreased fluorescence anisotropies in the hemoglobin-free erythrocyte membrane ($P < 0.001$). Reduced deformation of erythrocytes and improved membrane permeability were also observed.

Milk Production in Dairy Cows

Fifty-eight Holstein dairy cows were divided into two groups including one group receiving supplementation with a synbiotic consisting of *L. casei* subsp. *casei* and dextran (Yasuda et al., 2007). Significant improvements were observed in milk yields and in total amounts of fat, protein, and nonfat solids in the group receiving synbiotic supplementation.

CONCLUSIONS AND FUTURE PERSPECTIVES

The intestinal microbiota has unique features in each individual and is largely influenced by host genetics, environment, and lifestyle. Profound changes in our environment and lifestyles and altered exposures to chemical compounds including pharmaceuticals have likely affected the composition of the resident microbiota. Changes in our gut microbiota (microbiome) may be associated with altered environmental factors and trends in chronic diseases. Some studies have suggested that variations in the gut microbiota affect susceptibilities to various chronic diseases including diet-induced insulin resistance and type II diabetes mellitus (Dumas et al., 2006a, 2006b), type I diabetes (Brugman et al., 2006), and obesity (Backhed et al., 2007). Systemic inflammation in a variety of disorders may be difficult to manage with only probiotics or synbiotics. A multitude of treatments including different combinations of probiotics, prebiotics, nutrients, and antioxidants may be important in addition to fundamental changes of lifestyle and dietary habits.

Clearly the research linking our microbial composition and function with health status and susceptibility to disease is in its infancy. Each microbial species has unique functions, and conclusions cannot be generalized for members of the indigenous microbiota. Numerous food ingredients have specific effects on human health. Further scientific investigations are necessary in order to understand the unique interactions between the host-associated microbiota, diet, medical interventions with synbiotics, and aggregate effects on disease susceptibility, treatment, and prevention.

References

Aberra, F. 2005. Synergy in a synbiotic? *Inflamm. Bowel Dis.* 11:1024–1025.

Ahrne, S., S. Nobaek, B. Jeppsson, I. Adlerberth, A. E. Wold, and G. Molin. 1998. The normal *Lactobacillus* flora of healthy human rectal and oral mucosa. *J. Appl. Microbiol.* 85:88–94.

Armuzzi, A., F. Cremonini, F. Bartolozzi, F. Canducci, M. Candelli, V. Ojetti, G. Cammarota, M. Anti, A. De Lorenzo, P. Pola, G. Gasbarrini, and A. Gasbarrini. 2001a. The effect of oral administration of *Lactobacillus* GG on antibiotic-associated gastrointestinal side-effects during *Helicobacter pylori* eradication therapy. *Aliment. Pharmacol. Ther.* 15:163–169.

Armuzzi, A., F. Cremonini, V. Ojetti, F. Bartolozzi, F. Canducci, M. Candelli, L. Santarelli, G. Cammarota, A. De Lorenzo, P. Pola, G. Gasbarrini, and A. Gasbarrini. 2001b. Effect of *Lactobacillus* GG supplementation on antibiotic-associated gastrointestinal side effects during *Helicobacter pylori* eradication therapy: a pilot study. *Digestion* 63:1–7.

Backhed, F., J. K. Manchester, C. F. Semenkovich, and J. I. Gordon. 2007. Mechanisms underlying the resistance to diet-induced obesity in germ-free mice. *Proc. Natl. Acad. Sci. USA* 104:979–984.

Baqui, A. H., R. E. Black, S. El Arifeen, M. Yunus, J. Chakraborty, S. Ahmed, and J. P. Vaughan. 2002. Effect of zinc supplementation started during diarrhoea on morbidity and mortality in Bangladeshi children: community randomised trial. *BMJ* 325:1059.

Baron, J. H., A. M. Connell, and J. E. Lennard-Jones. 1964. Variation between observers in describing mucosal appearances in proctocolitis. *Br. Med. J.* 1:89–92.

Bengmark, S. 2007. Advanced glycation and lipoxidation end products–amplifiers of inflammation: the role of food. *JPEN J. Parenter. Enteral Nutr.* 31:430–440.

Bijkerk, C. J., J. W. Muris, J. A. Knottnerus, A. W. Hoes, and N. J. de Wit. 2004. Systematic review: the role of different types of fibre in the treatment of irritable bowel syndrome. *Aliment. Pharmacol. Ther.* 19:245–251.

Bommelaer, G., E. Dorval, P. Denis, P. Czernichow, J. Frexinos, A. Pelc, A. Slama, and A. El Hasnaoui. 2002. Prevalence of irritable bowel syndrome in the French population according to the Rome I criteria. *Gastroenterol. Clin. Biol.* 26:1118–1123.

Borody, T. J., E. F. Warren, S. Leis, R. Surace, and O. Ashman. 2003. Treatment of ulcerative colitis using fecal bacteriotherapy. *J. Clin. Gastroenterol.* 37:42–47.

Borody, T. J., E. F. Warren, S. M. Leis, R. Surace, O. Ashman, and S. Siarakas. 2004. Bacteriotherapy using fecal flora: toying with human motions. *J. Clin. Gastroenterol.* 38:475–483.

Brugman, S., F. A. Klatter, J. T. Visser, A. C. Wildeboer-Veloo, H. J. Harmsen, J. Rozing, and N. A. Bos. 2006. Antibiotic treatment partially protects against type 1 diabetes in the Bio-Breeding diabetes-prone rat. Is the gut flora involved in the development of type 1 diabetes? *Diabetologia* 49:2105–2108.

Caparros, T., J. Lopez, and T. Grau. 2001. Early enteral nutrition in critically ill patients with a high-protein diet enriched with arginine, fiber, and antioxidants compared with a standard high-protein diet. The effect on nosocomial infections and outcome. *JPEN J. Parenter. Enteral Nutr.* 25:299–308, 308–309.

Chermesh, I., A. Tamir, R. Reshef, Y. Chowers, A. Suissa, D. Katz, M. Gelber, Z. Halpern, S. Bengmark, and R. Eliakim. 2007. Failure of Synbiotic 2000 to prevent postoperative recurrence of Crohn's disease. *Dig. Dis. Sci.* 52:385–389.

Cook, I. J., E. J. Irvine, D. Campbell, S. Shannon, S. N. Reddy, and S. M. Collins. 1990. Effect of dietary fiber on symptoms and rectosigmoid motility in patients with irritable bowel syndrome. A controlled, crossover study. *Gastroenterology* 98:66–72.

de Felippe Junior, J., M. da Rocha e Silva Junior, F. M. Maciel, M. Soares Ade, and N. F. Mendes. 1993. Infection prevention in patients with severe multiple trauma with the immunomodulator beta 1-3 polyglucose (glucan). *Surg. Gynecol. Obstet.* 177:383–388.

Dumas, M. E., R. H. Barton, A. Toye, O. Cloarec, C. Blancher, A. Rothwell, J. Fearnside, R. Tatoud, V. Blanc, J. C. Lindon, S. C. Mitchell, E. Holmes, M. I. McCarthy, J. Scott, D. Gauguier, and J. K. Nicholson. 2006a. Metabolic profiling reveals a contribution of gut microbiota to fatty liver phenotype in insulin-resistant mice. *Proc. Natl. Acad. Sci. USA* 103:12511–12516.

Dumas, M. E., E. C. Maibaum, C. Teague, H. Ueshima, B. Zhou, J. C. Lindon, J. K. Nicholson, J. Stamler, P. Elliott, Q. Chan, and E. Holmes. 2006b. Assessment of analytical reproducibility of ¹H NMR spectroscopy based metabonomics for large-scale epidemiological research: the INTERMAP Study. *Anal. Chem.* 78:2199–2208.

Fernandez-Banares, F., J. Hinojosa, J. L. Sanchez-Lombrana, E. Navarro, J. F. Martinez-Salmeron, A. Garcia-Puges, F. Gonzalez-Huix, J. Riera, V. Gonzalez-Lara, F. Dominguez-Abascal, J. J. Gine, J. Moles, F. Gomollon, M. A. Gassull, et al. 1999. Randomized clinical trial of Plantago ovata seeds (dietary fiber) as compared with mesalamine in maintaining remission in ulcerative colitis. *Am. J. Gastroenterol.* 94:427–433.

Finegold, S. M., and V. L. Sutter. 1978. Fecal flora in different populations, with special reference to diet. *Am. J. Clin. Nutr.* 31:S116–S122.

Fujiwara, D., S. Inoue, H. Wakabayashi, and T. Fujii. 2004. The anti-allergic effects of lactic acid bacteria are strain dependent and mediated by effects on both Th1/Th2 cytokine expression and balance. *Int. Arch. Allergy Immunol.* 135:205–215.

Furrie, E., S. Macfarlane, A. Kennedy, J. H. Cummings, S. V. Walsh, D. A. O'Neil, and G. T. Macfarlane. 2005. Synbiotic therapy (*Bifidobacterium longum*/Synergy 1) initiates resolution of inflammation in patients with active ulcerative colitis: a randomised controlled pilot trial. *Gut* 54:242–249.

Gasche, C., M. C. Lomer, I. Cavill, and G. Weiss. 2004. Iron, anaemia, and inflammatory bowel diseases. *Gut* 53:1190–1197.

Gilliland, S. E., and M. L. Speck. 1977. Antagonistic action of *Lactobacillus acidophilus* towards intestinal and food-borne pathogens in associative cultures. *J. Food Prot.* 40:820–823.

Goldberg, T., W. Cai, M. Peppa, V. Dardaine, B. S. Baliga, J. Uribarri, and H. Vlassara. 2004. Advanced glycoxidation end products in commonly consumed foods. *J. Am. Diet Assoc.* 104:1287–1291.

Gotteland, M., L. Poliak, S. Cruchet, and O. Brunser. 2005. Effect of regular ingestion of *Saccharomyces boulardii* plus inulin or *Lactobacillus acidophilus* LB in children colonized by *Helicobacter pylori*. *Acta Paediatr.* 94:1747–1751.

Hallert, C., I. Bjorck, M. Nyman, A. Pousette, C. Granno, and H. Svensson. 2003. Increasing fecal butyrate in ulcerative colitis patients by diet: controlled pilot study. *Inflamm. Bowel Dis.* 9:116–121.

Henke, J. M., and B. L. Bassler. 2004. Bacterial social engagements. *Trends Cell Biol.* 14:648–656.

Hill, A. V. 1999. Immunogenetics. Defence by diversity. *Nature* 398:668–669.

Howarth, N. C., E. Saltzman, M. A. McCrory, A. S. Greenberg, J. Dwyer, L. Ausman, D. G. Kramer, and S. B. Roberts. 2003. Fermentable and nonfermentable fiber supplements did not alter hunger, satiety or body weight in a pilot study of men and women consuming self-selected diets. *J. Nutr.* 133:3141–3144.

Hylander, B., and S. Rossner. 1983. Effects of dietary fiber intake before meals on weight loss and hunger in a weight-reducing club. *Acta Med. Scand.* 213:217–220.

Ilkgul, O., H. Aydede, Y. Erhan, S. Surocuoglu, H. Gazi, S. Vatansever, F. Taneli, C. Ulman, C. Kose, and S. Bengmark. 2005. Subcutaneous administration of live *Lactobacillus* prevents sepsis-induced lung organ failure in rats. *Br. J. Intern. Care* 15:52–57.

Jain, P. K., C. E. McNaught, A. D. G. Anderson, J. MacFie, and C. J. Mitchell. 2004. Influence of synbiotic containing *Lactobacillus acidophilus* LA5, *Bifidobacterium lactis* BP12, *Streptococcus thermophilus*, *Lactobacillus bulgaricus* and oligofructose on gut barrier function and sepsis in critically ill patients: a randomized controlled trial. *Clin. Nutr.* 23:467–475.

Kanamori, Y., M. Sugiyama, K. Hashizume, N. Yuki, M. Morotomi, and R. Tanaka. 2004. Experience of long-term synbiotic therapy in seven short bowel patients with refractory enterocolitis. *J. Pediatr. Surg.* 39:1686–1692.

Kanauchi, O., T. Iwanaga, and K. Mitsuyama. 2001. Germinated barley foodstuff feeding. A novel neutraceutical therapeutic strategy for ulcerative colitis. *Digestion* 63(Suppl. 1):60–67.

Kaplan, H., and R. W. Hutkins. 2000. Fermentation of fructooligosaccharides by lactic acid bacteria and bifidobacteria. *Appl. Environ. Microbiol.* 66:2682–2684.

Knight, D., K. Girling, A. Banks, S. Snape, W. Weston, and S. Bengmark. 2004. The effect of enteral synbiotics on the incidence of ventilator associated pneumonia in mechanically ventilated critically ill patients. *Br. J. Anaesth.* 92:307P–308P.

Kotzampassi, K., E. J. Giamarellos-Bourboulis, A. Voudouris, P. Kazamias, and E. Eleftheriadis. 2006. Benefits of a synbiotic formula (Synbiotic 2000Forte) in critically ill trauma patients: early results of a randomized controlled trial. *World J. Surg.* 30:1848–1855.

Koutroubakis, I. E., E. Dilaveraki, I. G. Vlachonikolis, E. Vardas, G. Vrentzos, E. Ganotakis, I. A. Mouzas, A. Gravanis, D. Emmanouel, and E. A. Kouroumalis. 2000. Hyperhomocysteinemia in Greek patients with inflammatory bowel disease. *Dig. Dis. Sci.* 45:2347–2351.

Kruszewska, D., J. Lan, G. Lorca, N. Yanagisawa, I. Marklinder, and A. Ljungh. 2002. Selection of lactic acid bacteria as probiotic strains by *in vitro* tests. *Microecol. Ther.* 29:37–49.

Le Leu, R. K., I. L. Brown, Y. Hu, A. R. Bird, M. Jackson, A. Esterman, and G. P. Young. 2005. A synbiotic combination of resistant starch and *Bifidobacterium lactis* facilitates apoptotic deletion of carcinogen-damaged cells in rat colon. *J. Nutr.* **135:**996–1001.

Lesniewska, V., I. Rowland, P. D. Cani, A. M. Neyrinck, N. M. Delzenne, and P. J. Naughton. 2006. Effect on components of the intestinal microflora and plasma neuropeptide levels of feeding *Lactobacillus delbrueckii*, *Bifidobacterium lactis*, and inulin to adult and elderly rats. *Appl. Environ. Microbiol.* **72:**6533–6538.

Liong, M. T., F. R. Dunshea, and N. P. Shah. 2007. Effects of a synbiotic containing *Lactobacillus acidophilus* ATCC 4962 on plasma lipid profiles and morphology of erythrocytes in hypercholesterolaemic pigs on high- and low-fat diets. *Br. J. Nutr.* **98:**736–744.

Liu, Q., Z. P. Duan, D. K. Ha, S. Bengmark, J. Kurtovic, and S. M. Riordan. 2004. Synbiotic modulation of gut flora: effect on minimal hepatic encephalopathy in patients with cirrhosis. *Hepatology* **39:**1441–1449.

Ljungh, A., J. Lan, and N. Yanagisawa. 2002. Isolation, selection and characteristics of *Lactobacillus paracasei* subsp. *paracasei* F19. *Microb. Ecol. Health Dis.* **14:**4–6.

Luhrs, H., T. Gerke, J. G. Muller, R. Melcher, J. Schauber, F. Boxberge, W. Scheppach, and T. Menzel. 2002. Butyrate inhibits NF-κB activation in lamina propria macrophages of patients with ulcerative colitis. *Scand. J. Gastroenterol.* **37:**458–466.

Madden, J. A., and J. O. Hunter. 2002. A review of the role of the gut microflora in irritable bowel syndrome and the effects of probiotics. *Br. J. Nutr.* **88**(Suppl. 1):S67–S72.

Marteau, P. 2006. Probiotics, prebiotics, synbiotics: ecological treatment for inflammatory bowel disease? *Gut* **55:**1692–1693.

Miettinen, M., M. Alander, A. von Wright, J. Vuopio-Varkila, P. Marteau, and J. Huis in't Veld. 1998. The survival of and cytokine induction by lactic acid bacteria after passage through a gastrointestinal model. *Microb. Ecol. Health Dis.* **10:**141–147.

Moore, N., C. Chao, L. P. Yang, H. Storm, M. Oliva-Hemker, and J. M. Saavedra. 2003. Effects of fructo-oligosaccharide-supplemented infant cereal: a double-blind, randomized trial. *Br. J. Nutr.* **90:**581–587.

Murch, S. H. 2000. The immunologic basis for intestinal food allergy. *Curr. Opin. Gastroenterol.* **16:**552–557.

Naaber, P., I. Smidt, J. Stsepetova, T. Brilene, H. Annuk, and M. Mikelsaar. 2004. Inhibition of *Clostridium difficile* strains by intestinal *Lactobacillus* species. *J. Med. Microbiol.* **53:**551–554.

Nakano, E., C. J. Taylor, L. Chada, J. McGaw, and H. J. Powers. 2003. Hyperhomocystinemia in children with inflammatory bowel disease. *J. Pediatr. Gastroenterol. Nutr.* **37:**586–590.

Nobaek, S., M. L. Johansson, G. Molin, S. Ahrne, and B. Jeppsson. 2000. Alteration of intestinal microflora is associated with reduction in abdominal bloating and pain in patients with irritable bowel syndrome. *Am. J. Gastroenterol.* **95:**1231–1238.

Ogawa, T., S. Hashikawa, Y. Asai, H. Sakamoto, K. Yasuda, and Y. Makimura. 2006. A new synbiotic, *Lactobacillus casei* subsp. *casei* together with dextran, reduces murine and human allergic reaction. *FEMS Immunol. Med. Microbiol.* **46:**400–409.

Olah, A., T. Belagyi, L. Poto, L. Romics, Jr., and S. Bengmark. 2007. Synbiotic control of inflammation and infection in severe acute pancreatitis: a prospective, randomized, double blind study. *Hepatogastroenterology* **54:**590–594.

Parisi, G. C., M. Zilli, M. P. Miani, M. Carrara, E. Bottona, G. Verdianelli, G. Battaglia, S. Desideri, A. Faedo, C. Marzolino, A. Tonon, M. Ermani, and G. Leandro. 2002. High-fiber diet supplementation in patients with irritable bowel syndrome (IBS): a multicenter, randomized, open trial comparison between wheat bran diet and partially hydrolyzed guar gum (PHGG). *Dig. Dis. Sci.* **47:**1697–1704.

Passeron, T., J. P. Lacour, E. Fontas, and J. P. Ortonne. 2006. Prebiotics and synbiotics: two promising approaches for the treatment of atopic dermatitis in children above 2 years. *Allergy* **61:**431–437.

Pathmakanthan, S., M. Walsh, S. Bengmark, P. J. A. Willemse, and K. D. Bardhan. 2002. Efficacy and tolerability treating acute distal ulcerative colitis with synbiotic enemas: a pilot trial. *Gut* **51:**A307.

Peuranen, S., K. Tiihonen, J. Apajalahti, A. Kettunen, M. Saarinen, and N. Rautonen. 2004. Combination of polydextrose and lactitol affects microbial ecosystem and immune responses in rat gastrointestinal tract. *Br. J. Nutr.* **91:**905–914.

Pironi, L., G. L. Cornia, M. A. Ursitti, M. A. Dallasta, R. Miniero, F. Fasano, M. Miglioli, and L. Barbara. 1988. Evaluation of oral administration of folic and folinic acid to prevent folate deficiency in patients with inflammatory bowel disease treated with salicylazosulfapyridine. *Int. J. Clin. Pharmacol. Res.* **8:**143–148.

Rabbani, G. H., T. Teka, B. Zaman, N. Majid, M. Khatun, and G. J. Fuchs. 2001. Clinical studies in persistent diarrhea: dietary management with green banana or pectin in Bangladeshi children. *Gastroenterology* **121:**554–560.

Rafter, J., M. Bennett, G. Caderni, Y. Clune, R. Hughes, P. C. Karlsson, A. Klinder, M. O'Riordan, G. C. O'Sullivan, B. Pool-Zobel, G. Rechkemmer, M. Roller, I. Rowland, M. Salvadori, H. Thijs, J. Van Loo, B. Watzl, and J. K. Collins. 2007. Dietary synbiotics reduce cancer risk factors in polypectomized and colon cancer patients. *Am. J. Clin. Nutr.* **85:**488–496.

Rayes, N., D. Seehofer, T. Theruvath, R. A. Schiller, J. M. Langrehr, S. Jonas, S. Bengmark, and P. Neuhaus. 2005. Supply of pre- and probiotics reduces bacterial infection rates after liver transplantation–a randomized, double-blind trial. *Am. J. Transplant.* **5:**125–130.

Rayes, N., D. Seehofer, T. Theruvath, M. Mogl, J. M. Langrehr, N. C. Nussler, S. Bengmark, and P. Neuhaus. 2007. Effect of enteral nutrition and synbiotics on bacterial infection rates after pylorus-preserving pancreatoduodenectomy: a randomized, double-blind trial. *Ann. Surg.* **246:**36–41.

Riordan, S. M., N. A. Skinner, C. J. McIver, Q. Liu, S. Bengmark, D. Bihari, and K. Visvanathan. 2007. Synbiotic-associated improvement in liver function in cirrhotic patients: relation to changes in circulating cytokine messenger RNA and protein levels. *Microb. Ecol. Health Dis.* **19:**7–16.

Roma, E., D. Adamidis, R. Nikolara, A. Constantopoulos, and J. Messaritakis. 1999. Diet and chronic constipation in children: the role of fiber. *J. Pediatr. Gastroenterol. Nutr.* 28:169–174.

Rushdi, T. A., C. Pichard, and Y. H. Khater. 2004. Control of diarrhea by fiber-enriched diet in ICU patients on enteral nutrition: a prospective randomized controlled trial. *Clin. Nutr.* 23:1344–1352.

Rutgeerts, P., G. D'Haens, F. Baert, G. Van Assche, I. Noman, S. Vermeire, and S. Bengmark. 2004. Randomized placebo controlled trial of pro- and prebiotics (Synbiotics cocktail) for maintenance of infliximab induced remission of luminal Crohn's disease (CD). *Gastroenterology* 126:T1310.

Sansonetti, P. J. 2004. War and peace at mucosal surfaces. *Nat. Rev. Immunol.* 4:953–964.

Sartor, R. B. 2004. Therapeutic manipulation of the enteric microflora in inflammatory bowel diseases: antibiotics, probiotics, and prebiotics. *Gastroenterology* 126:1620–1633.

Sen, S., M. Mullan, T. J. Parker, J. Woolner, S. A. Tarry, and J. O. Hunter. 2001. Effects of *Lactobacillus plantarum* 299V on symptoms and colonic fermentation in irritable bowel syndrome (IBS). *Gut* 48:A57.

Spindler-Vesel, A., S. Bengmark, I. Vovk, O. Cerovic, and L. Kompan. 2007. Synbiotics, prebiotics, glutamine, or peptide in early enteral nutrition: a randomized study in trauma patients. *JPEN J. Parenter. Enteral Nutr.* 31:119–126.

Thomas, M. R., S. C. Litin, D. R. Osmon, A. P. Corr, A. L. Weaver, and C. M. Lohse. 2001. Lack of effect of *Lactobacillus* GG on antibiotic-associated diarrhea: a randomized, placebo-controlled trial. *Mayo Clin. Proc.* 76:883–889.

Timmerman, H. M., C. J. Koning, L. Mulder, F. M. Rombouts, and A. C. Beynen. 2004. Monostrain, multistrain and multispecies probiotics—a comparison of functionality and efficacy. *Int. J. Food Microbiol.* 96:219–233.

Tok, D., O. Ilkgul, S. Bengmark, H. Aydede, Y. Erhan, F. Taneli, C. Ulman, S. Vatansever, C. Kose, and G. Ok. 2007. Pretreatment with pro- and synbiotics reduces peritonitis-induced acute lung injury in rats. *J. Trauma* 62:880–885.

Tsuchiya, J., R. Barreto, R. Okura, S. Kawakita, E. Fesce, and F. Marotta. 2004. Single-blind follow-up study on the effectiveness of a symbiotic preparation in irritable bowel syndrome. *Chin. J. Dig. Dis.* 5:169–174.

Tucker, K. L., M. T. Hannan, H. Chen, L. A. Cupples, P. W. Wilson, and D. P. Kiel. 1999. Potassium, magnesium, and fruit and vegetable intakes are associated with greater bone mineral density in elderly men and women. *Am. J. Clin. Nutr.* 69:727–736.

Tucker, K. L., H. Chen, M. T. Hannan, L. A. Cupples, P. W. Wilson, D. Felson, and D. P. Kiel. 2002. Bone mineral density and dietary patterns in older adults: the Framingham Osteoporosis Study. *Am. J. Clin. Nutr.* 76:245–252.

Venturi, A., P. Gionchetti, F. Rizzello, R. Johansson, E. Zucconi, P. Brigidi, D. Matteuzzi, and M. Campieri. 1999. Impact on the composition of the faecal flora by a new probiotic preparation: preliminary data on maintenance treatment of patients with ulcerative colitis. *Aliment. Pharmacol. Ther.* 13:1103–1108.

Wegkamp, A., M. Starrenburg, W. M. de Vos, J. Hugenholtz, and W. Sybesma. 2004. Transformation of folate-consuming *Lactobacillus gasseri* into a folate producer. *Appl. Environ. Microbiol.* 70:3146–3148.

Welters, C. F., E. Heineman, F. B. Thunnissen, A. E. van den Bogaard, P. B. Soeters, and C. G. Baeten. 2002. Effect of dietary inulin supplementation on inflammation of pouch mucosa in patients with an ileal pouch-anal anastomosis. *Dis. Colon Rectum* 45:621–627.

Wischmeyer, P. E., J. Riehm, K. D. Singleton, H. Ren, M. W. Musch, M. Kahana, and E. B. Chang. 2003. Glutamine attenuates tumor necrosis factor-alpha release and enhances heat shock protein 72 in human peripheral blood mononuclear cells. *Nutrition* 19:1–6.

Woodcock, N. P., C. E. McNaught, D. R. Morgan, K. L. Gregg, and J. MacFie. 2004. An investigation into the effect of a probiotic on gut immune function in surgical patients. *Clin. Nutr.* 23:1069–1073.

Yang, H. 2002. Central and peripheral regulation of gastric acid secretion by peptide YY. *Peptides* 23:349–358.

Yasuda, K., S. Hashikawa, H. Sakamoto, Y. Tomita, S. Shibata, and T. Fukata. 2007. A new synbiotic consisting of *Lactobacillus casei* subsp. *casei* and dextran improves milk production in Holstein dairy cows. *J. Vet. Med. Sci.* 69:205–208.

Young, P., and B. D. Cash. 2006. Probiotic use in irritable bowel syndrome. *Curr. Gastroenterol. Rep.* 8:321–326.

Therapeutic Microbiology in Veterinary Medicine

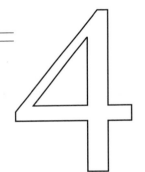

Therapeutic Microbiology: Probiotics and Related Strategies
Edited by J. Versalovic and M. Wilson
© 2008 ASM Press, Washington, DC

Sergey R. Konstantinov
Jerry Wells

25

Strategies for Altering the Intestinal Microbiota of Animals

HISTORY AND BACKGROUND

Considerable efforts have been devoted to the understanding of infectious diseases, including the biology of pathogens, vaccination, host resistance, and antimicrobial therapy in production animals. In contrast, relatively little is known about the prevention of diseases through dietary strategies. To date, stress-related gastrointestinal (GI) tract disorders have been overcome by adding subtherapeutic doses of antibiotics and elevated levels of metal trace elements (zinc and copper) in animal feed. However, given the desire for sustainable agriculture on a global scale without the use of production enhancers and chemotherapeutics, functional foods are seen as increasingly important strategies for maintaining animal health and improving animal performance. A better understanding of the composition and activity of a beneficial microbiota in different animals will be instrumental in this field.

Under normal conditions the large intestine of farm animals comprises a highly evolved and complex microbial ecosystem. Many of the microorganisms are considered beneficial and are able to prevent infection through competition for nutrients and/or exert positive effects on host nutrition by fermenting substrates that would otherwise not be digested. Abrupt changes in diet, stress, or the administration of antibiotics can unbalance this microbial ecosystem, thereby affecting the health status of the animal and increasing the risk of disease. Public concerns about antibiotic use in animal production and the spread of drug resistance, as well as the potential protective effects of beneficial microbes on the carriage of zoonotic pathogens, have given much impetus to probiotic research in agriculture and veterinary medicine. Fuller (Fuller, 1989) defined probiotics (Greek *pro*, for, and *bios*, life) as "a live microbial feed supplement, which beneficially affects the host animal by improving its intestinal microbial balance." This original definition, however, did not include the possibility of improving microbial conditions in both the rumen and the lower digestive tract and led to the definition of ruminal probiotics as "live cultures of microorganisms that are deliberately introduced into the rumen with the aim of improving animal health or nutrition" (Kmet et al., 1993). The term "probiotic" is generic and is often

Sergey R. Konstantinov, Duke University Medical Center, 272 Jones Bldg., Durham, NC 27710. **Jerry Wells,** Host-Microbcrobe-Interactomics Group, University of Wageningen, Marijkeweg 40, 6709 PG Wageningen, The Netherlands.

used in its broader sense to describe the effects of different microbial cultures, extracts, and enzyme preparations. In some studies, different terms such as "direct-fed microbials" or "microbial dietary adjuvants" have been used when referring to feed products that contain a source of live, naturally occurring microorganisms. In this chapter the term probiotics is used in a broad sense to include the use of various different microbes in veterinary strategies aimed at manipulation or replacement of intestinal microbes.

A wide variety of probiotic preparations have been patented throughout the world for cattle, goats, horses, pigs, poultry, sheep, and domestic animals to prevent infections and support growth and development. Most of these preparations contain different strains of the genus *Bacillus*, lactic acid bacteria (LAB), and yeasts. It is generally recognized that the probiotic strains should be nontoxic and nonpathogenic microorganisms that are able to withstand passage through the host's stomach and the small intestine and exert antipathogenic or/and immunomodulatory activities or deliver enzymes important for host physiology. Currently, our knowledge of the mode of action of probiotics in farm animals is very limited. Most research has been carried out on the effects of probiotics in rodents as model animals. Although some lactobacilli are commonly used in the production of fermented foods and human probiotic products and as additives in animal feed (Bernardeau et al., 2006), their applications as probiotics for farm animals are often difficult due to their instability during feed processing and storage (Simon et al., 2003). Although the development of probiotics is still in its early stages, a better understanding of the normal microbiota and its interactions with the animal host will aid the discovery of previously uncharacterized beneficial microorganisms and uncover novel targets for dietary manipulations.

MICROBIAL COMMUNITIES AS TARGETS FOR MANIPULATION

The diverse GI tract microbiota provides important stimuli for the development of the host mucosal immune system and physiology, while remaining in a truly mutualistic relationship with the host. The intestinal commensal microbiota interacts with a wide range of physiological functions of the host, as evidenced by the abnormal development of the intestinal functions of germfree animals. Germfree rodents, for instance, require a higher calorific intake to maintain their weight than those with an intestinal microbiota, have a lower rate of epithelial cell turnover, and have deficiencies in the numbers and distribution of certain immune cells in

the mucosal tissues (Wostmann et al., 1983; Cebra, 1999; Gaskins, 2001). The resident bacterial community stimulates the development of the intestinal epithelium and lymphoid tissue and also makes a profound contribution to host nutrition and the phenomenon of colonization resistance (Van der Waaij, 1989; Stokes et al., 2004). Since the intestinal microbiota interacts ultimately with the animal host, insight into its temporal, spatial, and functional development is needed. This information is required for the development of nutritional strategies aimed at preventing GI tract infections while improving host performance. To date there are only a few published studies on when and how the intestinal microbial communities are shaped in relation to animal host immunology and physiology, and more research is clearly needed on this topic.

Although in the past the microbial community composition in the GI tract of animals has been studied intensively, most attention has been paid to easily cultivable commensal bacteria and a number of opportunistic pathogens (Ewing and Cole, 1994). Many of the strictly anaerobic GI tract bacteria are still difficult to cultivate and, therefore, remained undetectable with conventional microbiological cultivation techniques. This drastically changed following the introduction of molecular detection techniques based on species-specific gene sequences. After the introduction of the 16S rRNA gene as a molecular marker in microbial taxonomy by Woese (Woese, 1987) and the first attempts to apply this DNA sequence information in microbial ecology (Olsen et al., 1986), a rapidly increasing number of applications of this approach have been published. Remarkably, these new approaches were first applied in marine and terrestrial ecosystems and later in studies on the GI tract of farm animals (Pryde et al., 1999; Leser et al., 2002; Zhu et al., 2002; Konstantinov et al., 2006) and humans (Suau et al., 1999). The 16S rRNA gene-based taxonomic studies on cattle, humans, horses, rodents, and pigs have revealed that the majority of recovered sequences are phylogenetically affiliated to several known groups of anaerobic bacteria of which only a few species have been cultivated (Konstantinov et al., 2005a, 2005b).

The crucial role of the mammalian GI tract microbiota in host health and performance is apparent during the neonatal and weaning period of farm animals. Starting at birth, the microbiota must ultimately develop from a simple, unstable community into a complex and climax community, a process that can be influenced by diet, environmental factors, and the host itself (Konstantinov et al., 2004a, 2004b). In contrast to the slow weaning process of human infants, monogastric animals, including piglets in the commercial animal production settings, experience an early and critical transition from mother's milk onto a solid diet rich in plant polysaccharides. In piglets, this transition is between 21 and 28 days of life. As weaning progresses, piglets become vulnerable to a higher incidence of gastrointestinal and respiratory diseases. Often, the presence of a pathogen alone is not sufficient to cause disease since the host's defense mechanisms are able to resist the effects of the pathogen. However, some factors can adversely influence the host and thus result in disease. The changes in the composition and activity of the GI tract microbial community after birth have been suggested to be among the factors that predispose the animals to infectious diseases, due to the reduced ability of the resident gut microbiota to exert a barrier effect against pathogens via the phenomenon of colonization resistance (Van der Waaij, 1987). This has been clearly demonstrated in domestic fowls where during the first week posthatch the chicks are most susceptible to *Salmonella* infections, whereas adult chickens are resistant to *Salmonella enterica* serovar Infantis (Nurmi and Rantala, 1973). It has also been reported that *Escherichia coli*, one of the first bacterial species to colonize the intestine of humans, mice, and piglets, displays antimicrobial activity against the *Salmonella* spp. able to cause infections (Hudault et al., 2001). Other species of the endogenous human and animal microbiota such as *Bifidobacterium* and *Lactobacillus* spp. are known to exert antimicrobial activity in vitro, and this has been proposed as a protective mechanism (Tannock, 2004).

Bacterial colonization starts at birth and follows a rapid succession during the first few weeks of life. The trend in the development of the microbiota is remarkably similar in the alimentary tract of most mammals (Mackie et al., 1999). Using conventional cultivation-based techniques, it has been shown that the first porcine intestinal colonizers are LAB, enterobacteria, and streptococci (Stewart, 1997). The neonatal microbiota is relatively stable and dominated by LAB throughout the first week of life. The recent application of molecular techniques to studying the microbial ecology of neonatal piglets has unveiled new trends in bacterial colonization (Konstantinov et al., 2006). As demonstrated by sequence analysis of 16S rRNA amplicons combined with fingerprinting and real-time PCR techniques, the ileal samples of 2-day-old piglets harbored a consortium of *E. coli*, *Shigella flexneri*, *Lactobacillus sobrius*, *Lactobacillus reuteri*, and *Lactobacillus acidophilus*-related sequences. Remarkable stability was encountered in the populations of the early colonizers such as *L. sobrius*, *L. reuteri*, and *L. acidophilus*-related populations, as long as the piglets remained with their sows. In the immediate postweaning period, shifts in the microbiota composition and metabolic activities were found for both the ileal and the colonic microbiota. When individual fecal samples were examined over a period of time, daily fluctuations in the predominant bacterial communities were also observed after weaning (Konstantinov et al., 2003). Taken together, the data suggest that the early postweaning period of piglets is characterized by instability in the predominant gut microbiota and its metabolic activities. Moreover, the populations of some potentially beneficial lactobacilli are significantly suppressed during the weaning transition. The data are consistent with other reports that the lactobacillus composition is age dependent and changes successively (Tannock, 1990; Sghir et al., 1998), which is likely to be due to several dietary, environmental, or host factors.

In humans, conditions such as diarrhea and inflammatory bowel diseases have been associated with changes in the composition of the intestinal microbiota (Guarner and Malagelada, 2003), whereas the microbiota of healthy adult individuals remains stable over time (Zoetendal et al., 1998). In piglets, it has often been hypothesized that an allergy to dietary proteins and/or postweaning anorexia (McCracken et al., 1999) may play a significant role in the GI tract disturbances during weaning. Recently, it has been demonstrated that weaning is associated with a significant up-regulation in gene expression of many inflammatory cytokines in the gut during the first 2 days postweaning (Pie et al., 2004). To what extent the early and acute inflammatory response, suggested as a primary factor in postweaning gut disorders in piglets, is related to the disturbance of specific beneficial bacterial populations remains to be determined. It is also possible that some key members of the farm animal microbiota attenuate inflammatory responses in the intestinal mucosa and contribute to intestinal homeostasis, and examples of anti-inflammatory effects of some nonpathogenic bacteria have already been published (Neish et al., 2000; Kelly et al., 2004).

There are several possible explanations of how probiotic microorganisms displace pathogens and enhance the development and stability of the microbial balance in farm animals. Some of the proposed mechanisms include competition with pathogens for nutrients and adhesion sites. Other probiotic effects may rely on the inactivation of pathogenic bacterial toxins or metabolites, the production of substances that inhibit pathogen growth, and the stimulation of nonspecific immunity. The adverse effects of stress and/or antibiotics often lead to instability in microbial communities followed by the rapid decrease of previously abundant beneficial members such as lactobacilli. Thus, the microbial community can be seen to be an important potential target in therapeutic and preventive interventions.

PROBIOTIC STRATEGIES IN VETERINARY MEDICINE

As early as the 1960s, decreased incidences of infections were among the claims attributed to the feeding of different microorganisms to farm animals. Based on their origin, three categories of probiotics were distinguished: (i) LAB (lactobacilli, enterococci, or streptococci), which naturally occur in the digestive tract; (ii) spore-forming bacteria belonging to the genus *Bacillus* with the soil as their natural habitat; and (iii) *Saccharomyces* yeasts, which normally grow on plant materials (Simon et al., 2003).

With the ban of antibiotics as growth promoters in the European Union, over 20 microbial cultures have been provisionally or finally authorized as feed additives for farm animals (Simon et al., 2003). This is in contrast to the U.S. Department of Agriculture (USDA), which has approved only two probiotic formulations that decrease pathogen levels when fed to poultry (Anonymous, 1998).

The reduction in the incidence of diarrhea by probiotics has frequently been studied because this problem is of the utmost importance for farm animals (Table 1). In piglets, bacteria that are associated with diarrheal disease after weaning include enterotoxigenic *E. coli* (ETEC) and other *E. coli* strains (postweaning colibacillosis) and *Salmonella* spp. (Hopwood and Hampson, 2003). The attachment of ETEC to the enterocytes lining the small intestinal villi is mediated by adhesins known as K88 (or F4). The degree of microbial adhesion is variable due to individual differences in the presence of intestinal receptors for the fimbriae of ETEC (Van den Broeck et al., 1999). After attachment to, and colonization of, the small intestinal enterocytes, ETEC provokes hypersecretory diarrhea through the release of specific enterotoxins. Thus far, no effective vaccines are available to control postweaning colibacillosis, and many pathogenic *E. coli* strains show resistance to multiple antibiotics (Amezcua et al., 2002). Although pathogen prevalence has been identified as the primary determinant of the incidence of infections in postweaning colibacillosis, there is abundant evidence to suggest that other factors are necessary for the manifestation of the disease. Changes in the composition and activity of the microbial community of the small intestine after weaning may be among the factors that predispose the animals to infections. A significant decrease in the number of LAB and an increase in coliforms have consistently been observed in the GI tract of piglets during the first weeks after weaning (Franklin et al., 2002; Konstantinov et al., 2006). The probiotic application of specific probiotic strains may therefore confer resistance to pathogen-induced intestinal challenges and restore homeostasis in the microbiota (Isolauri et al., 2002).

Although the results of attempts to use probiotic bacteria to reduce colonization of pathogenic bacteria are not always clear-cut, there is a general trend to use these feed additives for the prophylaxis of diarrhea. Some authors have found that oral administration of *Streptococcus faecium* to gnotobiotic piglets challenged with various pathogenic strains of *E. coli* induced an increased weight gain, less-severe diarrhea, and reduced colonization by pathogenic bacteria in the gut compared to control animals (Underdahl et al., 1982). A protective effectiveness of *Bifidobacterium lactis* has also been found in piglets, as the probiotic was able to lower the numbers of fecal rotavirus and *E. coli* and reduce the severity of diarrhea (Shu et al., 2001). Moreover, the application of *Bacillus cereus* and *Bacillus licheniformis* has been shown to protect against diarrhea caused by ETEC in piglets (Kyriakis et al., 1999). The results of other studies, however, demonstrated that probiotics had no influence on the clinical symptoms, mortality, or excretion of hemolytic *E. coli* in piglets (De Cupere et al., 1992) and that *B. cereus* was unable to reduce colonization by pathogenic *E. coli* (Goebel et al., 2000).

Recent attempts to understand some of the possible mechanisms involved in the beneficial effect of probiotics in piglets prompted experiments using a porcine-derived cell line (IPEC-1) (Roselli et al., 2007). The study found that ETEC induces up-regulation of interleukin-8 (IL-8), which correlates with the disruption of tight junctions. When added in vitro, a newly isolated porcine commensal bacterium, *Lactobacillus sobrius* DSM 16698[T], was able to reduce the ETEC attachment, up-regulate IL-10 expression, and protect the cytoskeleton and tight-junction organization. These results partly agree with other in vitro studies demonstrating that a mixture of lactobacilli, bifidobacteria, and streptococci (VSL#3) or *L. acidophilus* was able to stabilize tight junctions (Montalto et al., 2004; Otte and Podolsky, 2004). The results, however, need to be confirmed in animal experiments, where the gut epithelium is covered by mucins and direct bacterial access may be limited. Nonetheless, the in vitro data support the notion that certain probiotics can counteract the harmful effects of ETEC by mechanisms including pathogen adhesion inhibition and maintenance of membrane barrier integrity through IL-10 regulation.

It has been suggested that probiotic products decrease the need for antibiotics in poultry production and pathogen levels on farms, and the USDA has already designated a probiotic *Bacillus* strain for use with chickens as "Generally Recognized As Safe." Feeding chickens a strain of *Bacillus subtilis* resulted in increased body weight and feed conversion. In addition, *Salmonella* was successfully controlled by spraying a patented blend of 29 bacteria, isolated from the chicken cecum, on day-old chickens (Prescott et al., 2002). As they preen themselves, the chicks ingest the bacterial mixture, establishing a

Table 1 Overview of beneficial effects of some microorganisms in different animal species

Animals	Microbial species	Reported effects[a]	Reference(s)
Pigs			
Suckling and weaning piglets	B. cereus, B. licheniformis, B. lactis, E. faecium, L. acidophilus, Lactobacillus fermentum, S. cerevisiae	Reduced incidence of diarrhea	Conway, 1989; Jadamus et al., 2002; Kyriakis et al., 1999; Manner and Spieler, 1997; Redmond and Moore, 1965; Shu et al., 2001; Simon et al., 2003; Zani et al., 1998
Pigs	Lactobacillus bulgaricus	Neutralizes E. coli toxins	Mitchell and Kenworth, 1976
	L. casei (Shirota)	Affects fermentation in the large intestine	Ohashi et al., 2004
	L. johnsonii, L. pentosus	Reduction of Salmonella carriage	Casey et al., 2004
	L. murinus	Decreases Enterobacteriaceae counts in fecal samples	Gardiner et al., 2004
Poultry			
Chicken	B. cereus var. toyoii	Improves feed efficiency in Salmonella enterica serovar Enteritidis-infected broilers	Gil de los Santos et al., 2005
	B. subtilis	Reduces Clostridium perfringens in young chickens	La Ragione et al., 2003
	E. faecium	Enhances broiler chick performance with respect to weight gain and FC	Samli et al., 2007
	L. johnsonii FI9785	Controls endemic necrotic enteritis due to C. perfringens	La Ragione et al., 2004
	Saccharomyces boulardii	Reduces serovar Enteritidis in young chickens; improves feed efficiency	Line et al., 1998; Gil de los Santos et al., 2005
	Lactobacillus species	Inhibition of Eimeria tenella in vitro	Tierney et al., 2004
	Lactobacillus species	Reduction in mortality	Timmerman et al., 2006
	Lactobacillus-based probiotic	Effects on local cell-mediated immunity of chickens	Dalloul et al., 2003
Hens	Lactobacillus species	Increases egg production, decreases mortality, improves FC but not egg quality	Yoruk et al., 2004
Cattle			
Beef cattle	L. acidophilus	Reduces E. coli O157:H7 levels	Younts-Dahl et al., 2005
	L. acidophilus strain NP 51	Reduces E. coli O157:H7 prevalence in both fecal and hide samples	Younts-Dahl et al., 2004
Veal calves	Six Lactobacillus species	Enhances growth rate, BWG, FC, and tends to decrease mortality	Timmerman et al., 2005
Calves	L. rhamnosus GG	Survives GI tract transit without producing D-lactate	Ewaschuk et al., 2004
Cattle	Lactobacillus species	Decreases, but does not eliminate, fecal shedding of E. coli O157:H7	Brashears et al., 2003
Holstein calves	L. gallinarum LCB 12 and S. bovis	Reduces or stops carriage of E. coli O157	Ohya et al., 2000, 2001
	L. acidophilus and other genera	Improves DWG and FC, decreases diarrhea	Isik et al., 2004
Fish			
Rainbow trout	L. rhamnosus JCM 1136	Increases cellular innate immune responses	Panigrahi et al., 2004
	Lactobacillus species	Adhesion to mucus	Nikoskelainen et al., 2001
	L. rhamnosus GG	Increases serum immunoglobulin levels	Nikoskelainen et al., 2003
	L. rhamnosus GG	Increases survival	Verschuere et al., 2000
Nile tilapia	L. acidophilus, S. faecium, S. cerevisiae	Promotes growth	Lara-Flores et al., 2003

(Continued)

Table 1 Overview of beneficial effects of some microorganisms in different animal species *(Continued)*

Animals	Microbial species	Reported effects[a]	Reference(s)
Other species			
Horses, foals	*L. rhamnosus* GG	More consistent intestinal colonization in foals	Weese et al., 2003
Rabbits	*E. faecium* and *L. jugurti*	Reduction in total cholesterol	Rossi et al., 2000
Lambs	*Lactobacillus* species, *L. acidophilus, S. faecium, L. casei, L. fermentum, L. plantarum*	Stimulates feed intake and DWG; reduces fecal shedding of *E. coli* O157:H7	Umberger et al., 1989; Lema et al., 2001
Dogs	*Lactobacillus* strain AD1	Colonizes the GI tract during transit	Strompfovà et al., 2004
	L. acidophilus DSM13241	Survives transit through the canine GI tract	Baillon et al., 2004
Cats	*L. acidophilus* DSM13241	Exerts systemic and immunomodulatory effects	Marshall-Jones et al., 2006

[a]DWG, daily weight gain; BWG, body weight gain; FC, feed conversion.

functional microbial community in the cecum and limiting *Salmonella* colonization of the gut by so-called "competitive exclusion" (Nurmi and Rantala, 1973). Edens et al. (1997) reported that in ovo and ex ovo administration of *L. reuteri* resulted in an increased villus height, indicating that probiotics are potentially able to enhance nutrient absorption and thereby improve growth performance and feed efficiency. Via "competitive exclusion," probiotics are potentially able to reduce mortality from enteric pathogens, but the effects are not always consistent with this concept in reported trials with broilers (Timmerman et al., 2006). In challenge experiments with pathogens such as *E. coli, Salmonella enterica* serovar Typhimurium, and *Staphylococcus aureus*, there was a probiotic-induced reduction in mortality (Watkins and Miller, 1983). However, in another challenge trial with *Salmonella pullorum*, it was shown that the application of a probiotic *Enterococcus faecium* strain prevented mortality, but only if the probiotic was administered before the challenge (Audisio et al., 2000). This is in accordance with other reports that probiotics might reduce the colonization of pathogenic bacteria in chickens (Table 1).

Prevention of diarrhea is also important for baby calves. Huber (1997) summarized the effects of probiotic feeding to baby calves and, next to greater feed intake and improved weight gain, the reduction of diarrhea was one of the most prominent results observed. However, the authors also mentioned that most studies showed only nonsignificant beneficial effects. Reduction of pathogenic *E. coli* O157:H7 has also been reported following the administration of a probiotic preparation containing *Streptococcus bovis, Lactobacillus gallinarum,* or *Saccharomyces cerevisiae* as the active ingredients (Zhao et al., 1998; Ohya et al., 2000). However, the probiotic had to be administered before challenge with the pathogen. In a feeding trial with two different probiotic preparations (*E. faecium* and *B. cereus*) added to the milk replacer for calves (50- to 85-kg

body weight), a nonsignificant increase in live weight gain was observed, together with a significant decrease in the frequency of diarrhea (Simon et al., 2001). From these and other studies, it can be concluded that probiotics can also achieve a reduction in the frequency of diarrhea in calves.

Concomitant with the situation in different animal species, some protective effects of probiotics have also been reported in preventing infectious diarrhea in human infants. In a double-blind placebo-controlled trial, it has been shown that the administration of *Lactobacillus paracasei* ameliorates the outcome of diarrhea in nonrotavirus-infected infants (Sarker et al., 2005). In addition, a recent meta-analysis revealed that the use of *Lactobacillus* strain GG is associated with moderate clinical benefits in the treatment of acute diarrhea in children (Szajewska et al., 2007).

Disease outbreaks are being increasingly recognized as a significant threat in aquaculture production, and this has accelerated research on probiotics for the improvement of aquatic environmental quality and disease control in aquaculture. After the first publications on biological control in aquaculture in the 1980s, the research effort has steadily increased. Generally, probiotics are applied in the feed or added to the culture tank or pond as preventive agents against infection by pathogenic bacteria, although nutritional effects are also often attributed to probiotics, especially for filter feeders. Most probiotics proposed as biological control agents in aquaculture are LAB or yeasts, although other genera or species have also been mentioned by Verschuere (Verschuere et al., 2000) and are listed in Table 1.

FERMENTED LIQUID FEED AND LAB
Neonatal farmhouse animals including piglets often have an insufficiency of stomach acid, which is the first line of defense against bacterial invasion. Manipulation

of stomach acidity through lactic acid supplementation of the feed has been used to reduce gastric pH and the number of coliforms, because at high levels (>100 mM), lactic acid has a bactericidal effect (Ratcliffe et al., 1985, 1986). Unfortunately, natural fermentations cannot be relied upon to produce these concentrations of lactic acid. This problem can be overcome by the use of fermented liquid feed (FLF) inoculated with different LAB species that are used as preservatives in the human food industry or for the production of forage silage. Several workers (Russell et al., 1996; Geary et al., 1999) have shown that a *Lactobacillus* population develops in ad libitum liquid feeding systems for weaning pigs and that this is accompanied by a reduction of pH and the coliform population. These organisms produce lactic acid rapidly and to a high concentration. A number of LAB species have been identified that in 24 h are capable of producing in excess of 100 mM lactic acid with less than 30 mM acetic acid. Under these conditions, *S. enterica* serovar Typhimurium was rapidly excluded when introduced into feed that had been fermented for 48, 72, or 96 h (Beal et al., 2002). In another study (van Winsen et al., 2000), it was found that feed fermented with *L. plantarum* had a bacteriostatic effect on *Salmonella* during the first 2 h following inoculation and a bactericidal effect thereafter. Six hours after inoculation, serovar Typhimurium could not be detected in FLF. In contrast, serovar Typhimurium added to nonfermented feed survived and multiplied. It has also been shown that it is the lactic acid concentration of the fermented feed that is responsible for this effect (van Winsen et al., 2001). Studies have demonstrated that when serovar Typhimurium DT104:30 and *Pediococcus pentosaceus* are coinoculated into liquid feed, *P. pentosaceus* rapidly dominates the fermentation and reduces serovar Typhimurium to undetectable levels (Beal et al., 2002). FLF has also been implicated as being effective in reducing the incidence of pathogenic *E. coli* (Beal et al., 2001). In addition, feeding FLF does not appear to produce any significant effect on the number of LAB throughout the gut but it does dramatically reduce the number of coliforms in the lower small intestine, cecum, and colon. The ratio of LAB to coliforms in the lower gut of piglets weaned onto liquid diets has been found to be very similar to that of piglets that continued to suckle the sow (Jensen, 1998). This suggests that FLF might have a valuable role as part of a strategy for improving the animals' health in the absence of antibiotic growth promoters.

PLANT EXTRACTS AS FEED ADDITIVES?

The use of a diverse range of plant extracts to enhance animal health, growth, and performance has been advocated by a variety of sources for a very long time. Although diverse plant extracts have been suggested as alternatives to in-feed antibiotics, most of these claims have been evaluated only under in vitro conditions (Dorman and Deans, 2000; Friedman et al., 2002; Faleiro et al., 2003; Lis-Balchin, 2003).

Plants have evolved a wide range of low-molecular-weight metabolites. Generally these compounds enable the plants to interact with the environment and may act as a defense system against physiological and environmental stress as well as predators or pathogens. Beside compounds with toxic properties, several of these secondary plant metabolites have been reported to show beneficial effects in food products and also in mammalian metabolism. Beneficial effects of herbs or botanicals in pigs and poultry may arise from stimulation of feed intake (flavor) and secretion of digestive secretions, immune stimulation, and antibacterial, antiviral, or anti-inflammatory activity. Most of these active plant metabolites belong to the classes of isoprene derivatives, flavonoids, and glucosinolates. The antibiotic and anti-oxidant effects of these compounds have been extensively reviewed (Lis-Balchin, 2003). However, a major concern of much of this work is that it is based upon either in vitro studies or animal feeding performance trials and little is known about the mechanisms of their effects in vivo. Moreover, there are suggestions of little or no beneficial impact of these feed additives in feeding trials (Muhl and Liebert, 2007).

SOME BENEFICIAL EFFECTS OF NONDIGESTIBLE BUT FERMENTABLE CARBOHYDRATES

Fermentation in the GI tract is increasingly being recognized as having important implications for the health of the GI tract and thus of the host animal. It has been hypothesized that addition of fermentable carbohydrates to the feed is a comparatively straightforward way to improve the microbial balance in both the small and large intestines of farmhouse animals. Established more than 1 decade ago, the concept of dietary modulation of the microbiota composition through the addition of nondigestible but fermentable carbohydrates (NDC), introduced as prebiotics, was first studied in humans. Prebiotics have been defined as nondigestible food ingredients that beneficially affect the host by selectively stimulating the growth and/or activity of one of a limited number of bacteria in the colon (Gibson and Roberfroid, 1995). Using various techniques, it has been shown that some NDC can indeed selectively stimulate the growth and/or activity of LAB, with concomitant improvement of host colonization resistance (Roberfroid and Slavin, 2000). In vitro fermentation experiments showed that short-chain carbohydrates are fermented faster than long-chain carbohydrates. Similarly, linear chains are fermented faster than branched chains and soluble carbohydrates are fermented more rapidly than insoluble carbohydrates (Bauer et al., 2001). From these data it can be concluded that the fermentation rate of different NDC depends on their molecular structure; polysaccharides like cellulose and wheat fiber are non- or low-fermentable NDC, resistant starch is well fermentable, and inulin, fructo-oligosaccharides (FOS), and lactulose are rapidly fermentable (Ten Bruggencate et al., 2004).

Animal parameters such as growth and feed intake are usually not altered by the inclusion of NDC in the diet (Houdijk et al., 1998; Konstantinov et al., 2003; Konstantinov et al., 2004a, 2004b). This is in contrast to the expectation that such inclusion will negatively affect the growth of the animal, as it is supposed to reduce the proportion of enzymatically degradable ingredients. Until recently, any part of the diet which was fermented was considered to have been wasted (Williams et al., 2001).

Using cultivation-based approaches, the effects of NDC on the colonic microbiota in humans (Rastall and Gibson, 2002) and in mice have been reported with respect to their ability to confer resistance to some pathogenic challenges via the enhanced growth of specific LAB (Ten Bruggencate et al., 2004). Further characterization of the stimulated lactobacilli, however, has not been achieved beyond the genus level (Rastall and Gibson, 2002). In pigs, the recent application of molecular ecological tools revealed that the microbiota composition is susceptible to dietary NDC interventions (Leser et al., 2000; Konstantinov et al., 2004a, 2004b). A strong diet effect was also found in weaning piglets consuming a diet supplemented with sugar beet pulp (SBP) alone or mixed with FOS (Konstantinov, 2003). An increase in diversity and stability of the fecal bacterial community, as measured by denaturing gel gradient electrophoresis analysis of 16S rRNA gene PCR amplicons, was shown for the piglets fed NDC-enriched diets compared to a group fed a control diet. Furthermore, the bacterial community composition in the guts of weaning piglets was significantly affected by the dietary addition of SBP, inulin, lactulose, and wheat starch (Konstantinov, 2004a). Such a diet containing a mixture of fast (inulin and lactulose) and slow fermentable ingredients (wheat starch and SBP components) was specifically designed to stimulate the fermentation along the entire GI tract (Williams et al., 2001). Inulin and lactulose are two prebiotic oligosaccharides that have previously been reported to stimulate that part of the human colonic microbiota related to lactobacilli (Rycroft et al., 2001). However, dietary addition of FOS that can be derived from inulin has been also reported to increase colonization of the cecal mucosa and lumen of rats by *Salmonella* in challenge studies (Ten Bruggencate et al., 2004). Moreover, studies of pathogen survival in healthy animals fed NDC have shown beneficial, inconsistent, or adverse effect. By using in vitro techniques, SBP has been shown to be readily fermentable by porcine fecal bacteria (Bauer et al., 2001; Zhu et al., 2003). It has also been demonstrated to stimulate the bacterial diversity and result in higher short-chain fatty acid and lower ammonia concentrations than those of some other potential feed ingredients (Bauer et al., 2001). Furthermore, the addition of SBP to the diet of pigs was reported to reduce the populations of coliforms (Roberfroid, 1998). Other studies, however, suggested an increased proliferation of pathogenic *E. coli* when the piglets were fed with a fiber-enriched diet (McDonald et al., 2001). Overall, results concerning the role of NDC in the development of swine dysentery are often contradictory (Jensen and Jorgensen, 1994; Jensen et al., 2003). As shown by some research groups, diets with low fiber and resistant starches protect the pigs from infection with *Brachyspira hyodysenteriae* (Durmic et al., 1998; Pluske et al., 1998), while others were not able to confirm these findings (Leser et al., 2000; Lindecrona et al., 2003). In addition, it has been suggested that the combination of fermentable dietary fiber and oligosaccharides may specifically stimulate the *Lactobacillus amylovorus*-like population and lead to a higher bacterial diversity in the gut of weaning piglets (Konstantinov et al., 2004a). This implies that the response of the bacterial community needs to be thoroughly examined in respect to the in vivo growth of specific species in particular intestinal compartments following the introduction of NDC-enriched diets.

CURRENT DEVELOPMENTS AND FUTURE PROSPECTS

Compositional Analysis

Microbes of all types, including bacteria, viruses, archaea, fungi, and protozoans, colonize and persist in the intestinal tract of farm animals. Although the composition of these communities varies greatly between different animal species, it has been assumed that a stable and complex community is a prerequisite of a healthy ecosystem (Akkermans et al., 2003). A recent phylogenetic analysis of 16S rRNA genes from porcine intestinal samples (Leser et al., 2002) and chicken intestinal samples (Zhu et al., 2002) revealed that the majority of sequences retrieved from obligate anaerobic microorganisms are yet to be cultivated. This agrees with the results of published 16S rRNA gene-based cultivation-independent studies of the human intestinal microbiota (Suau et al., 1999; Eckburg et al., 2005). Further cultivation and molecular studies are needed to assess the spatial and temporal composition of the GI tract microbiota in different animal species. Although extensive studies of the diversity of gut ecosystems are still lacking, it can be expected that, when fully described, the species richness in the GI tract of farm animals will be measured in thousands. Techniques for fingerprinting microbial communities, including temperature/denaturing gradient gel electrophoresis and terminal restriction fragment length polymorphism, are useful for a rapid assessment of the predominant microbiota (Leser et al., 2000; Simpson et al., 2000; Konstantinov et al., 2003) but can detect only populations that exceed 10^8 CFU per g of sample (Zoetendal et al., 1998). Many of the species that establish smaller populations in the GI tract, including *E. coli* and *Campylobacter jejuni*, are known to play significant roles in health. In order to detect these minority groups by fingerprinting methods, specific primers for each targeted group of microorganisms need to be developed.

Beneficial Microorganisms and Assessment of Their Functionality

Studies of the taxonomic diversity of the microbiota have revealed the identity of the species present, but they provide only limited information with regard to the potential functional roles of these microorganisms. In addition, it may be argued that the physiology of commensal bacteria is more relevant to the issue of animal health than is the phylogeny of those organisms. Characterization of the in vivo functions of the bacteria present in the gut is highly challenging but may be more useful than methods that classify them phylogenetically. Often the immune effects of probiotic organisms are strain specific, and closely related microorganisms may have distinct impacts on the immune system. By extension, pattern recognition receptors of the host recognize structural details in the peptidoglycan backbone of the cell walls of gram-positive bacteria, and these structures can be shared among taxonomically different pathogenic and commensal bacteria. Hence, the results of phylogenic and physiological studies need to be thoroughly examined when considering claims of possible probiotic effects.

The functional efficacy of a particular organism in the complex microbial environment of the GI tract is dependent on its numerical abundance, survival, competitiveness, location, and metabolic activity. The fate of the ingested probiotic is of utmost importance, because it is generally supposed that the metabolic activity of the probiotic in the GI tract is essential for its action.

Specific monitoring of probiotic LAB such as lactobacilli or enterococci, however, is not possible with conventional methods but can be achieved by the use of, for instance, real-time PCR detection of strain-specific genomic fragments (Konstantinov et al., 2005a, 2005b) or other molecular ecological techniques. In contrast, probiotic bacilli can be detected more easily due to their spore-forming and facultative anaerobic growth. Since the number of facultative anaerobic spore-forming bacteria is negligible in the GI tract (except in the crop of poultry), the cultivation of heat-treated intestinal samples yields the spore content of the probiotic strain. This approach has been used in the detection of *B. cereus* var. *toyoi* in poultry and piglets (Jadamus et al., 2002; Gil de los Santos et al., 2005).

One approach to study the functionality of a particular microorganism in the GI milieu necessitates the use of molecular approaches to specifically detect gene expression. The development of techniques to detect in vivo bacterial gene expression is under way: in vivo expression technology (Bron et al., 2004) or the green fluorescent protein gene from *Aequoria victoria* as a marker can be used to detect, for example, in vivo expression and location of a *Lactobacillus* strain in the mouse GI tract (Geoffroy et al., 2000). However, there is a need to develop additional methods to detect prokaryotic gene expression in complex ecosystems. Examples of new approaches that have been used to achieve this include the determination of the expression pattern of *Helicobacter pylori* during its infection of the gastric mucosae using real-time reverse transcription-PCR (Rokbi et al., 2001) and the use of differential fluorescence induction reporter systems to study host-induced pathogen genes (Bumann and Valdivia, 2007). A molecular protocol has also been developed to assess the activity of *L. acidophilus* by detecting mRNA by reverse transcription-PCR in GI tract samples (Fitzsimons et al., 2003). These methodologies have potential applicability to the localization and the monitoring of the in vivo gene expression/activity of a specific microbe in a complex ecosystem, such as a probiotic culture in the GI tract.

Genomic analysis of differential gene expression in microbes and higher organisms has been greatly facilitated by the development of DNA microarrays. This technology has been exploited to monitor global intestinal transcriptional responses to the colonization of germfree mice with *Bacteroides thetaiotaomicron*, a prominent member of the normal murine and human intestinal microbiota (Hooper and Gordon, 2001). This study showed that this commensal was able to modulate expression of host genes participating in diverse and fundamental physiological functions, including nutrient absorption, mucosal barrier fortification, xenobiotic metabolism, angiogenesis, and postnatal intestinal maturation. In a later study, when mice were cocolonized with *B. thetaiotaomicron* and the probiotic *Bifidobacterium longum*, the host elicited a different gene expression profile from that obtained with *B. thetaiotaomicron* alone (Sonnenburg et al., 2006). These results highlight how the host response can be affected by changes in the composition of the intestinal microbiota.

The development of ultrafast genome-sequencing techniques in combination with single-cell analysis has already enabled the monitoring of uncultivated minority members of a microbial community (Marcy et al., 2007). This can be further applied to study the efficacy and functionality of beneficial intestinal microbes with low abundance in the GI tract. Furthermore, the recently developed metagenomic approach provides the opportunity to assess the gene content, and its encoded metabolic potential, of any microbial community. This has already been used to study the microbiota in healthy humans (Gill et al., 2006) and in individuals with Crohn's disease (Manichanh et al., 2006). Future metagenomic studies in farm animals may provide a more detailed description of the taxonomic diversity of their indigenous microbial communities and reveal the effects of the host genotype, diet, and pathogenic challenges on these communities. The further expansion of functional genomics may also aid in the unraveling of the mechanisms underlying the postulated health-promoting effects of probiotics and help to uncover novel activities of indigenous microbial communities.

Future Perspectives

Recent in vitro studies have suggested that probiotics can have protective effects on cytokine-induced apoptosis or permeability changes, attenuate epithelial inflammatory responses, and reduce invasion or adherence of pathogens (Madsen et al., 2001; Lievin-Le Moal et al., 2002; Resta-Lenert and Barrett, 2006). Additionally, certain probiotics and commensals have the capacity to induce tolerance in the host immune system following their interaction with dendritic cells and other antigen-presenting cells in vitro by elevating the levels of anti-inflammatory cytokines produced (Mohamadzadeh et al., 2005; Smits et al., 2005; Foligne et al., 2007). Further evidence of the beneficial activities of probiotics comes from their application in models of inflammatory bowel disease or allergic sensitization (Grangette et al., 2005; Fitzpatrick et al., 2007; Geier et al., 2007). Nevertheless, in vitro data and the results of studies using rodents as model animals are often criticized as potential artifacts and unrepresentative of the conditions in

different farm animals. Conclusive data concerning the specific mechanisms of probiotic functionality from different animal species are lacking. Although challenging, this is clearly a topic that warrants further research.

The relationship that exists between probiotic microorganisms and their host may be symbiotic (both partners benefit) when pathogenic challenges are avoided and the habitat of the bacterial communities is preserved. The host could benefit in several ways from probiotic bacteria during stress or antibiotic treatment. Under these conditions, which are characterized by great compositional flux in the microbiota, probiotics could provide colonization resistance. Additional benefits may include the provision of critical metabolic activities and the shaping of the underlying mucosal immune system by the induction of host genes involved in immunity. We anticipate that the achievement of such effects in order to improve animal health will be an important aspect of the use of probiotics in the future.

References

Akkermans, A. D. L., S. R. Konstantinov, W. Y. Zhu, C. F. Favier, and B. A. Williams. 2003. Postnatal development of the intestinal microbiota of the pig, p. 49–57. *In* R. O. Ball (ed.), *Proceedings of the 9th International Symposium on Digestive Physiology in Pigs.* University of Alberta, Banff, Canada.

Amezcua, R., R. M. Friendship, C. E. Dewey, C. L. Gyles, and J. R. Fairbrother. 2002. Presentation of postweaning *Escherichia coli* diarrhea in southern Ontario, prevalence of hemolytic *E. coli* serogroups involved, and their antimicrobial resistance patterns. *Can. J. Vet. Res.* **66:**73–78.

Anonymous. 1998. New product reduces salmonellae in chickens. *J. Am. Vet. Med. Assoc.* **212:**1358.

Audisio, C. M., G. Oliver, and M. C. Apella. 2000. Protective effect of *Enterococcus faecium* J96, a potential probiotic strain, on chicks infected with *Salmonella pullorum*. *J. Food Prot.* **63:**1333–1337.

Baillon, M. L., Z. V. Marshall-Jones, and R. F. Butterwick. 2004. Effects of probiotic *Lactobacillus acidophilus* strain DSM13241 in healthy adult dogs. *Am. J. Vet. Res.* **65:**338–343.

Bauer, E., B. A. Williams, C. Voigt, R. Mosenthin, and M. W. A. Verstegen. 2001. Microbial activities of faeces from unweaned and adult pigs, in relation to selected fermentable carbohydrates. *Anim. Sci.* **73:**313–322.

Beal, J. D., C. A. Moran, A. Campbell, and P. H. Brooks. 2001. The survival of potentially pathogenic *E. coli* in fermented liquid feed, p. 351–353. *In* B. Ogle (ed.), *Digestive Physiology of Pigs.* CABI Publishing, Wallingford, Oxford, United Kingdom.

Beal, J. D., S. J. Niven, A. Campbell, and P. H. Brooks. 2002. The effect of temperature on the growth and persistence of *Salmonella* in fermented liquid pig feed. *Int. J. Food Microbiol.* **79:**99–104.

Bernardeau, M., M. Guguen, and J. P. Vernoux. 2006. Beneficial lactobacilli in food and feed: long-term use, biodiversity and proposals for specific and realistic safety assessments. *FEMS Microbiol. Rev.* 30:487–513.

Brashears, M. M., M. L. Galyean, G. H. Loneragan, J. E. Mann, and K. Killinger-Mann. 2003. Prevalence of *Escherichia coli* O157:H7 and performance by beef feedlot cattle given *Lactobacillus* direct-fed microbials. *J. Food Prot.* 66:748–754.

Bron, P. A., C. Grangette, A. Mercenier, W. M. de Vos, and M. Kleerebezem. 2004. Identification of *Lactobacillus plantarum* genes that are induced in the gastrointestinal tract of mice. *J. Bacteriol.* 186:5721–5729.

Bumann, D., and R. H. Valdivia. 2007. Identification of host-induced pathogen genes by differential fluorescence induction reporter systems. *Nat. Protoc.* 2:770–777.

Casey, P. G., G. D. Casey, G. E. Gardiner, M. Tangney, C. Stanton, R. P. Ross, C. Hill, and G. F. Fitzgerald. 2004. Isolation and characterization of anti-*Salmonella* lactic acid bacteria from the porcine gastrointestinal tract. *Lett. Appl. Microbiol.* 39:431–438.

Cebra, J. J. 1999. Influences of microbiota on intestinal immune system development. *Am. J. Clin. Nutr.* 69(Suppl.):1046S–1051S.

Conway, P. L. 1989. Lactobacilli: fact or fiction, p. 263–281. *In* R. Grubb (ed.), *The Regulatory and Protective Role of the Normal Microflora*. Macmillan Press, Basingstoke, United Kingdom.

Dalloul, R. A., H. S. Lillehoj, T. A. Shellem, and J. A. Doerr. 2003. Intestinal immunomodulation by vitamin A deficiency and *Lactobacillus*-based probiotic in *Eimeria acervulina*-infected broiler chickens. *Avian Dis.* 47:1313–1320.

De Cupere, F., P. Deprez, D. Demeulenaere, and E. Muylle. 1992. Evaluation of the effect of 3 probiotics on experimental *Escherichia coli* enterotoxaemia in weaning piglets. *J. Vet. Med. Bull.* 39:277–284.

Dorman, H. J. D., and S. G. Deans. 2000. Antimicrobial agents from plants: antibacterial activity of plant volatile oils. *J. Appl. Microbiol.* 88:308–316.

Durmic, Z., D. W. Pethick, J. R. Pluske, and D. J. Hampson. 1998. Changes in bacterial populations in the colon of pigs fed different sources of dietary fibre, and the development of swine dysentery after experimental infection. *J. Appl. Microbiol.* 85:574–582.

Eckburg, P. B., E. M. Bik, C. N. Bernstein, E. Purdom, L. Dethlefsen, M. Sargent, S. R. Gill, K. E. Nelson, and D. A. Relman. 2005. Diversity of the human intestinal microbial flora. *Science* 308:1635–1638.

Edens, F. W., C. R. Parkhurst, I. A. Casas, and W. J. Dobrogosz. 1997. Principles of ex ovo competitive exclusion and in ovo administration of *Lactobacillus reuteri*. *Poult. Sci.* 76:179–196.

Ewaschuk, J. B., J. M. Naylor, M. Chirino-Trejo, and G. A. Zello. 2004. *Lactobacillus rhamnosus* strain GG is a potential probiotic for calves. *Can. J. Vet. Res.* 68:249–253.

Ewing, W. N., and D. J. A. Cole. 1994. *The Living Gut*. Context, Dungannon, Ireland.

Faleiro, M. L., M. G. Miguel, F. Ladeiro, F. Venancio, R. Tavares, J. C. Brito, A. C. Figueiredo, J. G. Barroso, and L. G. Pedro. 2003. Antimicrobial activity of essential oils isolated from Portuguese endemic species of Thymus. *Lett. Appl. Microbiol.* 36:35–40.

Fitzpatrick, L. R., K. L. Hertzog, A. L. Quatse, W. A. Koltun, J. S. Small, and K. Vrana. 2007. Effects of the probiotic formulation VSL#3 on colitis in weanling rats. *J. Pediatr. Gastroenterol. Nutr.* 44:561–570.

Fitzsimons, N. A., A. D. L. Akkermans, W. M. de Vos, and E. E. Vaughan. 2003. Bacterial gene expression detected in human faeces by reverse transcription-PCR. *J. Microbiol. Methods* 55:133–140.

Foligne, B., G. Zoumpopoulou, J. Dewulf, A. B. Younes, F. Chareyre, J.-C. Sirard, B. Pot, and C. Grangette. 2007. A key role of dendritic cells in probiotic functionality. *PLoS One* 3:e313.

Franklin, M. A., A. G. Mathew, J. R. Vickers, and R. A. Clift. 2002. Characterization of microbial populations and volatile fatty acid concentrations in the jejunum, ileum, and cecum of pigs weaned at 17 vs 24 days of age. *J. Anim. Sci.* 80:2904–2910.

Friedman, M., P. R. Henika, and R. E. Mandrell. 2002. Bactericidal activities of plant essential oils and some of their isolated constituents against *Campylobacter jejuni*, *Escherichia coli*, *Listeria monocytogenes*, and *Salmonella enterica*. *J. Food Prot.* 65:1545–1560.

Fuller, R. 1989. Probiotics in man and animals. *J. Appl. Bacteriol.* 66:365–378.

Gardiner, G. E., P. G. Casey, G. D. Casey, P. B. Lynch, P. G. Lawlor, C. Hill, G. F. Fitzgerald, C. Stanton, and R. P. Ross. 2004. Relative ability of orally administered *Lactobacillus murinus* to predominate and persist in the porcine gastrointestinal tract. *Appl. Environ. Microbiol.* 70:1895–1906.

Gaskins, H. R. 2001. Intestinal bacteria and their influence on swine growth, p. 585–608. *In* A. J. Lewis and L. L. Southern (ed.), *Swine Nutrition*. CRC Press, Boca Raton, FL.

Geary, T. M., P. H. Brooks, J. D. Beal, and A. Campbell. 1999. Effect on weaner pig performance and diet microbiology of feeding a liquid diet acidified to pH 4 with either lactic acid or through fermentation with Pediococcus acidilactici. *J. Sci. Food Agric.* 79:633–640.

Geier, M. S., R. N. Butler, P. M. Giffard, and G. S. Howarth. 2007. *Lactobacillus fermentum* BR11, a potential new probiotic, alleviates symptoms of colitis induced by dextran sulfate sodium (DSS) in rats. *Int. J. Food Microbiol.* 114:267.

Geoffroy, M.-C., C. Guyard, B. Quatannens, S. Pavan, M. Lange, and A. Mercenier. 2000. Use of green fluorescent protein to tag lactic acid bacterium strains under development as live vaccine vectors. *Appl. Environ. Microbiol.* 66:383–391.

Gibson, G. R., and M. B. Roberfroid. 1995. Dietary manipulation of the human colonic microbiota: introducing the concept of prebiotics. *J. Nutr.* 125:1401–1412.

Gil de los Santos, J. R., O. B. Storch, and C. Gil-Turnes. 2005. *Bacillus cereus* var. toyoii and *Saccharomyces boulardii* increased feed efficiency in broilers infected with *Salmonella enteritidis*. *Br. Poult. Sci.* 46:494–497.

Gill, S. R., M. Pop, R. T. DeBoy, P. B. Eckburg, P. J. Turnbaugh, B. S. Samuel, J. I. Gordon, D. A. Relman, C. M. Fraser-Liggett, and K. E. Nelson. 2006. Metagenomic analysis of the human distal gut microbiome. *Science* 312:1355–1359.

Goebel, S., W. Vahjen, A. Jadamus, and O. Simon. 2000. PCR assay for detection of porcine pathogenic *Escherichia coli* virulence factors in the gastrointestinal tract of piglets fed a spore forming probiotic. *Proc. Soc. Nutr. Physiol.* 9:64.

Grangette, C., S. Nutten, E. Palumbo, S. Morath, C. Hermann, J. Dewulf, B. Pot, T. Hartung, P. Hols, and A. Mercenier. 2005. Enhanced antiinflammatory capacity of a *Lactobacillus plantarum* mutant synthesizing modified teichoic acids. *Proc. Natl. Acad. Sci. USA* 102:10321–10326.

Guarner, F., and J. R. Malagelada. 2003. Gut flora in health and disease. *Lancet* 361:512–519.

Hooper, L. V., and J. I. Gordon. 2001. Commensal host-bacterial relationships in the gut. *Science* 292:1115–1118.

Hopwood, D. E., and D. J. Hampson. 2003. Interactions between the intestinal microflora, diet and diarrhoea, and their influences on the piglet health in the immediate post-weaning period, p. 199–219. *In* J. R. Pluske, J. L. Dividich, and M. W. A. Verstegen (ed.), *Weaning the Pig.* Wageningen Academic Publishers, Wageningen, The Netherlands.

Houdijk, J. G. M., M. W. Bosch, M. W. A. Verstegen, and E. J. Berenpas. 1998. Effect of dietary oligosaccharides on the growth performance and fecal characteristics of young growing pigs. *Anim. Feed Sci. Technol.* 71:35–48.

Huber, J. T. 1997. Probiotics in cattle, p. 162–180. *In* R. Fuller (ed.), *Probiotics 2—Applications and Practical Aspects.* Chapman & Hall, London, United Kingdom.

Hudault, S., J. Guignot, and A. L. Servin. 2001. *Escherichia coli* strains colonising the gastrointestinal tract protect germ-free mice against *Salmonella typhimurium* infection. *Gut* 49:47–55.

Isik, M., F. Ekumler, N. Özen, and M. Z. Firat. 2004. Effects of using probiotics on the growth performance and health of dairy calves. *Türk Veterinerlik ve Hayvancilik Dergisi* 28:63–69.

Isolauri, E., P. V. Kirjavainen, and S. Salminen. 2002. Probiotics: a role in the treatment of intestinal infection and inflammation? *Gut* 50:54–59.

Jadamus, A., W. Vahjen, K. Schaefer, and O. Simon. 2002. Influence of the probiotic strain *Bacillus cereus* var. *toyoi* on the development of enterobacterial growth and on selected parameters of bacterial metabolism in digesta samples of piglets. *J. Anim. Physiol. Anim. Nutr.* 86:42–54.

Jensen, B., and H. Jorgensen. 1994. Effect of dietary fiber on microbial activity and microbial gas production in various regions of the gastrointestinal tract of pigs. *Appl. Environ. Microbiol.* 60:1897–1904.

Jensen, B. B. 1998. The impact of feed additives on the microbial ecology of the gut in young pigs. *J. Anim. Feed Sci.* 7:45–64.

Jensen, B. B., O. Hojberg, L. L. Mikkelsen, M. S. Hedemann, and N. Canibe. 2003. Enhancing intestinal function to treat and prevent intestinal disease, p. 103–121. *Proceedings of the 9th International Symposium on Digestible Physiology in Pigs.* University of Alberta, Banff, Alberta, Canada.

Kelly, D., J. I. Campbell, T. P. King, G. Grant, E. A. Jansson, A. G. Coutts, S. Pettersson, and S. Conway. 2004. Commensal anaerobic gut bacteria attenuate inflammation by regulating nuclear-cytoplasmic shuttling of PPAR-gamma and RelA. *Nat. Immunol.* 5:104–112.

Kmet, V., H. J. Flint, and R. J. Wallace. 1993. Probiotics and manipulation of rumen development and function. *Arch. Anim. Nutr.* 44:1–10.

Konstantinov, S. R., A. Awati, H. Smidt, B. A. Williams, A. D. L. Akkermans, and W. M. de Vos. 2004a. Specific response of a novel and abundant *Lactobacillus amylovorus*-like phylotype to dietary prebiotics in the guts of weaning piglets. *Appl. Environ. Microbiol.* 70:3821–3830.

Konstantinov, S. R., A. A. Awati, B. A. Williams, B. G. Miller, P. Johns, C. R. Stokes, A. D. L. Akkermans, H. Smidt, and W. M. de Vos. 2006. Postnatal development of the porcine microbiota composition and activities. *Environ. Microbiol.* 8:1191–1199.

Konstantinov, S. R., C. F. Favier, W. Y. Zhu, B. A. Williams, J. Kluss, W.-B. Souffrant, W. M. de Vos, A. D. L. Akkermans, and H. Smidt. 2004b. Microbial diversity study of the porcine GI tract during the weaning transition. *Anim. Res.* 53:317–324.

Konstantinov, S. R., H. Smidt, and A. D. L. Akkermans. 2005a. Ecology and activity of clostridia in the intestine of mammals, p. 787–796. *In* P. Durre (ed.), *Handbook of Clostridia.* CRC Press, Boca Raton, FL.

Konstantinov, S. R., H. Smidt, and W. M. de Vos. 2005b. Representational difference analysis and real-time PCR for strain-specific quantification of *Lactobacillus sobrius* sp. nov. *Appl. Environ. Microbiol.* 71:7578–7581.

Konstantinov, S. R., W.-Y. Zhu, B. A. Williams, S. Tamminga, W. M. de Vos, and A. D. L. Akkermans. 2003. Effect of fermentable carbohydrates on piglet faecal bacterial communities as revealed by denaturing gradient gel electrophoresis analysis of 16S ribosomal DNA. *FEMS Microbiol. Ecol.* 43:225–235.

Kyriakis, S. C., V. K. Tsiloyiannis, J. Vlemmas, K. Sarris, A. C. Tsinas, C. Alexopoulus, and L. Jansegers. 1999. The effect of probiotic LSP 122 on the control of post-weaning diarrhoea syndrome of piglets. *Res. Vet. Sci.* 67:223–228.

Lara-Flores, M., M. A. Olvera-Novoa, B. E. Guzman-Mendez, and W. Lopez-Madrid. 2003. Use of the bacteria *Streptococcus faecium* and *Lactobacillus acidophilus*, and the yeast *Saccharomyces cerevisiae* as growth promoters in Nile tilapia (*Oreochromis niloticus*). *Aquaculture* 216:193.

La Ragione, R. M., A. Narbad, M. J. Gasson, and M. J. Woodward. 2004. *In vivo* characterization of *Lactobacillus johnsonii* FI9785 for use as a defined competitive exclusion agent against bacterial pathogens in poultry. *Lett. Appl. Microbiol.* 38:197–205.

La Ragione, R. M., and M. J. Woodward. 2003. Competitive exclusion by *Bacillus subtilis* spores of *Salmonella enterica* serotype enteritidis and *Clostridium perfringens* in young chickens. *Vet. Microbiol.* 17:245–256.

Lema, M., L. Williams, and D. R. Rao. 2001. Reduction of fecal shedding of enterohemorrhagic *Escherichia coli* O157: H7 in lambs by feeding microbial feed supplement. *Small Rumin. Res.* 39:31.

Leser, T. D., J. Z. Amenuvor, T. K. Jensen, R. H. Lindecrona, M. Boye, and K. Moller. 2002. Culture-independent analysis of gut bacteria: the pig gastrointestinal tract microbiota revisited. *Appl. Environ. Microbiol.* 68:673–690.

Leser, T. D., R. H. Vindecrona, T. K. Jensen, B. B. Jensen, and K. Moller. 2000. Changes in bacterial community structure in the colon of pigs fed different experimental diets and after infection with *Brachyspira hyodysenteriae*. *Appl. Environ. Microbiol.* 66:3290–3296.

Lievin-Le Moal, V., R. Amsellem, A. L. Servin, and M.-H. Coconnier. 2002. *Lactobacillus acidophilus* (strain LB) from the resident adult human gastrointestinal microflora exerts activity against brush border damage promoted by a diarrhoeagenic *Escherichia coli* in human enterocyte-like cells. *Gut* 50:803–811.

Lindecrona, R. H., T. J. Jensen, B. B. Jensen, T. Leser, M. Jiufeng, and K. Moller. 2003. The influence of diet on the development of swine dysentery upon experimental infection. *Anim. Sci.* 76:81–87.

Line, J. E., J. S. Bailey, N. A. Cox, N. J. Stern, and T. Tompkins. 1998. Effect of yeast-supplemented feed on *Salmonella* and *Campylobacter* populations in broilers. *Poult. Sci.* 77:405–410.

Lis-Balchin, M. 2003. Feed additives as alternatives to antibiotic growth promotors: botanicals, p. 333–352. *In* R. O. Ball (ed.), *Proceedings of the 9th International Symposium on Digestive Physiology in Pigs.* University of Alberta, Banff, Alberta, Canada.

Mackie, R. I., A. Sghir, and H. R. Gaskins. 1999. Developmental microbial ecology of the neonatal gastrointestinal tract. *Am. J. Clin. Nutr.* 69(S):1035S–1045S.

Madsen, K. L., A. Cornish, P. Soper, C. McKaigney, H. Jijon, C. Yachimec, J. Doyle, L. Jewell, and C. De Simone. 2001. Probiotic bacteria enhance murine and human intestinal epithelial barrier function. *Gastroenterology* 121:580–591.

Manichanh, C., L. Rigottier-Gois, E. Bonnaud, K. Gloux, E. Pelletier, L. Frangeul, R. Nalin, C. Jarrin, P. Chardon, P. Marteau, J. Roca, and J. Dore. 2006. Reduced diversity of faecal microbiota in Crohn's disease revealed by a metagenomic approach. *Gut* 55:205–211.

Manner, K., and A. Spieler. 1997. Probiotics in piglets—an alternative to traditional growth promoters. *Microecol. Ther.* 26:243–256.

Marcy, Y., C. Ouverney, E. M. Bik, T. Losekann, N. Ivanova, H. G. Martin, E. Szeto, D. Platt, P. Hugenholtz, D. A. Relman, and S. R. Quake. 2007. Dissecting biological "dark matter" with single-cell genetic analysis of rare and uncultivated TM7 microbes from the human mouth. *Proc. Natl. Acad. Sci. USA* 104:11889–11894.

Marshall-Jones, Z. V., M. L. Baillon, J. M. Croft, and R. F. Butterwick. 2006. Effects of *Lactobacillus acidophilus* DSM13241 as a probiotic in healthy adult cats. *Am. J. Vet. Res.* 67:1005–1012.

McCracken, B. A., M. E. Spurlock, M. A. Roos, F. A. Zuckermann, and H. R. Gaskins. 1999. Weaning anorexia may contribute to local inflammation in the piglet small intestine. *J. Nutr.* 129:613–619.

McDonald, D. E., D. W. Pethick, B. P. Mullan, and D. J. Hampson. 2001. Increasing viscosity of the intestinal contents alters small intestinal structure and intestinal growth, and stimulates proliferation of enterotoxigenic *Escherichia coli* in newly-weaned pigs. *Br. J. Nutr.* 86:487–498.

Mitchell, I., and R. Kenworth. 1976. Investigations on a metabolite from *Lactobacillus bulgaricus* which neutralizes the effect of enterotoxin from *Escherichia coli* pathogenic for pigs. *J. Appl. Bacteriol.* 41:163–174.

Mohamadzadeh, M., S. Olson, W. V. Kalina, G. Ruthel, G. L. Demmin, K. L. Warfield, S. Bavari, and T. R. Klaenhammer. 2005. Lactobacilli activate human dendritic cells that skew T cells toward T helper 1 polarization. *Proc. Natl. Acad. Sci. USA* 102:2880–2885.

Montalto, M., N. Maggiano, R. Ricci, V. Curigliano, L. Santoro, F. Di Nicuolo, F. M. Vecchio, A. Gasbarrini, and G. Gasbarrini. 2004. *Lactobacillus acidophilus* protects tight junctions from aspirin damage in HT-29 cells. *Digestion* 69:225–228.

Muhl, A., and F. Liebert. 2007. Growth and parameters of microflora in intestinal and faecal samples of piglets due to application of a phytogenic feed additive. *J. Anim. Physiol. Anim. Nutr.* 91:411–418.

Neish, A. S., A. T. Gewirtz, H. Zeng, A. N. Young, M. E. Hobert, V. Karmali, A. S. Rao, and J. L. Madara. 2000. Prokaryotic regulation of epithelial responses by inhibition of IkB-alfa ubiquitination. *Science* 289:1560–1563.

Nikoskelainen, S., A. C. Ouwehand, G. Bylund, S. Salminen, and E.-M. Lilius. 2003. Immune enhancement in rainbow trout (*Oncorhynchus mykiss*) by potential probiotic bacteria (*Lactobacillus rhamnosus*). *Fish Shellfish Immunol.* 15:443.

Nikoskelainen, S., S. Salminen, G. Bylund, and A. C. Ouwehand. 2001. Characterization of the properties of human- and dairy-derived probiotics for prevention of infectious diseases in fish. *Appl. Environ. Microbiol.* 67:2430–2435.

Nurmi, E., and M. Rantala. 1973. New aspects of *Salmonella* infection in broiler production. *Nature* 241:210–211.

Ohashi, Y., M. Tokunaga, and K. Ushida. 2004. The effect of *Lactobacillus casei* strain Shirota on the cecal fermentation pattern depends on the individual cecal microflora in pigs. *J. Nutr. Sci. Vitaminol.* (Tokyo) 50:399–403.

Ohya, T., T. Marubashi, and H. Ito. 2000. Significance of fecal volatile fatty acids in shedding of *Escherichia coli* O157 from calves: experimental infection and preliminary use of a probiotic product. *J. Vet. Med. Sci.* 62:1151–1155.

Ohya, T., M. Akiba, and H. Ito. 2001. Use of a trial probiotic product in calves experimentally infected with *Escherichia coli* O157. *Jpn. Agric. Res. Q.* 35:189–194.

Olsen, G., D. Lane, S. Giovannoni, N. Pace, and D. Stahl. 1986. Microbial ecology and evolution: a ribosomal RNA approach. *Annu. Rev. Microbiol.* 40:337–365.

Otte, J.-M., and D. K. Podolsky. 2004. Functional modulation of enterocytes by gram-positive and gram-negative microorganisms. *Am. J. Physiol. Gastrointest. Liver Physiol.* 286:G613–G626.

Panigrahi, A., V. Kiron, T. Kobayashi, J. Puangkaew, S. Satoh, and H. Sugita. 2004. Immune responses in rainbow trout *Oncorhynchus mykiss* induced by a potential probiotic bacteria *Lactobacillus rhamnosus* JCM 1136. *Vet. Immunol. Immunopathol.* 102:379–388.

Pie, S., J. P. Lalles, F. Blazy, J. Laffitte, B. Seve, and I. P. Oswald. 2004. Weaning is associated with an upregulation of expression of inflammatory cytokines in the intestine of piglets. *J. Nutr.* **134**:641–647.

Pluske, J. R., Z. Durmic, D. W. Pethick, B. P. Mullan, and D. J. Hampson. 1998. Confirmation of the role of rapidly fermentable carbohydrates in the expression of swine dysentery in pigs after experimental infection. *J. Nutr.* **128**:1737–1744.

Prescott, L. M., J. P. Harley, and D. A. Klein (ed.). 2002. *Microbiology*, 5 ed. McGraw-Hill, New York, NY.

Pryde, S. E., A. J. Richardson, C. S. Stewart, and H. J. Flint. 1999. Molecular analysis of the microbial diversity present in the colonic wall, colonic lumen, and cecal lumen of a pig. *Appl. Environ. Microbiol.* **65**:5372–5377.

Rastall, R. A., and G. R. Gibson. 2002. Prebiotic oligosaccharides: evaluation of biological activities and potential future develpments, p. 107–148. *In* G. W. Tannock (ed.), *Probiotics and Prebiotics: Where Are We Going?* Caiser Academic Press, Wymondham, United Kingdom.

Ratcliffe, B., C. B. Cole, R. Fuller, and M. J. Newport. 1985. The effect of yogurt on performance and the gut microflora of baby pigs. *Proc. Nutr. Soc.* **44**:A88.

Ratcliffe, B., C. B. Cole, R. Fuller, and M. J. Newport. 1986. The effect of yoghurt and milk fermented with a porcine strain of *Lactobacillus reuteri* on the performance and gastrointestinal flora of pigs weaned at two days of age. *Food Microbiol.* **3**:203–211.

Redmond, H. E., and R. W. Moore. 1965. Biologic effect of introducing *Lactobacillus acidophilus* into a large swine herd experiencing enteritidis. *Southw. Vet.* **18**:287–288.

Resta-Lenert, S., and K. E. Barrett. 2006. Probiotics and commensals reverse TNF-alfa- and IFN-gamma-induced dysfunction in human intestinal epithelial cells. *Gastroenterology* **130**:731.

Roberfroid, M., and J. Slavin. 2000. Nondigestible oligosaccharides. *Crit. Rev. Food Sci. Nutr.* **40**:461–480.

Roberfroid, M. B. 1998. Prebiotics and synbiotics: concepts and nutritional properties. *Br. J. Nutr.* **80**:S197–S202.

Rokbi, B., D. Seguin, B. Guy, V. Mazarin, E. Vidor, F. Mion, M. Cadoz, and M. J. Quentin-Millet. 2001. Assessment of *Helicobacter pylori* gene expression within mouse and human gastric mucosae by real-time reverse transcriptase PCR. *Infect. Immun.* **69**:4759–4766.

Roselli, M., A. Finamore, M. S. Britti, S. R. Konstantinov, H. Smidt, W. M. de Vos, and E. Mengheri. 2007. The novel porcine *Lactobacillus sobrius* strain protects intestinal cells from enterotoxigenic *Escherichia coli* K88 infection and prevents membrane barrier damage. *J. Nutr.* **137**:2709–2716.

Rossi, E. A., R. C. Vendramini, I. Z. Carlos, I. S. Ueiji, M. M. Squinzari, S. I. Silva Junior, and G. F. Valdez. 2000. Effects of a novel fermented soy product on the serum lipids of hypercholesterolemic rabbits. *Arq. Bras. Cardiol.* **74**:209–216.

Russell, P. J., T. M. Geary, P. H. Brooks, and A. Campbell. 1996. Performance, water use and effluent output of weaner pigs fed ad libitum with either dry pellets or liquid feed and the role of microbial activity in the liquid feed. *J. Sci. Food Agric.* **72**:8–16.

Rycroft, C. E., M. R. Jones, G. R. Gibson, and R. A. Rastall. 2001. A comparative in vitro evaluation of the fermentation properties of prebiotic oligosaccharides. *J. Appl. Microbiol.* **91**:878–887.

Samli, H. E., N. Senkoylu, F. Koc, M. Kanter, and A. Agma. 2007. Effects of *Enterococcus faecium* and dried whey on broiler performance, gut histomorphology and intestinal microbiota. *Arch. Anim. Nutr.* **61**:42–49.

Sarker, S. A., S. Sultana, G. J. Fuchs, N. H. Alam, T. Azim, H. Brussow, and L. Hammarstrom. 2005. *Lactobacillus paracasei* strain ST11 has no effect on rotavirus but ameliorates the outcome of nonrotavirus diarrhea in children from Bangladesh. *Pediatrics* **116**:221–228.

Sghir, A., D. Antonopoulos, and R. I. Mackie. 1998. Design and evaluation of a *Lactobacillus* group-specific ribosomal RNA-targeted hybridisation probe and its application to the study of intestinal microecology in pigs. *Syst. Appl. Microbiol.* **21**:291–296.

Shu, Q., F. Qu, and H. S. Gill. 2001. Probiotic treatment using *Bifidobacterium lactis* HN019 reduces weaning diarrhea associated with rotavirus and *Escherichia coli* infection in a piglet model. *J. Pediatr. Gastroenterol. Nutr.* **33**:171–177.

Simon, O., A. Jadamus, and W. Vahjen. 2001. Probiotic feed additives—effectiveness and expected modes of action. *J. Anim. Feed Sci.* **10**:51–67.

Simon, O., W. Vahjen, and L. Scharek. 2003. Micro-organisms as feed additives—probiotics, p. 295–318. *In* R. O. Ball (ed.), *Proceedings of 9th International symposium on Digestive Physiology in Pigs*. University of Alberta, Banff, Alberta, Canada.

Simpson, J. M., V. J. McCracken, H. R. Gaskins, and R. I. Mackie. 2000. Denaturing gradient gel electrophoresis analysis of 16S ribosomal DNA amplicons to monitor changes in fecal bacterial populations of weaning pigs after introduction of *Lactobacillus reuteri* strain MM53. *Appl. Environ. Microbiol.* **66**:4705–4714.

Smits, H. H., A. Engering, D. van der Kleij, E. C. de Jong, K. Schipper, T. M. M. van Capel, B. A. J. Zaat, M. Yazdanbakhsh, E. A. Wierenga, Y. van Kooyk, and M. L. Kapsenberg. 2005. Selective probiotic bacteria induce IL-10-producing regulatory T cells in vitro by modulating dendritic cell function through dendritic cell-specific intercellular adhesion molecule 3-grabbing noninteprin. *J. Allergy. Clin. Immunol.* **115**:1260–1267.

Sonnenburg, J. L., C. T. Chen, and J. I. Gordon. 2006. Genomic and metabolic studies of the impact of probiotics on a model gut symbiont and host. *PLoS Biol.* **4**:e413.

Stewart, C. S. 1997. Microorganisms in hindgut fermentors, p. 142-186. *In* R. I. Mackie, B. A. White and R. E. Isaacson (ed.), *Gastrointestinal Microbiology*. Chapman and Hall, New York, NY.

Stokes, C. R., M. Bailey, K. Haverson, C. Harris, P. Johes, C. Inman, S. Pie, I. P. Oswald, B. A. Williams, A. D. L. Akkermans, E. Sowa, H.-J. Rothoetter, and B. G. Miller. 2004. Postnatal development of intestinal immune system in piglets: implications for the process of weaning. *Anim. Res.* **53**:1–10.

Strompfovà, V., A. Laukovà, and A. C. Ouwehand. 2004. *Lactobacilli* and *enterococci* - potential probiotics for dogs. *Folia Microbiol.* **49**:203–208.

Suau, A., R. Bonnet, M. Sutren, J.-J. Godon, G. R. Gibson, M. D. Collins, and J. Dore. 1999. Direct analysis of genes encoding 16S rRNA from complex communities reveals many novel molecular species within the human gut. *Appl. Environ. Microbiol.* 65:4799–4807.

Szajewska, H., A. Skorka, M. Ruszczynski, and D. Gieruszczak-Bialek. 2007. Meta-analysis: *Lactobacillus* GG for treating acute diarrhoea in children. *Aliment. Pharmacol. Ther.* 25:871–881.

Tannock, G. W. 1990. The microecology of lactobacilli inhabiting the gastrointestinal tract. *Adv. Microb. Ecol.* 11:147–171.

Tannock, G. W. 2004. A special fondness for lactobacilli. *Appl. Environ. Microbiol.* 70:3189–3194.

Ten Bruggencate, S. J. M., I. M. J. Bovee-Oudenhoven, M. L. G. Lettink-Wissink, M. B. Katan, and R. Van der Meer. 2004. Dietary fructo-oligosaccharides and inulin decrease resistance of rats to salmonella: protective role of calcium. *Gut* 53:530–535.

Tierney, J., H. Gowing, D. Van Sinderen, S. Flynn, L. Stanley, N. McHardy, S. Hallahan, and G. Mulcahy. 2004. In vitro inhibition of *Eimeria tenella* invasion by indigenous chicken *Lactobacillus* species. *Vet. Parasitol.* 122:171–182.

Timmerman, H. M., L. Mulder, H. Everts, D. C. van Espen, E. van der Wal, G. Klaassen, S. M. G. Rouwers, R. Hartemink, F. M. Rombouts, and A. C. Beynen. 2005. Health and growth of veal calves fed milk replacers with or without probiotics. *J. Dairy Sci.* 88:2154–2165.

Timmerman, H. M., A. Veldman, E. van den Elsen, F. M. Rombouts, and A. C. Beynen. 2006. Mortality and growth performance of broilers given drinking water supplemented with chicken-specific probiotics. *Poult. Sci.* 85:1383–1388.

Umberger, S. H., D. R. Notter, K. E. Webb, and W. H. McClure. 1989. Evaluation of *Lactobacillus* inoculant on feedlot lamb performance. *Anim. Sci. Res. Rep.* 8:40–45.

Underdahl, N. R., A. Torres-Medina, and A. R. Doster. 1982. Effect of *Streptococcus faecium* C-68 in control of *Escherichia coli* induced diarrhea in gnotobiotic pigs. *Am. J. Vet. Res.* 43:2227–2232.

Van den Broeck, W., E. Cox, and B. M. Goddeeris. 1999. Receptor-dependent immune responses in pigs after oral immunization with F4 fimbriae. *Infect. Immun.* 67:520–526.

Van der Waaij, D. 1987. Colonization resistance of the digestive tract: mechanism and clinical consequences. *Nahrung* 31:507–517.

Van der Waaij, D. 1989. The ecology of the human intestine and its consequences for the overgrowth of pathogens such as *Clostridium difficile*. *Annu. Rev. Microbiol.* 43:69–87.

van Winsen, R. L., L. Lipman, S. Biesterveld, B. A. P. Urlings, J. M. A. Snijders, and F. van Knapen. 2000. Mechanism of *Salmonella* reduction in fermented pig feed. *J. Sci. Food Agric.* 81:342–346.

van Winsen, R. L., B. A. P. Urlings, L. J. A. Lipman, J. M. A. Snijders, D. Keuzenkamp, J. H. M. Verheijden, and F. van Knapen. 2001. Effect of fermented feed on the microbial population of the gastrointestinal tracts of pigs. *Appl. Environ. Microbiol.* 67:3071–3076.

Verschuere, L., G. Rombaut, P. Sorgeloos, and W. Verstraete. 2000. Probiotic bacteria as biological control agents in aquaculture. *Microbiol. Mol. Biol. Rev.* 64:655–671.

Watkins, B. A., and B. F. Miller. 1983. Competitive gut exclusion of avian pathogens by *Lactobacillus acidophilus*. *Poult. Sci.* 62:1772–1779.

Weese, J. S., M. E. Anderson, A. Lowe, and G. J. Monteith. 2003. Preliminary investigation of the probiotic potential of *Lactobacillus rhamnosus* strain GG in horses: fecal recovery following oral administration and safety. *Can. Vet. J.* 44:299–302.

Williams, B. A., M. W. A. Verstegen, and S. Tamminga. 2001. Fermentation in the monogastric large intestine: its relation to animal health. *Nutr. Res. Rev.* 14:207–227.

Woese, C. R. 1987. Bacterial evolution. *Microbiol. Rev.* 51:221–271.

Wostmann, B. S., C. Larkin, A. Moriarty, and E. Bruckner-Kardoss. 1983. Dietary intake, energy metabolism, and excretory losses of adult male germfree Wistar rats. *Lab. Anim. Sci.* 33:46–50.

Yoruk, M. A., M. Gul, A. Hayirli, and M. Macit. 2004. The effects of supplementation of humate and probiotic on egg production and quality parameters during the late laying period in hens. *Poult. Sci.* 83:84–88.

Younts-Dahl, S. M., M. L. Galyean, G. H. Loneragan, N. A. Elam, and M. M. Brashears. 2004. Dietary supplementation with *Lactobacillus*- and *Propionibacterium*-based direct-fed microbials and prevalence of *Escherichia coli* O157 in beef feedlot cattle and on hides at harvest. *J. Food Prot.* 67:889–893.

Younts-Dahl, S. M., G. D. Osborn, M. L. Galyean, J. D. Rivera, G. H. Loneragan, and M. M. Brashears. 2005. Reduction of *Escherichia coli* O157 in finishing beef cattle by various doses of *Lactobacillus acidophilus* in direct-fed microbials. *J. Food Prot.* 68:6–10.

Zani, J. L., F. Weykamp da Cruz, A. Freitas dos Santos, and C. Gil-Turnes. 1998. Effect of probiotic CenBiot on the control of diarrhoea and feed efficiency in pigs. *J. Appl. Microbiol.* 84:68–71.

Zhao, T., M. P. Doyle, B. G. Harmon, C. A. Brown, P. O. Mueller, and A. H. Parks. 1998. Reduction of carriage of enterohemorrhagic *Escherichia coli* O157:H7 in cattle by inoculation with probiotic bacteria. *J. Clin. Microbiol.* 36:641–647.

Zhu, W.-Y., B. A. Williams, S. R. Konstantinov, S. Tamminga, W. M. De Vos, and A. D. L. Akkermans. 2003. Analysis of 16S rDNA reveals bacterial shift during in vitro fermentation of fermentable carbohydrate using piglet faeces as inoculum. *Anaerobe* 9:175–180.

Zhu, X. Y., T. Zhong, Y. Pandya, and R. D. Joerger. 2002. 16S rRNA-based analysis of microbiota from the cecum of broiler chickens. *Appl. Environ. Microbiol.* 68:124–137.

Zoetendal, E. G., A. D. Akkermans, and W. M. de Vos. 1998. Temperature gradient gel electrophoresis analysis of 16S rRNA from human fecal samples reveals stable and host-specific communities of active bacteria. *Appl. Environ. Microbiol.* 64:3854–3859.

Therapeutic Microbiology: Probiotics and Related Strategies
Edited by J. Versalovic and M. Wilson
© 2008 ASM Press, Washington, DC

J. Scott Weese
Shayan Sharif
Alex Rodriguez-Palacios

Probiotics in Veterinary Medicine

26

Probiotic therapy is becoming increasingly popular in veterinary medicine, both for therapeutic uses and for growth promotion. The increase in interest in probiotic therapy is likely being driven by multiple factors. For food animals, measures to improve production and food safety are continually being evaluated and probiotic therapy is one of many possible approaches. Additionally, as there is increased scrutiny regarding the use of antimicrobial agents in food animals, evaluation of probiotics is a logical approach. In companion animals, the focus is typically on prevention or treatment of disease in individual animals. As society gains greater understanding and interest in alternative therapies and as concerns over emergence of antimicrobial resistance increase, the attraction of probiotic therapy is obvious. The diverse nature of the intestinal tract and intestinal microbiota in different animal species means that each individual animal species should be considered separately when evaluating probiotics, rather than dividing probiotics into human and veterinary categories.

PROBIOTICS IN FOOD-PRODUCING ANIMALS

The general objectives of probiotic therapy in food animals differ somewhat from those for humans and companion animals. Probiotics may be used in food animal species to prevent or treat disease, but this is typically focused on the herd, not individual animal, level. Other objectives include increasing growth rate, improving feed conversion, stimulating the immune system, and decreasing shedding of zoonotic pathogens. The potential for probiotics to be effective in these areas is particularly useful for food animals because of concerns regarding the use of antimicrobial agents, both therapeutically and as growth promoters.

Poultry

The two main areas of emphasis in poultry research include enteropathogen control and immune stimulation.

Probiotics for Control of Enteric Pathogens in Chickens

Nurmi and Rantala were the first to demonstrate that feeding the microbiota of adult chickens to young chicks

J. Scott Weese and Shayan Sharif, Dept. of Pathobiology, Ontario Veterinary College, University of Guelph, Guelph, Ontario, N1G 2W1, Canada.
Alex Rodriguez-Palacios, Dept. of Preventive Veterinary Medicine, Food Animal Health Research Program, Ohio Agricultural Research and Development Center, The Ohio State University, Wooster, OH 44691.

can protect them from colonization with *Salmonella* spp. (Nurmi and Rantala, 1973). The term "competitive exclusion" was subsequently coined by these authors. More recently, several studies have confirmed and extended the initial findings of Nurmi and Rantala by demonstrating the efficacy of probiotics to control other enteric infections in chickens, such as those caused by *Clostridium* (Hofacre et al., 1998), *Eimeria* (Dalloul et al., 2005), and *Campylobacter* spp. (Hakkinen and Schneitz, 1999). In general, probiotics may be classified into two broad categories: defined and undefined (Stavric and D'Aoust, 1993). Undefined probiotics refer to those products that are derived from the ceca and colons of adult animals and may contain several characterized or uncharacterized members of the microbiota. Therefore, the actual number of bacteria or the number of different genera or species in these mixtures is usually not known (Mead, 2000). In contrast, defined cultures contain characterized probiotic bacteria and are developed based on several criteria, including lack of pathogenicity, absence of plasmid-borne antimicrobial resistance genes, and the presence of bacteria belonging to the main commensal bacterial genera in the chicken gut (Klose et al., 2006; Mead, 2000). Consistent with other probiotics, the two most commonly represented genera in poultry probiotics are *Lactobacillus* spp. and *Bifidobacterium* spp. Although undefined probiotics may be more efficacious than defined probiotics, their use is restricted in some countries because of the potential risks associated with the presence of pathogenic or antimicrobial-resistant bacteria.

Probiotics are usually administered to poultry in drinking water or feed or are sometimes sprayed on newly hatched chicks in the hatchery. In some cases, treatment may involve a spray in the hatchery followed by administration of probiotics in drinking water upon arrival to the farm (Mead, 2000). Using various undefined probiotics, promising results have been obtained with respect to reduction of intestinal colonization with *Salmonella* and other enteric pathogens in the chicken. The first commercially available undefined probiotic was Broilact. This product was effective against cecal colonization by *Salmonella enterica* serovar Enteritidis and *S. enterica* Typhimurium (Cameron and Carter, 1992; Methner et al., 1997; Nuotio et al., 1992; Palmu and Camelin, 1997). Efficacy of Broilact against cecal colonization by *Campylobacter* has also been shown (Hakkinen and Schneitz, 1999). Mucosal Starter Culture (MSC), an undefined probiotic, has been tested in chickens. MSC significantly reduced cecal colonization by *Salmonella* (Bailey et al., 2000; Ferreira et al., 2003) and *Clostridium perfringens* (Craven et al., 1999). Aviguard, another undefined

probiotic product, was effective for the reduction of *Salmonella* in the chicken intestine and other organs (Ferreira et al., 2003; Nakamura et al., 2002). This product also significantly reduced mucosal lesions caused by *C. perfringens* in the chicken intestine (Hofacre et al., 1998). PREEMPT is a defined probiotic containing 29 different types of commensal bacteria of the broiler intestine that has been tested in commercial and experimental settings (Nisbet, 2002). Treatment of chickens with PREEMPT or its predecessor, CF3, reduced colonization of chickens with *S. enterica* serovar Enteritidis, *S. enterica* serovar Gallinarum, *Listeria monocytogenes*, and *Escherichia coli* O157:H7 (Nisbet, 2002). Another defined probiotic is Interbac, which contains *Lactobacillus acidophilus*, *Bifidobacterium bifidum*, and *Enterococcus faecalis*. In a study using oral gavage, administration of Interbac to day-old chicks was followed by *S. enterica* serovar Typhimurium challenge 24 h later. The cecal *Salmonella* load was significantly reduced in probiotic-treated chickens compared to untreated controls (Haghighi et al., 2008). The dose of probiotics was correlated with the reduction in *Salmonella* load. The high probiotic dose reduced the *Salmonella* load by 3 $\log_{10}$, and the low probiotic dose reduced the *Salmonella* load by 1.2 $\log_{10}$. Overall, probiotics offer a safe and effective approach for control of enteric pathogens in chickens.

Probiotics as Immune Enhancers in Chickens
In addition to competitive exclusion, other mechanisms including production of antibacterial substances, quorum sensing, and induction of innate and immune responses may be involved in mediation of probiotic effects (Lebeer et al., 2007; Revolledo et al., 2006; Santosa et al., 2006). The underlying immunomodulatory mechanisms of probiotic effects are emphasized in the discussion below.

Commensal bacteria in the intestine are in close proximity to, and in constant interaction with, the gut-associated lymphoid tissue (GALT). Microbial-host interactions may result in the modulation of mucosal and systemic immune responses (Macpherson et al., 2000). Dendritic cells (DCs) present in the gut lamina propria play a critical role in the uptake of microbial products and their presentation to other cells of the immune system (Rescigno et al., 2001). Lamina propria DCs have been demonstrated to project their dendrites through the tight junctions of epithelial cells to sample the microbial components of the gut lumen (Rescigno et al., 2001). Intestinal DCs express a repertoire of Toll-like receptors (TLRs) that are involved in the recognition of various microbial molecular patterns (Rakoff-Nahoum et al., 2004). Importantly, TLR2, TLR4, and TLR9 bind to microbial ligands, such as peptidoglycan, lipopolysaccharide, and unmethylated DNA, respectively (Rakoff-Nahoum et al., 2004). Interactions between these TLRs and their ligands may lead to maturation of DCs, marked by enhanced expression of CD80, CD86, CD40, and major histocompatibility complex class II (Janssens and Beyaert, 2003; Ratajczak et al., 2007). Lactobacilli, which constitute one of the major bacterial types of the gut microbiota, have been demonstrated to promote maturation of DCs and stimulate production of cytokines, including interleukin (IL)-10 and IL-12, by these cells (Christensen et al., 2002; Lammers et al., 2003; Ratajczak et al., 2007). IL-10 has a role in polarization and regulation of T-cell responses, while IL-12 promotes the differentiation of naïve T cells to T-helper (Th)1 cells. Thus, stimulation of intestinal DCs by microbial products may lead to activation and regulation of T cells (Ratajczak et al., 2007; Smits et al., 2005).

Cells of the avian GALT, which includes cecal tonsils, Peyer's patches, the bursa of Fabricius, and lymphoid aggregates alongside the digestive tract (Befus et al., 1980), may be involved in interactions with enteric microbes and microbial products. Although the molecular mechanisms of these interactions in the chicken are not well understood, it is known that GALT cells respond to antigens and may mount protective responses to pathogens (Lillehoj and Trout, 1996). The chicken GALT develops after hatching and reaches functional maturity by week 2 posthatching (Amit-Romach et al., 2004). The functional chicken GALT consists of T and B cells, macrophages, and natural killer (NK) cells (Lillehoj and Trout, 1996; Muir et al., 2000). Functional maturation of the chicken GALT may be correlated with the establishment of the intestinal microbiota. Since colonization of the small intestine in the chicken starts immediately after hatching and continues until week 2 posthatch, when the microbiota of the small intestine is established (Amit-Romach et al., 2004), it is possible that commensal bacteria of the microbiota have a role in the development of the chicken GALT.

Similar to the immune-system-enhancing activities of probiotics in humans and laboratory animal models, probiotics have also been shown to enhance adaptive immune and innate defenses in chickens. Administration of probiotics to chickens enhances systemic antibody responses to soluble and cellular antigens, including trinitrophenyl-keyhole limpet hemocyanin (TNP-KLH), KLH, and sheep red blood cells (Huang et al., 2004; Koenen et al., 2004). Koenen and coworkers (2004) reported that feeding chickens fermented liquid feed supplemented with various lactobacilli followed by immunization with TNP-KLH resulted in enhanced antibody responses to TNP. In another study, feeding

L. acidophilus and *Lactobacillus casei* to chickens enhanced serum immunoglobulin A (IgA), but not IgG, response to KLH (Huang et al., 2004). Administration of a defined probiotic prior to immunization with sheep red blood cells can result in enhanced antibody responses, primarily of the IgM isotype, to this antigen (Haghighi et al., 2005). However, no enhancement of mucosal antibody responses was observed in the latter study.

In a different context, the production of natural antibodies in chickens after treatment with probiotics has been evaluated. Commensal bacteria in the intestine may be involved in the development and diversification of the preimmune antibody repertoire in some species, such as rabbits. The evidence comes from germfree animals, which, in addition to limited antibody repertoire, have only a small number of plasma cells in their intestinal lamina propria (Jiang et al., 2004; Kroese et al., 1996; Rhee et al., 2004). Interestingly, lamina propria plasma cells produce T-cell-independent antibodies and possibly natural antibodies. Administration of a defined probiotic product on the day of hatching resulted in significantly increased serum antibodies reactive to tetanus toxoid, *C. perfringens* α-toxin, and bovine serum albumin in probiotic-treated chickens at 14 days of age compared to untreated controls (Haghighi et al., 2006). Moreover, there were more antibodies reactive to the same antigens in the intestinal contents of probiotic-treated compared to untreated control birds (Haghighi et al., 2006). Natural antibodies are produced by CD5[+] B-1 lymphocytes (Berland and Wortis, 2002). Therefore, it is possible that commensal bacteria in the intestine or their products activate the B-1 cells present in the intestinal lamina propria (Macpherson et al., 2000), leading to production of natural antibodies. Although the importance of natural antibodies in the protection of the host against pathogens has been shown, the significance of these antibodies in the chicken requires further investigations. Furthermore, the exact mechanisms of enhancement of immune responsiveness conferred by probiotics in these studies remain to be delineated.

Although probiotics may primarily act through competitive exclusion to reduce intestinal colonization by pathogens, immune-mediated mechanisms may also be involved in mediating resistance to gut colonization. Treatment of cells with commensal bacteria or their products results in modulation of cytokine production by host cells (Christensen et al., 2002; Lammers et al., 2003). Probiotics may reduce proinflammatory cytokine production by host cells after infection with pathogens. For example, in vitro treatment of an epithelial cell line with *Lactobacillus* or *Bifidobacterium* results in inhibition of *Salmonella*-induced IL-8 production (O'Hara et al., 2006; Silva et al., 2004). Also, in vivo treatment of mice with *Bifidobacterium longum* leads to reduced gamma interferon (IFN-γ) production following infection with *S. enterica* serovar Typhimurium (Silva et al., 2004). Recent studies have indicated that protection against *S. enterica* serovar Typhimurium was associated with reduced quantities of IFN-γ and IL-12 in cecal tonsils of probiotic-treated chickens (Haghighi et al., 2008). Importantly, *Salmonella* infection of chickens was associated with the production of proinflammatory and Th1 cytokines, such as IFN-γ (Beal et al., 2004; Withanage et al., 2004, 2005). Altogether, these findings raise the possibility that probiotics may exert their functions partly by modulating the cytokine milieu of host tissues.

Innate immune mechanisms are also affected by probiotics. A recent study examined the effects of probiotics on oxidative burst and degranulation in chicken heterophils and concluded that some probiotic bacteria had the capacity to increase both of these parameters in heterophils (Farnell et al., 2006). In laboratory animal models, it has been demonstrated that probiotics engage TLRs for mediation of their effects. Using TLR2 and TLR4 knockout mice, Grabig and coworkers concluded that *E. coli* strain Nissle 1917 mediates its control of experimental colitis via these two receptors (Grabig et al., 2006). In another study, administration of DNA, a ligand for TLR9, from probiotic bacteria resulted in amelioration of colitis (Rachmilewitz et al., 2004). Recently, the effects of various structural constituents of *L. acidophilus*, including DNA and peptidoglycan, on spatial and temporal gene expression of chicken lymphoid cells, have been studied, and DNA from probiotic bacteria activate STAT2 and STAT4 pathways leading to the induction of IFN-α, IFN-γ, and IL-18 genes (Brisbin et al., 2007). These findings suggest that probiotic bacteria and their structural constituents may regulate the adaptive immunity by induction of innate immunity in chickens.

Cattle
Probiotic therapy has received attention in cattle from many different perspectives, including increased production, decreased gastrointestinal disease, and decreased shedding of zoonotic enteropathogens.

Effects of Probiotics on Production
Production of offspring, milk, or meat involves a variety of factors, many of which are closely linked to the gastrointestinal tract. Accordingly, various aspects of production may be amenable to probiotic therapy. Improved ruminal digestion of dry matter is desirable in dairy cows during the peripartum transition period, when the risk of having a negative energy balance and

associated metabolic diseases is high. During this time, cows also experience a rapid increase of milk production, which enhances nutritional demands. Many early studies evaluated yeast supplements, particularly *Saccharomyces cerevisiae*, on milk production and milk composition (Dann et al., 2000; McGilliard and Stallings, 1998; Soder and Holden, 1999; Williams et al., 1991); however, studies using commercial yeast products have produced contradictory (Dann et al., 2000; Williams et al., 1991) or unpredictable (McGilliard and Stallings, 1998) results. The last study, a large clinical trial involving 3,417 milking cows and 46 dairy herds, showed that supplementation with a product containing *Bacillus subtilis*, *L. acidophilus*, *S. cerevisiae*, and *Aspergillus oryzae* improved the milk yield in 31 herds while decreasing it in the remaining 15 herds, highlighting the complex nature of production and health. There were minimal effects on milk composition.

Other studies involving *A. oryzae* have also produced contradictory results. A review of trials involving *A. oryzae* reported an increase in milk production in only 5 (35.7%) of 14 studies published before 1994 (Huber et al., 1994). In the review, Huber et al. pooled the raw mean values of milk production reported in 14 trials (representing 823 cows) and found that the average of means for supplemented cows was 1 liter of milk/day higher than the overall mean of the control cows. However, crude pooling of results has inherent limitations and conclusions must be interpreted with caution. Another study with high-yielding cows maintained in hot weather and involving *A. oryzae* reported no effect on productivity (Yu et al., 1997).

Dann et al. reported an increased dry matter intake (DMI) in the absence of changes in milk production with postparturient *S. cerevisiae* supplementation (Dann et al., 2000), while Williams et al. described an increase in both DMI and milk production (Williams et al., 1991). A more pronounced beneficial effect was documented for animals supplemented on high starch diets (McGilliard and Stallings, 1998). Administration of a combination of *S. cerevisiae* and two *Enterococcus faecium* strains had no effect on milk production parameters; however, there was a significant decrease in antimicrobial treatment of second-parturition cows in the treatment group, suggesting a health benefit in that particular subgroup (Oetzel et al., 2007). Interestingly, earlier studies using the same organisms reported an increase in milk production and DMI (Nocek et al., 2003) and increased milk production but lower milk fat percentage (Nocek and Kautz, 2006). In contrast, deleterious metabolic and microbiologic effects have been attributed to administration of an *E. faecium* strain in a digestibility study in feedlot cattle (Beauchemin et al., 2003). In that study, supplementation with *E. faecium* strain EF212 increased propionate production in the rumen but concurrently induced undesirable ruminal changes with reduction of lactate-utilizing protozoa and a moderate increase in the number of fecal coliforms. Interestingly, when the *E. faecium* was fed with *S. cerevisiae* most of the undesirable effects were no longer observed.

Lactobacilli have also been evaluated in bovine studies. An increase in milk production of 0.8 kg/day occurred in cows supplemented with *Lactobacillus buchneri* 40788-treated alfalfa silage (Kung et al., 2003). Later, Yasuda et al. tested a specific *L. casei* subsp. *casei* strain as a feed additive in combination with dextran (Yasuda et al., 2007). A positive effect on milk production and milk quality was reported, but the cause of this effect is unclear because dextran can have independent effects on the intestinal microbiota and digestibility parameters (Yasuda and Fukata, 2004).

Propionibacterium spp. have also been evaluated for their ability to modify the ruminal environment (Aleman et al., 2007; Ghorbani et al., 2002). Dietary supplementation with *Propionibacterium* strain P15 increased the number of ruminal protozoa with a concomitant increase of the ammonia concentration and a significant reduction in the number of amylolytic bacteria in supplemented steers (Ghorbani et al., 2002). Another study showed a transient change of parameters suggestive of improved energy balance in Holstein cows during the transition period (Francisco et al., 2002).

Production parameters have been evaluated in calves to a lesser degree, with mixed results. Administration of probiotic preparations has enhanced body weight gain in calves in some studies (Khuntia and Chaudhary, 2002; Timmerman et al., 2005), while no statistical differences have been observed in others (Higginbotham et al., 1994; Morrill et al., 1995; Peterson et al., 2007).

Results from the aforementioned studies are promising, but further research is warranted to verify the repeatability and external validity of the results. They also highlight the variability of results, even using similar or identical approaches, and the need to carefully define the study population for proper interpretation of results. Potentially complex management, production, and health factors must be considered when designing and evaluating studies.

Probiotics for Prevention of Diarrhea in Calves

Neonatal-calf diarrhea, most often caused by enterotoxigenic strains of *E. coli*, is an important cause of morbidity and mortality. A review of 42 clinical trials published between 1973 and 2003 assessing the effect of probiotics on calf diarrhea and weight gain reported that only 55% of the clinical trials documented a beneficial effect on incidence or severity of calf diarrhea (Rodriguez-Palacios et al., 2004). This finding is consistent with a previous review stating that only 40% of the studies published before 1995 showed positive results (Yoon and Stern, 1995). Of concern, 5% of trials evaluated in one review reported adverse effects of probiotic therapy (Rodriguez-Palacios et al., 2004). In the same review, 40% of the clinical trials used nonspecific and inadequate terms to refer to the "probiotic" inoculum tested, such as mixed lactic acid bacteria, lactobacilli, and gut-active microbes.

Two studies have evaluated *Lactobacillus rhamnosus* strain GG (LGG) (Ewaschuk et al., 2004, 2006). Survival of LGG following oral administration to neonatal calves was demonstrated (Ewaschuk et al., 2004); however, there was no effect of LGG supplementation on mortality or fecal dry matter in hospitalized diarrheic calves (Ewaschuk et al., 2006). The sample size may have limited the power of the latter study. Other studies have involved combinations of lactobacilli. Two commercial preparations containing six *Lactobacillus* spp. of bovine or human origin were shown to enhance the rate of growth and feed efficiency in veal calves, particularly during the first 2 weeks of the trials (Timmerman et al., 2005). The growth-promoting effects were still present at week 8 in some cases. The overall mortality rate and incidence of diarrhea were reduced, and animals with a lower general health score appeared to respond better to probiotics. A study of calves fed milk fermented with either mixed lactic acid bacteria, *L. acidophilus* 15, or *S. cerevisiae* NCDC49 reported a reduction in the incidence of diarrhea (Agarwal et al., 2002). A lack of effect on the incidence of cryptosporidiosis was reported in another study (Harp et al., 1996).

Control of *E. coli* O157 Shedding

E. coli O157:H7 is an important zoonotic pathogen, and cattle are considered the major reservoir (LeJeune and Wetzel, 2007). The prevalence of *E. coli* O157 carriage in cattle is variable and often high (up to 80%) (Khaitsa et al., 2003). *E. coli* O157 fecal shedding in finished beef cattle determines the risk of carcass contamination (Arthur et al., 2002), and preharvest strategies have been tested with variable results on modification of *E. coli* O157 shedding (Callaway et al., 2004). Some consider probiotic therapy to be a promising preharvest strategy (LeJeune and Wetzel, 2007), and numerous clinical or experimental trials have been conducted to investigate, with some evidence of success, the role of feeding probiotics to calves and feedlot steers for the control of fecal *E. coli* O157 shedding or hide contamination (Brashears et al., 2003; Ohya et al., 2000; Tkalcic et al., 2003; Zhao et al., 1998, 2003). Different microbiologic approaches have been pursued in order to minimize shedding of enterohemorrhagic *E. coli*. Modification of the shedding pattern of Shiga toxin-producing *E. coli* O157 and O111:NM, but not O26:H11, was achieved by treatment of calves with a mixture of three selected *E. coli* strains (Tkalcic et al., 2003). Similarly, administration of a mixture of 17 non-Shiga toxin-producing *E. coli* isolates and one *Proteus mirabilis* strain resulted in reduced fecal shedding and ruminal residence of *E. coli* O157 in a similar group of calves (Zhao et al., 1998). Another study described testing a selected group of *E. coli* strains in 12 calves based on their ability to produce colicins (Schamberger and Diez-Gonzalez, 2002). Oral administration of a mixture of eight colicinogenic *E. coli* strains (human, bovine, duck, and sheep origin) resulted in reduction of *E. coli* O157 counts and recovery from intestinal samples of experimentally infected calves (Schamberger et al., 2004). Other studies have been conducted to test lactobacilli or *Streptococcus bovis* of bovine origin. Administration of *S. bovis* LCB6 and *Lactobacillus gallinarum* LCB12, with an inhibitory effect on *E. coli* O157 in vitro, to 4-month-old calves resulted in complete inhibition of *E. coli* O157 fecal shedding (Ohya et al., 2000). However, the potential role of *S. bovis* in the pathogenesis of ruminal acidosis should be considered as a possible complication.

Perhaps the best-studied *Lactobacillus* species in cattle for prevention of *E. coli* carriage is *L. acidophilus*. Numerous studies have been published describing the selection of inhibitory lactobacilli for reduction of *E. coli* shedding (Brashears et al., 2003; Elam et al., 2003; Peterson et al., 2007; Stephens et al., 2007; Younts-Dahl et al., 2004, 2005) with encouraging results. For example, one study of 240 feedlot steers reported a reduction of *E. coli* O157 fecal shedding by 57%, with a corresponding reduction of hide contamination, but no effects on weight gain, grain consumption, and feed efficiency parameters (Younts-Dahl et al., 2004). Thus, it appears that probiotics offer a realistic, practical, and microbe-based approach for control of this important zoonotic pathogen.

Prevention of Ruminal Acidosis

Ruminal acidosis is a metabolic condition that arises from excessive fermentation of high-carbohydrate diets that can result in microbial imbalances and significant effects on production and health. Prevention and treatment goals include the reduction of lactic acid-producing bacteria, promotion of lactate-utilizing propionate-producing

organisms, and enhancement of bacterial and protozoal cellulolytic activity. Although there is currently no scientific evidence to recommend the use of probiotics for ruminal acidosis, some studies describing nutritional or fermentative effects in the rumen highlight the potential benefits of probiotic therapy. At a crude level, probiotic therapy has been used with anecdotal success for years in the form of ruminal transfaunation, i.e., the oral inoculation of fresh rumen fluid from a healthy cow to the rumen of a cow with poor rumen function. Whether this is an effect of bacteria, protozoa, or substrate is unclear, but the apparent clinical response indicates that administration of defined or undefined probiotics may be beneficial for cattle.

Yeast cultures may have potential applications in ruminal acidosis because of their ability to buffer deleterious effects of reduced ruminal pH. Administration of yeasts may provide benefits because these eukaryotic microbes utilize oxygen bound to newly masticated fibers, allowing anaerobic cellulolytic bacteria to proliferate and digest dietary fiber (Jouany, 2006). However, a study with sheep indicated that the ruminal inoculation of *S. cerevisiae* and *A. oryzae* reduced numbers of cellulolytic bacteria despite an increase in the total number of intestinal bacteria (Mathieu et al., 1996). A study of postpartum dairy cows that were fed a mixed commercial product containing *S. cerevisiae*, *E. faecium*, and *Lactobacillus plantarum* reported diurnal ruminal pH variability depending on the inoculum dose (Nocek et al., 2002). The lowest dose yielded the most optimal digestibility parameters and a more stable ruminal pH in cannulized cows. At the same time, the study concluded that high doses of the product (10^6 to 10^7 CFU/ml of rumen fluid) were detrimental to the ruminal environment. Overall, the potential for probiotic therapies in the context of ruminal acidosis remains to be fully evaluated.

Pigs

Probiotics are used in pigs for two main reasons: increased feed utilization efficiency with consequent weight gain and reduced frequency of diarrhea. Most of the focus is on postweaning diarrhea, which is a significant cause of morbidity, mortality, and production losses in commercial swine operations. Another potential use of probiotics is to decrease the numbers of potentially zoonotic bacteria in pigs, which could reduce the likelihood of contamination of meat during slaughter and processing.

Prevention of disease has been evaluated in experimental animal models, particularly with enterotoxigenic *E. coli*. Pretreatment of challenged piglets with *E. coli* Nissle 1917 protected all piglets from diarrhea in one study (Schroeder et al., 2006). However, the sample size was very small ($n = 4$) and, as with all experimental studies, extrapolation to actual meat or dairy production situations must be done cautiously. Better information is obtained from clinical trials in a standard production environment. Most studies have included prevention of postweaning diarrhea, which is mainly caused by enterotoxigenic *E. coli*. A variety of probiotic organisms have been evaluated, alone and in combination, with promising results. Administration of *Bacillus licheniformis* LSP 122 (10^7 spores/g of feed) resulted in reduced incidence and severity of diarrhea, reduced mortality, and improved weight gain when compared to untreated controls (Kyriakis et al., 1999). Similarly, administration of 10^9 CFU of *Bifidobacterium lactis* HN019 per day resulted in decreased severity of diarrhea, greater feed conversion, and lower concentrations of fecal rotavirus and *E. coli* shedding (Shu et al., 2001). Reduction in postweaning diarrhea was reported in a different study involving *Bacillus cereus* strain Toyoi (Taras et al., 2005). Administration of a combination of *B. licheniformis* and *B. subtilis* spores resulted in decreased overall morbidity and mortality from weaning until finishing, as well as decreased postweaning diarrhea and increased weight gain, feed conversion, and carcass quality (Alexopoulos et al., 2004). Increases in feed conversion and weight gain were reported with porcine-derived *Lactobacillus reuteri* BSA131 (Chang et al., 2001), and both *L. acidophilus* and *Bifidobacterium pseudolongum* had beneficial effects on weight gain in piglets during suckling and weaning periods (Abe et al., 1995). However, *B. cereus* Toyoi, *Lactobacillus* spp., or *E. faecium* did not have an effect on postweaning morbidity and mortality or *E. coli* shedding in one study (De Cupere et al., 1992). Neither *E. faecium* SF68 (Broom et al., 2006) nor *E. faecium* EK13 (Strompfova et al., 2006b) had any effect on feed intake, average daily gain, or feed conversion following postweaning administration.

Prevention of diarrhea in younger piglets has also been evaluated. Administration of a pig cecum-derived "competitive exclusion culture" reduced mortality and *E. coli* shedding in neonatal piglets (Genovese et al., 2000), although use of a crude culture meant that the organism or organisms responsible for the effect could not be identified. Clearer information can be obtained from studies using specific organisms or defined combinations of organisms. Piglets treated with *E. faecium* DSM 10663 (NCIMB 10415) from birth until weaning had a lower incidence of diarrhea, lower diarrhea scores, and greater weight gain (Zeyner and Boldt, 2006). Similar results have been obtained with *B. cereus* CIP5832 (Alexopoulos et al., 2001), *L. acidophilus* (Abe et al., 1995), and *B. pseudolongum* (Abe et al., 1995).

Production performance is closely related to animal health, yet the influences of probiotic therapy may extend beyond prevention and treatment of disease. Administration of *E. faecium* DSM during gestation and lactation can result in increased feed intake, litter size, and body weight (Bohmer et al., 2006). Similar improvements were reported with *B. cereus* Toyoi (Taras et al., 2005). Beneficial effects may reflect improved reproductive performance because of better feed intake and body condition rather than a direct influence on reproduction.

Because of the increasing scrutiny and restriction being placed on antimicrobial agents in feed, the use of probiotics as a replacement strategy for routine antimicrobial administration for prevention of disease or growth promotion has received attention. Results have been mixed, and no clear answer has emerged with respect to whether probiotics can replace antimicrobial agents in meat production environments. *B. subtilis* MA139 supplementation of feed resulted in increased feed conversion in piglets compared to the control group, with no difference compared to the antimicrobial-treated group (Guo et al., 2006). Similarly, pigs treated with *B. subtilis* and *B. licheniformis* during the postweaning period had the same mortality rate, daily gain, daily feed intake, and feed conversion as pigs treated with antimicrobials in feed during the same period (Kritas and Morrison, 2005). No differences were noted in the growth of pigs fed liquid feed fermented with *L. plantarum* strains versus dry feeding with antibiotics following experimental challenge with *E. coli* O149:K91:F4 (Amezcua, 2006). Evidence supports the use of probiotics as a valid replacement strategy for routine antimicrobial administration. However, the ability of probiotics to replace antimicrobial agents will likely depend on the management system, prominent pathogens, and geographic region. The responses to probiotics in herds with suboptimal overall health status or management may not be equally favorable.

An alternative approach is the use of fermented liquid feeds, in contrast to the studies involving probiotic supplementation of dry diets. Liquid feeds can be prepared using probiotic lactic acid bacteria and have the advantages of being cost-effective and facile delivery systems for relatively large numbers of organisms. Administration of fermented liquid feed has been associated with decreased enterobacterial levels in the gastrointestinal tracts of piglets and older pigs (van der Wolf et al., 2001; van Winsen et al., 2001). Decreased shedding of *Brachyspira hyodysenteriae* has also been reported (Hojberg et al., 2003). A reduced incidence of postweaning diarrhea has also been reported (van Winsen et al., 2002). However, it is unclear whether these protective effects occur as a result of probiotic organisms or large amounts of organic acids present in the feed, as the organic acids could have an independent effect on enterobacteria. As with probiotic supplementation of dry diets, not all studies with fermented liquid feeds have reported positive results. One recent study reported that pigs fed a traditional dry diet with antimicrobial agents had enhanced average daily weight gain compared to pigs fed fermented liquid diets and that fermented liquid diets had no beneficial effects on either experimental or natural enterotoxigenic *E. coli* infection in postweaning pigs (Amezcua, 2006). Interestingly, pigs fed a liquid diet with lactobacilli of porcine origin performed better than those fed a liquid diet fermented with lactobacilli of human origin, providing support to the notion that probiotics indigenous to host species may be more effective. No effect was apparent on *Brachyspira pilosicoli* shedding or disease following experimental infection (Lindecrona et al., 2004), consistent with a lack of improved production during the weaning-to-slaughter period (Lawlor et al., 2002). One aspect that should be scrutinized when reviewing information about fermented liquid feeds is the type of starter inoculum that was used, as not all studies specify the use of potential probiotic organisms in fermented feeds.

It is clear that potential benefits may result from probiotic therapy in pigs for both health and production purposes. However, the variability of results, even when the same probiotic organism is used, and the potentially large impact of animal management on responses to probiotic therapies indicate that clear guidelines for probiotic therapies cannot be developed yet for porcine applications. Further studies are required to better understand the optimal use of probiotics in pigs.

PROBIOTICS IN COMPANION ANIMALS

Probiotics are becoming increasingly popular for treatment and prevention of diseases in companion animals, particularly horses, dogs, and cats. The approaches to probiotic therapies in companion animals differ in many aspects from that in food production animals. Production parameters such as feed conversion are largely irrelevant, and individual animal health is the main priority. The infectious disease burden is also typically lower in companion animal management versus intensive food animal management, although high infection pressure and intensity of rearing can be present in some companion animal operations. The economic aspects of companion animal medicine are also much different. Because of the greater degree of emotional attachment and potentially high economic value of individual animals (especially race horses), cost issues are not as restrictive in these

species. Unfortunately, despite the widespread use of probiotics in these species, minimal objective investigations of efficacy or safety have been performed.

Horses

Gastrointestinal diseases are common in horses, ranging from sporadic mild disease to large outbreaks involving widespread mortality. Therefore, measures to decrease the burden of enteric diseases are desirable. These measures involve reductions of enteric infections such as salmonellosis or *Clostridium difficile*-associated diarrhea, as well as modifications of the intestinal environment to reduce the incidence of colic. Further, horses are particularly prone to development of antimicrobial-associated diarrhea, so therapeutic options that decrease the use of antimicrobial agents or reduce the risk of antimicrobial-associated diarrhea would be highly desirable.

Initial reports including clinical trials with commercial probiotic products were disappointing. Parraga et al. reported no apparent effects of two commercial probiotics on *Salmonella* shedding following gastrointestinal surgery (Parraga et al., 1997). One product contained 10^7 CFU of *L. plantarum*, *L. casei*, *L. acidophilus*, and *Streptococcus faecium* per g, while the other contained *L. acidophilus*, *E. faecium*, *Bifidobacterium thermophilum*, and *B. longum*. A similar study reported no effect of administration of a commercial product containing *E. faecium* and *Lactococcus lactis* (5×10^9 CFU) and "yeast" (10^8 CFU/day) on *Salmonella* spp. shedding in horses with colic at a veterinary teaching hospital (Kim et al., 2001). Possible reasons for lack of effect include improper organism selection and inadequate dosage. Further, quality control testing was not performed by the investigators, and based on studies of commercial veterinary probiotics (Weese, 2002), it is unclear whether the horses actually received the intended numbers of organisms. A study of an unspecified yeast product reported no effect on cardiorespiratory, hematological, and biochemical parameters during exercise (Art et al., 1994). A plausible mechanism for the intended effect was not clearly explained.

Colonization by *L. rhamnosus* strain GG (LGG), a human-derived organism, of both adult horses and foals was evaluated (Weese et al., 2003). Fecal recovery of LGG was rare in adult horses receiving 10^8 and 10^9 CFU/day. Even with a higher dose (5×10^{10} CFU/day), recovery was variable. It is plausible that non-equine-derived probiotics such as LGG might poorly colonize the intestinal tract of horses. LGG quantities in foal feces were higher and more consistent, which may reflect a less complex and less stable endogenous microbiota. Overall, survival of LGG was less than that reported for humans with similarly scaled doses, possibly reflecting the human origin of LGG (Goldin et al., 1992). The hypothesis that equine-derived organisms may be more likely to survive gastrointestinal passage in horses resulted in screening of equine feces for LAB with potentially beneficial in vitro properties (Weese et al., 2004a). One equine *Lactobacillus pentosus* strain was evaluated in vivo in a small colonization and safety trial and was recovered in feces of foals following oral administration (Weese and Rousseau, 2005). However, a randomized, blinded, placebo-controlled trial using this organism (2×10^{11} CFU/day) for prevention of neonatal foal diarrhea reported an association between probiotic administration and diarrhea, diarrhea plus other clinical signs (i.e., depression and anorexia), and the need for veterinary treatment (Weese and Rousseau, 2005). The reason for the negative effect of probiotic administration was not determined but could be due to the manner of screening and functional selection of such strains. Possibly, the elevated probiotic dosage combined with an immature intestinal microbiota resulted in excessive growth of *L. pentosus*. Results of this study highlight the need for safety studies of adequate size to identify potential problems, especially in neonatal animals.

Saccharomyces spp. have been evaluated as equine probiotics and are widely used in horses. Most studies involving yeast have focused on nutritional aspects and have not clearly evaluated other health benefits. In 1993, a study testing a commercial preparation containing a mixed yeast culture stated that "the probiotic improved the health of 4 of the 6 horses with hepatic-digestive disorders and that of all those with renal disorders" (Benoit, 1993). The study design and the diversity of nonspecific medical conditions in a limited number of horses ($n = 17$) make the validity of the conclusions questionable. A recent study that reported decreased duration of diarrhea following administration of "*Saccharomyces boulardii*" (10^{10} cells every 12 h for 14 days) to horses with enterocolitis (Desrochers et al., 2005) yielded encouraging results. However, this report used a small study population (14 horses in total) and did not report a difference in clinical outcome and duration of hospitalization. Larger studies are needed to assess the clinical efficacy of this yeast formulation.

Dogs

Studies on probiotics in dogs have been relatively superficial, although the depth of research is increasing. Probiotic therapy in dogs is typically directed at prevention and treatment of enteric disease.

Colonization studies have been performed with various lactic acid bacteria. *L. rhamnosus* GG (LGG)

was recovered in feces following oral administration, but organism recovery was sporadic in all except dogs receiving the highest dose (5×10^{11} CFU/day) (Weese and Anderson, 2002). When similar dosing regimens were compared, fecal LGG levels in dogs were much lower than those reported in humans (Goldin et al., 1992), perhaps indicative of a degree of species specificity of human-derived LGG. Thus, canine-derived organisms may have enhanced beneficial properties in dogs. A canine-derived strain of *Lactobacillus fermentum* (AD1) that was demonstrated to survive pH 3.0 and 1% bile in vitro and adhered to canine intestinal mucus was recovered from the feces of healthy adult dogs after oral administration at a dose of 10^9 CFU/day (Strompfova et al., 2006a). Significant elevations of fecal lactobacilli and enterococci in treated dogs were noted, but clinical efficacy was not reported. A significant increase in lactobacilli following administration of *Lactobacillus animalis* LA4 was reported, and organisms were recovered from several dogs up to 5 days following cessation of administration (Biagi et al., 2007). Another study of canine-derived probiotics including *L. fermentum* LAB8, *Lactobacillus salivarius* LAB12, *Weissella confusa* LAB10, *L. rhamnosus* LAB11, and *Lactobacillus mucosae* LAB 12 reported survival of upper gastrointestinal tract passage and modification of the jejunal lactic acid bacteria (Manninen et al., 2006). Following cessation of probiotic administration, inoculated organisms could not be detected, but the lactic acid bacteria that reemerged differed from the baseline microbiota, with a predominance of *L. acidophilus*. Although a significant modification of the gastrointestinal microbiota indicates survival of probiotics with local effects, demonstration of health benefits in dogs will need to be established in future studies.

One of the few published clinical trials evaluated the effect of a combination of two strains of *L. acidophilus* and one strain of *Lactobacillus johnsonii* (10^{10} CFU/day) for food-responsive diarrhea in a blinded placebo-controlled trial (Sauter et al., 2006). No effect was noted as all dogs improved similarly when placed on an elimination diet with or without probiotic supplementation. Weight gain and feed conversion are a lesser concern in companion animals than in food production animals. However, one study reported increased feed intake and average daily gain in puppies supplemented with *L. acidophilus* (10^7 CFU/day) from 10 to 19 weeks of age, with no effect later in life (Pasupathy et al., 2001).

Another popular approach to probiotic therapy in dogs is feeding commercial diets containing probiotics. Supplementation with probiotics is feasible only with dry (as opposed to canned) food because the high temperature produced during the canning process would render probiotic organisms nonviable. The main advantage of food supplementation is ease of administration. The extruding process used to produce dry pet foods can affect bacterial numbers, but survival of probiotics in food has been documented (Baillon et al., 2004; Biourge et al., 1998). Similar to studies involving probiotic supplements, studies with probiotic-containing foods have demonstrated encouraging preliminary data, although demonstrated health benefits are lacking to date. Biourge et al. reported transient fecal colonization with *Bacillus* sp. strain CIP5832 administered at a dose of approximately 1.5×10^6 CFU/g of diet (Biourge et al., 1998). Administration of *L. acidophilus* DSM 13241 ($>10^9$ CFU/day) to healthy adult dogs was reported to have resulted in increased numbers of fecal lactobacilli and decreased numbers of clostridia (Baillon et al., 2004). Changes in hematological parameters that purportedly indicated improved immune function were also reported, but the relevance of these findings is unclear.

Minimal evaluation of immunomodulatory effects of probiotics has been performed in dogs. Supplementation with 5×10^8 CFU of *E. faecium* SF68 per day in dogs was reported to yield increased fecal IgA concentrations and canine distemper virus vaccine-specific circulating IgG and IgA concentrations (Benyacoub et al., 2003). These results may demonstrate enhanced specific immune function, but the reported difference in fecal IgA concentration was not statistically significant and the clinical relevance of these findings is unclear.

Some discussion of potential safety concerns, particularly involving enterococci, has been documented. A study evaluating the effects of different probiotic strains on adhesion of selected pathogens to canine intestinal mucus reported that *E. faecium* caused a marked increase in adhesion of *Campylobacter jejuni* (Rinkinen et al., 2003). Concern was expressed that enterococcal probiotics could facilitate colonization of this canine and zoonotic pathogen, although this risk has not been clarified further. Other concerns regarding enterococcal probiotics in dogs include the opportunistically pathogenic nature of many enterococci and the theoretical potential for antimicrobial resistance acquisition and transmission. One *E. faecium* supplement is currently marketed by a major pet food manufacturer in North America. Promotional materials for this product claim that this strain is not pathogenic and cannot acquire or transmit antimicrobial resistance, but objective data have not been produced.

Limited evaluation of probiotics for nongastrointestinal disorders in dogs has been performed. Degradation of oxalate by lactic acid bacteria in vitro was reported in one study (Weese et al., 2004b), but the relevance of these findings for calcium oxalate urolithiasis is unclear.

Overall, while some encouraging studies have been reported, probiotics have not yet demonstrated beneficial effects in dogs. Further studies are needed to understand in vitro and in vivo properties required for successful probiotic treatment.

Cats

Minimal information exists regarding probiotic applications in cats, and no clinical studies have indicated a beneficial effect of probiotic therapy for any feline disease. Despite this limitation, probiotics are widely available as supplements and probiotic-containing foods.

L. acidophilus DSM13241 (2×10^8 CFU/day) was recovered from feces after administration to healthy adult cats, and significant reductions in clostridia and coliforms were noted (Marshall-Jones et al., 2006). Immunomodulatory effects were reported based on decreased lymphocyte and increased eosinophil populations and increased activities of peripheral blood phagocytes. The relevance of these findings, however, is unclear, and results cannot yet be extrapolated into evidence of beneficial health effects.

QUALITY CONTROL

As with probiotics marketed for human use, concerns about the quality of probiotics marketed for veterinary species, particularly companion animals, have been expressed. A microbiologic study of commercial veterinary probiotics identified numerous quality concerns (Weese, 2002). In this study, it was reported that no veterinary products contained the number of probiotic organisms stated on the label, and all products contained less than 2% of the stated bacterial numbers. Only 38% of commercial products listed specific organisms that were supposed to be present, and 50% of products lacked species and quantitative information on the product label. The product with the highest concentration of viable bacteria contained only 1.2×10^7 CFU/g.

A study of labeling of probiotic supplements identified similar deficiencies (Weese, 2003). Organisms listed on the label were improperly identified in 35% of veterinary products, organism names were misspelled in 18% of products, and one product claimed to contain an organism that does not formally exist. Only 22% of products provided quantitative information regarding numbers of organisms. Adequate identification, involving proper nomenclature and spelling of organisms, was present on only 12% of product labels.

Only one study has described commercial pet foods that claim to contain probiotics (Weese and Arroyo, 2003). Sixty-three percent of products that claimed to contain probiotics listed only fermentation products on the label, and no products contained all of the stated microorganisms. Only 53% of pet foods contained one or more of the organisms stated on the label. No growth of the stated contents or related organisms was identified in 26% of products. Average bacterial growth ranged from zero to only 1.8×10^5 CFU/g.

Apparently, the overall quality of most commercial veterinary probiotic supplements is questionable. The derivation of useful clinical information in animals is difficult because observers cannot be assured that animals are receiving the intended probiotic organisms at appropriate doses.

FUTURE NEEDS

Probiotic therapy is an area with attractive potential to improve animal health and improve economic production. Other potential benefits include decreasing zoonotic pathogen burdens, diminishing concerns about antimicrobial residues in food, and reducing antimicrobial use. As a result, antimicrobial resistance among zoonotic pathogens and the commensal microflora may be reduced. However, a glaring need for further objective studies is apparent, particularly studies involving companion animals. Ongoing evaluation of efficacy and safety of current commercial products and proper development of new probiotic formulations are warranted. Probiotics derived from animal species of interest should be considered carefully for specific applications. While it would be easier to simply transfer findings from one species to other veterinary species, this approach should be addressed with caution until animal-derived probiotics are fully evaluated. Public health issues related to administration of enterococci also need clarification, as concerns about dissemination of vancomycin-resistant enterococci in animals have increased. Regardless, probiotic therapy remains a promising option as parallel pressures to reduce antimicrobial use in animals, produce safe food cost-effectively, reduce environmental contamination with zoonotic pathogens, and maintain health in companion animals continue to be important priorities.

References

Abe, F., N. Ishibashi, and S. Shimamura. 1995. Effect of administration of bifidobacteria and lactic acid bacteria to newborn calves and piglets. *J. Dairy Sci.* **78**:2838–2846.

Agarwal, N., D. N. Kamra, L. C. Chaudhary, I. Agarwal, A. Sahoo, and N. N. Pathak. 2002. Microbial status and rumen enzyme profile of crossbred calves fed on different microbial feed additives. *Lett. Appl. Microbiol.* **34**:329–336.

Aleman, M. M., D. R. Stein, D. T. Allen, E. Perry, K. V. Lehloenya, T. G. Rehberger, K. J. Mertz, D. A. Jones, and L. J. Spicer. 2007. Effects of feeding two levels of propionibacteria to dairy cows on plasma hormones and metabolites. *J. Dairy Res.* **74**:146–153.

Alexopoulos, C., I. E. Georgoulakis, A. Tzivara, S. K. Kritas, A. Siochu, and S. C. Kyriakis. 2004. Field evaluation of the efficacy of a probiotic containing *Bacillus licheniformis* and *Bacillus subtilis* spores, on the health status and performance of sows and their litters. *J. Anim. Physiol. Anim. Nutr.* (Berlin) **88**:381–392.

Alexopoulos, C., A. Karagiannidis, S. K. Kritas, C. Boscos, I. E. Georgoulakis, and S. C. Kyriakis. 2001. Field evaluation of a bioregulator containing live *Bacillus cereus* spores on health status and performance of sows and their litters. *J. Vet. Med. A* **48**:137–145.

Amezcua, R. 2006. Post-weaning diarrhea caused by *Escherichia coli*: prevalence, antibiotic resistance, investigation of risk factors and control methods. Ph.D. thesis. University of Guelph, Guelph, Ontario, Canada.

Amit-Romach, E., D. Sklan, and Z. Uni. 2004. Microflora ecology of the chicken intestine using 16S ribosomal DNA primers. *Poult. Sci.* **83**:1093–1098.

Art, T., D. Votion, K. McEntee, H. Amory, A. Linden, R. Close, and P. Lekeux. 1994. Cardio-respiratory, haematological and biochemical parameter adjustments to exercise: effect of a probiotic in horses during training. *Vet. Res.* **25**:361–370.

Arthur, T. M., G. A. Barkocy-Gallagher, M. Rivera-Betancourt, and M. Koohmaraie. 2002. Prevalence and characterization of non-O157 Shiga toxin-producing *Escherichia coli* on carcasses in commercial beef cattle processing plants. *Appl. Environ. Microbiol.* **68**:4847–4852.

Bailey, J. S., N. J. Stern, and N. A. Cox. 2000. Commercial field trial evaluation of mucosal starter culture to reduce *Salmonella* incidence in processed broiler carcasses. *J. Food Prot.* **63**:867–870.

Baillon, M. L., Z. V. Marshall-Jones, and R. F. Butterwick. 2004. Effects of probiotic *Lactobacillus acidophilus* strain DSM13241 in healthy adult dogs. *Am. J. Vet. Res.* **65**:338–343.

Beal, R. K., C. Powers, P. Wigley, P. A. Barrow, and A. L. Smith. 2004. Temporal dynamics of the cellular, humoral and cytokine responses in chickens during primary and secondary infection with *Salmonella enterica* serovar Typhimurium. *Avian Pathol.* **33**:25–33.

Beauchemin, K. A., W. Z. Yang, D. P. Morgavi, G. R. Ghorbani, W. Kautz, and J. A. Leedle. 2003. Effects of bacterial direct-fed microbials and yeast on site and extent of digestion, blood chemistry, and subclinical ruminal acidosis in feedlot cattle. *J. Anim Sci.* **81**:1628–1640.

Befus, A. D., N. Johnston, G. A. Leslie, and J. Bienenstock. 1980. Gut-associated lymphoid tissue in the chicken. I. Morphology, ontogeny, and some functional characteristics of Peyer's patches. *J. Immunol.* **125**:2626–2632.

Benoit, P. 1993. Clinical trial of a probiotic. Clinical and nutritional follow-up of 17 horses. *Pract. Vet. Equine* **25**:61–64.

Benyacoub, J., G. L. Czarnecki-Maulden, C. Cavadini, T. Sauthier, R. E. Anderson, E. J. Schiffrin, and T. von der Weid. 2003. Supplementation of food with *Enterococcus faecium* (SF68) stimulates immune functions in young dogs. *J. Nutr.* 133:1158–1162.

Berland, R., and H. H. Wortis. 2002. Origins and functions of B-1 cells with notes on the role of CD5. *Annu. Rev. Immunol.* 20:253–300.

Biagi, G., I. Cipollini, A. Pompei, G. Zaghini, and D. Matteuzzi. 2007. Effect of a *Lactobacillus animalis* strain on composition and metabolism of the intestinal microflora in adult dogs. *Vet. Microbiol.* 124:160–165.

Biourge, V., C. Vallet, A. Levesque, R. Sergheraert, S. Chevalier, and J. L. Roberton. 1998. The use of probiotics in the diet of dogs. *J. Nutr.* 128:2730S–2732S.

Bohmer, B. M., W. Kramer, and D. A. Roth-Maier. 2006. Dietary probiotic supplementation and resulting effects on performance, health status, and microbial characteristics of primiparous sows. *J. Anim. Physiol. Anim. Nutr.* (Berlin) 90:309–315.

Brashears, M. M., M. L. Galyean, G. H. Loneragan, J. E. Mann, and K. Killinger-Mann. 2003. Prevalence of *Escherichia coli* O157:H7 and performance by beef feedlot cattle given *Lactobacillus* direct-fed microbials. *J. Food Prot.* 66:748–754.

Brisbin, J. T., H. Zhou, J. Gong, P. Sabour, M. R. Akbari, H. R. Haghighi, H. Yu, A. Clarke, A. J. Sarson, and S. Sharif. 2008. Gene expression profiling of chicken lymphoid cells after treatment with *Lactobacillus acidophilus* cellular components. *Dev. Comp. Immunol.* 32:563–574.

Broom, L. J., H. M. Miller, K. G. Kerr, and J. S. Knapp. 2006. Effects of zinc oxide and *Enterococcus faecium* SF68 dietary supplementation on the performance, intestinal microbiota and immune status of weaned piglets. *Res. Vet. Sci.* 80:45–54.

Callaway, T. R., R. C. Anderson, T. S. Edrington, K. J. Genovese, R. B. Harvey, T. L. Poole, and D. J. Nisbet. 2004. Recent pre-harvest supplementation strategies to reduce carriage and shedding of zoonotic enteric bacterial pathogens in food animals. *Anim. Health Res. Rev.* 5:35–47.

Cameron, D. M., and J. N. Carter. 1992. Evaluation of the efficacy of Broilact in preventing infection of broiler chicks with *Salmonella enteritidis* PT4. *Int. J. Food Microbiol.* 15:319–326.

Chang, Y. H., J. K. Kim, H. J. Kim, W. Y. Kim, Y. B. Kim, and Y. H. Park. 2001. Selection of a potential probiotic *Lactobacillus* strain and subsequent *in vivo* studies. *Antonie Leeuwenhoek* 80:193–199.

Christensen, H. R., H. Frokiaer, and J. J. Pestka. 2002. Lactobacilli differentially modulate expression of cytokines and maturation surface markers in murine dendritic cells. *J. Immunol.* 168:171–178.

Craven, S. E., N. J. Stern, N. A. Cox, J. S. Bailey, and M. Berrang. 1999. Cecal carriage of *Clostridium perfringens* in broiler chickens given Mucosal Starter Culture. *Avian Dis.* 43:484–490.

Dalloul, R. A., H. S. Lillehoj, N. M. Tamim, T. A. Shellem, and J. A. Doerr. 2005. Induction of local protective immunity to *Eimeria acervulina* by a *Lactobacillus*-based probiotic. *Comp. Immunol. Microbiol. Infect. Dis.* 28:351–361.

Dann, H. M., J. K. Drackley, G. C. McCoy, M. F. Hutjens, and J. E. Garrett. 2000. Effects of yeast culture (*Saccharomyces cerevisiae*) on prepartum intake and postpartum intake and milk production of Jersey cows. *J. Dairy Sci.* 83:123–127.

De Cupere, F., P. Deprez, D. Demeulenaere, and E. Muylle. 1992. Evaluation of the effect of 3 probiotics on experimental *Escherichia coli* enterotoxaemia in weaned piglets. *Zentrbl. Veterinarmed.* B 39:277–284.

Desrochers, A. M., B. A. Dolente, M. F. Roy, R. Boston, and S. Carlisle. 2005. Efficacy of *Saccharomyces boulardii* for treatment of horses with acute enterocolitis. *J. Am. Vet. Med. Assoc.* 227:954–959.

Elam, N. A., J. F. Gleghorn, J. D. Rivera, M. L. Galyean, P. J. Defoor, M. M. Brashears, and S. M. Younts-Dahl. 2003. Effects of live cultures of *Lactobacillus acidophilus* (strains NP45 and NP51) and *Propionibacterium freudenreichii* on performance, carcass, and intestinal characteristics, and *Escherichia coli* strain O157 shedding of finishing beef steers. *J. Anim. Sci.* 81:2686–2698.

Ewaschuk, J. B., J. M. Naylor, M. Chirino-Trejo, and G. A. Zello. 2004. *Lactobacillus rhamnosus* strain GG is a potential probiotic for calves. *Can. J. Vet. Res.* 68:249–253.

Ewaschuk, J. B., G. A. Zello, and J. M. Naylor. 2006. *Lactobacillus* GG does not affect D-lactic acidosis in diarrheic calves, in a clinical setting. *J. Vet. Intern. Med.* 20:614–619.

Farnell, M. B., A. M. Donoghue, F. S. de Los Santos, P. J. Blore, B. M. Hargis, G. Tellez, and D. J. Donoghue. 2006. Upregulation of oxidative burst and degranulation in chicken heterophils stimulated with probiotic bacteria. *Poult. Sci.* 85:1900–1906.

Ferreira, A. J., C. S. Ferreira, T. Knobl, A. M. Moreno, M. R. Bacarro, M. Chen, M. Robach, and G. C. Mead. 2003. Comparison of three commercial competitive-exclusion products for controlling *Salmonella* colonization of broilers in Brazil. *J. Food Prot.* 66:490–492.

Francisco, C. C., C. S. Chamberlain, D. N. Waldner, R. P. Wettemann, and L. J. Spicer. 2002. Propionibacteria fed to dairy cows: effects on energy balance, plasma metabolites and hormones, and reproduction. *J. Dairy Sci.* 85:1738–1751.

Genovese, K. J., R. C. Anderson, R. B. Harvey, and D. J. Nisbet. 2000. Competitive exclusion treatment reduces the mortality and fecal shedding associated with enterotoxigenic *Escherichia coli* infection in nursery-raised neonatal pigs. *Can. J. Vet. Res.* 64:204–207.

Ghorbani, G. R., D. P. Morgavi, K. A. Beauchemin, and J. A. Leedle. 2002. Effects of bacterial direct-fed microbials on ruminal fermentation, blood variables, and the microbial populations of feedlot cattle. *J. Anim Sci.* 80:1977–1985.

Goldin, B. R., S. L. Gorbach, M. Saxelin, S. Barakat, L. Gualtieri, and S. Salminen. 1992. Survival of *Lactobacillus* species (strain GG) in human gastrointestinal tract. *Dig. Dis. Sci.* 37:121–128.

Grabig, A., D. Paclik, C. Guzy, A. Dankof, D. C. Baumgart, J. Erckenbrecht, B. Raupach, U. Sonnenborn, J. Eckert, R. R. Schumann, B. Wiedenmann, A. U. Dignass, and A. Sturm. 2006. *Escherichia coli* strain Nissle 1917 ameliorates experimental colitis via toll-like receptor 2- and toll-like receptor 4-dependent pathways. *Infect. Immun.* 74:4075–4082.

Guo, X., D. Li, W. Lu, X. Piao, and X. Chen. 2006. Screening of *Bacillus* strains as potential probiotics and subsequent confirmation of the *in vivo* effectiveness of *Bacillus subtilis* MA139 in pigs. *Antonie Leeuwenhoek* 90:139–146.

Haghighi, H. R., M. F. Abdul-Careem, R. A. Dara, J. R. Chambers, and S. Sharif. 2008. Cytokine gene expression in chicken cecal tonsils following treatment with probiotics and *Salmonella* infection. *Vet. Microbiol.* 126:225–233.

Haghighi, H. R., J. Gong, C. L. Gyles, M. A. Hayes, B. Sanei, P. Parvizi, H. Gisavi, J. R. Chambers, and S. Sharif. 2005. Modulation of antibody-mediated immune response by probiotics in chickens. *Clin. Diagn. Lab. Immunol.* 12:1387–1392.

Haghighi, H. R., J. Gong, C. L. Gyles, M. A. Hayes, H. Zhou, B. Sanei, J. R. Chambers, and S. Sharif. 2006. Probiotics stimulate production of natural antibodies in chickens. *Clin. Vaccine Immunol.* 13:975–980.

Hakkinen, M., and C. Schneitz. 1999. Efficacy of a commercial competitive exclusion product against *Campylobacter jejuni. Br. Poult. Sci.* 40:619–621.

Harp, J. A., P. Jardon, E. R. Atwill, M. Zylstra, S. Checel, J. P. Goff, and C. De Simone. 1996. Field testing of prophylactic measures against *Cryptosporidium parvum* infection in calves in a California dairy herd. *Am. J. Vet. Res.* 57:1586–1588.

Higginbotham, G. E., C. A. Collar, M. S. Aseltine, and D. L. Bath. 1994. Effect of yeast culture and *Aspergillus oryzae* extract on milk yield in a commercial dairy herd. *J. Dairy Sci.* 77:343–348.

Hofacre, C. L., R. Froyman, B. Gautrias, B. George, M. A. Goodwin, and J. Brown. 1998. Use of Aviguard and other intestinal bioproducts in experimental *Clostridium perfringens*-associated necrotizing enteritis in broiler chickens. *Avian Dis.* 42:579–584.

Hojberg, O., N. Canibe, B. Knudsen, and B. B. Jensen. 2003. Potential rates of fermentation in digesta from the gastrointestinal tract of pigs: effect of feeding fermented liquid feed. *Appl. Environ. Microbiol.* 69:408–418.

Huang, M. K., Y. J. Choi, R. Houde, J. W. Lee, B. Lee, and X. Zhao. 2004. Effects of Lactobacilli and an acidophilic fungus on the production performance and immune responses in broiler chickens. *Poult. Sci.* 83:788–795.

Huber, J. T., G. Higginbotham, R. A. Gomez-Alarcon, R. B. Taylor, K. H. Chen, S. C. Chan, and Z. Wu. 1994. Heat stress interactions with protein, supplemental fat, and fungal cultures. *J. Dairy Sci.* 77:2080–2090.

Janssens, S., and R. Beyaert. 2003. Role of Toll-like receptors in pathogen recognition. *Clin. Microbiol. Rev.* 16:637–646.

Jiang, H. Q., M. C. Thurnheer, A. W. Zuercher, N. V. Boiko, N. A. Bos, and J. J. Cebra. 2004. Interactions of commensal gut microbes with subsets of B- and T-cells in the murine host. *Vaccine* 22:805–811.

Jouany, J. P. 2006. Optimizing rumen functions in the close-up transition period and early lactation to drive dry matter intake and energy balance in cows. *Anim. Reprod. Sci.* 96:250–264.

Khaitsa, M. L., D. R. Smith, J. A. Stoner, A. M. Parkhurst, S. Hinkley, T. J. Klopfenstein, and R. A. Moxley. 2003. Incidence, duration, and prevalence of *Escherichia coli* O157:H7

fecal shedding by feedlot cattle during the finishing period. *J. Food Prot.* 66:1972–1977.

Khuntia, M. L., and L. C. Chaudhary. 2002. Performance of male crossbred calves as influenced by substitution of grain by wheat bran and the addition of lactic acid bacteria to the diet. *Asian-Australian J. Anim. Sic.* 15:188–194.

Kim, L., P. S. Morley, J. L. Traub-Dargatz, M. D. Salman, and C. Gentry-Weeks. 2001. Factors associated with *Salmonella* shedding among colic patients at a veterinary teaching hospital. *J. Am. Vet. Med. Assoc.* 218:740–748.

Klose, V., M. Mohnl, R. Plail, G. Schatzmayr, and A. P. Loibner. 2006. Development of a competitive exclusion product for poultry meeting the regulatory requirements for registration in the European Union. *Mol. Nutr. Food Res.* 50:563–571.

Koenen, M. E., J. Kramer, R. van der Hulst, L. Heres, S. H. Jeurissen, and W. J. Boersma. 2004. Immunomodulation by probiotic lactobacilli in layer- and meat-type chickens. *Br. Poult. Sci.* 45:355–366.

Kritas, S. K., and R. B. Morrison. 2005. Evaluation of probiotics as a substitute for antibiotics in a large pig nursery. *Vet. Rec.* 156:447–448.

Kroese, F. G., R. de Waard, and N. A. Bos. 1996. B-1 cells and their reactivity with the murine intestinal microflora. *Semin. Immunol.* 8:11–18.

Kung, L., Jr., C. C. Taylor, M. P. Lynch, and J. M. Neylon. 2003. The effect of treating alfalfa with *Lactobacillus buchneri* 40788 on silage fermentation, aerobic stability, and nutritive value for lactating dairy cows. *J. Dairy Sci.* 86:336–343.

Kyriakis, S. C., V. K. Tsiloyiannis, J. Vlemmas, K. Sarris, A. C. Tsinas, C. Alexopoulos, and L. Jansegers. 1999. The effect of probiotic LSP 122 on the control of post-weaning diarrhoea syndrome of piglets. *Res. Vet. Sci.* 67:223–228.

Lammers, K. M., P. Brigidi, B. Vitali, P. Gionchetti, F. Rizzello, E. Caramelli, D. Matteuzzi, and M. Campieri. 2003. Immunomodulatory effects of probiotic bacteria DNA: IL-1 and IL-10 response in human peripheral blood mononuclear cells. *FEMS Immunol. Med. Microbiol.* 38:165–172.

Lawlor, P. G., P. B. Lynch, G. E. Gardiner, P. J. Caffrey, and J. V. O'Doherty. 2002. Effect of liquid feeding weaned pigs on growth performance to harvest. *J. Anim. Sci.* 80:1725–1735.

Lebeer, S., S. C. De Keersmaecker, T. L. Verhoeven, A. A. Fadda, K. Marchal, and J. Vanderleyden. 2007. Functional analysis of luxS in the probiotic strain *Lactobacillus rhamnosus* GG reveals a central metabolic role important for growth and biofilm formation. *J. Bacteriol.* 189:860–871.

LeJeune, J. T., and A. N. Wetzel. 2007. Preharvest control of *Escherichia coli* O157 in cattle. *J. Anim. Sci.* 85:E73–E80.

Lillehoj, H. S., and J. M. Trout. 1996. Avian gut-associated lymphoid tissues and intestinal immune responses to *Eimeria* parasites. *Clin. Microbiol. Rev.* 9:349–360.

Lindecrona, R. H., T. K. Jensen, and K. Moller. 2004. Influence of diet on the experimental infection of pigs with *Brachyspira pilosicoli. Vet. Rec.* 154:264–267.

Macpherson, A. J., D. Gatto, E. Sainsbury, G. R. Harriman, H. Hengartner, and R. M. Zinkernagel. 2000. A primitive T cell-independent mechanism of intestinal mucosal IgA responses to commensal bacteria. *Science* 288:2222–2226.

Manninen, T. J., M. L. Rinkinen, S. S. Beasley, and P. E. Saris. 2006. Alteration of the canine small-intestinal lactic acid bacterium microbiota by feeding of potential probiotics. *Appl. Environ. Microbiol.* 72:6539–6543.

Marshall-Jones, Z. V., M. L. Baillon, J. M. Croft, and R. F. Butterwick. 2006. Effects of *Lactobacillus acidophilus* DSM13241 as a probiotic in healthy adult cats. *Am. J. Vet. Res.* 67:1005–1012.

Mathieu, F., J. P. Jouany, J. Senaud, J. Bohatier, G. Bertin, and M. Mercier. 1996. The effect of *Saccharomyces cerevisiae* and *Aspergillus oryzae* on fermentation in the rumen of faunated and defaunated sheep; protozoal and probiotic interactions. *Reprod. Nutr. Dev.* 36:271–287.

McGilliard, M. L., and C. C. Stallings. 1998. Increase in milk yield of commercial dairy herds fed a microbial and enzyme supplement. *J. Dairy Sci.* 81:1353–1357.

Mead, G. C. 2000. Prospects for 'competitive exclusion' treatment to control salmonellas and other foodborne pathogens in poultry. *Vet. J.* 159:111–123.

Methner, U., P. A. Barrow, G. Martin, and H. Meyer. 1997. Comparative study of the protective effect against *Salmonella* colonisation in newly hatched SPF chickens using live, attenuated *Salmonella* vaccine strains, wild-type *Salmonella* strains or a competitive exclusion product. *Int. J. Food Microbiol.* 35:223–230.

Morrill, J. L., J. M. Morrill, A. M. Feyerherm, and J. F. Laster. 1995. Plasma proteins and a probiotic as ingredients in milk replacer. *J. Dairy Sci.* 78:902–907.

Muir, W. I., W. L. Bryden, and A. J. Husband. 2000. Immunity, vaccination and the avian intestinal tract. *Dev. Comp. Immunol.* 24:325–342.

Nakamura, A., Y. Ota, A. Mizukami, T. Ito, Y. B. Ngwai, and Y. Adachi. 2002. Evaluation of Aviguard, a commercial competitive exclusion product for efficacy and after-effect on the antibody response of chicks to Salmonella. *Poult. Sci.* 81:1653–1660.

Nisbet, D. 2002. Defined competitive exclusion cultures in the prevention of enteropathogen colonisation in poultry and swine. *Antonie Leeuwenhoek* 81:481–486.

Nocek, J. E., and W. P. Kautz. 2006. Direct-fed microbial supplementation on ruminal digestion, health, and performance of pre- and postpartum dairy cattle. *J. Dairy Sci.* 89:260–266.

Nocek, J. E., W. P. Kautz, J. A. Leedle, and J. G. Allman. 2002. Ruminal supplementation of direct-fed microbials on diurnal pH variation and *in situ* digestion in dairy cattle. *J. Dairy Sci.* 85:429–433.

Nocek, J. E., W. P. Kautz, J. A. Leedle, and E. Block. 2003. Direct-fed microbial supplementation on the performance of dairy cattle during the transition period. *J. Dairy Sci.* 86:331–335.

Nuotio, L., C. Schneitz, U. Halonen, and E. Nurmi. 1992. Use of competitive exclusion to protect newly-hatched chicks against intestinal colonisation and invasion by *Salmonella enteritidis* PT4. *Br. Poult. Sci.* 33:775–779.

Nurmi, E., and M. Rantala. 1973. New aspects of *Salmonella* infection in broiler production. *Nature* 241:210–211.

Oetzel, G. R., K. M. Emery, W. P. Kautz, and J. E. Nocek. 2007. Direct-fed microbial supplementation and health and performance of pre- and postpartum dairy cattle: a field trial. *J. Dairy Sci.* 90:2058–2068.

O'Hara, A. M., P. O'Regan, A. Fanning, C. O'Mahony, J. Macsharry, A. Lyons, J. Bienenstock, L. O'Mahony, and F. Shanahan. 2006. Functional modulation of human intestinal epithelial cell responses by *Bifidobacterium infantis* and *Lactobacillus salivarius. Immunology* 118:202–215.

Ohya, T., T. Marubashi, and H. Ito. 2000. Significance of fecal volatile fatty acids in shedding of *Escherichia coli* O157 from calves: experimental infection and preliminary use of a probiotic product. *J. Vet. Med. Sci.* 62:1151–1155.

Palmu, L., and I. Camelin. 1997. The use of competitive exclusion in broilers to reduce the level of *Salmonella* contamination on the farm and at the processing plant. *Poult. Sci.* 76:1501–1505.

Parraga, M. E., S. J. Spier, M. Thurmond, and D. Hirsh. 1997. A clinical trial of probiotic administration for prevention of *Salmonella* shedding in the postoperative period in horses with colic. *J. Vet. Intern. Med.* 11:36–41.

Pasupathy, K., A. Sahoo, and N. N. Pathak. 2001. Effect of lactobacillus supplementation on growth and nutrient utilization in mongrel pups. *Arch. Tierernahr.* 55:243–253.

Peterson, R. E., T. J. Klopfenstein, G. E. Erickson, J. Folmer, S. Hinkley, R. A. Moxley, and D. R. Smith. 2007. Effect of *Lactobacillus acidophilus* strain NP51 on *Escherichia coli* O157:H7 fecal shedding and finishing performance in beef feedlot cattle. *J. Food Prot.* 70:287–291.

Rachmilewitz, D., K. Katakura, F. Karmeli, T. Hayashi, C. Reinus, B. Rudensky, S. Akira, K. Takeda, J. Lee, K. Takabayashi, and E. Raz. 2004. Toll-like receptor 9 signaling mediates the anti-inflammatory effects of probiotics in murine experimental colitis. *Gastroenterology* 126:520–528.

Rakoff-Nahoum, S., J. Paglino, F. Eslami-Varzaneh, S. Edberg, and R. Medzhitov. 2004. Recognition of commensal microflora by toll-like receptors is required for intestinal homeostasis. *Cell* 118:229–241.

Ratajczak, C., C. Duez, C. Grangette, P. Pochard, A. B. Tonnel, and J. Pestel. 2007. Impact of lactic acid bacteria on dendritic cells from allergic patients in an experimental model of intestinal epithelium. *J. Biomed. Biotechnol.* 2007:71921.

Rescigno, M., M. Urbano, B. Valzasina, M. Francolini, G. Rotta, R. Bonasio, F. Granucci, J. P. Kraehenbuhl, and P. Ricciardi-Castagnoli. 2001. Dendritic cells express tight junction proteins and penetrate gut epithelial monolayers to sample bacteria. *Nat. Immunol.* 2:361–367.

Revolledo, L., A. J. Ferreira, and G. C. Mead. 2006. Prospects of Salmonella control: competitive exclusion, probiotics, and enhancement of avian intestinal immunity. *J. Appl. Poult. Res.* 15:341–351.

Rhee, K. J., P. Sethupathi, A. Driks, D. K. Lanning, and K. L. Knight. 2004. Role of commensal bacteria in development of gut-associated lymphoid tissues and preimmune antibody repertoire. *J. Immunol.* 172:1118–1124.

Rinkinen, M., K. Jalava, E. Westermarck, S. Salminen, and A. C. Ouwehand. 2003. Interaction between probiotic lactic acid bacteria and canine enteric pathogens: a risk factor for intestinal *Enterococcus faecium* colonization? *Vet. Microbiol.* 92:111–119.

Rodriguez-Palacios, A., J. S. Weese, T. Duffield, and H. R. Staempfli. 2004. Effect of oral probiotics on calf diarrhea: clinical trials published between 1973-2003. *J. Vet. Intern. Med.* **18**:395–396.

Santosa, S., E. Farnworth, and P. J. Jones. 2006. Probiotics and their potential health claims. *Nutr. Rev.* **64**:265–274.

Sauter, S. N., J. Benyacoub, K. Allenspach, F. Gaschen, E. Ontsouka, G. Reuteler, C. Cavadini, R. Knorr, and J. W. Blum. 2006. Effects of probiotic bacteria in dogs with food responsive diarrhoea treated with an elimination diet. *J. Anim. Physiol. Anim. Nutr.* (Berlin) **90**:269–277.

Schamberger, G. P., and F. Diez-Gonzalez. 2002. Selection of recently isolated colicinogenic *Escherichia coli* strains inhibitory to *Escherichia coli* O157:H7. *J. Food Prot.* **65**:1381–1387.

Schamberger, G. P., R. L. Phillips, J. L. Jacobs, and F. Diez-Gonzalez. 2004. Reduction of *Escherichia coli* O157:H7 populations in cattle by addition of colicin E7-producing *E. coli* to feed. *Appl. Environ. Microbiol.* **70**:6053–6060.

Schroeder, B., S. Duncker, S. Barth, R. Bauerfeind, A. D. Gruber, S. Deppenmeier, and G. Breves. 2006. Preventive effects of the probiotic *Escherichia coli* strain Nissle 1917 on acute secretory diarrhea in a pig model of intestinal infection. *Dig. Dis. Sci.* **51**:724–731.

Shu, Q., F. Qu, and H. S. Gill. 2001. Probiotic treatment using *Bifidobacterium lactis* HN019 reduces weanling diarrhea associated with rotavirus and *Escherichia coli* infection in a piglet model. *J. Pediatr. Gastroenterol. Nutr.* **33**:171–177.

Silva, A. M., F. H. Barbosa, R. Duarte, L. Q. Vieira, R. M. Arantes, and J. R. Nicoli. 2004. Effect of *Bifidobacterium longum* ingestion on experimental salmonellosis in mice. *J. Appl. Microbiol.* **97**:29–37.

Smits, H. H., A. Engering, D. van der Kleij, E. C. de Jong, K. Schipper, T. M. van Capel, B. A. Zaat, M. Yazdanbakhsh, E. A. Wierenga, Y. van Kooyk, and M. L. Kapsenberg. 2005. Selective probiotic bacteria induce IL-10-producing regulatory T cells *in vitro* by modulating dendritic cell function through dendritic cell-specific intercellular adhesion molecule 3-grabbing nonintegrin. *J. Allergy Clin. Immunol.* **115**:1260–1267.

Soder, K. J., and L. A. Holden. 1999. Dry matter intake and milk yield and composition of cows fed yeast prepartum and postpartum. *J. Dairy Sci.* **82**:605–610.

Stavric, S., and J.-Y. D'Aoust. 1993. Undefined and defined bacterial preparations for the competitive exclusion of *Salmonella* in poultry—a review. *J. Food Prot.* **56**:173–180.

Stephens, T. P., G. H. Loneragan, L. M. Chichester, and M. M. Brashears. 2007. Prevalence and enumeration of *Escherichia coli* O157 in steers receiving various strains of *Lactobacillus*-based direct-fed microbials. *J. Food Prot.* **70**:1252–1255.

Strompfova, V., M. Marcinakova, M. Simonova, B. Bogovic-Matijasic, and A. Laukova. 2006a. Application of potential probiotic *Lactobacillus fermentum* AD1 strain in healthy dogs. *Anaerobe* **12**:75–79.

Strompfova, V., M. Marcinakova, M. Simonova, S. Gancarcikova, Z. Jonecova, L. Scirankova, J. Koscova, V. Buleca, K. Cobanova, and A. Laukova. 2006b. *Enterococcus faecium* EK13—an enterocin a-producing strain with probiotic character and its effect in piglets. *Anaerobe* **12**:242–248.

Taras, D., W. Vahjen, M. Macha, and O. Simon. 2005. Response of performance characteristics and fecal consistency to long-lasting dietary supplementation with the probiotic strain *Bacillus cereus* var. toyoi to sows and piglets. *Arch. Anim. Nutr.* **59**:405–417.

Timmerman, H. M., L. Mulder, H. Everts, D. C. van Espen, E. van der Wal, G. Klaassen, S. M. Rouwers, R. Hartemink, F. M. Rombouts, and A. C. Beynen. 2005. Health and growth of veal calves fed milk replacers with or without probiotics. *J. Dairy Sci.* **88**:2154–2165.

Tkalcic, S., T. Zhao, B. G. Harmon, M. P. Doyle, C. A. Brown, and P. Zhao. 2003. Fecal shedding of enterohemorrhagic *Escherichia coli* in weaned calves following treatment with probiotic *Escherichia coli*. *J. Food Prot.* **66**:1184–1189.

van der Wolf, P. J., W. B. Wolbers, A. R. Elbers, H. M. van der Heijden, J. M. Koppen, W. A. Hunneman, F. W. van Schie, and M. J. Tielen. 2001. Herd level husbandry factors associated with the serological *Salmonella* prevalence in finishing pig herds in The Netherlands. *Vet. Microbiol.* **78**:205–219.

van Winsen, R. L., D. Keuzenkamp, B. A. Urlings, L. J. Lipman, J. A. Snijders, J. H. Verheijden, and F. van Knapen. 2002. Effect of fermented feed on shedding of *Enterobacteriaceae* by fattening pigs. *Vet. Microbiol.* **87**:267–276.

van Winsen, R. L., B. A. Urlings, L. J. Lipman, J. M. Snijders, D. Keuzenkamp, J. H. Verheijden, and F. van Knapen. 2001. Effect of fermented feed on the microbial population of the gastrointestinal tracts of pigs. *Appl. Environ. Microbiol.* **67**:3071–3076.

Weese, J. S. 2002. Microbiologic evaluation of commercial probiotics. *J. Am. Vet. Med. Assoc.* **220**:794–797.

Weese, J. S. 2003. Evaluation of deficiencies in labeling of commercial probiotics. *Can. Vet. J.* **44**:982–983.

Weese, J. S., and M. E. Anderson. 2002. Preliminary evaluation of *Lactobacillus rhamnosus* strain GG, a potential probiotic in dogs. *Can. Vet. J.* **43**:771–774.

Weese, J. S., M. E. Anderson, A. Lowe, and G. J. Monteith. 2003. Preliminary investigation of the probiotic potential of *Lactobacillus rhamnosus* strain GG in horses: fecal recovery following oral administration and safety. *Can. Vet. J.* **44**:299–302.

Weese, J. S., M. E. Anderson, A. Lowe, R. Penno, T. M. da Costa, L. Button, and K. C. Goth. 2004a. Screening of the equine intestinal microflora for potential probiotic organisms. *Equine Vet. J.* **36**:351–355.

Weese, J. S., and L. Arroyo. 2003. Bacteriological evaluation of dog and cat diets that claim to contain probiotics. *Can. Vet. J.* **44**:212–216.

Weese, J. S., and J. Rousseau. 2005. Evaluation of *Lactobacillus pentosus* WE7 for prevention of diarrhea in neonatal foals. *J. Am. Vet. Med. Assoc.* **226**:2031–2034.

Weese, J. S., H. E. Weese, L. Yuricek, and J. Rousseau. 2004b. Oxalate degradation by intestinal lactic acid bacteria in dogs and cats. *Vet. Microbiol.* **101**:161–166.

Williams, P. E., C. A. Tait, G. M. Innes, and C. J. Newbold. 1991. Effects of the inclusion of yeast culture (*Saccharomyces cerevisiae* plus growth medium) in the diet of dairy cows on milk yield and forage degradation and fermentation patterns in the rumen of steers. *J. Anim. Sci.* **69**:3016–3026.

Withanage, G. S., P. Kaiser, P. Wigley, C. Powers, P. Mastroeni, H. Brooks, P. Barrow, A. Smith, D. Maskell, and I. McConnell. 2004. Rapid expression of chemokines and proinflammatory cytokines in newly hatched chickens infected with *Salmonella enterica* serovar Typhimurium. *Infect. Immun.* 72:2152–2159.

Withanage, G. S., P. Wigley, P. Kaiser, P. Mastroeni, H. Brooks, C. Powers, R. Beal, P. Barrow, D. Maskell, and I. McConnell. 2005. Cytokine and chemokine responses associated with clearance of a primary *Salmonella enterica* serovar Typhimurium infection in the chicken and in protective immunity to rechallenge. *Infect. Immun.* 73:5173–5182.

Yasuda, K., and T. Fukata. 2004. Mixed feed containing dextran improves milk production of Holstein dairy cows. *J. Vet. Med. Sci.* 66:1287–1288.

Yasuda, K., S. Hashikawa, H. Sakamoto, Y. Tomita, S. Shibata, and T. Fukata. 2007. A new synbiotic consisting of *Lactobacillus casei* subsp. *casei* and dextran improves milk production in Holstein dairy cows. *J. Vet. Med. Sci.* 69:205–208.

Yoon, I. K., and M. D. Stern. 1995. Influence of direct-fed microbials on ruminal microbial fermentation and performance of ruminants: a review. *Asian-Australian J. Anim. Sci.* 8:533–555.

Younts-Dahl, S. M., M. L. Galyean, G. H. Loneragan, N. A. Elam, and M. M. Brashears. 2004. Dietary supplementation with *Lactobacillus*- and *Propionibacterium*-based direct-fed microbials and prevalence of *Escherichia coli* O157 in beef feedlot cattle and on hides at harvest. *J. Food Prot.* 67:889–893.

Younts-Dahl, S. M., G. D. Osborn, M. L. Galyean, J. D. Rivera, G. H. Loneragan, and M. M. Brashears. 2005. Reduction of *Escherichia coli* O157 in finishing beef cattle by various doses of *Lactobacillus acidophilus* in direct-fed microbials. *J. Food Prot.* 68:6–10.

Yu, P., J. T. Huber, C. B. Theurer, K. H. Chen, L. G. Nussio, and Z. Wu. 1997. Effect of steam-flaked or steam-rolled corn with or without *Aspergillus oryzae* in the diet on performance of dairy cows fed during hot weather. *J. Dairy Sci.* 80:3293–3297.

Zeyner, A., and E. Boldt. 2006. Effects of a probiotic *Enterococcus faecium* strain supplemented from birth to weaning on diarrhoea patterns and performance of piglets. *J. Anim. Physiol. Anim. Nutr.* (Berlin) 90:25–31.

Zhao, T., M. P. Doyle, B. G. Harmon, C. A. Brown, P. O. Mueller, and A. H. Parks. 1998. Reduction of carriage of enterohemorrhagic *Escherichia coli* O157:H7 in cattle by inoculation with probiotic bacteria. *J. Clin. Microbiol.* 36:641–647.

Zhao, T., S. Tkalcic, M. P. Doyle, B. G. Harmon, C. A. Brown, and P. Zhao. 2003. Pathogenicity of enterohemorrhagic *Escherichia coli* in neonatal calves and evaluation of fecal shedding by treatment with probiotic *Escherichia coli*. *J. Food Prot.* 66:924–930.

Therapeutic Microbiology: Probiotics and Related Strategies
Edited by J. Versalovic and M. Wilson
© 2008 ASM Press, Washington, DC

David Hernot, Eva Ogué,
George Fahey, Robert A. Rastall

27

Prebiotics and Synbiotics in Companion Animal Science

There is now considerable evidence to suggest that the colonic microbiota is susceptible to manipulation through diet (Salminen et al., 1998). Certain foods, recognized as colonic functional foods, confer additional health benefits by improving the composition and activities of the gastrointestinal microbiota (Bellisle et al., 1998). Dietary components used for this purpose include probiotics, prebiotics, and synbiotics. Infections of the gastrointestinal tract (GIT) have an impact on the entire organism (Salminen et al., 1995) and are a major health problem that accounts for a large percentage of veterinary admissions. Lately, it has been of increasing interest to pet food manufacturers, as an alternative to antibiotics, to incorporate these approaches into the diet of dogs and cats in order to prevent disease or to reduce the incidence of common pathogenic bacteria. In addition, pet owners are progressively becoming more aware of the important role of diet in the health and well-being of their pets. Aside from its role in nutrition, pet food manufacturers have recently begun to exploit diet as a tool to manage host health (Tzortzis et al., 2003a).

THE CANINE AND FELINE GIT

Even though dogs and cats present anatomical and morphological differences in their GIT, the structure and the functionality in the two mammals are comparable (O'Brien, 2005). The GIT is an extremely complex organ having multiple functions directed toward the digestion and absorption of nutrients and the control of potentially harmful pathogens and the commensal microbiota (Buddington, 1996; Stokes and Waly, 2006). In both dogs and cats, the colon is the main site of microbial colonization, resulting in a complex ecosystem that can influence the overall health of the host animal (Bornside and Cohn, 1965; Strombeck, 1990; Buddington and Paulsen, 1998). In addition to their role in gastrointestinal immunity, commensal microbial populations are critically important in pathogen resistance, production of short-chain fatty acids (SCFA), mucosal barrier fortification, and angiogenesis (Banta et al., 1979; Gibson and Macfarlane, 1995; Swanson et al., 2002a; McManus et al., 2002). Nevertheless, comprehensive studies of the feline and canine intestinal microbiota are scarce, as much of the information presently available is from

David Hernot and George Fahey, Dept. of Animal Sciences, University of Illinois, 1207 W. Gregory Dr., Urbana, IL 61801. **Eva Ogué and Robert A. Rastall,** Dept. of Food Biosciences, P.O. Box 226, The University of Reading, Whiteknights, Reading, RG6 6AP, United Kingdom.

studies which have used standard culture techniques (Itoh et al., 1984; Osbaldiston and Stowe, 1971; Davis et al., 1977; Benno et al., 1992a, 1992b). The culturing technique has several drawbacks for use in enumeration and diversity studies, mainly due to the poor selectivity of nutrient media and the recovery of only cultivable bacteria. Consequently, information on the bacterial diversity and bacterial populations derived from such studies is not totally reliable (Greetham et al., 2002).

Previous studies have shown common bacterial groups isolated from different regions of the GIT and from the feces of dogs and cats; however, there is variation between these studies concerning the population numbers (Mitsuoka, 1969, 1992; Davis et al., 1977; Balish et al., 1977; Benno et al., 1992b; Buddington, 2003; Mentula et al., 2005). The most common bacterial groups isolated from dogs include clostridia, bacteroides, streptococci, coliforms, enterococci, lactobacilli, and bifidobacteria with counts increasing towards the large intestine (Bornside and Cohn, 1965; Davis et al., 1977; Mentula et al., 2005). The main bacterial groups found so far (by both culturing and molecular techniques) in the feline fecal contents are enterococci, *Escherichia coli*, lactobacilli, clostridia, eubacteria, and bacteroides (Osbaldiston and Stowe, 1971; Itoh et al., 1984; Inness et al., 2007). Nevertheless, the predominant bacterial groups differ between studies, particularly with regard to bifidobacteria, which appear to be very inconsistent between individuals, mainly in cats (Mitsuoka, 1969; Davis et al., 1977; Balish et al., 1977; Itoh et al., 1984; Benno et al., 1992b; Buddington, 2003; Rinkinen et al., 2004; Mentula et al., 2005; Inness et al., 2007). More recently, two different studies have described the canine colonic microbiota by using molecular techniques. Simpson et al. (2002) enumerated bacterial groups from feces of healthy adult German shepherd dogs by selective media and confirmed their identity by denaturing gradient gel electrophoresis. Tzortzis et al. (2004b) used fluorescence in situ hybridization (FISH) to enumerate the fecal microbiota of one Labrador dog. In both studies *Eubacterium* spp. and *Bacteroides* spp. were the predominant groups while *Bifidobacterium* spp. levels were much lower. The two studies also showed discrepancies with regard to the predominance of lactobacilli—these were 100-fold higher (10^9 log cells/g of feces) when enumerated by selective media than by the FISH method (10^7 log cells/g of feces).

Regardless of the limitations of culture-dependent techniques, different factors can alter the relative proportions and metabolic activities of the various bacterial groups (Buddington, 1996). Factors such as environment, breed, age, and, of course, diet can influence the

canine and feline gut microbiota (Balish et al., 1977; Itoh et al., 1984; Benno and Mitsuoka, 1992; Benno et al., 1992a, 1992b; Czarnecki-Maulden and Russell, 2000; Patil et al., 2000; Simpson et al., 2002). There are many different breeds of dogs, each of which differs considerably in body size. The beagle has been the most extensively studied breed in terms of intestinal microbiology and anatomy (Clapper and Meade, 1963; Clapper, 1970; Davis et al., 1977). It has been demonstrated that there is a relationship between total transit time and fecal quality in dogs differing in body size (Hernot et al., 2005), and it would not be surprising if this factor also had an impact on the gut microbiota. Although different breeds of cats exist, differences in body size are not as distinguishable as in dogs and it may be that the variations in bacterial populations would be less significant. Unfortunately, to our knowledge, no studies on the effect of breed on the feline colonic microbiota have been published. Previous studies with humans have shown that variations in the gut microbiota occur with aging. Species such as bifidobacteria, which are regarded as beneficial, are thought to decline in numbers, whereas clostridial and enterobacterial populations, which are viewed as being detrimental to health, increase (Mitsuoka, 1992; Hopkins and Macfarlane, 2002). Benno et al. (1992a) characterized the changes in microbial populations of dogs with aging, reporting a decrease in lactobacillus and bidifobacterial levels in the cecum and colon of elder dogs and an increase in the numbers of *Clostridium perfringens*. These results are in disagreement with a study carried out by Simpson et al. (2002), who reported that the numbers of lactobacilli and bifidobacteria were not influenced by the age of dogs. Only bacteroides were significantly higher ($P < 0.01$) in younger dogs. Further studies are required in order to obtain a more comprehensive picture of the various species that colonize the intestine of dogs and cats and thereby to explain the effect that different intrinsic or extrinsic factors may have on their intestinal microbiota.

Under certain circumstances (antibiotic intake, stress, or poor diet), the microbial balance can be perturbed, resulting in increased numbers of pathogenic species that can cause acute or chronic gut problems (Guilford and Matz, 2003). Species such as *E. coli*, *Salmonella* spp., *Clostridium* spp., or *Campylobacter* spp. are pathogens associated with enteric infections in canines and felines (Nair et al., 1985; Beaudry et al., 1996; Beutin et al., 1999). Although the role of the endogenous microbiota in feline and canine gastrointestinal disorders has not been thoroughly evaluated, it is believed that enteropathogenic bacteria produce colonic disease by invading the epithelium or by attaching to the mucosa, producing enterotoxins that are cytotoxic or that promote fluid and electrolyte secretion (Cave, 2003; Jergens and Zoran, 2005). Intestinal diseases in dogs and cats include small intestinal bacteria overgrowth, inflammatory bowel disease, chronic small bowel diarrhea, chronic large bowel diarrhea, and colon cancer (Kirk et al., 2000; Debraekeleer et al., 2000; Guilford and Matz, 2003; Jergens and Zoran, 2005).

The present contribution focuses on how the addition of prebiotics and synbiotics to the diets of dogs and cats can be viewed as a tool to manage the GIT ecosystem and enhance the health of these companion animals.

Carbohydrates Used as Prebiotics in Companion Animals

The main category of compound with prebiotic activity is the oligosaccharide, although selected dietary fibers and resistant starches may demonstrate prebiotic activity as well (Swanson et al., 2002a; Topping et al., 2003). Of all the oligosaccharides, the fructans have been the most widely tested in companion animals, including chicory (a natural source of long-chain fructan), inulin (a long-chain fructan), oligofructose (OF) (fructan chains with 8 to 10 units), and short-chain fructo-oligosaccharides (scFOS) (fructan chains with three to five units). The effects of lactosucrose, lactulose, maltodextrin-like oligosaccharides, α-gluco-oligosaccharides, mannanoligosaccharides (MOS), isomalto-oligosaccharides (IMO), and galacto-oligosaccharides also have been tested in companion animals (mostly in dogs). Nevertheless, not all of these carbohydrates may satisfy the Gibson and Roberfroid (1995) definition of a prebiotic. Finally, two glucose-based nonstructural carbohydrates, pullulan and γ-cyclodextrin, have recently been described as prebiotics in a canine study (Spears et al., 2005). Most of the prebiotics have been tested in only a limited number of studies, and the primary outcomes were confined to nutrient digestibility, stool quality, or selective microbiota changes. It appears that prebiotic supplementation has several beneficial effects in the GIT of dogs and cats. However, relatively little information exists as regards their inclusion in companion animal diets.

Prebiotic Concentrations in Dietary Ingredients

The practice of dietary supplementation of fructans or other oligosaccharides will depend, in part, on the contribution of natural prebiotics in pet food ingredients. Because of the lack of a database on the concentrations of fructans or other oligosaccharides in pet food ingredients, 25 common pet food ingredients were selected and analyzed for fructan concentration (Hussein et al., 1998). In this study, the concentrations of three

major subcomponents of fructans (1-kestotriose [GF$_2$], 1,1-kestotetraose [GF$_3$], and 1,1,1-kestopentaose [GF$_4$]) were assayed using anion-exchange high-performance liquid chromatography. No fructans were detected in corn, corn distiller's solubles, hominy, milo, brown rice, white rice, brewer's rice, rice hulls, seaweed, or soybean meal. On a dry matter (DM) basis, wheat coproducts (bran, germ, and middlings) contained the highest concentrations of total fructans, followed by peanut hulls, alfalfa meal, barley, and wheat grain. The remaining ingredients contained very low concentrations (<0.4 mg/g). In another study, Van Loo et al. (1995) reported the concentrations of inulin and oligofructose in common dietary ingredients (Table 1). Their analyses quantified glucose and fructose released by enzymatic hydrolysis of the food or plant material and assayed oligofructose (degree of polymerization [DP], up to 10) and inulin contents with a DP of 2 to 60 (Quemener et al., 1994). Values were reported on an "as-is" basis and indicated the range of concentrations determined due to variation in sources of each food or plant material. Garlic contained the highest concentration of oligofructose. Wheat and dried onion contained similar amounts of oligofructose, while rye flour and barley contained the lowest

Table 1 Fructan content of selected feeds, pet foods, and food ingredients

Item	Fructan content (mg/g)	
	DM basis[a]	"As is" basis[b]
Alfalfa meal	2.24	
Barley	1.92	0.05–0.10
Beet pulp	0.05	
Canola meal	0.04	
Corn gluten feed	0.09	
Corn gluten meal	0.34	
Garlic		0.98–1.60
Oats	0.36	
Oat groats	0.12	
Onion, dried		0.11–0.75
Peanut hulls	2.40	
Rice bran	0.14	
Rye flour		0.05–0.10
Soybean hulls	0.12	
Wheat	1.36	0.10–0.40
Wheat bran	4.00	
Wheat germ	4.68	
Wheat middlings	5.07	

[a]As defined by Hussein et al. (1998), i.e., sum of 1-kestotriose, 1,1-kestotetraose, and 1,1,1-kestopentaose.

[b]As defined by van Loo et al. (1995), i.e., sum of inulin and oligofructose with DP of 2 to 60.

concentrations. The authors concluded that oligofructose and inulin were present in measurable quantities in a wide variety of common foods and food ingredients. Other oligosaccharides have been studied to a lesser extent than fructans.

Prebiotic Intake by Companion Animals

The use of fructan-containing ingredients in diet formulations provides an intrinsic source of oligosaccharides. However, wheat, wheat coproducts, alfalfa meal, barley, and peanut hulls may not commonly be incorporated into diets at high rates. Corn gluten meal, oats, oat groats, soybean hulls, and rice bran, containing lesser amounts of fructans, are more widely utilized in companion animal diets. As regards garlic and onion, they are not commonly included in companion animal diets. Unless supplements are employed, fructans intake by companion animals is dependent on their concentration in dietary ingredients and the quantity of fructan-containing ingredients included in a given diet (Flickinger et al., 2003a). Nevertheless, very little information is known about the natural fructan content of pet foods, and their contribution to the dietary fiber fraction is not taken into account in any nutritional recommendations. This is also true for other oligosaccharides.

Safety Considerations

It is well established that high concentrations of prebiotics (e.g., 3 to 6% of diet DM) result in significant positive changes in most of the response criteria tested in canine and feline experiments. However, these high concentrations are impractical both from physiological and economic points of view. Very little research conducted to date has addressed the issue of low-level inclusion of prebiotics in companion animal diets. Our experience suggests that concentrations of active ingredient (i.e., the oligosaccharide exclusive of carrier or associated substances) ranging from 0.1 to 0.75% of diet DM are efficacious.

IN VITRO FERMENTATION EXPERIMENTS USING CANINE AND FELINE FECAL INOCULUM

Numerous in vitro fermentation experiments using a canine or feline fecal inoculum have evaluated the fermentation profiles of carbohydrates, quantified as SCFA production. Vickers et al. (2001) used an in vitro fermentation system to test prebiotic fermentability. In this study, yeast cell wall (YCW) containing MOS, scFOS, and four inulin sources were compared to beet pulp, cellulose, and soy fiber, which are common fiber sources

used in pet diets. Substrates were fermented at 39°C for 6, 12, and 24 h. Lactate and SCFA concentrations were determined and used as a measure of fermentability. Inulin sources varied as regards DP and solubility, as follows: (i) DP = 2 to 8; (ii) DP = 9, but insoluble in water; (iii) DP = 9, but soluble in water; and (iv) DP > 12. Fermentation of MOS resulted in moderate concentrations of total SCFA after 6 h (0.49 mmol/g of organic matter), 12 h (1.45 mmol/g), and 24 h (2.40 mmol/g) of in vitro fermentation. All inulin sources and scFOS were highly fermentable. In comparison, scFOS produced 0.97, 3.60, and 4.60 mmol of SCFA/g. Very low concentrations of lactate were produced as a result of YCW fermentation. In contrast, fermentation of scFOS and all inulin sources resulted in greater ($P < 0.05$) lactate concentrations than YCW and control fiber sources. Fructan chain length (DP) also affected SCFA production over time, with scFOS resulting in greater ($P < 0.05$) lactate concentrations than three of the four inulin sources after 12 and 24 h of fermentation. The results of this study demonstrate the prebiotic nature of fructans, with rapid production of SCFA and lactate. YCW, however, was only moderately fermentable and lacked the ability to promote growth of lactic acid bacteria.

In addition to fermentability, two other in vitro studies tested the prebiotic potential of carbohydrates by evaluating their effects on bacterial populations (Tzortzis et al., 2004a, 2004b). In the first study, the authors evaluated the effects of various carbohydrate sources on the production of extracellular antagonistic compounds against two E. coli strains and Salmonella enterica serotype Typhimurium by three canine-derived lactobacilli strains. In a second study, the same researchers evaluated in vitro fermentation properties of prebiotics by using a canine fecal inoculum (Tzortzis et al., 2004b). Primary outcomes included bacterial growth as measured by FISH and SCFA production after 10 and 24 h of fermentation. The probes used in this study were Bif164, Bac303, Lab158, His150, Ec1531, and Erec482, specific for Bifidobacterium spp., Bacteroides/Prevotella group, Lactobacillus/Enterococcus group, Clostridium clusters I and II (including C. perfringens/Clostridium histolyticum), E. coli, and Clostridium coccoides/Eubacterium rectale group, respectively. Compared to baseline values, all substrates increased the total bacterial counts as well as the bifidobacterial and lactobacillus concentrations. In addition, FOS fermentation decreased ($P < 0.05$) E. coli concentration and increased ($P < 0.05$) clostridial concentrations. As expected, all substrates increased SCFA and lactate concentrations compared to baseline. In the first study, some substrates were reported to induce an inhibitory effect on the growth of certain pathogenic bacteria. Overall, these results demonstrate the ability of certain carbohydrates to aid in resistance to pathogens. Because these studies included combinations of bacteria and carbohydrates, further details of the results obtained are described in the synbiotic section.

CANINE PREBIOTIC EXPERIMENTS

Although the canine and feline prebiotic literature is not as robust as that of humans, their use has gained steady support over the past decade. In contrast to many of the prebiotic experiments using rodents, most canine experiments have tested prebiotics at low dietary concentrations ($\leq 1\%$). Concentrations greater than 1% are not relevant to canine nutrition and health from the perspective of both digestive physiology and economics (Swanson and Fahey, 2006).

Effects on Fecal Characteristics

Stool consistency and volume produced are important criteria used by pet owners when selecting a food. Thus, food intake and fecal characteristics are important outcomes of prebiotic supplementation and have been reported in most experiments. When prebiotics are provided in the diet at concentrations of 1 to 2%, as occurs in most of the canine prebiotic experiments, food intake is generally unaffected (Swanson et al., 2002b, 2002c; Verlinden et al., 2006; Middelbos et al., 2007). Nevertheless, one study reported an increased trend in food intake with MOS and chicory + MOS supplementation in senior dogs (Grieshop et al., 2004). However, even at constant food intake across treatments, prebiotic supplementation may result in greater wet fecal volume, decreased fecal DM percentage, and decreased fecal pH. Although prebiotic consumption may result in production of softer feces (Twomey et al., 2003; Grieshop et al., 2004), canine experiments have generated mixed results (Zentek et al., 2003; Flickinger et al., 2002). In general, effects on fecal characteristics may vary depending on the concentration and the nature of the prebiotic and the type of diet fed (Flickinger et al., 2003a). Prebiotics have been reported to increase stool frequency and moisture content in humans, thereby effectively preventing and treating constipation (Hidaka et al., 1986; Kleessen et al., 1997). Similar benefits apply to dogs when supplemented at low concentrations (1 to 2%).

Effect on Nutrient Digestibility

Macronutrient digestibility is a primary contributor to fecal characteristics and was a primary outcome measured in the canine prebiotic experiments. While the majority of the experiments measured total tract digestibility, a few also measured nutrient digestibility at the terminal ileum (Propst et al., 2003; Flickinger et al., 2003b; Middelbos et al., 2007). The literature suggests that prebiotic consumption decreases total tract macronutrient (e.g., organic matter [OM], crude protein [CP]) digestibility by dogs. Propst et al. (2003) tested three concentrations (0.3, 0.6, and 0.9% of diet, as-fed basis) of two fructans, OF and inulin, against a 0% supplemental fructan control. Total tract digestibilities of DM, OM, and CP decreased ($P < 0.05$) as a result of dietary OF and inulin supplementation. These effects of OF supplementation on total tract macronutrient digestibility were confirmed by Flickinger et al. (2003b), and similar results were observed with MOS, IMO, and FOS (Zentek et al., 2002; Hesta et al., 2003; Middelbos et al., 2007). It is of interest that in the Propst et al. (2003) study, total tract digestibilities of CP exhibited a trend toward a quadratic decrease when dogs were supplemented with OF ($P < 0.10$) and inulin ($P < 0.06$) and that total tract CP digestibility decreased linearly with OF inclusion in the diet (from 81.7% with the control diet to 79.5% with 0.9% OF concentration; $P < 0.05$). Like other fermentable fiber sources, prebiotic supplementation often increases fecal nitrogen (bacterial mass) concentrations (Cummings et al., 1979; Cummings and Bingham, 1987). Ileal CP digestibility, a more accurate measure of protein availability to the host, has not been found to be affected in the canine studies published thus far. Because fermentable substrates are known to influence N metabolism, some canine experiments focused on the effect of prebiotic supplementation on fecal N excretion. In general, prebiotic consumption resulted in increased fecal N excretion in the form of bacterial N (Hesta et al., 2003; Karr-Lilienthal et al., 2004). The increased use of colonic N for bacterial protein synthesis, resulting in greater fecal N and decreased total tract N digestibility, is not a negative outcome of prebiotic consumption. As is discussed below, these outcomes may, in fact, prove to be beneficial as regards the overall health of the colon.

Rodent studies have reported improved mineral absorption in animals fed prebiotics. This effect is believed to be due to an increased production of SCFA, which improve colonic absorption of Na^+, Ca^{2+} and Cl^- (Binder and Mehta, 1989; Lutz and Scharrer, 1991). Increased absorption is thought to be due to exchange mechanisms (e.g., Na^+-H^+ exchange) present in the colon. The work of Beynen et al. (2002) has been the only canine study to evaluate prebiotic effects on mineral absorption. As in rodent studies, increased Ca and Mg absorption was reported in dogs consuming 1% OF. As mineral absorption efficiency is important in several canine life stages, physiological states, and/or breeds, more research on this topic is needed.

Effect on Microbial Populations

By definition, a nondigestible carbohydrate is considered to be a prebiotic only if it stimulates the activity or number of one or a select number of microorganisms (Gibson and Roberfroid, 1995). Therefore, intestinal microbial populations have been one of the most common outcome variables measured in canine studies. Lactate-producing bacteria such as *Lactobacillus* spp. and *Bifidobacterium* spp. are believed to be beneficial members of the colonic microbiota of dogs and cats; however, more research is needed to substantiate this. Even though *Clostridium* spp. and *E. coli* are members of the intestinal microbiota and may reside in healthy animals without disease for years, they are considered to be potential pathogens and often are viewed as examples of detrimental bacteria. Similar to the human literature (Gibson et al., 1995; Bouhnik et al., 1999), canine studies often have reported beneficial outcomes of prebiotic supplementation on microbial populations. Most of the canine experiments reported greater fecal bifidobacterial and lower fecal clostridial concentrations in dogs consuming prebiotics. This beneficial effect on bacterial populations was particularly verified with MOS and scFOS (<2% supplementation), chicory (from 1 to 4% supplementation), and inulin (3% supplementation) (Russell, 1998; Strickling et al., 2000; Swanson et al., 2002b; Zentek et al., 2003) (Table 2). Although not measured in all experiments, lactobacillus concentrations also were reported to increase in the feces of prebiotic-fed dogs. In two studies, lactobacillus concentrations were reported to increase in both ileal and fecal samples (Swanson et al., 2002d; Spears et al., 2005). Spears et al. (2005) tested the prebiotic potential of high-molecular-weight pullulan and γ-cyclodextrin fed to dogs at low concentrations. Increasing pullulan tended ($P < 0.10$) to linearly increase bifidobacteria and lactobacilli and quadratically increase fecal lactobacilli. A similar response was noted for ileal bifidobacteria and lactobacilli with γ-cyclodextrin. γ-Cyclodextrin resulted in a quadratic decrease ($P < 0.05$) in fecal *C. perfringens*. The authors concluded that pullulan and

γ-cyclodextrin supplementation may have beneficial effects on the microbial ecology of dogs. The responses of other microbial species to prebiotic supplementation have been inconsistent (Terada et al., 1992; Beynen et al., 2002), but the ability of prebiotics, fructans in particular, to influence the bacterial composition of the gut microbiota in dogs is now evident (Vanhoutte et al., 2005). Given these results, it appears that prebiotics beneficially manipulate intestinal microbial populations in dogs. With the increased use of molecular techniques to identify bacterial species and evaluate dietary responses on the colonic microbiota, this line of research will continue to increase our understanding of microbe-host interactions and the influences of dietary manipulation.

Effect on Fermentation Products

While bacterial numbers alone may indicate some degree of intestinal health status, fermentative end product concentrations also are important criteria when evaluating prebiotic potential. Acetate, propionate, and butyrate are the primary SCFA produced from carbohydrate fermentation, and butyrate is the main energy source for colonocytes (Roediger, 1980). Along with lactate, an intermediary product of bacterial fermentation, these organic acids decrease luminal pH and assist in pathogen resistance. In vitro experiments suggest that SCFA increase the expression of intestinal heat shock proteins, a highly conserved family of stress proteins crucial to the integrity of the GIT (Ren et al., 2001). Because of their demonstrated importance, the majority of canine prebiotic studies measured fecal SCFA and/or lactate concentrations. Several of these studies reported increased fecal concentrations in dogs consuming prebiotics (Flickinger et al., 2003b; Propst et al., 2003; Twomey et al., 2003; Middelbos et al., 2007). In these studies, fecal acetate, propionate, butyrate, total SCFA, and lactate concentrations followed a common trend, increasing as a result of prebiotic consumption. For example, Flickinger et al. (2003b) showed a 40% increase in fecal total SCFA with 0.9% OF concentration in the diet. Although the

Table 2 Summary of effects of prebiotics on microbial populations of dogs[a]

Reference	Diet	Prebiotic	Level	Lactobacilli	Bifidobacteria	*E. coli*	Clostridia
Russell, 1998	Dry	Chicory	3% diet	NR	↑	NR	↓
		scFOS	1% diet	NR	↑	NR	↓
Swanson et al., 2002b	Dry	scFOS	4 g/day	↑	↑	↔	↓
Zentek et al., 2003	Dry	Inulin	1.5% diet	NR	↑	NR	↓
Grieshop et al., 2004	Dry	MOS	1% diet	↔	↑	↓	↔

[a]NR, not reported; ↑, increased; ↓, decreased; ↔, no change. Adapted from Swanson et al., 2006.

measurement of SCFA concentrations in the proximal colon would be useful, sample collection in this part of the GIT is usually not possible in canine studies. Because SCFA are rapidly absorbed by the host (von Englehardt et al., 1989), it is not known how well fecal SCFA concentrations correlate with luminal SCFA concentrations. Nevertheless, fecal SCFA are reflective of descending colon SCFA concentrations, and it is in the descending colon that the majority of bowel disease occurs. As a consequence, the increase in fecal SCFA and lactate concentrations is a potentially beneficial outcome of prebiotic supplementation.

Effect on Protein Catabolites

In contrast to the benefits that occur from carbohydrate fermentation, the outcomes of microbial breakdown of proteins in the colon are usually detrimental. Increasing protein flow to the colon provides more substrates for potential pathogens such as *C. perfringens*, which is known for its ability to degrade amino acids and produce fecal odor. In addition to being responsible for fecal odor, protein catabolites are harmful to the intestinal epithelia. For example, high ammonia concentrations are suspected to contribute to colon carcinogenesis (Visek, 1978), while phenols have been positively associated with intestinal disease (Ramakrishna et al., 1991). Fermentable carbohydrates, including prebiotics, may decrease colonic protein catabolite concentrations by providing the gut microbiota with an additional energy supply. In the colon, bacteria act as N sinks, utilizing undigested proteins and their metabolites in the presence of energy for protein synthesis (Cummings et al., 1979). Bacteria use ammonia as a major source of N, and other forms of protein or amino acids are deaminated to ammonia before being used metabolically (Jackson, 1995). Thus, by providing sufficient energy in the form of fermentable carbohydrates, bacteria are able to use available amino acids for their own protein synthesis rather than using them for energy, a process that results in the production of putrefactive compounds.

Fecal ammonia concentrations determined in different studies appear to be highly variable and do not indicate any clear response to prebiotic supplementation (Zentek et al., 2002; Swanson et al., 2002c; Hesta et al., 2003; Middelbos et al., 2007). Branched-chain fatty acid concentrations followed a similar pattern, resulting in contradictory data. The most convincing evidence related the positive effects of prebiotics on phenol and indole concentrations (Swanson et al., 2002b, 2002c; Propst et al., 2003), which were substantially decreased (up to 50% decrease in total fecal phenol and indole concentrations with FOS supplementation [Swanson et al., 2002b]), despite no changes being observed in certain studies (Middelbos et al., 2007). Given the popularity of high-protein diet feeding of canines, there is a need to identify ingredients capable of decreasing the putrefactive compounds produced from excess protein intake. The results of the studies performed thus far suggest a potential role for prebiotics in this regard.

Immune Effects

The GIT is the largest immune organ of the body (Jalkanen, 1990), with the gut-associated lymphoid tissues (GALT) possessing approximately 80% of the body's immunological-substance secreting cells (Brandtzaeg et al., 1989) and more than 50% of the immune effector cells (McKay and Perdue, 1993). It has been well established that the development of GALT is highly dependent on colonization by bacterial populations in the gut. Even after the gastrointestinal immune system is fully developed, immune cells are on constant guard against pathogenic invasion. Given the role of the microbiota on GALT and the potential for prebiotics to manipulate gut microbial ecology, it is logical to hypothesize enhanced gut immunity in response to prebiotic supplementation. The stimulation of the intestinal immune system by scFOS has already been described in dogs (Field et al., 1999). However, few canine studies have evaluated the effects of prebiotics on immune indices in the blood (white blood cell concentrations and serum immunoglobulin A [IgA]) and/or GIT (IgA concentrations in ileal digesta). IgA is important in mucosal immunity as it inhibits the attachment and penetration of bacteria in the lumen, increases mucus secretion (McKay and Perdue, 1993), and prevents inflammatory reactions that potentially would result in damage to the epithelial tissues (Russell et al., 1989). The presence of normal IgA concentrations may play a role in some intestinal diseases, as reduced IgA concentrations have been associated with Crohn's disease in humans (MacDermott et al., 1986) and with small intestinal bacterial overgrowth in dogs (Batt et al., 1991). In 2007, Adogony et al. (2007) evaluated the effect of dietary supplementation with scFOS on mucosal immunoglobulin concentration in mammary secretions. The results showed that in colostrum and in milk, during the whole lactation period, the level of IgM was constantly ($P < 0.01$) higher (as a mean, 1.4 times more) in scFOS-supplemented female dogs than in controls. Generally speaking, significant effects of prebiotics on immune cell populations were reported. Nevertheless, results across studies have been conflicting and no clear trends can be identified at this time for both ileal or serum IgA and blood cell concentrations (Swanson et al., 2002c, 2002d; Grieshop et al., 2004; Verlinden et al., 2006; Middelbos et al., 2007). Future experiments should not only determine immune cell numbers but also test their functional capacity (e.g., lymphocyte blastogenesis or phagocytic activity of neutrophils) to more accurately evaluate prebiotic effects on immune capacity.

Effects on Gastrointestinal Morphology

It appears that prebiotic supplementation increases intestinal length, weight, and surface area, colonic blood flow, and small intestinal carrier-mediated glucose uptake in dogs. Howard et al. (1999) evaluated the effects of different fiber sources on epithelial cell proliferation, intestinal weight, and colonic blood flow in dogs. Twenty-eight adult dogs surgically fitted with ultrasonic blood flow probes were randomly assigned to one of four treatments: beet pulp (6% of diet); scFOS (1.5% of diet); cellulose (6% of diet); and a fiber blend (composed of beet pulp [BP] [6% of diet], gum talha [2% of diet], and scFOS [1.5% of diet]). A transient increase ($P < 0.05$; increased blood flow at 6, but not at 12, 16.5, or 21 h) in colonic blood flow was observed with scFOS supplementation, which the authors suggested was likely due to SCFA absorption resulting from rapid fermentation of scFOS. In addition, scFOS consumption reduced cell proliferation (smaller proliferation zone [$P < 0.01$] and shorter leading edge [$P < 0.10$]) in the proximal colon, suggesting that more crypt cells underwent differentiation. Although this result was unexpected, enhanced rates of differentiation may protect against cancer by decreasing the number of proliferating colonocytes exposed to carcinogenic compounds present in colonic digesta. These results complement the observations in rats, where a probiotic and FOS reduced the presence of aberrant crypts and foci (Gallaher et al., 1996).

PREBIOTIC AND DIETARY FIBERS

In a canine study, Middelbos et al. (2007) evaluated the efficacy of blends of cellulose, FOS, and MOS from YCW as replacements for commonly used dietary fibers in dog foods. Five treatments (2.5% cellulose; 2.5% BP; 1.0% cellulose–1.5% scFOS [CF]; 1.0% cellulose–1.2% scFOS–0.3% YCW [CFY1]; and 1.0% cellulose–0.9% scFOS–0.6% YCW [CFY2]) were tested against a control diet not supplemented with dietary fiber. Total tract DM and OM digestibilities were lower ($P < 0.05$) for the cellulose treatment (83.2 and 88.7% versus 86.2 and 91.7% with the control diet, respectively). Crude protein digestibility was lower ($P < 0.05$) for the treatments containing carbohydrate blends (84.9, 84.7, and 84.8% with the CF, CFY1, and CFY2 diets) than for the control, cellulose, and BP treatment (86.9, 86.7, and 87.0%, respectively). Fecal bifidobacterial and fecal butyrate concentrations were significantly higher for the BP treatment and for all

treatments containing carbohydrate blends than for the cellulose and the control diets ($P < 0.05$). Lactobacillus concentrations tended to be higher ($P < 0.08$) in treatments containing fermentable fiber and BP than in the cellulose treatment. This is the first report that BP inclusion in dog diets is capable of sustaining bifidobacterial and lactobacillus populations in concentrations similar to those of diets containing fermentable oligosaccharides. Ileal nutrient digestibilities and immune indices were not affected by treatment. These results suggest that dog foods containing blends of fermentable and nonfermentable carbohydrates produce physiological responses similar to those of dog food containing BP as a fiber source. Blends of these carbohydrates could, therefore, be useful substitutes for BP in dog foods.

FELINE PREBIOTIC EXPERIMENTS

Although cats are strict carnivores and are metabolically different from dogs for many ways, the potential benefits from prebiotic supplementation also exist for this species. Given the small number of studies performed to date, it is evident that more research is needed in this area. In the feline prebiotic studies that have been published, inulin, lactosucrose, OF, and FOS have been tested (Terada et al., 1993; Sparkes et al., 1998; Groeneveld et al., 2001; Hesta et al., 2001, 2005). Because outcome variables were different in each of the four experiments, few trends can be drawn from this small data set. However, a few effects are similar to those observed in canine experiments and demonstrate potential in feline diets. First, prebiotic supplementation may lead to an increased number of defecations per day and wet fecal volume, decreased fecal DM percentage, and softer feces (Hesta et al., 2001). Second, prebiotics appear to decrease total tract nutrient digestibility. As in dogs, decreased CP digestibility corresponds with increased fecal N concentrations (Groeneveld et al., 2001; Hesta et al., 2001, 2005). Third, in some feline studies prebiotics have been shown to manipulate microbial populations in a beneficial manner, resulting in increased concentrations of bifidobacteria and/or lactobacilli and decreased C. perfringens and/or E. coli concentrations. Lastly, supplementation appears to result in greater fecal SCFA and lower fecal protein catabolites in cats fed prebiotics than in cats fed the control diet.

SYNBIOTICS IN COMPANION ANIMALS

There is clearly potential for exploiting the synergy between prebiotic and probiotic ingredients for increased effectiveness of functional foods. A synbiotic was first defined as a mixture of probiotics and prebiotics that beneficially affects the host by improving the survival and implantation of live microbial dietary supplements in the GIT by selectively stimulating the growth and/or by activating the metabolism of one or a limited number of health-promoting bacteria and thus improving host welfare (Gibson and Roberfroid, 1995). Synbiotics are believed to increase the persistence of the probiotic bacteria present in the GIT by offering an available selective substrate. Unfortunately, the development of synbiotics for application in companion animals is only in its infancy. There is only one in vivo study by Swanson et al. (2002b) in which 20 dogs were randomly assigned to one of four treatments: (i) 2 g of sucrose plus 80 mg of cellulose; (ii) 2 g of FOS plus 80 mg of cellulose; (iii) 2 g of sucrose plus 10^9 CFU of *Lactobacillus acidophilus* NCFM (Rhodi, Madison, WI); or (iv) 2 g of FOS plus 10^9 CFU of *L. acidophilus*. FOS supplementation increased bifidobacteria ($P < 0.05$) and lactobacilli ($P < 0.08$) and also increased fecal lactate ($P < 0.06$) and butyrate ($P < 0.05$) and decreased fecal ammonia ($P < 0.05$). FOS positively altered gut microbial ecology and fecal protein catabolites, whereas the supplementation of *L. acidophilus* was more effective when fed in combination with FOS rather than fed alone.

An exciting approach in the field of companion animals is that of synbiotics rationally targeted to particular species of probiotic. This has been attempted for the first time in a study conducted by Tzortzis et al. (2004a) in which three candidate lactobacilli, *L. acidophilus* NCIMB 41085, *L. reuteri* NCIMB 41152, and *L. mucosae* NCIMB 41149, isolated from a Labrador dog were evaluated for their growth on various carbohydrates (Table 3). The production of extracellular antagonistic compounds against *S. enterica* serotype Typhimurium, enteropathogenic *E. coli*, and a toxin-negative mutant of *E. coli* O157:H7 was also evaluated. An initial screening was performed using bacteria-carbohydrate combinations to identify those that inhibited pathogenic growth in 24-h batch coculture experiments. Each of the batch culture fermentors was inoculated with pure cultures of one of the *Lactobacillus* strains and one of the pathogens. Cell-free supernatants of cocultures that were found to decrease pathogen growth in the initial screening were tested further for pathogen inhibition in pure cultures at neutral or acidic pH. Substrates reported to induce an inhibitory effect on pathogen growth included Panorich and maltose for *L. mucosae*; Biotose for *L. acidophilus*; and Biotiose, glucose, and maltose for *L. reuteri*. Further analyses carried out using supernatants from these compounds resulted in pathogen inhibition. Overall, these results show that the growth substrate influences the production of antimicrobial compounds, suggesting

Table 3 List of carbohydrates (prebiotics and nonprebiotics) used as substrates for bacterial growth

Substrate	Carbohydrate composition
Cellobiose	Two glucose molecules linked in a β (1→4) bond
Gentiobiose	Disaccharide composed of two units of D-glucose with a β (1→6) linkage
Glucose	Monosaccharide
IMO	Oligosaccharide mixture containing predominantly α (1→6)-linked glucose residues and also some mixed α (1→4)- and α (1→6)-linked gluco-oligosaccharides
Lactose	Disaccharide consisting of β-D-galactose and β-D-glucose molecules bonded through a β (1→4) glycosidic linkage
Laevan	Polymer of β-D-fructose
Maltose	Disaccharide formed from two units of glucose joined with an α (1→4) linkage
Melezitose	Nonreducing trisaccharide sugar. One molecule of fructose joined with two molecules of glucose with a β (3→1) and an α (2→1) linkage
Melibiose	Disaccharide composed of one molecule of galactose and one molecule of glucose with an α (1→6) linkage
Palatinose	A disaccharide consisting of D-glucose and D-fructose in α (1→6) linkage
Panorich	30% panose, 23% glucose, 17% maltose, 16% branched oligosaccharides (DP ≥ 4), 9% isomaltose, 3% maltotriose, and 2% isomaltotriose
Raffinose	Trisaccharide composed of one molecule of galactose and one molecule of glucose with an α (1→6) and one molecule of fructose with a linkage and an α (1→4) linkage
scFOS	Polymers of D-fructose joined by β (1→2) bonds linked to a nonreducing α D-glucose
Stachyose	Tetrasaccharide consisting of two D-galactose units, one D-glucose unit, and one D-fructose unit sequentially linked
Biotose	41% glucose, 20% isomaltose, 9% isomaltotriose, 9% panose, 7% maltose, and 14% other sugars
Tagatose	Naturally occurring monosaccharide
Xylo-oligosaccharides	Oligosaccharides derived from xylan, predominantly linear linked XOS
Sucrose	Disaccharide consisting of one molecule of glucose and one molecule of fructose with a β (1→2) linkage
Xylan	Linear backbone structure consisting of β (1→4) linked xylosyl residues

a substrate specificity of the probiotic to combat specific pathogens. Because the results indicated that acidity is not the sole inhibitory agent, the authors suggested that the induction of bacteriocins is another possible mechanism of action.

The synbiotic concept was taken further by the same researchers (Tzortzis et al., 2003b) in an attempt to synthesize highly targeted synbiotics for canine application. The probiotic *L. reuteri*, described above, was selected for the extraction of the extracellular enzyme α-galactosidase from pure cultures of the probiotic and used to synthesize an oligosaccharide mixture by a glycosyl transfer reaction using melibiose as a glycosyl donor. A canine fecal inoculum was used to measure in vitro fermentability of the synthesized oligosaccharide versus three reference carbohydrates: FOS, melibiose, and raffinose (Tzortzis et al., 2004b). The addition of *L. acidophilus* (10^9 CFU/ml) was used as a control for the evaluation of the synbiotic properties of the galactosyl-melibiose mixture (GMM) with *L. reuteri* (10^9 CFU/ml). Populations of predominant gut bacterial groups were monitored over 24 h of batch culture by FISH, and SCFA production was also determined. GMM showed a greater increase ($P < 0.05$) in *Bifidobacterium* spp. and the *Lactobacillus/Enterococcus* group as well as a greater decrease ($P < 0.05$) in *Clostridium* spp. (clusters I and II) and *E. coli* population numbers than with the commercial prebiotics (FOS, melibiose, and raffinose). The prebiotic effect was further increased by the addition of *L. reuteri* followed by a change in the SCFA production pattern compared to GMM alone or GMM with *L. acidophilus*.

While the use of probiotics and prebiotics has been relatively well studied in companion animals, the synbiotic field is still not thoroughly explored. Although there is limited literature available, prebiotics appear to have a beneficial influence on the canine and feline intestinal ecosystem; however, synbiotic performance among different colonic bacterial groups and the health outcomes have not been extensively studied under either in vitro or in vivo conditions. There is, therefore, a need to study which effects are the intrinsic ones that a probiotic and a prebiotic exert when used in combination as a synbiotic mixture in companion animals.

GENERAL CONCLUSION

Recently research has focused upon the efficacy of various fibers as prebiotics in the canine and feline GIT. The increasing number of published studies assessing the potential of prebiotics suggests that the supplementation of prebiotics in companion animal diets has several beneficial effects in the GIT of dogs and cats such

as positive alteration of the microbial balance, decreases in fecal protein catabolites, better stool quality, and changes in immune status. Although some pet foods have been shown to contain traces of inulin and FOS, most of the studies with dogs and cats have been conducted by supplementing known doses of prebiotic; however, more research is required to identify optimal doses and potential side effects of prebiotics in companion animals. Prebiotics have been reported to increase the production of lactate and SCFA in the colon, which contribute to colonic health; nevertheless, the mechanisms of how prebiotics function in the large intestine are not totally understood. To completely understand these mechanisms, researchers must identify all microbial species that colonize the canine and feline GIT and determine the interactions among these as well as the interactions with the epithelial cells in the gut. Elucidation of such relationships should provide guidelines for the formulation of diets that support the health of companion animals. In order to accurately identify and quantify microbial species in the gut, greater use of molecular techniques is essential in view of the fact that, to date, most of the published studies of the canine and feline gut microbiota are based on culturing techniques with their well-known limitations. With the new generation of molecular microbiological techniques it will be possible to gain definitive information on the species that are influenced by the prebiotic intake.

Most of the studies performed to date have used healthy adult dogs and cats. It is important to know how age and health status (and breed) may influence the intestinal microbiota of these animals so that studies of the effects of prebiotic supplementation on animals of different breeds and life stages and suffering various disease states can be carried out. More well-designed trials are needed to establish the factors that may induce changes in the colonic microbiota.

In conclusion, research on prebiotics for companion animal applications is still in the early stages. Although prebiotics have shown positive effects on colonic microbial ecology, researchers must be careful not to overlook potential adverse effects of prebiotic supplementation. Before the use of synbiotics in animal nutrition is implemented, there is a need to define which bacterial species can be categorized as probiotics in companion animals. At the moment, the concept of probiotics is based on the outcomes of studies on human intestinal ecology. Taking into consideration the lack of knowledge of the canine and feline intestinal microbiota, it is rather premature to consider as probiotics, the same bacterial genera that are used in human applications. Certainly, more research remains to be done to determine the appropriate role of probiotics, prebiotics, and synbiotics in animal nutrition.

References

Adogony, V., F. Respondek, V. Biourge, F. Rudeaux, J. Delaval, J.-L. Bind, and H. Salmon. 2007. Effects of dietary scFOS on immunoglobulins in colostrums and milk of bitches. *J. Anim. Physiol. Anim. Nutr.* 91:169–174.

Balish, E., D. Cleven, J. Brown, and C. E. Yale. 1977. Nose, throat and fecal flora of beagle dogs housed in "locked" or "open" environments. *Appl. Environ. Microbiol.* 34:207–221.

Banta, C. A., E. T. Clemens, M. M. Krinsky, and B. E. Sheffy. 1979. Sites of organic acid production and patterns of digesta movement in the gastrointestinal tract of dogs. *J. Nutr.* 109:1592–1600.

Batt, R. M., A. Barnes, H. C. Rutgers, and S. C. Carter. 1991. Relative IgA deficiency and small intestinal bacterial overgrowth in German shepherd dogs. *Res. Vet. Sci.* 50:106–111.

Beaudry, M., C. Zhu, J. M. Fairbrother, and J. Harel. 1996. Genotypic and phenotypic characterization of *Escherichia coli* isolates from dogs manifesting attaching and effacing lesions. *J. Clin. Microbiol.* 34:144–148.

Bellisle, F., J. E. Blundell, L. Dye, M. Fantino, E. Fern, R. J. Fletcher, J. Lambert, M. Roberfroid, S. Specter, J. Westenhofer, and M. S. Westerterp-Plantenga. 1998. Functional food science and behaviour and psychological functions. *Br. J. Nutr.* 80:S173–S193.

Benno, Y., and T. Mitsuoka. 1992. Evaluation of the anaerobic method of analysis of faecal microflora of beagle dogs. *J. Vet. Med. Sci.* 54:1039–1041.

Benno, Y., H. Nakao, K. Uchida, and T. Mitsuoka. 1992a. Impact of the advances in age on the gastrointestinal microflora of beagle dogs. *J. Vet. Med. Sci.* 54:703–706.

Benno, Y., H. Nakao, K. Uchida, and T. Mitsuoka. 1992b. Individual and seasonal variations in the composition of fecal microflora of beagle dogs. *Bifido. Microflora* 11:69–76.

Beutin, L. 1999. *Escherichia coli* as a pathogen in dogs and cats. *Vet. Res.* 30:285–298.

Beynen, A. C., J. C. Baas, P. E. Hoekemeijer, H. J. Kappert, M. H. Bakker, J. P. Koopman, and A. G. Lemmens. 2002. Faecal bacterial profile, nitrogen excretion and mineral absorption in healthy dogs fed supplemental oligofructose. *J. Anim. Physiol. Anim. Nutr.* 86:298–305.

Binder, H. J., and P. Mehta. 1989. Short-chain fatty acids stimulate active sodium and chloride absorption in vitro in the rat distal colon. *Gastroenterology* 96:989–996.

Bornside, G. H., and I. Cohn. 1965. Comparative bacterial flora of animals and man. *Am. J. Dig. Dis.* 10:844–852.

Bouhnik, Y., K. Vahedi, L. Achour, A. Attar, J. Salfati, P. Pochart, P. Marteau, B. Flourié, F. Bornet, and J.-C. Rambaud. 1999. Short-chain fructo-oligosaccharide administration dose-dependently increases fecal bifidobacteria in healthy humans. *J. Nutr.* 129:113–116.

Brandtzaeg, P., T. S. Halstensen, and K. Kett. 1989. Immunobiology and immunopathology of human gut mucosa: humoral immunity and intraepithelial lymphocytes. *Gastroenterology* 97:1562–1584.

Buddington, R. K. 1996. Structure and functions of the dog and cat intestine, p. 61–78. *In* D. P. Carey, S. A. Norton, and S. M. Bolser (ed.), *Recent Advances in Canine and Feline Nutrition,* vol I. *Proceedings of the 1996 Iams Nutrition Symposium.* Orange Frazer Press, Wilmington, OH.

Buddington, R. K. 2003. Postnatal changes in bacterial populations in the gastrointestinal tract of dogs. *Am. J. Vet. Res.* 64:646–651.

Buddington, R. K., and D. B. Paulsen. 1998. Development of the canine and feline gastrointestinal tract, p. 195–215. *In* G. A. Reinhart and D. P. Carey (ed.), *Recent Advances in Canine and Feline Nutrition. 1998 IAMS Nutrition Symposium Proceedings.* Orange Frazer Press, Wilmington, OH.

Cave, N. J. 2003. Chronic inflammatory disorders of the gastrointestinal tract of companion animals. *N. Z. Vet. J.* 51:262–274.

Clapper, W. E. 1970. Microbiology: gastrointestinal tract, p. 469–473. *In* A. C. Andersen (ed.), *The Beagle as an Experimental Dog.* The Iowa State University Press, Ames, IA.

Clapper, W. E., and G. H. Meade. 1963. Normal flora of the nose, throat and lower intestine of dogs. *J. Bacteriol.* 85:643–648.

Cummings, J. H., M. J. Hill, E. S. Bones, W. J. Branch, and D. J. A. Jenkins. 1979. The effect of meat protein and dietary fiber on colonic function and metabolism. II. Bacterial metabolites in feces and urine. *Am. J. Clin. Nutr.* 32:2094–2101.

Cummings, J. H., and S. A. Bingham. 1987. Dietary fiber, fermentation and large bowel cancer. *Cancer Surv.* 6:601–621.

Czarnecki-Maulden, G. L., and T. J. Russell. 2000. Effect of diet type on fecal microflora in dogs. *FASEB J.* 14:A488.

Davis, C. P., D. Cleven, E. Balish, and C. E. Yale. 1977. Bacterial association in the gastrointestinal tract of beagle dogs. *Appl. Environ. Microbiol.* 34:194–206.

Debraekeleer, J., K. L. Gross, and S. C. Zicker. 2000. Normal dogs, p. 213–260. *In* M. S. Hand, C. D. Thatcher, R. L. Remillard, and P. Roudebush (ed.), *Small Animal Clinical Nutrition.* Mark Morris Institute, Topeka, KS.

Field, C. J., M. I. McBurney, S. Massimino, M. Hayek, and G. Sunvold. 1999. The fermentable fiber of the diet alters the function and composition of canine gut associated lymphoid tissue. *Vet. Immunol. Immunopathol.* 72:325–341.

Flickinger, E. A., T. F. Hatch, R. C. Wofford, C. M. Grieshop, S. M. Murray, and G. C. Fahey, Jr. 2002. In vitro fermentation properties of selected fructooligosaccharide-containing vegetables and in vivo colonic microbial populations are affected by diet in healthy human infants. *J. Nutr.* 132:2188–2194.

Flickinger, E. A., J. Van Loo, and G. C. Fahey, Jr. 2003a. Nutritional responses to the presence of inulin and oligofructose in the diets of domesticated animals: a review. *Crit. Rev. Food Sci. Nutr.* 43:19–60.

Flickinger, E. A., E. M. W. C. Schreijen, A. R. Patil, H. S. Hussein, C. M. Grieshop, N. R. Merchen, and G. C. Fahey, Jr. 2003b. Nutrient digestibilities, microbial populations, and protein catabolites as affected by fructan supplementation of dog diets. *J. Anim. Sci.* 81:2008–2018.

Gallaher, D. D., W. H. Stallings, L. L. Blessing, F. F. Busta, and L. J. Brady. 1996. Probiotics, cecal microflora, and aberrant crypts in the rat colon. *J. Nutr.* 126:1362–1371.

Gibson, G. R., E. R. Beatty, X. Wang, and J. H. Cummings. 1995. Selective stimulation of bifidobacteria in the human colon by oligofructose and inulin. *Gastroenterology* 108:975–982.

Gibson, G. R., and G. T. Macfarlane (ed.). 1995. *Human Colonic Bacteria: Role in Nutrition, Physiology and Pathology.* CRC Press, Boca Raton, FL.

Gibson, G. R., and M. B. Roberfroid. 1995. Dietary modulation of the human colonic microbiota: introducing the concept of prebiotics. *J. Nutr.* 125:1401–1412.

Greetham, H. L., C. Giffard, R. A. Hutson, M. D. Collins, and G. R. Gibson. 2002. Bacteriology of the Labrador dog gut: a cultural and genotypic approach. *J. Appl. Microbiol.* 93:640–646.

Grieshop, C. M., E. A. Flickinger, K. J. Bruce, A. R. Patil, G. L. Czarnecki-Maulden, and G. C. Fahey, Jr. 2004. Gastrointestinal and immunological responses of senior dogs to chicory and mannanoligosaccharides. *Arch. Anim. Nutr.* 58:483–493.

Groeneveld, E. A., H. J. Kappert, J. Van der Kuilen, and A. C. Beynen. 2001. Consumption of fructooligosaccharides and nitrogen excretion in cats. *Int. J. Vitam. Nutr. Res.* 71:254–256.

Guilford, W. G., and M. E. Matz. 2003. The nutritional management of gastrointestinal tract disorders in companion animals. *N. Z. Vet. J.* 51:284–291.

Hernot, D. C., V. C. Biourge, L. J. Martin, H. J. Dumon, and P. G. Nguyen. 2005. Relationship between total transit time and faecal quality in adult dogs differing in body size. *J. Anim. Physiol. Anim. Nutr.* 89:189–193.

Hesta, M., G. P. J. Janssens, J. Debraekeleer, and R. De Wilde. 2001. The effect of oligofructose and inulin on faecal characteristics and nutrient digestibility in healthy cats. *J. Anim. Physiol. Anim. Nutr.* 85:135–141.

Hesta, M., W. Roosen, G. P. J. Janssens, S. Millet, and R. De Wilde. 2003. Prebiotics affect nutrient digestibility but not faecal ammonia in dogs fed increased dietary protein levels. *Br. J. Nutr.* 90:1007–1014.

Hesta, M., E. Hoornaert, A. Verlinden, and G. P. J. Janssens. 2005. The effect of oligofructose on urea metabolism and faecal odour components in cats. *J. Anim. Physiol. Anim. Nutr.* 89:208–215.

Hidaka, H., T. Eida, T. Takizawa, T. Tokunaga, and Y. Tashiro. 1986. Effects of fructooligosaccharides on intestinal flora and human health. *Bifido Microflora* 5:37–50.

Hopkins, M. J., and G. T. Macfarlane. 2002. Changes in predominant bacterial populations in human faeces with age and with *Clostridium difficile* infection. *J. Med. Microbiol.* 51:448–454.

Howard, M. D., M. S. Kerley, F. A. Mann, G. D. Sunvold, and G. A. Reinhart. 1999. Blood flow and epithelial cell proliferation of the canine colon are altered by source of dietary fiber. *Vet. Clin. Nutr.* 6:8–15.

Hussein, H. S., J. M. Campbell, L. L. Bauer, G. C. Fahey, Jr., A. J. C. Lewis Hogarth, B. W. Wolf, and D. E. Hunter. 1998. Selected fructooligosaccharide composition of pet-food ingredients. *J. Nutr.* 128:2803S–2805S.

Inness, V. L., A. L. McCartney, C. Khoo, K. L. Gross, and G. R. Gibson. 2007. Molecular characterisation of the gut microflora of healthy and inflammatory bowel disease cats using fluorescence *in situ* hybridisation with special reference to *Desulfovibrio* spp. *J. Anim. Physiol. Anim. Nutr.* (Berlin) 91:48–53.

Itoh, K., T. Mitsuoka, K. Maejima, C. Hiraga, and K. Nakano. 1984. Comparison of faecal flora of cats based on different housing conditions with special reference to *Bifidobacterium. Lab. Anim.* 18:280–284.

Jackson, A. A. 1995. Salvage of urea-nitrogen and protein requirements. *Proc. Nutr. Soc.* 54:535–547.

Jalkanen, S. 1990. Lymphocyte homing into the gut. *Immunopathology* 12:153–164.

Jergens, A. E., and D. L. Zoran. 2005. Diseases of the colon and rectum, p. 203–221. *In* E. J. Small, J. W. Simpson, and D. A. Williams (ed.), *Canine and Feline Gastroenterology.* British Small Animal Veterinary Association, Gloucester, United Kingdom.

Karr-Lilienthal, L. K., C. M. Grieshop, J. K. Spears, A. R. Patil, G. L. Czarnecki-Maulden, N. R. Merchen, and G. C. Fahey, Jr. 2004. Estimation of the proportion of bacterial nitrogen in canine feces using diaminopimelic acid as an internal bacterial marker. *J. Anim. Sci.* 82:1707–1712.

Kirk, C. A., J. Debraekeleer, and P. J. Armstrong. 2000. Normal cats, p. 213–260. *In* M. S. Hand, C. D. Thatcher, R. L. Remillard, and P. Roudebush (ed.), *Small Animal Clinical Nutrition.* Mark Morris Institute, Topeka, KS.

Kleessen, B., B. Sykura, H. J. Zunft, and M. Blaut. 1997. Effects of inulin and lactose on fecal microflora, microbial activity, and bowel habit in elderly constipated persons. *Am. J. Clin. Nutr.* 65:1397–1402.

Lutz, T., and E. Scharrer. 1991. Effect of short-chain fatty acids on calcium absorption by the rat colon. *Exp. Physiol.* 76:615–618.

MacDermott, R. P., G. S. Nash, M. J. Bertovich, R. F. Mohrman, I. J. Kodner, D. L. Delacroix, and J. P. Vaerman. 1986. Altered patterns of secretion of monomeric IgA and IgA subclass 1 by intestinal mononuclear cells in inflammatory bowel disease. *Gastroenterology* 91:379–385.

McKay, D. M., and M. H. Perdue. 1993. Intestinal epithelial function: the case for immunophysiological regulation. *Dig. Dis. Sci.* 38:1377–1387.

Mcmanus, C. M., K. E. Michel, D. M. Simon, and R. J. Washabau. 2002. Effect of short-chain fatty acids on contraction of smooth muscle in the canine colon. *Am. J. Vet. Res.* 63:295–300.

Mentula, S., J. Harmoinen, M. Heikkila, E. Westermarck, M. Rautio, P. Huovinen, and E. Kononen. 2005. Comparison between cultured small intestinal and fecal microbiotas in beagle dogs. *Appl. Environ. Microbiol.* 71:4169–4175.

Middelbos, I. S., N. D. Fastinger, and G. C. Fahey, Jr. 2007. Evaluation of fermentable oligosaccharides in diets fed to dogs in comparison to fiber standards. *J. Anim. Sci.* 85:3033–3044.

Mitsuoka, T. 1969. Comparative studies on bifidobacteria isolated from the alimentary tract of man and animals (including descriptions of *Bifidobacterium thermophilum* nov. spec. and *Bifidobacterium pseudolongum* nov. spec). *Zentbl. Bakteriol.* 210:52–64.

Mitsuoka, T. 1992. Intestinal flora and aging. *Nutr. Rev.* 50:438–446.

Nair, G. B., R. K. Sarkar, S. Chowdhury, and S. C. Pal. 1985. *Campylobacter* infection in domestic dogs. *Vet. Rec.* 116:237–238.

O'Brien, R. T. 2005. Imaging the gastrointestinal tract, liver and pancreas, p. 203–221. *In* E. J. Hall, J. W. Simpson, and D. A. Williams (ed.), *Canine and Feline Gastroenterology*. British Small Animal Veterinary Association, Gloucester, United Kingdom.

Osbaldiston, G. W., and E. C. Stowe. 1971. Microflora of alimentary tract of cats. *Am. J. Vet. Res.* 32:1399–405.

Patil, A. R., G. L. Czarnecki-Maulden, and K. E. Dowling. 2000. Effect of advances in age on fecal microflora of cats. *FASEB J.* 14:A488.

Propst, E. L., E. A. Flickinger, L. L. Bauer, N. R. Merchen, and G. C. Fahey, Jr. 2003. A dose-response experiment evaluating the effects of oligofructose and inulin on nutrient digestibility, stool quality, and fecal protein catabolites in healthy adult dogs. *J. Anim. Sci.* 81:3057–3066.

Quemener, B., J.-F. Thibaut, and P. Coussement. 1994. Determination of inulin and oligofructose in food products, and integration in the AOAC method for measurement of total dietary fibre. *Lebensm. Wiss. Technol.* 27:125–132.

Ramakrishna, B. S., I. C. Roberts-Thomas, P. R. Pannall, and W. E. W. Roediger. 1991. Impaired sulphation of phenol by the colonic mucosa in quiescent and active colitis. *Gut* 32:46–49.

Ren, H., M. W. Musch, K. Kojima, D. Boone, A. Ma, and E. B. Chang. 2001. Short-chain fatty acids induce intestinal epithelial heat shock protein 25 expression in rats and IEC 18 cells. *Gastroenterology* 121:631–639.

Rinkinen, M. L., J. M. Koort, A. C. Ouwehand, E. Westermarck, and K. J. Bjorkroth. 2004. *Streptococcus alactolyticus* is the dominating culturable lactic acid bacterium species in canine jejunum and feces of four fistulated dogs. *FEMS. Microbiol. Lett.* 15:35–39.

Roediger, W. E. W. 1980. Role of anaerobic bacteria in the metabolic welfare of the colonic mucosa in man. *Gut* 21:793–798.

Russell, M. W., J. Reinholdt, and M. Kilian. 1989. Anti-inflammatory activity of human IgA antibodies and their Fab α fragments: inhibition of IgG-mediated complement activation. *Eur. J. Immunol.* 19:2243–2249.

Russell, T. J. 1998. The effect of natural source of nondigestible oligosaccharides on the fecal microflora of the dog and effects on digestion. Friskies R & D Center/Missouri, St. Joseph, MO.

Salminen, S., E. Isolauri, and T. Onnela. 1995. Gut flora in normal and disorder status. *Chemotherapy* 41(Suppl. 1): 5–15.

Salminen, S., C. Bouley, M. C. Boutron-Ruault, J. H. Cummings, A. Franck, G. R. Gibson, E. Isolauri, M. C. Moreau, M. Roberfroid, and I. Rowland. 1998. Functional food science and gastrointestinal physiology and function. *Br. J. Nutr.* 80:S147–Sl71.

Simpson, J. M., B. Martineau, W. E. Jones, J. M. Ballam, and R. I. Mackie. 2002. Characterization of fecal bacterial populations in canines: effects of age, breed and dietary fiber. *Microb. Ecol.* 44:186–197.

Sparkes, A. H., K. Papasouliotis, G. Sunvold, G. Werrett, E. A. Gruffydd-Jones, K. Egan, T. J. Gruffydd-Jones, and G. Reinhart. 1998. Effect of dietary supplementation with fructo-oligosaccharides on fecal flora of healthy cats. *Am. J. Vet. Res.* 59:436–440.

Spears, J. K., L. K. Karr-Lilienthal, and G. C. Fahey, Jr. 2005. Influence of supplemental high molecular weight pullulan or γ-cyclodextrin on ileal and total tract nutrient digestibility, fecal characteristics, and microbial populations in the dog. *Arch. Anim. Nutr.* 59:257–270.

Stokes, C., and N. Waly. 2006. Mucosal defence along the gastrointestinal tract of cats and dogs. *Vet. Rec.* 37:281–293.

Strickling, J. A., D. L. Harmon, K. A. Dawson, and K. L. Gross. 2000. Evaluation of oligosaccharide addition to dog diets: influences on nutrient digestion and microbial populations. *Anim. Feed Sci. Technol.* 86:205–219.

Strombeck, D. R. 1990. Small and large intestine: normal structure and function, p. 318–350. *In* D. R. Strombeck and W. G. Guildford (ed.), *Small Animal Gastroenterology*. Stonegate Publishing, Davis, CA.

Swanson, K. S., E. A. Flickinger, C. M. Grieshop, and G. C. Fahey, Jr. 2002a. Prebiotics and probiotics: definition, synergistic effects, and impact on nutritional and health status of companion animals. *Nestle White Paper* 2002:1–9.

Swanson, K. S., C. M. Grieshop, E. A. Flickinger, L. L. Bauer, J. Chow, B. W. Wolf, K. A. Garleb, and G. C. Fahey, Jr. 2002b. Fructooligosaccharides and *Lactobacillus acidophilus* modify gut microbial populations, total tract nutrient digestibilities, and fecal protein catabolite concentrations in healthy adult dogs. *J. Nutr.* 132:3721–3731.

Swanson, K. S., C. M. Grieshop, E. A. Flickinger, L. L. Bauer, H.-P. Healy, K. A. Dawson, N. R. Merchen, and G. C. Fahey, Jr. 2002c. Supplemental fructooligosaccharides and mannanoligosaccharides influence immune function, ileal and total tract nutrient digestibilities, microbial populations and concentrations of protein catabolites in the large bowel of dogs. *J. Nutr.* 132:980–989.

Swanson, K. S., C. M. Grieshop, E. A. Flickinger, H.-P. Healy, K. A. Dawson, N. R. Merchen, and G. C. Fahey, Jr. 2002d. Effects of supplemental fructooligosaccharides plus mannanoligosaccharides on immune function and ileal and fecal microbial populations in adult dogs. *Arch. Anim. Nutr.* 56:309–318.

Swanson, K. S., and G. C. Fahey, Jr. 2006. Prebiotic impacts on companion animals, p. 213–236. *In* G. R. Gibson and R. A. Rastall (ed.), *Prebiotics Development and Application*. John Wiley and Sons, Ltd, West Sussex, United Kingdom.

Terada, A., H. Hara, T. Oishi, S. Matsui, T. Mitsuoka, S. Nakajyo, I. Fujimori, and K. Hara. 1992. Effect of dietary lactosucrose on faecal flora and faecal metabolites of dogs. *Microb. Ecol. Health Dis.* 5:87–92.

Terada, A., H. Hara, S. Kato, T. Kimura, I. Fujimori, K. Hara, T. Maruyama, and T. Mitsuoka. 1993. Effect of lactosucrose (4^G-β-D-Galactosylsucrose) on fecal flora and fecal putrefactive products of cats. *J. Vet. Med. Sci.* 55:291–295.

Topping, D. L., M. Fukushima, and A. R. Bird. 2003. Resistant starch as a prebiotic and synbiotic: state of the art. *Proc. Nutr. Soc.* 62:171–176.

Twomey, L. N., J. R. Pluske, J. B. Rowe, M. Choct, W. Brown, and D. W. Pethick. 2003. The effects of added fructooligosaccharide (Raftilose® P95) and inulinase on faecal quality and digestibility in dogs. *Anim. Feed Sci. Technol.* 108:83–93.

Tzortzis, G., G. R. Gibson, and R. A. Rastall. 2003a. Canine functional foods. *Food Sci. Tech. Bull. Funct. Foods* 1(6): 1–10.

Tzortzis, G., A. J. Jay, M. L. Baillon, G. R. Gibson, and R. A. Rastall. 2003b. Synthesis of alpha-galactooligosaccharides with alpha-galactosidase from *Lactobacillus reuteri* of canine origin. *Appl. Microbiol. Biotechnol.* 63:286–292.

Tzortzis, G., M. L. A. Baillon, G. R. Gibson, and R. A. Rastall. 2004a. Modulation of anti-pathogenic activity in canine-derived *Lactobacillus* species by carbohydrate growth substrate. *J. Appl. Microbiol.* 96:552–559.

Tzortzis, G., A. K. Goulas, M. L. A. Baillon, G. R. Gibson, and R. A. Rastall. 2004b. *In vitro* evaluation of the fermentation properties of galactooligosaccharides synthesized by α-galactosidase from *Lactobacillus reuteri*. *Appl. Microbiol. Biotechnol.* 64:106–111.

Vanhoutte, T., G. Huys, E. De Brandt, G. C. Fahey, Jr., and J. Swings. 2005. Molecular monitoring and characterization of the faecal microbiota of healthy dogs during fructan supplementation. *FEMS Microbiol. Lett.* 249:65–71.

Van Loo, J., P. Coussement, L. de Leenheer, H. Hoebregs, and G. Smits. 1995. On the presence of inulin and oligofructose as natural ingredients in the western diet. *Crit. Rev. Food Sci. Nutr.* 35:525–552.

Verlinden, A., M. Hesta, J. M. Hermans, and G. P. J. Janssens. 2006. The effects of inulin supplementation of diets with or without hydrolysed protein sources on digestibility, faecal characteristics, haematology and immunoglobulins in dogs. *Br. J. Nutr.* 96:936–944.

Vickers, R. J., G. D. Sunvold, R. L. Kelley, and G. A. Reinhart. 2001. Comparison of fermentation of selected fructooligosaccharides and other fiber substrates by canine colonic microflora. *Am. J. Vet. Res.* 62:609–615.

Visek, W. J. 1978. Diet and cell growth modulation by ammonia. *Am. J. Clin. Nutr.* 31:S216–S220.

Von Englehardt, W., K. Ronnau, G. Rechkemmer, and T. Sakata. 1989. Absorption of short-chain fatty acids and their role in the hindgut of monogastric animals. *Anim. Feed Sci. Technol.* 23: 43–53.

Zentek, J., B. Marquart, and T. Pietrzak. 2002. Intestinal effects of mannan-oligosaccharides, transgalactooligosaccharides, lactose and lactulose in dogs. *J. Nutr.* 132:1682S–1684S.

Zentek, J., B. Marquart, T. Pietrzak, O. Ballèvre, and F. Rochat. 2003. Dietary effects on bifidobacteria and *Clostridium perfringens* in the canine intestinal tract. *J. Anim. Physiol. Anim. Nutr.* 87:397–407.

Viral Strategies

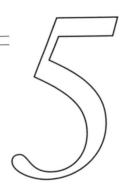

Therapeutic Microbiology: Probiotics and Related Strategies
Edited by J. Versalovic and M. Wilson
© 2008 ASM Press, Washington, DC

Mikael Skurnik
Saija Kiljunen
Maria Pajunen

28

Phage Therapy

HISTORY AND BACKGROUND

As a group, viruses are believed to be ancient and originate from the time before the divergence of the three domains of life, *Archaea*, *Bacteria*, and *Eucarya* (Hendrix et al., 1999, 2003). Tailed double-stranded (ds) DNA phages infect cyanobacteria and other gram-negative bacteria and have also been described for *Archaea*. These viruses are, however, assumed to have entered the *Archaea* by interdomain spread from *Bacteria*, which suggests that the emergence of this virus group succeeded the divergence of *Archaea* and *Bacteria* but preceded the split of cyanobacteria from other gram-negative bacteria. This gives a time estimation of 3 to 3.5 billion years (Hambly and Suttle, 2005; Prangishvili et al., 2006).

Bacteriophages (phages) are viruses that infect bacterial hosts and depend on bacterial processes to produce viral proteins and viral particles. They were discovered by Frederick W. Twort in London (1915) and by Felix d'Hérelle in Paris (1917), who named this invisible microbe bacteriophage. Naming of the bacteriophage has been subject to some misinterpretation as it has been assumed that

d'Hérelle meant to imply that the bacteriophage "devours" (derived from the Greek φαγειν [*phagein*], to eat or devour) the bacterium. Later on, however, he concluded that the suffix "phage" is not used in its strict sense "to eat," but in that of "developing at the expense of" (Summers, 1999).

Bacteriophages are the most abundant and the most versatile group of organisms on Earth. In environmental samples phages usually outnumber their bacterial hosts 3- to 10-fold, and the global phage population has been estimated to approach 10^{31} (Breitbart and Rohwer, 2005; Hendrix, 2002; Pedulla et al., 2003; Wommack and Colwell, 2000). Due to their abundance, phages are active components of their ecosystems and can liberate carbon and nutrients by virus-mediated lysis of planktonic organisms in the aquatic food webs; they also have important roles in biogeochemical cycles, gene transfer, and prokaryotic diversity (Weinbauer, 2004; Weinbauer and Rassoulzadegan, 2004; Wilhelm and Suttle, 1999; Wommack and Colwell, 2000).

Phages have been studied for a variety of reasons. In the decade following their discovery, research was driven

Mikael Skurnik, Infection Biology Research Program, Department of Bacteriology and Immunology, Haartman Institute, University of Helsinki, and Helsinki University Central Hospital Laboratory Diagnostics, 00014 Helsinki, Finland. **Saija Kiljunen**, Department of Virology, University of Turku, 00014 Turku, Finland. **Maria Pajunen**, Institute of Biotechnology, University of Helsinki, 00014 Helsinki, Finland.

by the hope that phages might prove useful in combating bacterial diseases. Later, phages became favored objects for basic experiments in molecular biology, and nowadays phages are used as cloning and display vehicles in genetic engineering and other molecular biology applications. Most recently, mainly due to the problem of increased antibiotic resistance, the use of phages as potential therapeutic agents has reemerged.

BACTERIOPHAGES

Phage Life Cycles

Phages can be divided into lytic and temperate based on their life cycles. Infection by a lytic, or virulent, phage results in the lysis of the bacterial cell and release of new phage progeny (Ackermann and DuBow, 1987b). The first step of a lytic cycle is the adsorption of the phage on the bacterial surface. The infection then proceeds by the entry of the phage nucleic acid into the bacterial cytoplasm and consequent transcription and translation of phage proteins as well as by synthesis of multiple copies of the phage genome. New phage particles are assembled and finally released upon lysis of the host bacterium. The common parameters used to describe the phage life cycle are eclipse period (the time required for the new phage progeny to be assembled), latent period (the time until the host cells are lysed), and burst size (the number of new phage particles released from an infected cell) (Ackermann and DuBow, 1987b).

Temperate phages are able to choose between lytic and lysogenic life cycles (Ackermann and DuBow, 1987b; Little, 2005). It has been claimed that more than 90% of the known phages are temperate (Freifelder, 1983). All known temperate phages contain dsDNA. They can be classified according to their prophage state, i.e., mode of association with the bacterial genome: (i) phages that insert their DNA into chromosomes by site-specific recombination (e.g., lambdoid phages) (Hendrix et al., 1983), (ii) phages that use DNA transposition to replicate and lysogenize (phage Mu and its relatives) (Harshey, 1988), and (iii) phages that lysogenize by plasmid formation (Yarmolinsky and Sternberg, 1988). The plasmid formed during the lysogenization may be linear, as in *Escherichia coli* phage N15 and *Yersinia enterocolitica* phage PY54 (Hertwig et al., 2003; Ravin et al., 2000), or circular, as exemplified by *E. coli* phage P1 and *Clostridium botulinum* phage c-st (Lobocka et al., 2004; Sakaguchi et al., 2005). The phage genome integrated into the bacterial chromosome replicates as part of it. The expression of phage lytic genes is repressed, but other genes in the phage genome may be expressed

in a state called lysogenic conversion. Indeed, the expression of these extra genes may benefit the fitness of the lysogenic bacterium and thus indirectly also the phage genome (Brüssow et al., 2004). The choice between lytic and lysogenic cycles, the so-called lysis-lysogeny decision, is a complex process and understood well for a few phages only (Little, 2005), the best-characterized example being the *E. coli* phage λ (Hendrix et al., 1983; Little, 2005).

Phage Receptors

Bacteriophages do not randomly attach to the surface of a host cell; rather, they adsorb to specific receptor sites. The ability of a phage to adsorb to its receptor is the major factor that determines the host specificity. This attachment seems to take place in two steps: a temperature-independent reversible step is followed by a temperature-dependent irreversible step (Lindberg, 1973). The primary antireceptor (or adhesin) of phages is usually the tail fiber, tail spike, or some other surface appendage. Presumably every structure exposed on the bacterial surface may serve as a bacteriophage receptor. For gram-negative bacteria, this means carbohydrates (LPS and capsule), outer membrane proteins (OMPs), or pilus and flagellum structures (Heller, 1992; Koebnik et al., 2000; Lindberg, 1973; Wright et al., 1980). For gram-positive bacteria, the phage-host interactions are generally less well known, but typically the phage adsorption occurs via cell wall carbohydrates like teichoic acids (Dupont et al., 2004; Wendlinger et al., 1996). Table 1 gives examples of phages and the types of receptors they have on gram-positive and gram-negative bacteria.

Capsule-specific phages often have capsule-degrading enzymatic activities associated with their tail spikes or fibers, examples of which are the endo-N-acylneuraminidases (which degrade α-1,8-linked polysialic acid chains) of K1-specific phages (Kwiatkowski et al., 1982; Pelkonen et al., 1989). Some temperate polysaccharide-specific phages in a prophage state modify their receptors and thus avoid superinfection. Serotype-converting phages and their enzymes in *Salmonella* (Vander Byl and Kropinski, 2000), *Shigella* (Allison and Verma, 2000), and *Pseudomonas* have been studied thoroughly (Newton et al., 2001).

Phage Taxonomy

The International Committee for Taxonomy of Viruses (ICTV) describes viruses as "elementary biosystems that possess some of the properties of living systems such as having a genome and being able to adapt to a changing environment" (van Regenmortel and Mahy, 2004). In

Table 1 Examples of phage receptors

Bacterial host	Phage	Receptor[a]	Reference(s)
Gram negative			
Salmonella	P22	**LPS O-antigen**	Baxa et al., 1996
Y. enterocolitica	φYeO3-12	**LPS O-antigen**	Pajunen et al., 2000
Vibrio cholerae	K139	**LPS O-antigen**	Nesper et al., 2000
Shigella flexneri	Sf6	**LPS O-antigen**	Chua et al., 1999
E. coli	T3, T4, T7	**LPS core**	Prehm et al., 1976; Lindberg, 1973
Y. entercolitica	φR1-37	**LPS core**	Kiljunen et al., 2005
P. aeruginosa	φCTX	**LPS core**	Yokota et al., 1994
E. coli	PK1A to E	**K1 capsule**	Gross et al., 1977; Kwiatkowski et al., 1982; Pelkonen et al., 1989
E. coli	K1F	**K1 capsule**	Scholl et al., 2005; Vimr et al., 1984
E. coli	K5	**K5 capsule**	Gupta et al., 1982
E. coli	K1-5 (2 tail fiber proteins)	**K1 and K5 capsules**	Scholl et al., 2001
E. coli	Several phages	OmpA	Morona et al., 1984, 1985; Schwarz et al., 1983
E. coli	T1, φ80, and T5	Ferrichrome transporter FhuA	Bonhivers et al., 1998; Endriss and Braun, 2004; Killmann et al., 1995; Plancon et al., 2002
E. coli	λ	Maltoporin LamB	Randall-Hazelbauer and Schwartz, 1973; Wang et al., 2000
E. coli	fd, M13, f1	F pilus	Holland et al., 2006; Lubkowski et al., 1999
P. aeruginosa	Pf1	Type IV PAK pilus	Holland et al., 2006; Lubkowski et al., 1999
P. aeruginosa	Pf3	Conjugative pilus	Holland et al., 2006; Lubkowski et al., 1999
V. cholerae	KSF-1φ	Mannose-sensitive hemagglutinin type IV pilus	Faruque et al., 2005
Gram-negative bacteria harboring a conjugative plasmid	PRD1, the broad-host-range enveloped phage	Conjugative pilus	Grahn et al., 1999; Olsen et al., 1974
Escherichia, Salmonella, and *Serratia*	Phage X	Flagellum	Samuel et al., 1999
Aeromonas	PM3	Flagellum	Merino et al., 1990
Gram positive			
Lactococcus lactis	KH, bIL170, φ645	**Carbohydrates**	Valyasevi et al., 1990
Lactobacillus delbrueckii	LL-H	**Lipoteichoic acid**	Räisänen et al., 2004, 2007
B. subtilis	SP50	**Teichoic acids**	Archibald and Coapes, 1976
Listeria monocytogens	A118 and A500	**Teichoic acids**	Wendlinger et al., 1996
B. subtilis	PBS1	Flagellum	
B. subtilis	SPP1	Integral membrane protein	Raimondo et al., 1968; Sao-Jose et al., 2004
Listeria	A511	Peptidoglycan moiety	Wendlinger et al., 1996

[a]Receptors in boldface type are carbohydrates; others are proteins.

1962, Lwoff, Horne, and Tournier introduced modern taxonomy, a classification system of viruses based on the properties of the virion and its nucleic acid (http://www.ncbi.nlm.nih.gov/ICTVdb/). In the present ICTV system, the hierarchy ranks are species, genus, family, and order. A virus species is defined as "a polyethic class of viruses that constitute a replicating lineage and occupy a particular ecological niche" (Büchen-Osmond, 2003; van Regenmortel and Mahy, 2004). Members of a particular species share a number of properties but do not necessarily have any single property in common. A viral family, instead, is "a universal class sharing a number of properties that are both necessary and sufficient for class membership" (van Regenmortel and Mahy, 2004).

Bacteriophages are divided into one order and 13 families (Table 2) (Ackermann, 2003; Ackermann and DuBow, 1987a, 1987b). The order *Caudovirales* (tailed phages) consists of three major structural types (families): *Podoviridae* (short tails), *Myoviridae* (long contractile tails), and *Siphoviridae* (long, noncontractile tails). The order *Caudovirales* comprises ca. 96% of known phages and is very likely the most abundant group of similar organisms in the biosphere. Within families, there are several genera that can be distinguished on the basis of host specificity and genetic relatedness. There are six genera in the family *Myoviridae*, six in the *Siphoviridae*, and three in the *Podoviridae* (Ackermann, 2001, 2003; Maniloff and Ackermann, 1998). Polyhedral, filamentous, and pleomorphic phages are classified into 10 families altogether (Table 2), each having one to four genera.

The present, morphology-based taxonomy has faced a major criticism during the past few years (Lawrence et al., 2002; Nelson, 2004). The ICTV taxonomy is dependent on electron microscopic images and does not take into account the rapidly increasing genomic and proteomic data. However, there are several phages for which there is no electron microscopic image available but whose genomes have been completely sequenced. This specially concerns lysogenic prophages and phages of nonculturable bacteria. It has been estimated that one-half of the phages whose genome had been deposited in databanks were not classified properly by the current taxonomic system (Nelson, 2004). In addition, looking only at phage morphology largely underestimates the diversity of phage genomes and may result in mistakes in classification. Phage genomes are highly mosaic (Campbell, 2003; Pedulla et al., 2003), and it is now becoming evident that a strictly hierarchical taxonomy cannot represent the complex relationships between viral species. There is thus an increasing consensus that in the future, phage classification should be based on genomic data (Lawrence et al., 2002; Nelson, 2004; Proux et al., 2002).

Phage Genomes and Evolution

Phages are not a homogeneous group. The extreme diversity of phages is manifested in the types and sizes

Table 2 Classification of bacteriophages[a]

Family	Shape	Schematic figure	Characteristics	Nucleic acid	Example
Myoviridae	Tailed		Contractile tail	dsDNA	T4
Siphoviridae	Tailed		Long, noncontractile tail	dsDNA	λ
Podoviridae	Tailed		Short tail	dsDNA	T7
Microviridae	Polyhedral		Small, no envelope	ssDNA	φX174
Corticoviridae	Polyhedral		Complex capsid, internal lipid membrane	dsDNA	PM2
Tectiviridae	Polyhedral		Protein shell and inner lipoprotein vesicle	dsDNA	PRD1
Leviviridae	Polyhedral		Icosahedral capsid	ssRNA	MS2
Cystoviridae	Polyhedral		Lipid envelope	dsRNA	φ6
Inoviridae	Filamentous		Filaments or rods	ssDNA	fd
Lipothrixviridae	Filamentous		Rods, lipid envelope	dsDNA	TTV1
Rudiviridae	Filamentous		Straight, rigid rods	dsDNA	SIRV1
Plasmaviridae	Pleomorphic		No capsid, lipid envelope	dsDNA	L2
Fuselloviridae	Pleomorphic		Lemon-shaped, lipid envelope, spikes at one pole	dsDNA	SSV1

[a]Data from Kiljunen, 2006. Modified from Ackermann, 2003 and Ackermann and DuBow, 1987b; http://www.ncbi.nlm.nih.gov/ICTVdb/index.htm. Families *Myoviridae*, *Siphoviridae*, and *Podoviridae* form the order *Caudovirales*.

of their genomes. While all cellular life forms possess a dsDNA genome, viruses may have genomic RNA or DNA, in either single-stranded (ss) or ds form (Table 2). Tailed phages, which constitute ca. 96% of known phages, all have dsDNA genomes (Ackermann, 2003; Ackermann and DuBow, 1987b). Phage genomes vary in size by at least 2 orders of magnitude, from four genes in RNA coli-phages, such as phage MS2, to more than 400 genes, as in a recently sequenced *Bacillus* phage G genome.

A number of phages have dsDNA genomes in which one of the normal nucleotides is completely substituted by a modified base (Gommers-Ampt and Borst, 1995; Warren, 1980). The most thoroughly studied example is T4 DNA, where cytosine is replaced by 5-hydroxymeth-ylcytosine (Wyatt and Cohen, 1953), which is further α- (70%) or β- (30%) glucosylated (Lehman and Pratt, 1960). Other examples are *Bacillus subtilis* phages φe, H1, SPO1, SP8, SP82G, 2C, and φ25, where thymine is replaced by 5-hydroxymethyluracil (Hemphill and Whiteley, 1975); and PBS1, PBS2, and yersiniophage φR1-37, where thymine is replaced by deoxyuridine (Kiljunen et al., 2005; Takahashi and Marmur, 1963). In some phages, only a fraction of certain base residues is chemically modified (Gommers-Ampt and Borst, 1995; Warren, 1980). These include *E. coli* phage Mu, in which ca. 15% of adenine residues are replaced by N^6-carboxymethyladenines (Swinton et al., 1983) and *B. subtilis* phage SP15, in which 62% of thymine residues are modified to phosphoglucuronated 5-dihy-droxypentyluracil (Ehrlich and Ehrlich, 1981). The role of modified nucleotides in phage DNA is in many cases to confer resistance to host- or phage-encoded nucle-ases (Gommers-Ampt and Borst, 1995; Warren, 1980), and many restriction endonucleases have been shown to digest modified DNA slowly if at all (Huang et al., 1982). Modified bases may also serve as signals for transcription by phage-encoded RNA polymerases and phage DNA packaging.

The molecular mechanisms driving evolution may be either vertical or horizontal. Vertical mechanisms cre-ate variation through mutations (nucleotide exchanges, deletions, and inversions), after which the new variant is inherited by the next generation. Horizontal mecha-nisms transfer the genetic information (ranging from single genes to complete functional units) within the whole population, and even through species barriers, to form novel combinations (Brüssow et al., 2004; Woese, 2000). Rapidly accumulating genomic data and in silico analyses of prophages, phage remnants, and functional phages have clearly demonstrated that the genomes of modern phages are highly mosaic (Brüssow and Desiere, 2001; Juhala et al., 2000; Pedulla et al., 2003). Tailed

phages are thought to comprise a single large evolu-tionary group, for which horizontal evolution provides access to a common gene pool, but in which access is not uniform (Hendrix et al., 1999).

Genetic mosaicism in lambdoid and T-even phages has actually been known already since the 1950s by heteroduplex mapping, and this led to the "modular theory" of phage evolution (Botstein, 1980). The modu-lar theory has dominated the ideas on the evolution of bacteriophages for more than 2 decades. The theory pro-poses that recombination between different members of the family of phages takes place in homologous regions that mark the positions of the mosaic boundaries. In other words, the product and unit of phage evolution is not a given virus, but a family of interchangeable ele-ments (modules), each of which is multigenic and can be considered as a functional unit (Casjens et al., 1992). The current view is that nonhomologous recombina-tion actually occurs indiscriminately across the whole genome (Brüssow et al., 2004; Hendrix, 2002), but most such recombination events disrupt an essential gene or regulatory function and result in a nonviable phage that is rapidly eliminated. Sometimes, however, such recom-bination events lead to gene products producing viable bacteriophages, and the new genes and combinations of genes initially acquired by nonhomologous recombina-tion can be distributed throughout the population by homologous recombination. Comparative analysis of phage genomes has led to the identification of genetic elements called "morons" (Juhala et al., 2000) that are typically transcribed autonomously and have often a GC content clearly different from that of the surround-ing genes. A moron that benefits its new host gradually becomes fully integrated into the phage genome and its regulatory circuit (Hendrix, 2002, 2003; Hendrix et al., 2000; Juhala et al., 2000).

THE IMPACT OF PHAGES ON BACTERIAL EVOLUTION

The relatedness of phages reflects to some extent the relatedness of their bacterial hosts, suggesting coevo-lution of phages and the host bacteria (Desiere et al., 2001). Phages have a fundamental influence on bac-terial evolution and diversification (Brüssow et al., 2004; Weinbauer and Rassoulzadegan, 2004). The struggle for survival between phage and bacteria pro-vokes an "arms race," whereby bacteria develop defense mechanisms like restriction enzymes or changes in their phage receptor molecules. Phages then circumvent these by chemically modified nucleotides and avoidance of restriction enzyme recognition sequences or mutating antireceptors, respectively (Comeau and Krisch, 2005; Weitz et al., 2005).

Bacteriophages can promote bacterial diversity in several ways. In the lytic state they may do so by "killing the winner"—that is, infecting and lysing the most abundant bacterial species, thus allowing less competitive species to coexist (Weinbauer and Rassoulzadegan, 2004). Phages are the main mediators of horizontal evolution of prokaryotes (Canchaya et al., 2003) either via (generalized) transduction or lysogenic conversion. In generalized transduction, the fragments of host DNA are accidentally packaged into the phage head and delivered into a new host cell (Brüssow et al., 2004; Weinbauer and Rassoulzadegan, 2004).

Lysogenic conversion is a feature of temperate phages; however, the prophage would be rapidly eliminated unless its presence increased the fitness of the lysogen. Lysogenic conversion genes may confer immunity to superinfection by similar or closely related phages or the genes may enhance the survival of the lysogen in its ecological niche; e.g., genes enhancing virulence of pathogenic bacteria may encode toxins, adhesins, invasions, or resistance to innate immunity (Brüssow et al., 2004; Canchaya et al., 2003; Wagner and Waldor, 2002). Examples of lysogenic conversion are toxin genes expressed by *Pseudomonas aeruginosa* phage φCTX (Nakayama et al., 1999), *E. coli* O:157:H7 phage 933W (Plunkett et al., 1999), and *C. botulinum* phage c-st (Sakaguchi et al., 2005) and *Vibrio cholerae* phage CTXφ (Miller, 2003; Waldor and Mekalanos, 1996).

Pathogenicity islands are large chromosomal regions that encode several virulence factors and may share characteristics with bacteriophages, e.g., they encode virulence factors and integrases, their GC content differs from the rest of the host genome, and they are flanked by repeat sequences (Hacker et al., 1997). These similarities have led to the hypothesis that many pathogenicity islands might have a phage origin and have been acquired by new hosts via transduction.

Interestingly, bacteriophage-bacteriophage interactions, by providing a helper function, have been shown to play a role in the evolution of pathogenic bacteria. One example is the case of two *Vibrio* phages, where one phage VPIφ encodes for the receptor of the second phage CTXφ (Karaolis et al., 1999). Furthermore, a complex interaction network of VPI genes and *V. cholerae* chromosomal genes regulates gene expression from both VPI and CTX prophages.

On the evolutionary time scale, the nature of prophage genomes in bacterial chromosomes is ephemeral. Mutations and deletions accumulate gradually in the genes coding for phage lytic functions, resulting in a defective prophage that can no longer be induced. Often, most of the original prophage genome is lost, and only the remnants of the phage sequences remain in the bacterial genome. In such cases the prophage origin of the remaining genes may be difficult to interpret (Brüssow et al., 2004; Canchaya et al., 2003).

BACTERIOPHAGE THERAPY

Early bacteriophage research was largely driven by the desire to use phages to combat bacterial diseases—phage therapy. Felix d'Hérelle and other early phage therapy researchers used phages to cure shigellosis, cholera, and staphylococcal infections. The results obtained were often promising but hampered by improper understanding of bacteriophage biology. Also, the experimental settings used, the crude and inefficient phage preparations, and the lack of proper controls generated contradictions (Carlton, 1999; Merril et al., 1996; Stone, 2002; Sulakvelidze et al., 2001; Summers, 1999, 2001). Despite the efforts of d'Hérelle and other scientists, the use of bacteriophages as antibacterial therapy was generally abandoned soon after the introduction of antibiotics in the 1940s in the Western world, but it was continued actively in the Former Soviet Union and Eastern Europe, especially Poland (McKinstry and Edgar, 2005; Stone, 2002; Summers, 2001). The institutions most actively involved in therapeutic phage research and production were the Eliava Institute in Tbilisi, Georgia (http://www.eliava-ibmv.caucasus.net/), and the Hirszfeld Institute in Wroclaw, Poland (http://www.iitd.pan.wroc.pl/). Unfortunately, the studies carried out in these countries were not well reported in the western hemisphere (Summers, 1999, 2001). Now, however, due to the increasing problem of antibiotic-resistant bacteria, interest in phage therapy is reemerging also in the West. The major concerns of phage therapy include efficacy, pharmacokinetics, and safety issues. These aspects are discussed below in more detail.

Prerequisites for Phage Therapy

Levin and Bull (Levin and Bull, 2004) suggest that phage therapy needs only to decrease the numbers of infecting bacteria to a level where the host defenses can take care of the remaining bacteria. They also comment that it is difficult to understand why a phage that replicates extremely well in the target bacteria fails when it is used for treatment. Understanding this requires a quantitative appreciation of the dynamics of the phage infection process, especially in vivo.

Before attempting phage therapy several, sometimes rather demanding, prerequisites should be met (Skurnik and Strauch, 2006):

1. Phage therapy should not be attempted before the biology of the therapeutic phage is well understood.

Since the phage-host systems are extremely complicated, this prerequisite has to be faced with some common sense.

2. Phage preparations should meet all the safety requirements; the preparations should be free of bacteria and their components.

3. Phage preparations contain infective phage particles; thus, storage of the preparations should be validated.

4. The phage receptor should be known. In a bacterial population of 10^6 to 10^8 bacteria, there is a high possibility of spontaneous phage-resistant mutants in which the receptor is either missing or altered. It can be assumed that a mutation eliminating the receptor that functions as a virulence factor of a pathogen (such as lipopolysaccharide) would attenuate the bacterium, making it easier for the host immune system to eliminate the bacteria.

5. The efficacy of phage therapy should be tested in an animal model. Each phage may behave differently in vivo.

Even when the above prerequisites are properly met, many bureaucratic and regulatory obstacles need to be settled before a therapeutic phage preparation can reach the end user.

Specific Features of Phage Therapy

Phage therapy and antibiotic treatment of bacterial infections differ from each other in several fundamental aspects. One of the most significant differences is the narrow host specificity of bacteriophages, which often makes it necessary to diagnose the bacteria involved in the infection before the appropriate phage treatment can be initiated. This requirement is in contrast to antibiotics, which have a broader target range and are often used to treat undiagnosed bacterial infections. On the other hand, the narrow host specificity minimizes the side effects of the phage treatment on the normal microbiota.

Phages are superior to antibiotics in that they are effective against multidrug-resistant pathogenic bacteria. The appearance of phage-resistant mutants is not as common as that of antibiotic resistance, and it is relatively easy to isolate a phage variant that is capable of infecting the mutated strain. This also holds true in a more general manner, since one of the advantages of phage therapy is the possibility of isolating new phages for hard-to-treat bacterial infections, in other words, to perform custom treatments. Furthermore, phage-associated side effects are uncommon since phages or their products do not affect eukaryotic cells (Matsuzaki et al., 2005).

The benefits listed above also hold true in the context of prophylactic treatment of food products: phages will not harm necessary bacteria in foods (e.g., starter cultures) or the accompanying bacterial biota in the environment. Moreover, since phages are generally composed entirely of proteins and nucleic acids, their eventual breakdown products consist exclusively of amino acids and nucleic acids. Thus, they are not xenobiotics and, unlike antibiotics and antiseptic agents, their introduction into, and distribution within, a given environment may be seen as a natural process (Carlton et al., 2005).

From a commercial viewpoint, due to the 90-year tradition of phage therapy, it is difficult to obtain clear intellectual property rights and this causes general reluctance to develop and use phage therapy in the West (Clark and March, 2006). This also prevents the technology from receiving much-needed funding. On the other hand, the development of a new therapeutic phage is cost-effective in comparison with the development of a new antibiotic (Brüssow, 2005; Matsuzaki et al., 2005; Skurnik and Strauch, 2006). A more difficult problem may be that, as we have seen during the last decade, there has been a shift in the focus of the major pharmaceutical companies toward therapeutics for chronic diseases. Drugs used to treat chronic diseases provide a long-term financial benefit for the companies, while agents such as antibiotics and phage are generally used briefly for acute illness.

Safety of Phage Therapy Products

When considering the criteria for the application of phage in the control of bacteria in food, feed, or medical therapy, all phages intended for therapy should be characterized in detail. This should encompass (i) determination of genome sequence and structure, (ii) bioinformatic analyses including all relevant databases, and, of course, (iii) proof of the applicability of the phage(s) for a specified application (Carlton et al., 2005). A more general safety requirement is that the phage preparation used for any therapeutic purpose should be extensively purified and free of contaminating endotoxins and other bacterial components.

As discussed earlier, phages may carry genes whose products promote bacterial virulence. This specially concerns temperate phages and phages capable of transduction; thus, the minimal requirement to ensure safety could be that phages considered for therapy should be lytic and nontransducing (Bruttin and Brüssow, 2005; Brüssow, 2005). As the genomes of temperate phages often have distinct elements (like integrases), sequencing and analyzing the genome may be enough to identify lytic phages. The latter requirement may be more complicated, since, for example, the phage life cycle does not correlate with transducing capability. As an example, many temperate *Listeria* phages are able to transduce genetic markers (Hodgson, 2000), but this has not been reported for strictly virulent *Listeria* phages (Carlton et al., 2005). On the other hand, phage φR1-37, a virulent yersiniophage (Kiljunen et al., 2005), is able to transduce genetic material at a low frequency (unpublished observations). One could of course argue that a very low transduction frequency might not have any practical consequences. There are, however, indications that in vivo conditions might be more favorable for transduction than in vitro conditions (Toth et al., 2003). The possibility of transduction should therefore be taken seriously, and methods for its detection should be developed. One such method could be the PCR-based screen introduced by Sander and Schmieger (Sander and Schmieger, 2001). Many phages break down bacterial DNA to recycle the bacterial host genome for their own DNA synthesis and thus lack the molecular basis for coexistence with the host. Such phages usually carry genes encoding enzymes involved in nucleotide metabolism, which could therefore be a desirable property of therapeutic phages (Carlton et al., 2005).

If infecting bacteria are present in large quantities in the human body, phage therapy may pose an additional risk of liberating substantial amounts of endotoxins upon lysis of the bacterial cells. Such a problem was recently targeted by Hagens and coworkers, who used nonreplicating, genetically modified filamentous phage Pf3R to kill *P. aeruginosa* in a mouse model. They removed an export protein gene from the phage genome and replaced it with the gene coding for restriction endonuclease BglIIR. The modified phage infected the host bacterium and expressed BglII, which cut the host but not the phage genomic DNA (the phage genome does not have the recognition site). The host was killed, and clearly less endotoxin was released in vitro than after infection by the lytic phage. In addition, in vivo experiments with infected mice demonstrated a protective effect against three to five times the median lethal dose of bacteria (Hagens et al., 2004).

It is also important to bear in mind that humans are constantly consuming significant amounts of phages in their foods; thus, in general, phages can be considered to be safe.

Selection of the Effective Therapeutic Phage

To ensure the effectiveness of the therapeutic phage, the bacterial strain causing the infection needs to be identified and the ability of the phage to kill the organism should be tested. The identification of bacteria by conventional culturing methods may often be too time-consuming, and thus, one could envision that in the future, different modern high-throughput screening methods might be useful. These could include DNA-based bacterial identification systems, like PCR and microarrays, but also various phage-based screens. For the latter, Merril suggests the use of reporter phages for rapid identification of the pathogen (Merril et al., 2006). A reporter bacteriophage has a reporter gene integrated into its genome, and the gene is expressed only when the phage infects a live host cell. Reporter phages would at once allow the selection of efficient phages from therapeutic phage banks; however, this approach is hampered by the fact that genetic engineering of some bacteriophages is difficult or almost impossible. As an alternative, an array of immobilized phages or phage antireceptors representing the repertoire of therapeutic phages could be used to fish out susceptible bacteria from the patient samples. The detection of bacteria bound to the phage antireceptor array could be based on 16S rRNA probes or some other sophisticated method.

Testing the killing potential of each possible therapeutic phage against every infecting bacterial strain is not always feasible; however, a comprehensive library of therapeutically approved phages kept in standardized phage banks could cover this need.

The high specificity of most phage-host systems is a general limitation when using a limited number of characterized phages to attack a given target bacterium. The problem might be solved by careful selection and pooling of several phages with different lysis ranges and/or using a single broad-host-range phage able to infect all (or a majority of) the targeted organisms. The latter possibility is perhaps more attractive, as a single phage would be easier to characterize and get approved by the authorities (Carlton et al., 2005). However, due to the highly specialized nature of the phage-host systems, the existence of such omnipotent phages in nature is rare and the possibility of constructing one by genetic engineering cannot be regarded as good.

Phage Pharmacokinetics

For each phage, pharmacokinetic information is required to design the most effective way to apply the therapeutic phage product. In general, phage pharmacokinetics is still rather poorly understood, as surprisingly little detailed research has been performed on the fate of phages in animals and humans. Often, in vitro and in vivo situations are substantially different and a phage that lyses its host bacterium under laboratory conditions may fail to do so in the mammalian environment (Dabrowska et al., 2005; Kasman et al., 2002; Payne and Jansen, 2003).

Phage therapy challenges current pharmacokinetic studies because the phage can replicate in vivo when target bacteria are present; in other words, it behaves as a self-amplifying drug. This can lead to unfamiliar kinetic phenomena. The self-replicative nature of phage therapy means that compared to chemical drugs like antibiotics, there is a reduced need for multiple doses.

Critical parameters that affect phage therapy are the phage adsorption rate, burst size, latent period, and initial phage dose; density-dependent thresholds and associated critical times should also be considered (Payne and Jansen, 2001). Another critical parameter is the clearance rate of the phage particles from the body fluids by the reticuloendothelial system. On the other hand, bacteriophages able to persist in the tissues have been selected by in vivo passage; usually phage variants with altered surface properties emerge (Capparelli et al., 2007; Merril et al., 1996).

Payne has developed mathematical models to predict the behavior of phages in vivo taking into account population dynamics (Payne and Jansen, 2003). Two paradoxical observations should be mentioned here. It is certain that the timing of the phage treatment is critical and that phage administered too early may result in clearing of the phage from the body before it reaches the replication threshold. Similarly, addition of antibiotics in parallel with phage may hamper the phage efficacy. The replication threshold and proliferation threshold are expressions used to describe the situation where a low concentration of host bacteria is present in the culture and it takes some time before the bacteria reach a density at which a net increase in phage concentrations can be seen (Kasman et al., 2002). Apparently, the threshold depends on the rare encounters of the phage with the relatively few host cells. In vivo experiments should demonstrate also whether the physical and chemical conditions encountered in vivo support the phage life cycle. In some body compartments, bacteria may reside in an environment that does not provide phages with optimal conditions for infection.

Weld et al. studied mathematical models of phage growth and also tried to fit the formulae to experimental data (Weld et al., 2004). They used T4 and K1-5 phages, E. coli strains as host bacteria, and rats as the animal model. They concluded that their mathematical model failed to predict phage growth in the rats, demonstrating the complexity of phage growth in vivo. Coexistence of the host bacterium and its specific phage was studied by Fischer and coworkers (Fischer et al., 2004). They showed that within a bacterial population, a fraction of cells may exist in a phage-resistant form, thus indicating heterogeneity within the population. Bull et al. presented

an analysis of the now-classical Smith and Huggins phage therapy experiments (Smith and Huggins, 1982, 1983; Smith et al., 1987) and repeated some of their experiments (Bull et al., 2002). They also introduced and used a resistance competition assay and a phage replication assay to analyze the parameters involved in the phage treatment.

Phage Products

In addition to whole phages, purified phage products may also be used as therapeutic agents. The most attractive alternatives are the phage enzymes needed for cell lysis. Phages promote destruction of the bacterial cell wall and subsequent cell lysis by two distinct mechanisms. Most lytic dsDNA phages, E. coli phages T4 and T7 (Mathews et al., 1983; Molineux, 1999) being the most extensively studied examples, disrupt bacterial walls by encoding a holin-endolysin system. The holin protein permeabilizes the membrane and lets endolysin gain access to the periplasm where it can degrade the peptidoglycan matrix (Bernhardt et al., 2002; Wang et al., 2000). As an example, Bacillus anthracis is killed by the γ phage lysin PlyG, and PlyG can protect mice infected by B. anthracis (Schuch et al., 2002). Analogously, murein-degrading enzymes (lysozymes, amidases, or endopeptidases) of phages infecting Streptococcus pneumoniae have been used successfully in mouse infections (Jado et al., 2003; Loeffler et al., 2001, 2003). A combination of a lysozyme and amidase was found to have synergistic effect in vitro (Loeffler and Fischetti, 2003) and also in protecting mice (Jado et al., 2003). Additional studies revealed that combinations of a murein-degrading enzyme with conventional antibiotics showed synergistic activities in vitro. However, this has to be confirmed by in vivo studies (Djurkovic et al., 2005). In a mouse model, a single dose of a lysin significantly reduced bacterial colonization by group B streptococci (Streptococcus agalactiae) in both the vagina and the oropharynx (Cheng et al., 2005).

Phage tail-like bacteriocins are another group of phage products able to eliminate target bacteria. This special group of bacteriocins consists of high-molecular-weight particles composed of fragments of bacteriophages, and they are produced by a number of Enterobacteriaceae and other gram-negative bacteria (Bradley, 1967; Daw and Falkiner, 1996). A phage tail-like bacteriocin, enterocoliticin, was isolated from the culture supernatant of Y. enterocolitica strain 29930. Upon contact with susceptible Yersinia strains, the phage tails contract and kill the bacterial cell by forming pores in the cell wall, leading to a rapid loss of ions (Strauch et al., 2001). The efficacy of enterocoliticin as an antimicrobial agent against infections with pathogenic *Y. enterocolitica* O3 strains was recently assessed (Damasko et al., 2005). In cell cultures exposed to *Y. enterocolitica*, enterocoliticin killed bacteria adhering to the surface of eukaryotic cells whereas intracellularly located bacteria were not destroyed. In mice infected orally, an increase in *Y. enterocolitica* numbers was inhibited at time points shortly after the oral application of enterocoliticin, indicating that the particles were effective against recently introduced pathogens. Repeated application of enterocoliticin, however, did not prevent the colonization of the gastrointestinal tract by *Y. enterocolitica*, suggesting that the bacteria rapidly escaped out of the reach of the enterocoliticin in vivo. Based on this study, the use of phage tail-like bacteriocins as antimicrobial agents most likely will be limited to in vitro applications.

Lytic phages with smaller genomes, such as the ssRNA phage Qβ and the ssDNA phage φX174, interfere with the bacterial enzymes that make precursors of murein, a key component of bacterial cell walls, in a manner similar to penicillin. This has raised the attractive possibility that oligopeptide antibiotics might be designed on the basis of these lytic proteins (Bernhardt et al., 2001, 2002).

In Vivo Phage Studies

Due to the explosive increase of antibiotic-resistant bacteria and the urgent need for new antimicrobial strategies, phage therapy research has experienced a renaissance. During the last decade, several ambitious in vivo phage therapy studies have been published, some of which are discussed below.

Brüssow and colleagues conducted systematic experiments with *E. coli* phages (Chibani-Chennoufi et al., 2004). A collection of *E. coli*-specific phages isolated from various sources were tested against a collection of *E. coli* strains, both pathogenic (enteropathogenic *E. coli* and enterohemorrhagic *E. coli*) and nonpathogenic, the latter representing the ECOR collection (Ochman and Selander, 1984). Altogether four phages related to the well-characterized T4 coliphage, showing the widest and complementary infection range among the strains, were selected for the mouse experiments. The endogenous *E. coli* gut microbiotas of 10 conventional mice represented by 500 lactose-positive colonies were assayed for phage susceptibility. Practically all *E. coli* cells were lysed by at least one of the phages. The susceptibility of intestinal *E. coli* from the mice to the phages in vivo was determined by orally applying increasing doses of phages mixed in the drinking water. When lactose-positive colonies were counted from the stools, only a slight decrease in their numbers was seen (counts dropped from $10^{6.2}$ to $10^{5.7}$) at different time points. The recovered colonies were

sensitive to phage lysis, and the phages survived the passage through the gut, although they did not multiply significantly; thus, the survival of the bacteria in the gut during the phage passage could only be explained by some physiological reasons that prevented phage-induced lysis. The authors went further and gave phages orally to axenic mice that were infected with a single *E. coli* strain. In these mice the phage titers in the stools increased in 1 day from the input of 10^5/ml in the drinking water to 10^{10}/ml in the stool. At the same time, the numbers of *E. coli* in the stools dropped from 10^8 to 10^4, from where the numbers leveled off during the subsequent days to 10^5. Again, the recovered colonies were sensitive to the phages, suggesting that the bacteria had resided in gut sites protected from phage.

In a very thorough study Biswas et al. (Biswas et al., 2002) performed experiments using a mouse model of vancomycin-resistant *Enterococcus faecium* (VRE) infection. They isolated VRE-specific phages from raw sewage and selected for animal experiments one that showed an antibacterial effect against 79% of studied strains in vitro. They showed first that phage administered intraperitoneally (i.p.) 45 min postinfection was able to rescue mice from VRE bacteremia and that the rescue was associated with a significant decrease in bacterial numbers in blood. They also demonstrated that phage administration before 5 h postinfection still fully rescued the mice, while treatment delayed beyond 5 h rescued only some of the mice (Biswas et al., 2002).

Bacteriophage φMR11 was tested in mouse infections caused by *Staphylococcus aureus* (Matsuzaki et al., 2003). The temperate bacteriophage was isolated after induction of *S. aureus* strains by mitomycin and was selected for experimental studies due to its broad ability to infect and lyse the 75 *S. aureus* indicator strains. The 43-kb phage genome was completely sequenced and did not carry any known toxin, virulence factor, or antibiotic resistance genes. The authors also characterized the phage with regard to its biological features. Mice were infected i.p. with an *S. aureus* dose that killed 80% of the untreated mice in 24 h and all of them in 7 days. Most of the mice died between 6 and 7 h after infection. Mice receiving phage i.p. immediately following the bacterial challenge were protected. In an experimental design whereby mice were infected with the φMR11 lysogen strain, no protection was observed. This enabled the authors to conclude that the direct bactericidal effect of the phage was the principal determinant of the protective effect, and an indirect effect such as a phage-stimulated immune response (e.g., production of cytokines) did not play a role (Matsuzaki et al., 2003). Phages could rescue mice when administered 60 min later than the bacteria.

Phage and bacterial numbers in the circulation were determined after the infection and showed that the bacterial load was much lower in the blood of phage-treated mice than in the blood of those that received only bacteria. They also noticed that phage titers in mice infected with bacteria remained higher than the titers in mice that received only the phage, suggesting that the phage replicated in the infected mice and consumed the bacteria. This happened until the bacteria disappeared from the circulation, which was paralleled by elimination of the phage (Matsuzaki et al., 2003).

Capparelli et al. (2007) described an *S. aureus*-specific bacteriophage, M^{Sa}, a derivative of a wild-type phage "educated" to persist in mouse blood for 20 to 25 days. When inoculated into mice simultaneously with *S. aureus* A170, the phage rescued the mice in a dose-dependent manner. The phage also fully cleared the bacteria when applied to nonlethal 10-day infections. The authors found that a bacterial load of 10^4 CFU/ml was necessary to allow in vivo phage replication. The phage were also efficient when used in abscesses induced in the skin; it prevented abscess formation and reduced the bacterial number and abscess size. The phage M^{Sa} could be delivered inside macrophages by *S. aureus* and was able to kill intracellular staphylococci both in vivo and in vitro (Capparelli et al., 2007).

Watanabe et al. (2007) used a lytic phage KPP10 in a murine model of gut-derived sepsis caused by *P. aeruginosa* to evaluate the efficacy of phage therapy. They helped the establishment of *P. aeruginosa* colonization in the gut by disturbing the normal microbiota of the mice with ampicillin and invasion of tissues by disrupting the mucosal barrier with cyclophosphamide treatment. Mice treated this way started to succumb 14 days after the infection due to sepsis. Significant protection against the infection was obtained if the phage KPP10 was given orally 1 day after the bacterial infection, but not when given 1 day prior, or 6 days after, the bacterial infection. The authors analyzed the mouse tissues thoroughly both for bacterial and phage concentrations: the bacterial load was significantly lower in the blood, spleen, liver, and mesenteric lymph nodes in phage-treated mice than in saline-treated controls. Viable phage were recovered from both blood and liver. The authors also showed that phage protected i.p.-infected mice; for this, the phage had to be administered simultaneously to the infection since phage given 1 day before had no protective effect (Watanabe et al., 2007).

However, not all studies of phage therapy have had such promising outcomes; for example, some recent experiments performed with *Y. enterocolitica* O:3, an enteropathogen with pigs as the main source of human infections. This organism uses several virulence factors to colonize the intestinal tissue, and it invades via M cells of Peyer's patches into the lamina propria and mesenteric lymph nodes. Bacteriophages PY100 and φYeO3-12 were tested for their ability to eradicate this organism from the gut microbiota of 8-week-old female BALB/c mice (Skurnik and Strauch, 2006). Both *Yersinia* phages were administered orally in a single application and were active for at least 24 h within the gastrointestinal tract and, in some mice, even in deeper organs, indicating that particles had passed the gastrointestinal barrier. Even though in in vitro cultures the bacteria were efficiently killed by both phages, neither a single nor repeated applications (by administering the phage at 24-h intervals four times starting 1 h after the infection) inhibited the colonization of mice by *Y. enterocolitica* O:3 (Skurnik and Strauch, 2006). Thus, *Y. enterocolitica* colonization in mice could not be controlled by phage therapy, at least with the regimen investigated. Perhaps the aggressive tissue invasion and transient intracellular lifestyle of *Y. enterocolitica* hamper the efficiency of phage eradication. It would not be surprising if similar results are obtained with other bacterial pathogens.

Huff and colleagues have explored the possibilities of phage therapy using chicken challenged with a respiratory infection due to *E. coli* (Huff et al., 2005). Their first papers reported just the clinical signs of the infected birds, without analysis of the phage or bacterial loads (Huff et al., 2002a, 2002b). Phage mixed with *E. coli* prior to an air sac infection protected the chickens, but phage administered into the drinking water did not. They first showed that an aerosol spray was a promising way to administer the phage (Huff et al., 2002a, 2002b) and then compared the aerosol spray and an intramuscular injection of bacteriophage (Huff et al., 2003b). Phage given as an aerosol spray immediately after the *E. coli* infection, but not after 24 h, were protective, whereas the intramuscular phage were also protective when given immediately, or 24 or 48 h after challenge. The presence of phage in the blood was also monitored. Almost no birds had phage in the blood after aerosol spraying, while high numbers of phage were present after intramuscular administration (Huff et al., 2003b). Multiple intramuscular treatments proved to be more effective than a single dose (Huff et al., 2003a). Another clinical trial was conducted to evaluate a combination of the antibiotic enrofloxacin and intramuscularly administered bacteriophage (Huff et al., 2004). Even though both treatments individually provided effective treatments of the *E. coli* infection, the synergy between the two treatments led to a total protection of the birds. This suggested the significant value of the combined treatment.

The escape of invasive pathogens into closed tissue and organ compartments may block the effective use of bacteriophages, especially if the phages cannot actively follow the bacteria. Replicating phages may enter the compartment inside an invading bacterium in a manner analogous to that of the Trojan horse. It is, however, quite clear that many variations of this theme will be encountered among different bacteriophage/pathogen systems. In an attempt to utilize the Trojan horse concept, Broxmeyer et al. (2002) developed a system whereby *Mycobacterium smegmatis*, an avirulent mycobacterium, was used to deliver the lytic phage TM4 into macrophages in tissue cultures in which both *Mycobacterium avium* and *Mycobacterium tuberculosis* resided. The results showed that the treatment was able to reduce the numbers of viable intracellular bacilli (Broxmeyer et al., 2002).

Listeria Phage P100

The study of a *Listeria monocytogenes* phage P100 was conducted according to current guidelines that should accompany the application of phages in therapy. The authors provided a detailed characterization of the phage P100-encoded information, performed toxicity studies keeping the potential use of P100 as a biopreservation food additive in mind, and showed its usefulness in controlling *Listeria* in a model food system (Carlton et al., 2005). Phage P100 is a broad-host-range, strictly virulent phage, which infects and kills the majority of *L. monocytogenes* strains. The authors determined the 131-kb genome nucleotide sequence. The predicted 174 gene products contained no homologies to proteins which are known or suspected to be toxins, pathogenicity factors, antibiotic resistance determinants, or any known allergens. An oral toxicity study with rats revealed no abnormal histological changes, morbidity, or mortality. The authors concluded that no indications for any potential risk associated with using P100 as a food additive were present (Carlton et al., 2005). Largely based on this thorough safety analysis, LISTEX P100 (www.ebifoodsafety.com) is the first bacteriophage product to receive (in October 2006) the "Generally Recognized as Safe" status by the U.S. Food and Drug Administration.

CONCLUDING REMARKS

Based on the examples presented in this chapter, the use of bacteriophages to control bacterial infections is promising. The global increase of antibiotic-resistant organisms warrants the exploitation of alternative strategies to manage infectious diseases. The therapeutic use of bacteriophages, perhaps in combination with antibiotics

or other treatments, may work. At the same time, to obtain safe and controlled phage therapy products, there is a need for detailed information on the properties and behavior of the multitude of phage-bacterium systems, both in vitro and especially in vivo. The in vivo susceptibility of bacterial pathogens to bacteriophages is still largely poorly understood. Finally, clear-cut instructions and quality requirements for phage products should be made available.

References

Ackermann, H. W. 2001. Frequency of morphological phage descriptions in the year 2000. Brief review. *Arch. Virol.* **146:**843–857.

Ackermann, H. W. 2003. Bacteriophage observations and evolution. *Res. Microbiol.* **154:**245–251.

Ackermann, H. W., and M. S. DuBow. 1987a. Natural groups of bacteriophages, p. 85–100. *In* H. W. Ackermann and M. S. DuBow (ed.), *Viruses of Procaryotes.* CRC Press, Inc, Boca Raton, FL.

Ackermann, H. W., and M. S. DuBow. 1987b. *Viruses of Procaryotes.* CRC Press, Inc., Boca Raton, FL.

Allison, G. E., and N. K. Verma. 2000. Serotype-converting bacteriophages and O-antigen modification in *Shigella flexneri. Trends Microbiol.* **8:**17–23.

Archibald, A. R., and H. E. Coapes. 1976. Bacteriophage SP50 as a marker for cell wall growth in *Bacillus subtilis. J. Bacteriol.* **125:**1195–1206.

Baxa, U., S. Steinbacher, S. Miller, A. Weintraub, R. Huber, and R. Seckler. 1996. Interactions of phage P22 tails with their cellular receptor, *Salmonella* O-antigen polysaccharide. *Biophys. J.* **71:**2040–2048.

Bernhardt, T. G., I. N. Wang, D. K. Struck, and R. Young. 2001. A protein antibiotic in the phage Qβ: diversity in lysis targets. *Science* **292:**2326–2329.

Bernhardt, T. G., I. N. Wang, D. K. Struck, and R. Young. 2002. Breaking free: "protein antibiotics" and phage lysis. *Res. Microbiol.* **153:**493–501.

Biswas, B., S. Adhya, P. Washart, B. Paul, A. N. Trostel, B. Powell, R. Carlton, and C. R. Merril. 2002. Bacteriophage therapy rescues mice bacteremic from a clinical isolate of vancomycin-resistant *Enterococcus faecium. Infect. Immun.* **70:**204–210.

Bonhivers, M., L. Plancon, A. Ghazi, P. Boulanger, M. le Maire, O. Lambert, J. L. Rigaud, and L. Letellier. 1998. FhuA, an *Escherichia coli* outer membrane protein with a dual function of transporter and channel which mediates the transport of phage DNA. *Biochimie* **80:**363–369.

Botstein, D. 1980. A theory of modular evolution for bacteriophages. *Ann. N. Y. Acad. Sci.* **354:**484–490.

Bradley, D. E. 1967. Ultrastructure of bacteriophage and bacteriocins. *Bacteriol. Rev.* **31:**230–314.

Breitbart, M., and F. Rohwer. 2005. Here a virus, there a virus, everywhere the same virus? *Trends Microbiol.* **13:**278–284.

Broxmeyer, L., D. Sosnowska, E. Miltner, O. Chacon, D. Wagner, J. McGarvey, R. G. Barletta, and L. E. Bermudez. 2002.

Killing of *Mycobacterium avium* and *Mycobacterium tuberculosis* by a mycobacteriophage delivered by a nonvirulent mycobacterium: a model for phage therapy of intracellular bacterial pathogens. *J. Infect. Dis.* **186**:1155–1160.

Brüssow, H. 2005. Phage therapy: the *Escherichia coli* experience. *Microbiology* **151**:2133–2140.

Brüssow, H., C. Canchaya, and W. D. Hardt. 2004. Phages and the evolution of bacterial pathogens: from genomic rearrangements to lysogenic conversion. *Microbiol. Mol. Biol. Rev.* **68**:560–602.

Brüssow, H., and F. Desiere. 2001. Comparative phage genomics and the evolution of *Siphoviridae*: insights from dairy phages. *Mol. Microbiol.* **39**:213–222.

Bruttin, A., and H. Brüssow. 2005. Human volunteers receiving *Escherichia coli* phage T4 orally: a safety test of phage therapy. *Antimicrob. Agents Chemother.* **49**:2874–2878.

Büchen-Osmond, C. 2003. Taxonomy and classification of viruses, p. 1217–1226. *In* P. R. Murray, E. J. Baron, J. H. Jorgensen, M. A. Pfaller, and R. H. Yolken (ed.), *Manual of Clinical Microbiology*, 8th ed. ASM Press, Washington, DC.

Bull, J. J., B. R. Levin, T. DeRouin, N. Walker, and C. A. Bloch. 2002. Dynamics of success and failure in phage and antibiotic therapy in experimental infections. *BMC Microbiol.* **2**:35.

Campbell, A. 2003. The future of bacteriophage biology. *Nat. Rev. Gene.* **4**:471–477.

Canchaya, C., C. Proux, G. Fournous, A. Bruttin, and H. Brüssow. 2003. Prophage genomics. *Microbiol. Mol. Biol. Rev.* **67**:238–276.

Capparelli, R., M. Parlato, G. Borriello, P. Salvatore, and D. Iannelli. 2007. Experimental phage therapy against *Staphylococcus aureus* in mice. *Antimicrob. Agents Chemother.* **51**:2765–2773.

Carlton, R. M. 1999. Phage therapy: past history and future prospects. *Arch. Immunol. Ther. Exp.* **47**:267–274.

Carlton, R. M., W. H. Noordman, B. Biswas, E. D. de Meester, and M. J. Loessner. 2005. Bacteriophage P100 for control of *Listeria monocytogenes* in foods: genome sequence, bioinformatic analyses, oral toxicity study, and application. *Regul. Toxicol. Pharmacol.* **43**:301–312.

Casjens, S., G. F. Hatfull, and R. W. Hendrix. 1992. Evolution of dsDNA tailed bacteriophage genomes. *Semin. Virol.* **3**:383–397.

Cheng, Q., D. Nelson, S. Zhu, and V. A. Fischetti. 2005. Removal of group B streptococci colonizing the vagina and oropharynx of mice with a bacteriophage lytic enzyme. *Antimicrob. Agents Chemother.* **49**:111–117.

Chibani-Chennoufi, S., J. Sidoti, A. Bruttin, E. Kutter, S. Sarker, and H. Brüssow. 2004. In vitro and in vivo bacteriolytic activities of *Escherichia coli* phages: implications for phage therapy. *Antimicrob. Agents Chemother.* **48**:2558–2569.

Chua, J. E., P. A. Manning, and R. Morona. 1999. The *Shigella flexneri* bacteriophage Sf6 tailspike protein (TSP)/endorhamnosidase is related to the bacteriophage P22 TSP and has a motif common to exo- and endoglycanases, and C-5 epimerases. *Microbiology* **145**:1649–1659.

Clark, J. R., and J. B. March. 2006. Bacteriophages and biotechnology: vaccines, gene therapy and antibacterials. *Trends Biotechnol.* **24**:212–218.

Comeau, A. M., and H. M. Krisch. 2005. War is peace—dispatches from the bacterial and phage killing fields. *Curr. Opin. Microbiol.* **8**:488–494.

Dabrowska, K., K. Switala-Jelen, A. Opolski, B. Weber-Dabrowska, and A. Gorski. 2005. Bacteriophage penetration in vertebrates. *J. Appl. Microbiol.* **98**:7–13.

Damasko, C., A. Konietzny, H. Kaspar, B. Appel, P. Dersch, and E. Strauch. 2005. Studies of the efficacy of enterocoliticin, a phage-tail like bacteriocin, as antimicrobial agent against *Yersinia enterocolitica* serotype O3 in a cell culture system and in mice. *J. Vet. Med. B* **52**:1–9.

Daw, M. A., and F. R. Falkiner. 1996. Bacteriocins: nature, function and structure. *Micron* **27**:467–479.

Desiere, F., W. M. McShan, D. van Sinderen, J. J. Ferretti, and H. Brüssow. 2001. Comparative genomics reveals close genetic relationships between phages from dairy bacteria and pathogenic *Streptococci*: evolutionary implications for prophage-host interactions. *Virology* **288**:325–341.

Djurkovic, S., J. M. Loeffler, and V. A. Fischetti. 2005. Synergistic killing of *Streptococcus pneumoniae* with the bacteriophage lytic enzyme Cpl-1 and penicillin or gentamicin depends on the level of penicillin resistance. *Antimicrob. Agents Chemother.* **49**:1225–1228.

Dupont, K., T. Janzen, F. K. Vogensen, J. Josephsen, and B. Stuer-Lauridsen. 2004. Identification of *Lactococcus lactis* genes required for bacteriophage adsorption. *Appl. Environ. Microbiol.* **70**:5825–5832.

Ehrlich, M., and K. C. Ehrlich. 1981. A novel, highly modified, bacteriophage DNA in which thymine is partly replaced by a phosphoglucuronate moiety covalently bound to 5-(4′,5′-dihydroxypentyl)uracil. *J. Biol. Chem.* **256**:9966–9972.

Endriss, F., and V. Braun. 2004. Loop deletions indicate regions important for FhuA transport and receptor functions in *Escherichia coli*. *J. Bacteriol.* **186**:4818–4823.

Faruque, S. M., I. Bin Naser, K. Fujihara, P. Diraphat, N. Chowdhury, M. Kamruzzaman, F. Qadri, S. Yamasaki, A. N. Ghosh, and J. J. Mekalanos. 2005. Genomic sequence and receptor for the *Vibrio cholerae* phage KSF-1φ: evolutionary divergence among filamentous vibriophages mediating lateral gene transfer. *J. Bacteriol.* **187**:4095–4103.

Fischer, C. R., M. Yoichi, H. Unno, and Y. Tanji. 2004. The coexistence of *Escherichia coli* serotype O157:H7 and its specific bacteriophage in continuous culture. *FEMS Microbiol. Lett.* **241**:171–177.

Freifelder, D. 1983. *Molecular Biology: a Comprehensive Introduction to Prokaryotes and Eukaryotes*. Science Books Int., Boston, MA.

Gommers-Ampt, J. H., and P. Borst. 1995. Hypermodified bases in DNA. *FASEB J.* **9**:1034–1042.

Grahn, A. M., J. Caldentey, J. K. Bamford, and D. H. Bamford. 1999. Stable packaging of phage PRD1 DNA requires adsorption protein P2, which binds to the IncP plasmid-encoded conjugative transfer complex. *J. Bacteriol.* **181**:6689–6696.

Gross, R. J., T. Cheasty, and B. Rowe. 1977. Isolation of bacteriophages specific for the K1 polysaccharide antigen of *Escherichia coli*. *J. Clin. Microbiol.* **6**:548–550.

Gupta, D. S., B. Jann, G. Schmidt, J. R. Golecki, I. Orskov, F. Orskov, and K. Jann. 1982. Coliphage K5, specific for *E. coli* exhibiting the capsular K5 antigen. *FEMS Microbiol. Lett.* **14**:75–78.

Hacker, J., G. Blum-Oehler, I. Mühldorfer, and H. Tschäpe. 1997. Pathogenicity islands of virulent bacteria: structure, function and impact on microbial evolution. *Mol. Microbiol.* **23**:1089–1097.

Hagens, S., A. Habel, U. Von Ahsen, A. Von Gabain, and U. Bläsi. 2004. Therapy of experimental pseudomonas infections with a nonreplicating genetically modified phage. *Antimicrob. Agents Chemother.* **48**:3817–3822.

Hambly, E., and C. A. Suttle. 2005. The viriosphere, diversity, and genetic exchange within phage communities. *Curr. Opin. Microbiol.* **8**:444–450.

Harshey, R. M. 1988. Phage Mu, p. 193–234. *In* R. Calendar (ed.), *The Bacteriophages*. Plenum Press, New York, NY.

Heller, K. J. 1992. Molecular interaction between bacteriophage and the gram-negative cell envelope. *Arch. Microbiol.* **158**:235–248.

Hemphill, H. E., and H. R. Whiteley. 1975. Bacteriophages of *Bacillus subtilis*. *Bacteriol. Rev.* **39**:257–315.

Hendrix, R. W. 2002. Bacteriophages: evolution of the majority. *Theor. Popul. Biol.* **61**:471–480.

Hendrix, R. W. 2003. Bacteriophage genomics. *Curr. Opin. Microbiol.* **6**:506–511.

Hendrix, R. W., G. F. Hatfull, and M. C. Smith. 2003. Bacteriophages with tails: chasing their origins and evolution. *Res. Microbiol.* **154**:253–257.

Hendrix, R. W., J. G. Lawrence, G. F. Hatfull, and S. Casjens. 2000. The origins and ongoing evolution of viruses. *Trends Microbiol.* **8**:504–508.

Hendrix, R. W., J. W. Roberts, F. W. Stahl, and R. A. Weisberg. 1983. *Lambda II*. Cold Spring Harbor Laboratory, Cold Spring Harbor, NY.

Hendrix, R. W., M. C. Smith, R. N. Burns, M. E. Ford, and G. F. Hatfull. 1999. Evolutionary relationships among diverse bacteriophages and prophages: all the world's a phage. *Proc. Natl. Acad. Sci. USA* **96**:2192–2197.

Hertwig, S., I. Klein, R. Lurz, E. Lanka, and B. Appel. 2003. PY54, a linear plasmid prophage of *Yersinia enterocolitica* with covalently closed ends. *Mol. Microbiol.* **48**:989–1003.

Hodgson, D. A. 2000. Generalized transduction of serotype 1/2 and serotype 4b strains of *Listeria monocytogenes*. *Mol. Microbiol.* **35**:312–323.

Holland, S. J., C. Sanz, and R. N. Perham. 2006. Identification and specificity of pilus adsorption proteins of filamentous bacteriophages infecting *Pseudomonas aeruginosa*. *Virology* **345**:540–548.

Huang, L. H., C. M. Farnet, K. C. Ehrlich, and M. Ehrlich. 1982. Digestion of highly modified bacteriophage DNA by restriction endonucleases. *Nucleic. Acids Res.* **10**:1579–1591.

Huff, W. E., G. R. Huff, N. C. Rath, J. M. Balog, and A. M. Donoghue. 2005. Alternatives to antibiotics: utilization of bacteriophage to treat colibacillosis and prevent foodborne pathogens. *Poult. Sci.* **84**:655–659.

Huff, W. E., G. R. Huff, N. C. Rath, J. M. Balog, and A. M. Donoghue. 2002a. Prevention of *Escherichia coli* infection in broiler chickens with a bacteriophage aerosol spray. *Poult. Sci.* **81**:1486–1491.

Huff, W. E., G. R. Huff, N. C. Rath, J. M. Balog, and A. M. Donoghue. 2003a. Bacteriophage treatment of a severe *Escherichia coli* respiratory infection in broiler chickens. *Avian Dis.* **47**:1399–1405.

Huff, W. E., G. R. Huff, N. C. Rath, J. M. Balog, and A. M. Donoghue. 2003b. Evaluation of aerosol spray and intramuscular injection of bacteriophage to treat an *Escherichia coli* respiratory infection. *Poult. Sci.* **82**:1108–1112.

Huff, W. E., G. R. Huff, N. C. Rath, J. M. Balog, and A. M. Donoghue. 2004. Therapeutic efficacy of bacteriophage and Baytril (enrofloxacin) individually and in combination to treat colibacillosis in broilers. *Poult. Sci.* **83**:1944–1947.

Huff, W. E., G. R. Huff, N. C. Rath, J. M. Balog, H. Xie, P. A. Moore, Jr., and A. M. Donoghue. 2002b. Prevention of *Escherichia coli* respiratory infection in broiler chickens with bacteriophage (SPR02). *Poult. Sci.* **81**:437–441.

Jado, I., R. Lopez, E. Garcia, A. Fenoll, J. Casal, and P. Garcia. 2003. Phage lytic enzymes as therapy for antibiotic-resistant *Streptococcus pneumoniae* infection in a murine sepsis model. *J. Antimicrob. Chemother.* **52**:967–973.

Juhala, R. J., M. E. Ford, R. L. Duda, A. Youlton, G. F. Hatfull, and R. W. Hendrix. 2000. Genomic sequences of bacteriophages HK97 and HK022: pervasive genetic mosaicism in the lambdoid bacteriophages. *J. Mol. Biol.* **299**:27–51.

Karaolis, D. K., S. Somara, D. R. Maneval, Jr., J. A. Johnson, and J. B. Kaper. 1999. A bacteriophage encoding a pathogenicity island, a type-IV pilus and a phage receptor in cholera bacteria. *Nature* **399**:375–379.

Kasman, L. M., A. Kasman, C. Westwater, J. Dolan, M. G. Schmidt, and J. S. Norris. 2002. Overcoming the phage replication threshold: a mathematical model with implications for phage therapy. *J. Virol.* **76**:5557–5564.

Kiljunen, S. 2006. Molecular biology, genetics and applications of yersiniophages. Ph.D. thesis. University of Turku, Turku, Finland.

Kiljunen, S., K. Hakala, E. Pinta, S. Huttunen, P. Pluta, A. Gador, H. Lönnberg, and M. Skurnik. 2005. Yersiniophage φR1-37 is a tailed bacteriophage having a 270 kb DNA genome with thymidine replaced by deoxyuridine. *Microbiology* **151**:4093–4102.

Killmann, H., G. Videnov, G. Jung, H. Schwarz, and V. Braun. 1995. Identification of receptor binding sites by competitive peptide mapping: phages T1, T5, and phi 80 and colicin M bind to the gating loop of FhuA. *J. Bacteriol.* **177**:694–698.

Koebnik, R., K. P. Locher, and P. Van Gelder. 2000. Structure and function of bacterial outer membrane proteins: barrels in a nutshell. *Mol. Microbiol.* **37**:239–253.

Kwiatkowski, B., B. Boschek, H. Thiele, and S. Stirm. 1982. Endo-N-acetylneuraminidase associated with bacteriophage particles. *J. Virol.* **43**:697–704.

Lawrence, J. G., G. F. Hatfull, and R. W. Hendrix. 2002. Imbroglios of viral taxonomy: genetic exchange and failings of phenetic approaches. *J. Bacteriol.* **184**:4891–4905.

Lehman, I. R., and E. A. Pratt. 1960. On the structure of the glucosylated hydroxymethylcytosine nucleotides of coliphages T2, T4, and T6. *J. Biol. Chem.* **235**:3254–3259.

Levin, B. R., and J. J. Bull. 2004. Population and evolutionary dynamics of phage therapy. *Nat. Rev. Microbiol.* **2**:166–173.

Lindberg, A. A. 1973. Bacteriophage receptors. *Annu. Rev. Microbiol.* **27:**205–241.

Little, J. W. 2005. Lysogeny, prophage induction and lysogenic conversion. *In* M. K. Waldor, D. I. Friedman, and S. Adhya (ed.), *Phages: Their Role in Bacterial Pathogenesis and Biotechnology.* ASM Press, Washington, DC.

Lobocka, M. B., D. J. Rose, G. Plunkett III, M. Rusin, A. Samojedny, H. Lehnherr, M. B. Yarmolinsky, and F. R. Blattner. 2004. Genome of bacteriophage P1. *J. Bacteriol.* **186:**7032–7068.

Loeffler, J. M., S. Djurkovic, and V. A. Fischetti. 2003. Phage lytic enzyme Cpl-1 as a novel antimicrobial for pneumococcal bacteremia. *Infect. Immun.* **71:**6199–6204.

Loeffler, J. M., and V. A. Fischetti. 2003. Synergistic lethal effect of a combination of phage lytic enzymes with different activities on penicillin-sensitive and -resistant *Streptococcus pneumoniae* strains. *Antimicrob. Agents Chemother.* **47:**375–377.

Loeffler, J. M., D. Nelson, and V. A. Fischetti. 2001. Rapid killing of *Streptococcus pneumoniae* with a bacteriophage cell wall hydrolase. *Science* **294:**2170–2172.

Lubkowski, J., F. Hennecke, A. Plückthun, and A. Wlodawer. 1999. Filamentous phage infection: crystal structure of g3p in complex with its coreceptor, the C-terminal domain of TolA. *Structure* **7:**711–722.

Maniloff, J., and H. W. Ackermann. 1998. Taxonomy of bacterial viruses: establishment of tailed virus genera and the order Caudovirales. *Arch. Virol.* **143:**2051–2063.

Mathews, C. K., E. Kutter, G. Mosig, and P. B. Berget. 1983. *Bacteriophage T4.* American Society for Microbiology, Washington, DC.

Matsuzaki, S., M. Rashel, J. Uchiyama, S. Sakurai, T. Ujihara, M. Kuroda, M. Ikeuchi, T. Tani, M. Fujieda, H. Wakiguchi, and S. Imai. 2005. Bacteriophage therapy: a revitalized therapy against bacterial infectious diseases. *J. Infect. Chemother.* **11:**211–219.

Matsuzaki, S., M. Yasuda, H. Nishikawa, M. Kuroda, T. Ujihara, T. Shuin, Y. Shen, Z. Jin, S. Fujimoto, M. D. Nasimuzzaman, H. Wakiguchi, S. Sugihara, T. Sugiura, S. Koda, A. Muraoka, and S. Imai. 2003. Experimental protection of mice against lethal *Staphylococcus aureus* infection by novel bacteriophage φMR11. *J. Infect. Dis.* **187:**613–624.

McKinstry, M., and R. Edgar. 2005. Use of phages in therapy and bacterial detection, p. 430–440. *In* M. K. Waldor, D. I. Friedman, and S. Adhya (ed.), *Phages: Their Role in Bacterial Pathogenesis and Biotechnology.* ASM Press, Washington, DC.

Merino, S., S. Camprubi, and J. M. Tomas. 1990. Isolation and characterization of bacteriophage PM3 from *Aeromonas hydrophila* the bacterial receptor for which is the monopolar flagellum. *FEMS Microbiol. Lett.* **57:**277–282.

Merril, C. R., B. Biswas, R. Carlton, N. C. Jensen, G. J. Creed, S. Zullo, and S. Adhya. 1996. Long-circulating bacteriophage as antibacterial agents. *Proc. Natl. Acad. Sci. USA* **93:**3188–3192.

Merril, C. R., D. Scholl, and S. Adhya. 2006. Phage therapy, p. 725–741. *In* R. Calendar (ed.), *The Bacteriophages,* 2nd ed. Oxford University Press, New York, NY.

Miller, J. F. 2003. Bacteriophage and the evolution of epidemic cholera. *Infect. Immun.* **71:**2981–2982.

Molineux, I. J. 1999. The T7 family of bacteriophages, p. 2495–2507. *In* T. E. Creighton (ed.), *Encyclopedia of Molecular Biology.* John Wiley and Co, New York, NY.

Morona, R., M. Klose, and U. Henning. 1984. *Escherichia coli* K-12 outer membrane protein (OmpA) as a bacteriophage receptor: analysis of mutant genes expressing altered proteins. *J. Bacteriol.* **159:**570–578.

Morona, R., C. Kramer, and U. Henning. 1985. Bacteriophage receptor area of outer membrane protein OmpA of *Escherichia coli* K-12. *J. Bacteriol.* **164:**539–543.

Nakayama, K., S. Kanaya, M. Ohnishi, Y. Terawaki, and T. Hayashi. 1999. The complete nucleotide sequence of φCTX, a cytotoxin-converting phage of *Pseudomonas aeruginosa*: implications for phage evolution and horizontal gene transfer via bacteriophages. *Mol. Microbiol.* **31:**399–419.

Nelson, D. 2004. Phage taxonomy: we agree to disagree. *J. Bacteriol.* **186:**7029–7031.

Nesper, J., D. Kapfhammer, K. E. Klose, H. Merkert, and J. Reidl. 2000. Characterization of *Vibrio cholerae* O1 antigen as the bacteriophage K139 receptor and identification of *IS 1004* insertions aborting O1 antigen biosynthesis. *J. Bacteriol.* **182:**5097–5104.

Newton, G. J., C. Daniels, L. L. Burrows, A. M. Kropinski, A. J. Clarke, and J. S. Lam. 2001. Three-component-mediated serotype conversion in *Pseudomonas aeruginosa* by bacteriophage D3. *Mol. Microbiol.* **39:**1237–1247.

Ochman, H., and R. K. Selander. 1984. Standard reference strains of *Escherichia coli* from natural populations. *J. Bacteriol.* **157:**690–693.

Olsen, R. H., J. S. Siak, and R. H. Gray. 1974. Characteristics of PRD1, a plasmid-dependent broad host range DNA bacteriophage. *J. Virol.* **14:**689–699.

Pajunen, M., S. Kiljunen, and M. Skurnik. 2000. Bacteriophage φYeO3-12, specific for *Yersinia enterocolitica* serotype O:3, is related to coliphages T3 and T7. *J. Bacteriol.* **182:**5114–5120.

Payne, R. J., and V. A. Jansen. 2001. Understanding bacteriophage therapy as a density-dependent kinetic process. *J. Theor. Biol.* **208:**37–48.

Payne, R. J., and V. A. Jansen. 2003. Pharmacokinetic principles of bacteriophage therapy. *Clin. Pharmacokinet.* **42:**315–325.

Pedulla, M. L., M. E. Ford, J. M. Houtz, T. Karthikeyan, C. Wadsworth, J. A. Lewis, D. Jacobs-Sera, J. Falbo, J. Gross, N. R. Pannunzio, W. Brucker, V. Kumar, J. Kandasamy, L. Keenan, S. Bardarov, J. Kriakov, J. G. Lawrence, W. R. Jacobs, Jr., R. W. Hendrix, and G. F. Hatfull. 2003. Origins of highly mosaic mycobacteriophage genomes. *Cell* **113:**171–182.

Pelkonen, S., J. Pelkonen, and J. Finne. 1989. Common cleavage pattern of polysialic acid by bacteriophage endosialidases of different properties and origins. *J. Virol.* **63:**4409–4416.

Plancon, L., C. Janmot, M. le Maire, M. Desmadril, M. Bonhivers, L. Letellier, and P. Boulanger. 2002. Characterization of a high-affinity complex between the bacterial outer membrane protein FhuA and the phage T5 protein pb5. *J. Mol. Biol.* **318:**557–569.

Plunkett, G., III, D. J. Rose, T. J. Durfee, and F. R. Blattner. 1999. Sequence of Shiga toxin 2 phage 933W from *Escherichia coli* O157:H7: Shiga toxin as a phage late-gene product. *J. Bacteriol.* **181:**1767–1778.

Prangishvili, D., P. Forterre, and R. A. Garrett. 2006. Viruses of the Archaea: a unifying view. *Nat. Rev. Microbiol.* **4:**837–848.

Prehm, P., B. Jann, K. Jann, G. Schmidt, and S. Stirm. 1976. On a bacteriophage T3 and T4 receptor region within the cell wall lipopolysaccharide of *Escherichia coli* B. *J. Mol. Biol.* **101:**277–281.

Proux, C., D. van Sinderen, J. Suarez, P. Garcia, V. Ladero, G. F. Fitzgerald, F. Desiere, and H. Brüssow. 2002. The dilemma of phage taxonomy illustrated by comparative genomics of Sfi21-like *Siphoviridae* in lactic acid bacteria. *J. Bacteriol.* **184:**6026–6036.

Raimondo, L. M., N. P. Lundh, and R. J. Martinez. 1968. Primary adsorption site of phage PBS1: the flagellum of *Bacillus subtilis*. *J. Virol.* **2:**256–264.

Räisänen, L., C. Draing, M. Pfitzenmaier, K. Schubert, T. Jaakonsaari, S. von Aulock, T. Hartung, and T. Alatossava. 2007. Molecular interaction between lipoteichoic acids and *Lactobacillus delbrueckii* phages depends on D-alanyl and α-glucose substitution of poly(glycerophosphate) backbones. *J. Bacteriol.* **189:**4135–4140.

Räisänen, L., K. Schubert, T. Jaakonsaari, and T. Alatossava. 2004. Characterization of lipoteichoic acids as *Lactobacillus delbrueckii* phage receptor components. *J. Bacteriol.* **186:**5529–5532.

Randall-Hazelbauer, L., and M. Schwartz. 1973. Isolation of the bacteriophage lambda receptor from *Escherichia coli*. *J. Bacteriol.* **116:**1436–1446.

Ravin, V., N. Ravin, S. Casjens, M. E. Ford, G. F. Hatfull, and R. W. Hendrix. 2000. Genomic sequence and analysis of the atypical temperate bacteriophage N15. *J. Mol. Biol.* **299:**53–73.

Sakaguchi, Y., T. Hayashi, K. Kurokawa, K. Nakayama, K. Oshima, Y. Fujinaga, M. Ohnishi, E. Ohtsubo, M. Hattori, and K. Oguma. 2005. The genome sequence of *Clostridium botulinum* type C neurotoxin-converting phage and the molecular mechanisms of unstable lysogeny. *Proc. Natl. Acad. Sci. USA* **102:**17472–17477.

Samuel, A. D., T. P. Pitta, W. S. Ryu, P. N. Danese, E. C. Leung, and H. C. Berg. 1999. Flagellar determinants of bacterial sensitivity to chi-phage. *Proc. Natl. Acad. Sci. USA* **96:**9863–9866.

Sander, M., and H. Schmieger. 2001. Method for host-independent detection of generalized transducing bacteriophages in natural habitats. *Appl. Environ. Microbiol.* **67:**1490–1493.

Sao-Jose, C., C. Baptista, and M. A. Santos. 2004. *Bacillus subtilis* operon encoding a membrane receptor for bacteriophage SPP1. *J. Bacteriol.* **186:**8337–8346.

Scholl, D., S. Adhya, and C. Merril. 2005. *Escherichia coli* K1's capsule is a barrier to bacteriophage T7. *Appl. Environ. Microbiol.* **71:**4872–4874.

Scholl, D., S. Rogers, S. Adhya, and C. R. Merril. 2001. Bacteriophage K1-5 encodes two different tail fiber proteins, allowing it to infect and replicate on both K1 and K5 strains of *Escherichia coli*. *J. Virol.* **75:**2509–2515.

Schuch, R., D. Nelson, and V. A. Fischetti. 2002. A bacteriolytic agent that detects and kills *Bacillus anthracis*. *Nature* **418:**884–889.

Schwarz, H., I. Riede, I. Sonntag, and U. Henning. 1983. Degrees of relatedness of T-even type *E. coli* phages using different or the same receptors and topology of serologically cross-reacting sites. *EMBO J.* **2:**375–380.

Skurnik, M., and E. Strauch. 2006. Phage therapy: facts and fiction. *Int. J. Med. Microbiol.* **296:**5–14.

Smith, H. W., and M. B. Huggins. 1982. Successful treatment of experimental *Escherichia coli* infections in mice using phage: its general superiority over antibiotics. *J. Gen. Microbiol.* **128:**307–318.

Smith, H. W., and M. B. Huggins. 1983. Effectiveness of phages in treating experimental *Escherichia coli* diarrhoea in calves, piglets and lambs. *J. Gen. Microbiol.* **129:**2659–2675.

Smith, H. W., M. B. Huggins, and K. M. Shaw. 1987. The control of experimental *Escherichia coli* diarrhoea in calves by means of bacteriophages. *J. Gen. Microbiol.* **133:**1111–1126.

Stone, R. 2002. Bacteriophage therapy. Stalin's forgotten cure. *Science* **298:**728–731.

Strauch, E., H. Kaspar, C. Schaudinn, P. Dersch, K. Madela, C. Gewinner, S. Hertwig, J. Wecke, and B. Appel. 2001. Characterization of enterocoliticin, a phage tail-like bacteriocin, and its effect on pathogenic *Yersinia enterocolitica* strains. *Appl. Environ. Microbiol.* **67:**5634–5642.

Sulakvelidze, A., Z. Alavidze, and J. G. Morris, Jr. 2001. Bacteriophage therapy. *Antimicrob. Agents Chemother.* **45:**649–659.

Summers, W. C. 1999. *Felix d'Herelle and the Origins of Molecular Biology*. Yale University Press, New Haven, CT.

Summers, W. C. 2001. Bacteriophage therapy. *Annu. Rev. Microbiol.* **55:**437–451.

Swinton, D., S. Hattman, P. F. Crain, C. S. Cheng, D. L. Smith, and J. A. McCloskey. 1983. Purification and characterization of the unusual deoxynucleoside, α-N-(9-β-D-2'-deoxyribofuranosylpurin-6-yl)glycinamide, specified by the phage Mu modification function. *Proc. Natl. Acad. Sci. USA* **80:**7400–7404.

Takahashi, I., and J. Marmur. 1963. Replacement of thymidylic acid by deoxyuridylic acid in the deoxyribonucleic acid of a transducing phage for *Bacillus subtilis*. *Nature* **197:**794–795.

Toth, I., H. Schmidt, M. Dow, A. Malik, E. Oswald, and B. Nagy. 2003. Transduction of porcine enteropathogenic *Escherichia coli* with a derivative of a Shiga toxin 2-encoding bacteriophage in a porcine ligated ileal loop system. *Appl. Environ. Microb.* **69:**7242–7247.

Valyasevi, R., W. E. Sandine, and B. L. Geller. 1990. The bacteriophage kh receptor of *Lactococcus lactis* subsp. *cremoris* KH is the rhamnose of the extracellular wall polysaccharide. *Appl. Environ. Microbiol.* **56:**1882–1889.

Vander Byl, C., and A. M. Kropinski. 2000. Sequence of the genome of *Salmonella* bacteriophage P22. *J. Bacteriol.* **182:**6472–6481.

van Regenmortel, M. H., and B. W. Mahy. 2004. Emerging issues in virus taxonomy. *Emerg. Infect. Dis.* **10:**8–13.

Vimr, E. R., R. D. McCoy, H. F. Vollger, N. C. Wilkison, and F. A. Troy. 1984. Use of prokaryotic-derived probes to identify poly(sialic acid) in neonatal neuronal membranes. *Proc. Natl. Acad. Sci. USA* 81:1971–1975.

Wagner, P. L., and M. K. Waldor. 2002. Bacteriophage control of bacterial virulence. *Infect. Immun.* 70:3985–3993.

Waldor, M. K., and J. J. Mekalanos. 1996. Lysogenic conversion by a filamentous phage encoding cholera toxin. *Science* 272:1910–1914.

Wang, J., M. Hofnung, and A. Charbit. 2000. The C-terminal portion of the tail fiber protein of bacteriophage lambda is responsible for binding to LamB, its receptor at the surface of *Escherichia coli* K-12. *J. Bacteriol.* 182:508–512.

Warren, R. A. 1980. Modified bases in bacteriophage DNAs. *Annu. Rev. Microbiol.* 34:137–158.

Watanabe, R., T. Matsumoto, G. Sano, Y. Ishii, K. Tateda, Y. Sumiyama, J. Uchiyama, S. Sakurai, S. Matsuzaki, S. Imai, and K. Yamaguchi. 2007. Efficacy of bacteriophage therapy against gut-derived sepsis caused by *Pseudomonas aeruginosa* in mice. *Antimicrob. Agents Chemother.* 51:446–452.

Weinbauer, M. G. 2004. Ecology of prokaryotic viruses. *FEMS Microbiol. Rev.* 28:127–181.

Weinbauer, M. G., and F. Rassoulzadegan. 2004. Are viruses driving microbial diversification and diversity? *Environ. Microbiol.* 6:1–11.

Weitz, J. S., H. Hartman, and S. A. Levin. 2005. Coevolutionary arms races between bacteria and bacteriophage. *Proc. Natl. Acad. Sci. USA* 102:9535–9540.

Weld, R. J., C. Butts, and J. A. Heinemann. 2004. Models of phage growth and their applicability to phage therapy. *J. Theor. Biol.* 227:1–11.

Wendlinger, G., M. J. Loessner, and S. Scherer. 1996. Bacteriophage receptors on *Listeria monocytogenes* cells are the N-acetylglucosamine and rhamnose substituents of teichoic acids or the peptidoglycan itself. *Microbiology* 142:985–992.

Wilhelm, S. W., and C. A. Suttle. 1999. Viruses and nutrient cycles in the sea. *BioScience* 49:781–788.

Woese, C. R. 2000. Interpreting the universal phylogenetic tree. *Proc. Natl. Acad. Sci. USA* 97:8392–8396.

Wommack, K. E., and R. R. Colwell. 2000. Virioplankton: viruses in aquatic ecosystems. *Microbiol. Mol. Biol. Rev.* 64:69–114.

Wright, A., M. McConnell, and S. Kanegasaki. 1980. Lipopolysaccharide as a bacteriophage receptor. *In* L. L. Randall and L. Philipson (ed.), *Virus Receptors.* Chapman and Hall, London, United Kingdom.

Wyatt, G. R., and S. S. Cohen. 1953. The bases of the nucleic acids of some bacterial and animal viruses: the occurrence of 5-hydroxymethylcytosine. *Biochem. J.* 55:774–782.

Yarmolinsky, M. R., and N. A. Sternberg. 1988. Bacteriophage P1, p. 291–438. *In* R. Calendar (ed.), *The Bacteriophages.* Plenum Press, New York, NY.

Yokota, S., T. Hayashi, and H. Matsumoto. 1994. Identification of the lipopolysaccharide core region as the receptor site for a cytotoxin-converting phage, φCTX, of *Pseudomonas aeruginosa. J. Bacteriol.* 176:5262–5269.

Future Prospects

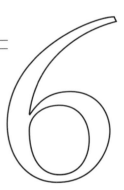

Therapeutic Microbiology: Probiotics and Related Strategies
Edited by J. Versalovic and M. Wilson
© 2008 ASM Press, Washington, DC

James Versalovic
Michael Wilson

29

The Road Ahead: a Look at the Future

With the launch of the international human microbiome project (Turnbaugh et al., 2007), fundamental concepts such as the microbiome and metagenome highlight the potential importance of complex microbial communities for health and disease. The microbiome refers to the aggregate genetic information, or metagenome, encoded by the collective genomes of the autochthonous microbiotas at different body sites. The analyses of such dynamic and complex cellular communities require new technologies such as high-throughput DNA sequencing in order to assemble aggregate genomic data. In addition to determining genome content, bacterial species will be defined by targeting specific genes and performing phylogenetic studies. Ultimately, a detailed understanding of the organisms constituting the indigenous microbiota and genes present in these metagenomes will create a foundation for discoveries of new prebiotics, probiotics, and their respective applications.

With the advancement of the microbiome initiative, the concept of probiotics is likely to evolve and include a much wider variety of microbes that could benefit the host. At this time, probiotics comprise a restricted set of microorganisms including lactic acid bacteria, bifidobacteria, *Escherichia coli*, and the yeast "*Saccharomyces boulardii.*" These beneficial microorganisms have been described in this volume, but many more genera and species may be isolated or identified in the next decade. Future descriptions of probiotics are likely to describe entirely novel classes of microbes as fundamental discoveries are made in the international microbiome project. The characterization of many more bacterial genomes and their respective metabolic pathways will facilitate the identification of key functions and species that encode these functions for the benefit of the host.

Beneficial effects of probiotics include the provision of key nutrients for the intestinal mucosa, regulation of cell proliferation and differentiation, and immunomodulation. While probiotics have been studied for the prevention of infections and the suppression of inflammation, new applications and refinements of existing strategies will be based on the science of systems biology. Synthesis and secretion of key nutrients such as vitamins and cofactors at different body sites may stimulate a reassessment of microbes as "nutrient factories" that could provide

James Versalovic, Department of Pathology, Baylor College of Medicine, and Department of Pathology, Texas Children's Hospital, 6621 Fannin Street, MC 1-2261, Houston, TX 77030. **Michael Wilson,** Division of Microbial Diseases, UCL Eastman Dental Institue, University College London, 256 Grays Inn Road, London WC1X 8LD, United Kingdom.

essential factors for the maintenance of human health. Advances in microbial genomics are uncovering interesting features of biochemical pathways including the production of B complex vitamins, essential amino acids, polyamines, antioxidants such as hydroxycinnamates, and fatty acids. Probiotics may be useful as part of a multipronged strategy to confront malnutrition in the developing world and may be combined with prebiotics, micronutrients, and other foods in global health programs. The inclusion of viable organisms in the diet may enhance the digestion and absorption of nutrients in a limited food supply and maximize the caloric intake and energy extraction from food in needy populations.

Nutraceuticals and functional foods are extending beyond nutrition to include properties such as the regulation of cell signaling and immunity (Penner et al., 2005). Regulation of epithelial cell proliferation may be important during infancy in order to facilitate complete maturation and development of the gastrointestinal tract and mucosal immunity. Promotion of apoptosis in response to specific immune signals may be a key feature to selectively delete activated immune cells during acute or chronic inflammation. Isomers of linoleic acid, or conjugated linoleic acids, are produced by bacterial combinations and confer proapoptotic effects on intestinal epithelial cells (Ewaschuk et al., 2006). Fatty acids may be converted by commensal microbes to produce bioactive compounds that regulate cell proliferation and affect relative susceptibilities to human cancers. Next-generation probiotics may be selected or engineered to contain such bioconversion features as part of solutions in preventative medicine and therapeutics.

Exciting new developments in the understanding of probiotics and the regulation of mucosal immunity are pointing to new directions with respect to selection and engineering of beneficial microbes. Proimmune effects of probiotics include the stimulation of innate and adaptive immune responses such as enhancement of proliferation of immunoglobulin A-producing cells in individuals receiving probiotics (Rautava et al., 2006). Immunomodulation may include the enhanced development and maturation of immunity early in life, resulting in improved vaccination strategies and protection against infectious diseases. Probiotics may also suppress immunity in disorders of chronic inflammation, and such effects may reflect the activation of different immune signaling pathways requiring different types of probiotics for disease amelioration. Next-generation immunoprobiotics may be optimized to stimulate immunity in the context of infection prevention and development in infancy and to suppress inflammation in the context of diagnosed inflammatory bowel disease or autoimmune diseases.

Natural or engineered probiotics may be included in future strategies to prevent or treat disease, but improved abilities to rigorously screen and manipulate candidate probiotics will be important for the selection of beneficial microbes. Highly parallel or high-throughput screening systems will enable a more comprehensive evaluation of candidate probiotics including novel organisms isolated from animal, human, or environmental sources. Advances in comparative and functional genomics are creating new opportunities for rational engineering of different probiotic species. Improvements in nucleic acid transfer, mutagenesis strategies, and plasmid-borne and chromosomal integration systems in lactic acid bacteria are providing opportunities for defining key genes contributing to probiosis. Characterization of gene regulatory sequences that are important in vivo has been defined in animal models and enables investigators to couple key genes with constitutive or inducible promoters that may be active within the mammalian host. Probiotics may also be engineered with particular nutritional requirements such that nutrient supplementation is required for maintenance of engineered bacteria in patients (Steidler and Rottiers, 2006).

This feature of obligatory nutrient supplementation may be important to allay regulatory concerns and promote patient safety. The refinement of signals for cell surface localization and protein secretion in commensal bacteria may facilitate the delivery of endogenous or heterologous bioactive molecules derived from mammals or other microbes. As scientists unravel basic mechanisms of intercellular communication between microbes and host cells, the composition and aggregate functions of the microbiome may be tailored to specific host genotypes for maximal benefit.

The concept of prebiotics is undergoing revision in order to encompass a wider variety of nutrients that may stimulate the selective proliferation and survival of beneficial microbes. Prebiotics currently include mostly oligosaccharides and more complex carbohydrates, and several classes of prebiotics have been described in the preceding chapters. New types of oligosaccharides are being discovered as human breast milk and its corresponding glycome are being explored with cutting-edge technologies. Techniques such as microchip liquid chromatography mass spectrometry (HPLC-Chip/MS) and matrix-assisted laser desorption ionization Fourier transform ion cyclotron resonance mass spectrometry (MALDI-FT ICR MS) are being applied towards the characterization and annotation of the human milk glycome (Ninonuevo et al., 2006). Current efforts to emulate human milk oligosaccharides as a part of new prebiotics development strategies include recombinant microbes for oligosaccharide production (Espinosa et al., 2007). Similar to probiotics, advances in food science, nutrition, and metabolomics may yield novel classes of organic compounds that may selectively stimulate beneficial bacteria and health-promoting microbial communities. Characterization of novel compounds in foods, host-derived factors, or commensal microbe-derived molecules may result in synbiotics that effectively match newly discovered probiotics with organic substrates that selectively promote their growth.

Functional genomics and metabolic pathway reconstruction of commensal bacteria may result in the identification of pathways fostering production of specific macromolecules that may be synthesized by particular bacteria for the benefit of microbial communities indigenous to humans and other animals. Specific microbes may have net abilities to provide important nutrients for fellow members of microbial communities. Other organisms may be adept at producing catabolic enzymes that promote effective scavenging of nutrients produced by neighboring organisms or the host. A more detailed understanding is emerging regarding the respective roles of different indigenous and symbiotic microbes in the gastrointestinal tract. Comparative genomics of symbiotic bacterial species has highlighted molecular evolution and its role in niche and habitat adaptation of *Bacteroidetes* in the distal human intestine (Xu et al., 2007). Knowledge of how microorganisms adapt in different host environments may be applied to tailor future combinations of probiotics. In concert with a wider diversity of prebiotics and probiotics in the future, novel functions or mechanisms of action will be uncovered as a result of functional metagenomics. The burgeoning area of metabolomics is creating new opportunities for high-throughput screening of novel organic compounds that may be produced by diverse bacteria. Techniques such as nuclear magnetic resonance and multistage mass spectrometry are facilitating the characterization of novel microbe-derived compounds. Specific metabolic profiles, or metabotypes, in the host have been correlated with the resident microbiome (Martin et al., 2007), suggesting how the microbiome may modulate nutrient absorption, storage, and energy harvest.

Advances in therapeutic microbiology including prebiotics and probiotics may provide opportunities for beneficial microbes to contribute to the development of personalized medicine (Burke and Psaty, 2007). As human genomics and systems biology surge forward, the linkage of human genotypes with disease susceptibilities will become more comprehensive. One component of the human microbiome project will include human genome sequencing of a subset of individuals sampled for metagenomics studies of their microbiomes at different body sites. The coupling of human genomics and the microbiome may enable future predictions of suitable prebiotics and probiotics for particular individuals or patient groups. As diseases are further stratified with advances in human genomics and molecular pathophysiology, relative deficiencies in resident microbial populations or aggregate microbial functions may point towards solutions that include specific types of prebiotics or probiotics. Future trends may include cost-effective whole-genome sequencing for human individuals, and such prognostic information may be combined with analyses of one's microbiome at multiple body sites. Aggregate disease risk may include knowledge of the microbiome, and disease risk may be modified by rational manipulation of resident microbial communities. The future of therapeutics in human and veterinary medicine may depend on advances in the science of therapeutic microbiology.

References

Burke, W., and B. M. Psaty. 2007. Personalized medicine in the era of genomics. *JAMA* **298:**1682–1684.

Espinosa, R. M., M. Tamez, and P. Prieto. 2007. Efforts to emulate human milk oligosaccharides. *Br. J. Nutr.* **98**(Suppl. 1): S74–S79.

Ewaschuk, J. B., J. W. Walker, H. Diaz, and K. L. Madsen. 2006. Bioproduction of conjugated linoleic acid by probiotic bacteria occurs *in vitro* and *in vivo* in mice. *J. Nutr.* **136:**1483–1487.

Martin, F. P., M. E. Dumas, Y. Wang, C. Legido-Quigley, I. K. Yap, H. Tang, S. Zirah, G. M. Murphy, O. Cloarec, J. C. Lindon, N. Sprenger, L. B. Fay, S. Kochhar, P. van Bladeren, E. Holmes, and J. K. Nicholson. 2007. A top-down systems biology view of microbiome-mammalian metabolic interactions in a mouse model. *Mol. Syst. Biol.* **3:**112.

Ninonuevo, M. R., Y. Park, H. Yin, J. Zhang, R. E. Ward, B. H. Clowers, J. B. German, S. L. Freeman, K. Killeen, R. Grimm, and C. B. Lebrilla. 2006. A strategy for annotating the human milk glycome. *J. Agric. Food Chem.* **54:**7471–7480.

Penner, R., R. N. Fedorak, and K. L. Madsen. 2005. Probiotics and nutraceuticals: non-medicinal treatments of gastrointestinal diseases. *Curr. Opin. Pharmacol.* **5:**596–603.

Rautava, S., H. Arvilommi, and E. Isolauri. 2006. Specific probiotics in enhancing maturation of IgA responses in formula-fed infants. *Pediatr. Res.* **60:**221–224.

Steidler, L., and P. Rottiers. 2006. Therapeutic drug delivery by genetically modified *Lactococcus lactis*. *Ann. N. Y. Acad. Sci.* **1072:**176–186.

Turnbaugh, P. J., R. E. Ley, M. Hamady, C. M. Fraser-Liggett, R. Knight, and J. I. Gordon. 2007. The human microbiome project. *Nature* **449:**804–810.

Xu, J., M. A. Mahowald, R. E. Ley, C. A. Lozupone, M. Hamady, E. C. Martens, B. Henrissat, P. M. Coutinho, P. Minx, P. Latreille, H. Cordum, A. Van Brunt, K. Kim, R. S. Fulton, L. A. Fulton, S. W. Clifton, R. K. Wilson, R. D. Knight, and J. I. Gordon. 2007. Evolution of symbiotic bacteria in the distal human intestine. *PLoS Biol.* **5:**e156.

Index